Pediatric Sports Medicine
for Primary Care

Pediatric Sports Medicine for Primary Care

Editors

Richard B. Birrer, M.D.

Senior Vice President and Chief Medical Officer
St. Joseph's Regional Medical Center
Paterson, New Jersey;
Professor of Medicine
Cornell University Medical Center
New York, New York

Bernard A. Griesemer, M.D.

Director, HealthTracks Center
Pediatrics and Adolescent Health
St. John's Health System
Springfield, Missouri

Mary B. Cataletto, M.D.

Associate Professor of Clinical Pediatrics
State University of New York, Stony Brook
Stony Brook, New York;
Associate Director, Pediatric Pulmonary Medicine
Winthrop University Hospital
Mineola, New York

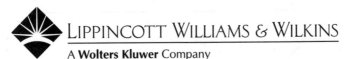

LIPPINCOTT WILLIAMS & WILKINS
A **Wolters Kluwer** Company
Philadelphia • Baltimore • New York • London
Buenos Aires • Hong Kong • Sydney • Tokyo

Acquisitions Editor: Timothy Y. Hiscock
Developmental Editor: Kerry B. Barrett
Production Editor: Christiana Sahl
Manufacturing Manager: Tim Reynolds
Cover Designer: Patricia Gast
Compositor: Lippincott Williams & Wilkins Desktop Division
Printer: Maple Press

Library of Congress Cataloging-in-Publication Data

Birrer, Richard B.
  Pediatric sports medicine for primary care / Richard B. Birrer, Bernard A. Griesemer, Mary B. Cataletto.
     p. ; cm.
Includes bibliographical references and index.
ISBN 0-7817-3159-3 (alk. papar)
  1. Pediatric sports medicine. I. Griesemer, Bernard. II. Cataletto, Mary B. III. Title.
[DNLM: 1. Sports Medicine—methods—Child. 2. Athletic Injuries—Child. 3. Child Development. 4. Primary Health Care—methods—Child. 5. Sports—Child.
QT 261 B619p 2002]
RC1218.C45 B575 2002
617.1′027′083—dc21

                                                                2002016288

10 9 8 7 6 5 4 3 2 1

To Thomas Shaffer and Joseph Findaro
and the families of all the participants in this text
without whose emotional support, patience, and understanding
this book could not have become a reality.

Contents

vii

Part III. Musculoskeletal Conditions and Young Athletes

Appendices

Contributing Authors

Marcia K. Anderson, Ph.D., L.A.T.C.   *Professor and Department Chair, Department of Movement Arts, Health Promotion, and Leisure Studies, Bridgewater State College, Bridgewater, Massachusetts*

David T. Bernhardt, M.D.   *Associate Professor, Department of Pediatrics; Fellowship Director of Sports Medicine, University of Wisconsin, Madison, Wisconsin*

Richard B. Birrer, M.D., F.A.A.F.P., F.A.C.S.M., F.A.C.P., F.A.C.E.P.   *Senior Vice President and Chief Medical Officer, St. Joseph's Regional Medical Center, Paterson, New Jersey; Professor of Medicine, Cornell University Medical Center, New York, New York*

Cora Collette Breuner, M.D., M.P.H.   *Assistant Professor, Department of Pediatrics, Section on Adolescent Medicine, University of Washington; Assistant Professor, Department of Pediatrics, Children's Hospital and Regional Medical Center, Seattle, Washington*

William Michael Brown, M.D., F.A.A.P.   *Assistant Director, Family Practice Residency; Chairman, Department of Pediatrics, Bayfront Medical Center, St. Petersburg, Florida*

J. C. Buller, M.D.   *Resident Physician, Department of Family Medicine, Loma Linda University Medical Center, Loma Linda, California*

Mary B. Cataletto, M.D.   *Associate Professor of Clinical Pediatrics, State University of New York, Stony Brook, Stony Brook, New York; Associate Director, Department of Pediatric Pulmonary Medicine, Winthrop University Hospital, Mineola, New York*

James R. Clugston, M.D.   *Sports Medicine Clinic, Student Health Care Center, University of Florida, Gainesville, Florida*

Kevin DeWeber, M.D.   *Major, United States Army; Director, Department of Family Practice, Evans Army Community Hospital, Fort Carson, Colorado; Team Physician, Army World Class Athlete Program*

Rachel A. Dunnagan, M.D.   *Attending Physician, Department of Family Practice, Bay Pines Veterans Administration Medical Center, St. Petersburg, Florida*

Robert C. Gambrell, M.D.   *Clinical Associate Professor, Department of Family Medicine and Surgery, Medical College of Georgia; Sports Medicine Associates of Augusta, Augusta, Georgia*

Edward R. Gillett, M.D.   *Clinical Assistant Professor, Department of Family Medicine, University of South Florida College of Medicine, Tampa, Florida; Associate Director, Family Practice Residency; Medical Director, Bayfront Medical Center, St. Petersburg, Florida*

Bernard A. Griesemer, M.D., F.A.A.P.   *Director, HealthTracks Center, St. John's Health System, Springfield, Missouri*

Kimberly G. Harmon, M.D.   *Clinical Assistant Professor, Department of Family Medicine and Department of Orthopaedics and Sports Medicine; Team Physician, University of Washington, Seattle, Washington*

George D. Harris, M.D., M.S.   *Clinical Associate Professor, Department of Family Medicine, University of South Florida, Tampa, Florida; Assistant Director, Family Practice Residency, Bayfront Medical Center, St. Petersburg, Florida*

Ken Honsik, M.D.   *Sports Medicine Fellow, Kaiser Permanente Medical Center; Fontana Medical Center, Fontana, California*

Charleen L. Isé, M.D.   *Assistant Clinical Professor, Department of Family Medicine, University of South Florida, Tampa, Florida; Associate Director, Bayfront Family Practice Residency, Bayfront Medical Center, St. Petersburg, Florida*

William Jih, M.D.   *Resident Physician, Chief Resident, Department of Family Medicine, Loma Linda University Medical Center, Loma Linda, California*

John P. Kugler, M.D., M.P.H.   *Colonel, United States Army; Assistant Clinical Professor, Department of Family Practice, Uniformed Services University of the Health Sciences, Bethseda, Maryland; Department Chief, Department of Primary Care and Community Medicine, Dewitt Army Community Hospital, Fort Belvoir, Virginia*

Beverly C. Land, D.O.   *Lieutenant Colonel, United States Army; Director of Sports Medicine, Department of Family Practice, Womack Army Medical Center, Fort Bragg, North Carolina*

Gregory L. Landry, M.D.   *Professor, Department of Pediatrics, University of Wisconsin, Madison, Wisconsin*

Mark E. Lavallee, M.D.   *Assistant Clinical Professor, Department of Family Medicine, Indiana University School of Medicine, Indianapolis, Indiana; USA Weightlifting Sports Medicine Board member; Director, Department of Sports Medicine, Memorial Hospital, South Bend, Indiana*

Kim Edward LeBlanc, M.D., Ph.D., F.A.A.F.P., F.A.C.S.M.   *Certificate of Added Qualifications in Sports Medicine; Professor, Department of Family Medicine, Louisiana State University Health Sciences Center, New Orleans, Louisiana; Head and Residency Program Director, Department of Family Practice, University Medical Center, Lafayette, Louisiana*

Jack M. Levine, M.D.   *Assistant Clinical Professor, Department of Pediatrics, Albert Einstein College of Medicine, Bronx, New York; Medical Director, Henry Viscardi School, Albertson, New York*

Brian L. Mahaffey, M.D., M.S.P.H.   *Adjunct Faculty and Team Physician, Department of Sports Medicine and Athletic Training, Southwest Missouri State University; Director, Midwest Sports Medicine Center, St. John's Clinics, Inc., Springfield, Missouri*

Robert M. Malina, Ph.D., F.A.C.S.M.   *Professor, Department of Kinesiology; Adjunct Professor, Department of Anthropology, Michigan State University, East Lansing, Michigan*

Eron Grant Manusov, M.D.   *Director, Family Care Center, First Health of Carolinas, Pinehurst, North Carolina*

William F. Miser, M.D., M.A.   *Associate Professor, Department of Family Medicine, The Ohio State University, Columbus, Ohio*

James L. Moeller, M.D., F.A.C.S.M.   *Chief, Division of Sports Medicine, William Beaumont Hospital, Troy, Michigan; Team Physician, Oakland University, Rochester, Michigan; Sports Medicine Associates PLC, Auburn Hills, Michigan*

Joseph L. Moore, M.D.   *Captain, United States Navy; Associate Professor, Uniformed Services University, University of California School of Medicine, San Diego, California; Commanding Officer, Naval Medical Clinic—Pearl Harbor, Pearl Harbor, Hawaii*

Francis G. O'Connor, M.D.   *Associate Professor, Department of Family Medicine, Uniformed Services University, Bethseda, Maryland; Director, Sports Medicine Fellowship, Department of Family Medicine, Uniformed Services University of the Health Sciences, Fairfax Station, Virginia*

Ralph G. Oriscello, M.D., F.A.C.C., F.A.C.P.   *Professor, Department of Medicine, Seton Hall University School of Postgraduate Medical Education; Director, Department of Critical Care Medicine, Trinitas Hospital, Elizabeth, New Jersey*

Charles S. Peterson, M.D. *Sports Medicine Fellow, Department of Family and Community Medicine, Medical College of Wisconsin, Milwaukee, Wisconsin; Department of Family Medicine, Mayo Clinic—Scottsdale, Scottsdale, Arizona*

Margot Putukian, M.D., F.A.C.S.M. *Associate Professor, Department of Orthopedics and Rehabilitation, Hershey Medical Center; Director, Department of Primary Care Sports Medicine, Centre Community Hospital; Team Physician, Penn State University, University Park, Pennsylvania*

Arnold M. Ramirez, M.D. *Assistant Professor, Department of Family Medicine, University of South Florida College of Medicine, Tampa, Florida*

Brent S. E. Rich, M.D., A.T.C. *University Sports Medicine, Phoenix, Arizona; Head Team Physician, 2002 United States ParaOlympic Team; Team Physician, 2000 United States Olympic Team; Team Physician, Arizona State University; Team Physician, Arizona Diamondbacks; Team Physician, Mountain Point and Desert Vista High Schools*

Sami F. Rifat, M.D. *Division of Sports Medicine, William Beaumont Hospital, Troy, Michigan; Head Team Physician, Oakland University, Rochester, Michigan; Sports Medicine Associates PLC, Auburn Hills, Michigan*

Robert Sallis, M.D. *Assistant Clinical Professor, Department of Family Medicine, University of California—Los Angeles, Riverside, California; Codirector of Sports Medicine Fellowship, Kaiser Permanente Medical Center, Fontana, California*

Joel L. Shaw, M.D. *Family Practice Resident, Dewitt Army Community Hospital, Fort Belvoir, Virginia*

Lauren M. Simon, M.D., M.P.H. *Director, Primary Care Sports Medicine; Assistant Director, Family Practice Residency Program; Assistant Professor, Department of Family Medicine, Loma Linda University School of Medicine, Loma Linda, California*

Stephen M. Simons, M.D., F.A.C.S.M. *Codirector, Sports Medicine Institute, St. Joseph's Regional Medical Center; Director of Sports Medicine, Department of Family Practice, St. Joseph's Regional Medical Center, South Bend, Indiana*

Brian K. Sloan, M.D. *Sports Medicine Fellow, Department of Family Practice, St. Joseph's Regional Medical Center, South Bend, Indiana*

Paul R. Stricker, M.D. *Associate Professor, Department of Pediatrics, Children's Hospital, University of California—San Diego; Staff Physician, Orthopedics and Sports Medicine, Scripps Clinic, La Jolla, California*

Keith A. Stuessi, M.D. *United States Navy*

Kenneth L. Taylor-Butler, M.D. *Faculty Physician, Trinity Family Practice Residency, Trinity Lutheran Hospital, Kansas City, Missouri*

Daniel J. Van Durme, M.D., F.A.A.F.P. *Associate Professor and Vice Chairman, Department of Family Medicine, University of South Florida College of Medicine, Tampa, Florida*

Jaci L. VanHeest, Ph.D. *Assistant Professor, Department of Kinesiology, University of Connecticut, Storrs, Connecticut*

Russell D. White, M.D. *Clinical Associate Professor, Department of Family Medicine, University of South Florida College of Medicine, Tampa, Florida; Director, Sports Medicine Fellowship; Associate Director, Family Practice Residency, Bayfront Medical Center, St. Petersburg, Florida*

Mark S. Williams, D.O. *Major, United States Army; Director, Primary Care Sports Medicine, Department of Family Practice and Community Medicine, Martin Army Community Hospital, Fort Benning, Georgia*

Foreword

This is the era of the child—no longer is it that of the miniature adult. Just as a caterpillar becomes a moth, so a child is transformed into an adult. Children live in different worlds and have quite different emotional and physical needs. Nowhere is this more evident than in the world of physical activity, development, and repair.

The individual child is a growing entity with open growth plates; relatively poor "thermostat" control; developing hormones; a thin body wall; muscles that ache from being pulled by the long bones, which are growing at a faster rate; and hypertrophied tibial tuberosities. Younger children, in particular, have relatively larger skulls (top-heavy) and more vulnerable trunk organs (i.e., heart, spleen, liver, and kidney) and "hollow" viscuses, such as the lungs, duodenum, and urinary bladder. The immature skeleton is like rubber, lacking the consistency of adult bone under stress, thus "squashing" much of what lies in between it and the external surface. Moreover, children display a growing mental and emotional awareness—a clean slate that is vulnerable to anything that an adult chooses to write upon it.

Girls and boys are quite alike until puberty, when definite differences appear—broad shoulders appear in boys, shifting their centers of gravity higher, while their shoulder girdles become heavier and more powerful; broad hips develop in girls, giving them a lower center of gravity. Teenaged girls also develop greater endurance, and they must understand and begin to cope with a change in hormonal physiology. Neither gender is better than the other, but they are different.

The first true recognition of this occurred more than 40 years ago when primary and secondary school coaches began discussing and understanding these differences, stimulated and assisted by forward-looking pediatricians like Thomas Shaffer and Joe Findaro (deceased). The American Academy of Pediatrics honored Thomas Shaffer for his pioneer work and leadership in Pediatric Sports Medicine in the millennium year.

Pediatric sports medicine has been engaged in a slow upward struggle that has achieved its rightful place and recognition only in the last decade. Many adults, unfortunately, are still unaware of the vast differences in the needs of the pediatric athlete, who ranges in age and potential from the toddler to the Olympic teen.

The primary care physician is the front line of pediatric sports medicine. As such, we guide and protect not only the physical, but also the emotional, growth of the child and balance these as this child advances along the rocky and often treacherous road to adulthood. We are the ones who recognize the child with "burn out" because he or she is forgetting his or her sneakers, missing practices, getting injured, or hanging out with the wrong crowd. Alternately, we realize that these may be the early symptoms of substance abuse or depression. We usually pick these clues up first.

The reasons for the existence of Pediatric Sports Medicine are multiple, including mental and physical health; happiness; and normal development and respect for oneself and for others, to name only a few. The ultimate goal of athletic pursuits should be having fun, not winning.

Similar to the teacher in primary and secondary education, the pediatrician and primary care physician share the responsibility for nurturing the world's most precious resource.

As clinicians, we must never forget that most children will not be great athletes. Many have disabilities, but all have the potential to become productive and happy world citizens. A physical activity or sport can be found for every child, and a child for every activity. Our job is to help to insure that a child's disabilities do not become his or her handicaps.

The goal of this book is to provide the primary care physician with a text that is devoted to the physical and mental growth, development, and care of these unique beings from a sports perspective, so that we may help them realize their full potential and happiness.

—*Elizabeth Coryllos*, M.D.

Preface

As the specialty of sports medicine has evolved, the world of the child and adolescent athlete has been relatively ignored, while their involvement in recreational and organized sports has exploded. As in all aspects of medical care, children cannot be considered "small adults" for the purposes of sports medicine. However, the basic and clinical science of adult sports medicine is readily applicable to the active child and adolescent. This then was the challenge presented to the authors in *Pediatric Sports Medicine for Primary Care*. This text focuses on the basic aspects of sports medicine, with a specific focus on the younger athlete.

The vast majority of active youngsters are under the care of primary care physicians in the specialties of pediatrics, internal medicine, and family practice. These physicians are best suited for integrating the patient's social, family, school, and athletic environment so that the child's maximum exercise potential can be achieved and he or she can function under the safest, healthiest conditions. Even with the importance that primary care physicians place on physical activity and proper nutrition, fewer than 50% of children in the United States regularly participate in appropriate physical activities. Primary care physicians, with the Surgeon General of the United States, are concerned about these low levels of physical activity and aerobic fitness, which may become lifelong habits. The task of the primary care physician is to promote wellness in his or her young patients. In this century, physical activity has been recognized as a main component of health promotion. As clinicians, we must realize that recreational and sports activities play an important role in helping our patients, whether children, adolescents, or young adults, to initiate and to maintain a healthy level of physical activity. Therefore, physicians also need to develop skills that allow their young patients to return to their physical activity programs as quickly and as safely as possible if an injury has occurred.

Thus, the purpose of this text is to provide a comprehensive, yet practical, reference source for the busy primary care physician involved with pediatric sports medicine, whether in the office or on the playing field. The chapters are written not only to provide basic sports medicine information to the primary care physician but also to relate information that is unique or critically important for the health of the young athlete under his or her care.

The scope of the text includes a thorough discussion of nonoperative medical problems encountered in the pediatric athlete. Part I covers the role and responsibilities of being a team physician, the preparticipation evaluation, growth and development, sports nutrition, drugs and sports, the psychosocial aspects of athletic activities, training, equipment, environmental concerns, legal guidelines, and common medical problems. Part II discusses the developmentally disabled athlete and athletes who are competing while managing acute, subacute, and chronic diseases, such as diabetic, renal, cardiopulmonary, infectious, dermatologic, gynecologic, and neurologic conditions.

Part III begins with the on-field management of injuries and progresses to the ongoing management and full rehabilitation of the young athlete who has sustained an injury. The core of the section handles overuse and acute trauma to the various anatomic parts of the body (e.g., head and face, spine, chest, abdomen, and upper and lower extremities). Each area utilizes the following standard format: introduction, epidemiology, mechanism of injury, symptoms and/or signs, differential diagnosis, management referral and consultation guidelines, return-to-play criteria, and prevention. The section concludes with a special discussion of specific problems that may have a higher incidence in certain sports (e.g., running, aquatics, gymnastics, and soccer). These special problems are discussed from both a training and prevention and an injury management prospective.

The three editors have reviewed every chapter, and they have given specific attention to streamlining the tables and figures, as well as liberally cross-referencing the material in order to maximize consistency and minimize duplication. All chapters have recent references from the peer-reviewed literature, and the appendices incorporate important position statements, guidelines, and websites, as well as supporting materials. This approach facilitates the reader's ability to seek further information as expeditiously as possible.

The contributing authors are mostly drawn from the specialties of family medicine and pediatrics, and many hold the Certificate of Added Qualification in Sports Medicine. A few authors are certified subspecialists with fellowship training in sports medicine or other pediatric subspecialties. All are actively engaged in the care of the active child and adolescent. In addition to being aggressively engaged in improving the health care of young athletes, the editors and authors of this textbook are striving to advance the field of primary care sports medicine, especially as it applies to the pediatric athlete.

—R. B. Birrer

—B. Griesemer

—M. B. Cataletto

Acknowledgments

This book has been the product of many devoted individuals dedicated to the well-being of the child, including secretaries, coaches, nurses, primary care physicians, professors, and our families. They number too many to name each here.

We give special thanks to Tim Hiscock, Kerry Barrett, Carol Barbera, Christiana Sahl, and the staff of Lippincott Williams & Wilkins and to Mary Carobene of St. Joseph's Regional Medical Center.

PART I

Sports Medicine Essentials

1

The Sports Medicine Physician

Richard B. Birrer

And is not bodily habit spoiled by rest and idleness but preserved for a long time by motion and exercise?

Plato, Theaetetus

One of the most enjoyable aspects of primary care is providing care to active children and encouraging young people who are not physically active to make physical activity a part of their lifestyle. The biology of the human organism requires physical activity for optimum performance. Primary care physicians see sport-related and recreational-related injuries throughout their clinical careers and thus need to participate actively in the care of these young athletes in order to sustain their physical activity levels for reasons of both health and performance. Family physicians, pediatricians, internists, adolescent medicine specialists, and generalists as team physicians are best suited to provide the full range of healthcare to the young athlete. Nonprimary care physicians (e.g., emergency medicine, orthopedics, obstetrics/gynecology) complement the medical team in order to provide comprehensive coverage. Balancing the needs of the athlete, the team, and the academic institution and its representatives is the ethical responsibility of the competent team physician. The "team doc" is prototypically pictured as competent clinician, an inveterate enthusiast, and the consummate diplomat. Sports medicine involvement for a local elementary school, middle school, high school, or university is a natural extension of the practice of a primary care physician. More than 30,000 physicians now serve as team physicians or medical consultants for teams or school systems. Estimates indicate that 85% of the physicians serving in this capacity are primary care physicians.

EPIDEMIOLOGY

Physical exercise at the pediatric level consists largely of recreational activity and organized sports. Sports and recreation are pleasurable activities that engage approximately 42 million Americans who are 18 years of age or younger, 7.5 million of whom participate in school sports (1). While much of this activity occurs at irregular intervals (i.e., weekend warriors) during picnics and family outings, structured programs span the spectrum of community-sponsored softball and bowling teams to fun-runs to school-based intramurals and varsity sports teams. Twenty million of the approximately 60 million adolescents who participate in high school sports sustain a sports-related injury annually. While most are minor, they occur predominately during practice rather than in actual competition. A catastrophic injury occurs in 1 out of 100,000 high school athletes (2). Highly competitive activities take place at the college, amateur, and Olympic levels. While the average age of participation is 11 years (range of 3 to 18 years), the 5-year-old to 14-year-old group, however, suffers the majority of injuries (1,3). Furthermore, children in this age group sustain 30% to 32% of sports-related injuries, with the highest rates of injury being observed in gymnastics and tetherball. Severe injuries are seen in activities associated with augmented speed, collision, and contact (e.g., skateboarding, bicycling, all-terrain vehicles, sleds, and gymnastics). Competitive sports have double the average rate of injuries for all sports combined at 16 per 1,000 hours of activity. Sprains and strains are the most frequent type of injury in all age groups. Contusions, abrasions, and lacerations account for an almost equal share of injuries in the 5-year-old to 14-year-old group (1). The head is injured most frequently in individuals who are less than 6 years old; upper extremities, particularly the fingers, in the 5- to 14-year-old group; and the lower extremity, in those over 15 years of age. Less than 2% of all treated victims require hospitalization (2). Determining the percentages of injuries that are acute, chronic, or due to overuse is difficult. However, reinjury rates of the same limb or body part appear to be 2 to 3 times higher than the risk of the initial injury.

The risk of injury for a given sport is also compounded by the significant risk of injury that accompanies cross-training or participation in other sports for off-season conditioning. Incidence rates in these sports-related activities range from 50 to 200 injuries per 1,000 participants (3). Unsupervised recreational activities (e.g., skateboarding, sledding, and sandlot sports) are associated with significantly higher rates of injury than organized sports events and games. Since the 1970s, female participation in sports has increased by 600% to 700%, whereas male participation has increased by a modest 20% to 30% (4). Female participation in organized sports has benefitted from the passage of Title IX in 1972, which prohibited sex discrimination in schools that receive federal funding. Sixty-nine percent of American women now participate in sports or fitness activities. Women predominate in skating, gymnastics, dancing, swimming, calisthenics, aerobics, exercise walking, biking, and exercising with equipment. They comprise nearly half of the new golfers and the majority of new participants in weight training, running, cycling, and basketball. While injury profiles for many sports indicate no gender-unique injuries, certain sports (e.g., basketball, volleyball, and gymnastics) are associated with higher injury rates and severity of injuries in female athletes (5). Presumably, the differences are due to the specific sports, the coaching techniques, and the athlete's readiness to participate, although additional research is needed to delineate further the factors associated with an injury pattern showing gender differentials.

THE SPORTS MEDICINE TEAM

The primary members of the sports medicine team are the athlete, physician, coach, and athletic trainer (Fig. 1.1). Secondary members include support systems for each, including the athlete's family, friends, teammates, clinical consultants (i.e., dentist, podiatrist, orthopedist, nutritionist, and psychologist), administrative support, and officials. The athlete is the focal point of the team. Viewing the sports team metaphorically as a family can be helpful. In this mobile, heterogeneous, changing industrial society, the sports team represents a valid surrogate family. The 1979 Pittsburgh Pirates, the World Championship baseball team that year, proudly termed itself The Family. The structure of most athletic organizations resembles the prototypical roles of the nuclear family and generates a strong emotional base. In a metaphoric sense, the manager or coach will be viewed as a father or other authority figure. The athletic trainer typically plays the role of a nurturing mother, and the assistant coaches assume the role of big brothers or big sisters. Team members represent siblings, and ancillary personnel and cheerleaders can be considered the extended family. Putting the team

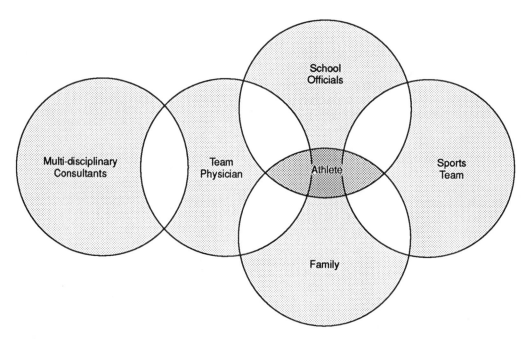

FIG. 1.1. The sports medicine team.

in this perspective is helpful in the following two ways: (a) it facilitates an understanding of the emotional and organizational relationships among team members and (b) it provides a working perspective for the physician.

Athletic Trainer

A certified athletic trainer is available in about 35% of high schools (6). The certified trainer fulfills a major role as a healthcare provider by working to prevent athletic injuries, assisting in the evaluation and rehabilitation of injuries when they occur, and coordinating the school's athletic program (7). The athletic trainer should hold certification from the National Athletic Trainers Association. American Red Cross first aid and basic life support (BLS) training and appropriate certification are also recommended. In conjunction with the physician, the trainer designs, coordinates, and implements the athletic training and injury prevention program; obtains pertinent medical history; and maintains current injury profiles. The team trainer should have a working knowledge of taping, wrapping, padding, and bracing; should be able to recognize and evaluate injuries; and should render the appropriate first aid if the physician is not present. The athletic trainer should participate in the decision-making process with regard to further athletic participation and should ensure that athletes with significant injuries receive appropriate care that complies with the return-to-play decisions of the medical team. The certified athletic trainer frequently coordinates transportation for the injured athlete. Trainers are also frequently the principal source of information for the team physician during the rehabilitation of injured athletes, and the trainer stays in close contact with the team physician at all times. The athletic trainer serves as the liaison among the team, athlete, athlete's family, physician, and coaching staff. Because the certified athletic trainer functions as a physician extender, compliance with treatment protocols and professional communication with the supervising physician are paramount since negligence on the part of the trainer will often be imputed to the doctor.

Coach

Responsibilities of the coaching staff also include the general care and well being of athletes. The responsibility is evident on a daily basis through solid leadership and sound coaching principles. Certifications in first aid from the American Red Cross and BLS are strongly recommended. In situations with no certified athletic trainer, the coach's role in the prevention and care of injuries is proportionately greater. A good coach reinforces the rules, reaffirms the value of sportsmanlike conduct, and encourages a playing environment that is conducive to fair competition. The responsibility of the coaching staff also extends to the preseason and postseason training programs. Proper preseason clearance, injury, and rehabilitation follow-up, as well as return-to-play criteria, are significant components of the yearlong coaching duties. Coaches and trainers can be taught to do yearly performance tests like flexibility, strength, agility, endurance, and speed. Preventive guidance includes weight training programs, fluid requirements, and equipment fitting. Coaches are often the first line of defense for healthcare providers in the ongoing efforts to reduce the use of unethical and unhealthy performance-enhancing practices. During the competitive season, the coaches are a major component of the medical team when they assess playing conditions (temperature and humidity) and appropriately adjust the scheduling of practices or competitions. Periodic inspection standards for equipment and training areas and emergency planning are the responsibilities of the coaching staff.

Officials

The officials are responsible for consistent implementation of the stipulated rules and regulations during competitive sports. Duties include pregame preparations (equipment, weigh-ins, and playing field) and game officiating (conditions, injuries). In nonprofessional sports, a liability policy may be appropriate.

Team Physician

The term sports physician is a general term that refers to a physician who cares for young athletes involved with any sporting or recreational activity. This involvement may entail only preparticipation clearance, weekend games, and/or the care of athletic injuries in a clinical setting. The term team physician is defined by specific requirements and responsibilities (*vide infra*) (8). The team physician plays an extremely influential role in the sports community, and he or she is expected to provide not only physical aid but also philosophical and psychologic counseling to young athletes who may be concerned about poor sports performance, difficulties with schoolwork, and the pressures that accompany the social adjustments of adolescence. The comprehensive continuous care provided by the primary care physician makes him or her uniquely qualified to be a natural complement to the sports team family, as well as the cornerstone of the sports medicine team. Team physicians serve an average of 11 years.

REQUIREMENTS

The team physician must have a medical degree (M.D. or D.O.) with an unrestricted license to practice medicine and surgery in the state of record, and he or she must be in good standing with the state Department of Health and the Licensing board (8). The physician must be certified in BLS and should have a working knowledge of emergency and trauma care, with particular proficiency in the management of musculoskeletal injuries, catastrophic injury management, and medical conditions encountered in sports. Additional training in sports medicine (e.g., fellowship, continuing medical education) is certainly advantageous in caring for young athletes. Also, a certification in sports medicine from an organization recognized by the American Board of Medical Specialties; a significant clinical practice of sports medicine (>50%); certification in advanced life support (ALS) and advanced trauma life support (ATLS); membership and participation in a sports medicine society; involvement in academic sports medicine (e.g., research, teaching, and scholarly publication); and a knowledge base of compensation, disability, and medicolegal issues are desirable. Continuing medical education (CME) is available from local, regional, and national sources, particularly the American Academy of Family Physicians, the American Academy of Pediatrics, the American Academy of Orthopaedic Surgeons, the American College of Sports Medicine, the American Medical Society of Sports Medicine, the American Orthopaedic Society for Sports Medicine, and the American Osteopathic Academy of Sports Medicine. Additional opportunities exist through medical societies, peer review journals, electronic media (CD-ROM and websites), and other organizations, such as the United States Olympic Committee, the National Basketball Association Professional Team Physicians' Society, the Association of Ringside Physicians, the National Football League Team Physicians' Society, or major league baseball.

Team physicians also contribute to the care of young athletes and the advancement of sports medicine by contributing to the information base in both the professional and lay literature. Identifying a researchable hypothesis, collecting data, and presenting the findings at any of the many sports medicine meetings promotes the continued evolution and refinement of the specialty.

The team physician plays a critical role in developing the medical team into a cohesive unit, which then allows better-integrated performance by and better healthcare for the athlete. Equanimity assures that professional judgment will prevail over personal enthusiasm. Availability (i.e., a personal and well-organized coverage system) through regular rounds on and off the field (i.e., sidelines, training room, office, nights, and weekends), as well as competitions—whether home or away—plus some unstructured time, is essential. Finally, personal involvement in a sporting activity, whether on a competitive or recreational basis, provides practical insights into the world of the athlete. Training and competition at a personal level helps one understand the athlete's mindset, in addition to promoting a healthy lifestyle.

RESPONSIBILITIES

The fundamental responsibilities of the job require that the athlete be allowed to participate in sport(s) activity through confidential healthcare that maximizes the prevention of and protection from injury and the risk of reinjury. The responsibility does not allow those needs to become subordinate to the team, coaching decisions, or the academic institution (9). Enjoyment, education, facilitation of success, and protection from liability are all goals of the coordinated sports medicine team at all levels—trainer, coach, and institution.

One of the many characteristics of a committed team physician is the amount of time and expertise that must be committed in order to optimize the potential of each athlete under his or her care. Duties fall under two broad categories—administrative and clinical. Administrative responsibilities include the definition of roles for involved parties; the establishment of a chain of command; emergency planning and training; event coverage protocols; medicolegal and malpractice responsibilities; environmental and/or playing conditions; equipment and/or supply assessments; and the regular education of and communication with athletes, athletic trainers, coaches, parents, and officials regarding athlete-related issues.

Clinical responsibilities include the implementation of a preparticipation physical examination and appropriate clearance. Clinical duties involve event coverage (e.g., elementary school, middle school, high school, college, amateur, Olympics), including on-field and off-field management of injuries, a rehabilitative and return-to-play process, assurance of proper medical record documentation and security, provision of the appropriate preventive counseling, and education about athletic problems (e.g., substance abuse, conditioning and training, ergogenic aids, nutrition, and medical problems). The team physician coordinates all aspects of the sports medicine team. This requires ultimately assuming the responsibility of clinical decision making for an athlete's safe participation in a sport.

Coaches and trainers can be taught to do yearly performance tests (e.g., flexibility, strength, agility, endurance, and speed). Preventive guidance includes weight-training programs, defining fluid requirements, and equipment fitting. The training room (the Athletic Medicine Unit) must have a separate area with controlled access and appropriate medical and rescue equipment (10). In addition, a crash kit for cardiopulmonary resuscitation (CPR) and a sports medicine bag should be prepared and maintained by the trainer and should be periodically checked by the physician. During away events, appropriate equipment and supplies must be available through either regular channels or the host facility.

PROBLEM AREAS

In defining the relationship of the physician to the team, league, or academic institution, an explicit formal agreement or contract, preferably in writing, should be made, particularly if a monetary arrangement is involved. A job description and performance criteria are desirable. At a minimum, the physician must have professional autonomy with respect to all clinical decisions. Relationships with colleagues, malpractice coverage, and financial incentives are common challenges facing the team physician. While medical-legal issues are specifically addressed in Chapter 10, the physician must ensure that his or her malpractice policy covers clinical sports medicine issues, including emergencies and trauma, outside of the office setting. One problem frequently encountered by team physicians is that, when traveling, for instance, they are not covered outside of their home state. Maintaining collegial relationships maximizes involvement and optimizes outcomes. For instance, failure to obtain a consultant's report or a lack of feedback to the athlete's primary care physician leaves a palpable gap in the athlete's care, as well as in the physician's own relationships with his or her colleagues. Playability issues especially require a clear, open discussion in advance of a decision.

Much of the team physician's work at the elementary, middle, and high school level will be *pro bono* on a volunteer basis (4). Reimbursement for preparticipation clearances and game coverage is usually nominal. Special support grants may be available in some programs. Professional charges, however, can be submitted for injury evaluation and management. At the college, amateur, and professional levels, insurance coverage is usually available. Community service and the ability to work with young motivated patients, however, provide immense personal satisfaction. Moreover, the prestige and credibility in the community's eyes afford significant marketing opportunities for practice building.

INJURY MANAGEMENT

Athletes are injured on and, even more frequently, off the playing field. Informed consent for treatment must be sought at the appropriate patient–athlete, parent, and/or guardian level, and an injury control contract, clearly delineating responsibility and chain of command, must be established early. Of utmost importance is the team physician's emergency plan, which should be in place, with arrangements made beforehand with the help of the trainer, coaches, officials, and opposing team's physician. The telephone numbers of ambulances, hospitals, physicians, and parents should be readily available, either in the training kit or the training room.

If the team physician has difficulty remembering the players and their health history, having medical records that are secured safely and taken along with the team is advisable.

The chain of command of the sports medicine team always begins with the physician, unless he or she has delegated authority to the certified athletic trainer or another member of the medical staff. The team physician must be alert to the action on the field, since injuries can be more easily assessed if the mechanism of injury is known. According to team protocol, only the trainer is allowed onto the field to assess an injury, which thus reduces parental apprehension, especially with many transitory minor injuries. If the physician is needed, the common protocol involves the trainer using a prepared signal to call the physician onto the field. The physician's initial responsibility involves assessing the extent of injury and deciding if, when, and how to move the player (Chapter 27). Because performance outcomes, scholarships, and professional opportunities for individuals and the team may hinge on a medical call, the decision timeline may be intense. If an injury is judged non–life-threatening according to accepted protocol, the player should be moved to the sidelines for further evaluation.

A prompt decision on diagnosis and treatment is essential before the specifics of the competition affects judgment about the athlete's playability. For a team physician to take the helmet away from an injured or overly anxious player in order to prevent the player from returning to the game is not unusual. On other hand, allowing the player to return to the game as soon as possible, if the injury is minor, is important. A good rule of thumb is "If in doubt, keep the athlete out!" The physician's decision concerning injuries and playability should be final.

The team physician should follow up on the injured athlete during halftime, immediately after the game, and the following day in the dressing room or his or her private office or by phone, depending on the seriousness of the injury and whether the player wishes to be seen (10). If a serious injury occurs, the team physician should try to accompany the injured athlete to the hospital. The physician for the opposing team, if available, should then be called upon to serve both teams during the game. All concerned parties—parents, coaches, and players—should be advised of the location of the hospital to which an injured athlete is taken in order to expedite the medical care and to reduce anxiety. A follow-up visit is appropriate. Careful documentation of all findings is essential. On the field, a portable dictation machine can be useful. Transcription and filing of important data, which are usually overseen by the athletic trainer, are a must.

A team physician must always bear in mind that an anxious crowd of parents and spectators is witnessing his or her demeanor. The ability to act immediately and with authority helps dispel the fear that often permeates the stands after an injury. Living with the media is a reality. Referral of the press to the team coach or trainer allows the physician to perform his or her professional duties better.

SUMMARY

Sports and recreational activities during the formative years help build character in youngsters, and the coordinated involvement by a primary care physician can favorably enhance a young athlete's appreciation of the possibilities and limitations of athletics in this and later life cycles. Specifically, a committed team physician can wield significant influence in this role and should use these strengths for the enrichment of the young athlete, as well as the good of the sport. Success can be measured by a lifelong commitment to sports and recreational activities. For the committed physician, this is an awesome challenge and special privilege.

REFERENCES

1. United States Consumer Product Safety Commission. *National Electronic Injury Surveillance System*, National Injury Clearinghouse, All Products, 1998.
2. Powell JW. National high school athletic injury registry. *Am J Sports Med* 1998; 16:134–135.
3. Mueller F, Blyth C. Epidemiology of sports injuries in children. *Clin Sports Med* 1982;3:343–352.
4. Howe WB. Primary care sports medicine: a part-timer's perspective. *The Physician and Sports Medicine* 1988; 16:103–114.
5. Dyment PG, ed. *Sports medicine: health care for young athletes*, 2nd ed. Elk Grove Village, IL: American Academy of Pediatrics, 1991.
6. Lyznicki JM, Riggs JA, Champion HC. Certified athletic trainers in secondary schools. *Journal of Athletic Training* 1999;34:272–276.
7. Certified Athletic Trainers in Secondary Schools. *Report 5 of the Council on Scientific Affairs* (A-98). Chicago, IL: American Medical Association, 2000.
8. *Team physician consensus statement*. American Academy of Family Physicians, American Academy of Orthopaedic Surgeons, American College of Sports Medicine, American Medical Society of Sports Medicine, American Orthopaedic Society of Sports Medicine and American Osteopathic Academy of Sports Medicine, 2000.
9. American Academy of Pediatrics. *A self-appraisal checklist for health supervision in scholastic athletic programs*. Elk Grove Village, IL: American Academy of Pediatrics, 1993.
10. Sideline preparedness for the team physician: a consensus statement. *Med Sci Sports Exerc* 2001;33:846–849.

2

The Preparticipation Physical Examination

Charles S. Peterson and Brent S.E. Rich

GOALS AND OBJECTIVES

Athletics plays a major role in the lives of many school-aged children. Participation in sports is an enjoyable means to establish lifelong habits for healthful living. Unfortunately, many sports may place participants at an increased risk of injury. The preparticipation physical examination (PPE) is a safety net to screen for life-threatening illnesses or injuries that would preclude participation in sports, and it establishes a pattern to assist athletes in surmounting potential obstacles.

This chapter provides physicians with the background and skills training necessary to perform the PPE effectively. In the ideal situation, the PPE is a tool for promoting safe participation in athletics. Health maintenance examinations provide the backdrop for medical care and preventive medicine. In the real world, the PPE often becomes a substitute for health maintenance examinations. As many as 78% of athletes use the PPE as their only health maintenance examination (1,2). Sports physicals, which are intended to ensure safe participation in sports, may inadvertently impose a negative impact on a young athlete's health when they replace health maintenance screening and become the only planned interaction with a physician (3). The PPE is a golden opportunity in the lives of many children and adolescents, and providers should take full advantage of this.

Occasionally, athletes mistakenly feel that the PPE is primarily used to search for a reason to disqualify them from participation. In the rare situation when clearance is not granted, the goal then shifts to a team effort among the athlete, physician, parents, trainers, and coaches to work toward possible participation. Of all athletes screened, only 0.3% to 1.9% fail to qualify for participation; of these, 3.2% to 13.5% require a follow-up examination, imaging, or testing (4–8). Many athletes not suited for a particular sport may qualify for another sport and should be accordingly redirected.

The main objective of the PPE is to detect any conditions or limitations that could place the athlete at risk for injury, disability, or death. The PPE has proved effective for detecting serious health problems that would preclude athletic participation (1,2,5–7,9). In one study, 89% of athletes believed that the PPE helped to prevent serious injury (10); however, contrary to this misconception, the examination poorly predicts or prevents injury in actuality (10,11), except for when fitness assessments and sport-specific counseling are part of the evaluation. In today's litigious society, providers also must satisfy legal, institutional, and insurance requirements.

The PPE also has secondary objectives. As time permits or limited access to healthcare requires, emphasis also must be placed on health maintenance, including counseling on dietary, behavioral, and family issues, and on addressing any questions that the athlete may have (12). Testing power, speed, agility, flexibility, and body composition may be of use for establishing baseline fitness for training or rehabilitation (12). Fitness assessment data also may be used in research to determine optimal training methods for various sports (13,14). Finally, the PPE must establish clearance for participation and provide avenues for follow-up and future health guidance.

SETTING UP THE EVALUATION

Who Should Perform the Examination?

Depending on the state or athletic governing body, the PPE may be performed by various health care professionals, including nurse practitioners, physician assistants, and physicians, both primary care and specialists. The physician, however, is responsible for the PPE, and he or she is best suited to address the various clinical situations that may arise. Nonphysician health care professionals often provide necessary assistance under the supervision of a physician (15).

Both primary care physicians and specialists may have the appropriate experience and devote the needed attention to the objectives of the PPE. Both should consult the other as necessary when they encounter situations that are outside of their training. Regardless of background, the most effective providers have an understanding of the demands and risks of sports, and thus they tailor the PPE to the needs of athletes (16).

When Should the Examination Be Performed?

Optimal timing sets the performance of the PPE 4 to 6 weeks before preseason practice (12,17–19). This helps to alleviate scheduling conflicts and affords the athlete and physician time to make adjustments or treatment plans for any injuries or concerns. A convenient time for evaluation might be at the end of the school year. The athlete must then touch base with the primary physician, coach, and trainer if he or she has any interval health concerns (15).

How Often Should the Examination Be Performed?

Opinions vary with regard to the frequency of PPEs. They range from multiple evaluations per year before each sport (20) to evaluations before starting a new school level, such as from junior high to high school (2,12,18,21,22). Annual PPEs are often considered the norm (18,19,23). The National Collegiate Athletic Association (NCAA), however, requires only one PPE when the individual enters a school's athletic program (24). If a periodic PPE is performed when entering a new level of schooling, an interim history generally suffices (see Appendix A) (25). Physical examinations then focus on any injuries or historical concerns.

Should the Examination Be Office-based or Station-based?

The ongoing debate over the most appropriate setting for the PPE continues. If the PPE is performed in an office setting by the athlete's primary physician, it may be more complete and cohesive because the primary care physician has access to the patient's history. The primary care physician is also the person who can most effectively address social issues. Disadvantages of the office-based PPE are that it can be costly, time-consuming, and inconvenient, especially when one considers the millions of student athletes who need examinations before the season begins.

An alternative setting to both mass examinations in the gymnasium and the private office setting is the station concept (Table 2.1). In this format, the athletes check in at various stations for vital signs, including height, weight, blood pressure, visual acuity, and hearing. The young athlete then moves to the history-taking step, which can either be taken at a separate station or can be performed in combination with the physical examination and determination of clearance for specific sports. Components of the examination can be further divided by systems: (a) head, eyes, ears, nose, and throat; (b) cardiovascular and pulmonary; (c) gastrointestinal, genitourinary, and der-

TABLE 2.1. *Required and optional stations and personnel for station-based preparticipation physical evaluations*

Station	Personnel
Required	
Sign-in	Ancillary personnel (coach, nurse, community volunteer)
Height, weight	Ancillary personnel
Vital signs	Ancillary personnel
Vision	Ancillary personnel
Physical examination[a]	Physician[a]
History review, assessment, and clearance	Physician
Optional	
Nutrition	Dietitian
Dental	Dentist
Injury evaluation[b]	Physician
Flexibility	Athletic trainer, physical therapist
Body composition	Athletic trainer, exercise physiologist, physical therapist
Strength	Athletic trainer, coach, exercise physiologist, physical therapist
Speed, agility, power, endurance, and balance	Athletic trainer, coach, exercise physiologist

[a]The physical examination can be subdivided, if more than one physician is present. Qualified medical personnel may perform the musculoskeletal examination under the direction of a physician.
[b]An evaluation station for musculoskeletal injury may be used to provide a more complete evaluation, if a musculoskeletal injury is detected during the required musculoskeletal screening examination.
From Smith DM, Kovan JR, Rich BSE, et al. *Preparticipation physical evaluation*, 2nd ed. Minneapolis: McGraw-Hill, 1997, with permission.

matologic; and (d) neuromusculoskeletal. Based on staff availability, elements of the examination can be done separately or in combination (4).

The station concept requires a large staff, a greater degree of staff coordination, and a large space. Athletes and providers often find this method more convenient because they are able to "batch" dozens to hundreds of athletes through the PPE in a timely manner. Station-based PPEs can incorporate the unique skills of physical therapists, athletic trainers, dietitians, dentists, and exercise physiologists, all of whom can add to the sports emphasis of the PPE (15).

What Routine Screening Tests Should Be Performed?

No particular screening test has been proved to be cost-effective for the standard PPE of the asymptomatic athlete (15). Studies show no benefit from laboratory screening, including complete blood count, ferritin, urinalysis, chemistry profile, lipid panel, or sickle cell trait (26–30). Routine testing by way of electrocardiography, echocardiography, stress test, and spirometry also fails to prove cost-effective (31–37). Even when cost is minimized, these tests are ineffective in asymptomatic athletes. In a 1995 study, Weidenbener et al. (38) incorporated echocardiography into the PPE through donated equipment and interpretation. Of nearly 3,000 examinations, no conditions were found that affected clearance.

A more common condition, exercise-induced asthma, remains undiagnosed in an estimated 3% to 14% of young athletes (36,39–41). History, examination, and resting spirometry are unreliable for diagnosing asthma (36,37,40,42). Exercise challenge tests are more effective in assisting the primary care physician in making the diagnosis of exercise-induced asthma (36–43). However, no reproducible studies have proved that exercise challenge tests for exercise-induced asthma are cost-effective in a PPE setting (15).

When illness or history indicates further investigation, testing becomes cost-effective and more reliable. For example, an athlete with a family history of type 2 diabetes may benefit from a fasting glucose test. In athletes with suspected eating disorders, fatigue, or heavy menstruation, a workup for anemia is warranted. Generally, provisional permission to participate in sports may be given pending test results (15).

Screening laboratory studies may be appropriate in certain situations. For example, on the collegiate level, many female athletes are required to be tested for anemia. Urine drug testing also has a place as a screening tool among professional athletes and elite amateurs (15). High-risk populations, such as boxers, may be required to have human immunodeficiency virus (HIV)

testing (43), although mandatory testing remains rare. The physician must be aware of the guidelines for various governing bodies and should provide for efficient collection and reporting of results.

Should the Examination Be Sport-Specific or Comprehensive?

Sport-specific examinations focus on areas of stress, based on the athlete's particular sport. For example, swimmers and baseball pitchers should have a more detailed examination of the shoulders and upper extremities. Runners may undergo a more thorough examination of the lower extremities. Assessments of biomechanics, strength, endurance, and flexibility can supplement examinations. In addition to looking for abnormalities, examiners who are familiar with sports may find potential ways for improvement of technique or training methods. Some sports medicine physicians recommend sport-specific physical examinations (13,14).

THE MEDICAL HISTORY OF THE PREPARTICIPATION PHYSICAL EXAMINATION

The history portion of the PPE is often regarded as the most important component. When it is used properly, obtaining a thorough history will usually detect recent injury or illness and any long-term problem that may affect performance or safety. Examiners who obtain a thorough history elicit about 75% of all problems that affect athletes (1,2,44). Alternatively, histories uniformly show inaccuracies when the sources of the history are compared. In one study (2), only 39% of histories provided by athletes corresponded to those given by their parents.

Care must be taken to ensure the accuracy of the history. This can be accomplished by having parents review and sign the completed form. Physicians must review items of concern and ask follow-up questions. The history form provided in the *Preparticipation Physical Evaluation* is an excellent example (see Appendix B) (15).

Past Medical History

Discussion of past medical history focuses on the potential for future risk of injury based on past illness and injury. Inquiry concerning prior hospitalizations can bring out impending concerns that might otherwise have been overlooked. Major illnesses, during which the athlete may have missed school or work or may have had a prolonged recovery, also should be addressed. Determination must also be made of chronic illness, such as diabetes, with an assessment of its management.

Discovery of recent illnesses or fevers helps the provider to look carefully for residual conditions, such as organomegaly or dehydration, which might limit or endanger an athlete's performance. Although such findings are unlikely to affect participation in the long run, follow-up might be necessary before clearance is offered.

Similarly, genetic syndromes may or may not affect participation, but knowledge of these helps in the evaluation. Depending on the nature of the condition, laboratory evaluation, close follow-up, or a more detailed examination may be necessary. Clearance should be based on the individual's risk for injury or illness, rather than on his or her disability.

Past Surgical History

The importance of surgical history centers on ensuring that the athlete has had appropriate rehabilitation or healing time. The nature of operations also may lead to a more detailed examination of the affected system.

Family History

Care must be taken with the family history because this may be the only indication for a potential problem in an apparently healthy athlete. Relatives with hypertrophic cardiomyopathy (HCM), arrhythmia, congenital heart disease, sudden death, or atherosclerotic disease at a relatively young age should be warnings for the examiner. Deaths among athletes generally occur as a result of these abnormalities. Genetic conditions, such as Marfan syndrome or Ehlers-Danlos syndrome, also are associated with a risk to the heart and other abnormalities.

Allergy History

A thorough list of allergies to medications must be maintained to avoid administration of these agents. A history of anaphylactic response, whether to envenomation or exercise-induced, should be reported to the team physician to ensure that emergency medications are available. A patient with chronic seasonal allergies should be evaluated for the presence of asthma.

Medication History

Current medications should be part of the record. This helps with following therapy and refills, but it can also alert the physician to medical conditions. Many athletes take over-the-counter nutritional supplements or herbal remedies, which should be included on the medication list as well.

Orthopedic History

The greatest risk for musculoskeletal injury is the history of previous injury. A history of musculoskeletal injury, most commonly an injury to the knee and ankle, remains the primary reason for the disqualification of athletes. Examiners must determine not only the type of injury, but also the treatment and rehabilitation. An injury that is inadequately treated puts the athlete at substantially greater risk for subsequent injury. Some athletes with prior injury wear braces, and this should be documented in the record (45). Any history of injury requires a more detailed examination and a determination of the need for further treatment or rehabilitation.

Cardiovascular History

In athletes younger than 30 years, more than 95% of all sudden deaths are due to structural cardiac abnormalities. Approximately 1,000 of 200,000 high school athletes per academic year are at risk, and at least one will have sudden cardiac death (32,46,47). The male to female ratio is approximately 5 to 1 (48). The cardiac evaluation and a thorough history and examination are thus of paramount importance in the PPE. To a certain degree, the PPE is an attempt to prevent such deaths, but the detection of the athletes at risk can be difficult.

Major concerns include arrhythmia, HCM, atherosclerotic disease, and congenital heart disease (Table 2.2)(47,49–56). Because no cost-effective screening

TABLE 2.2. *Cardiovascular abnormalities in young athletes*

Cardiac congenital abnormalities
Hypertrophic cardiomyopathy
Coronary artery abnormalities
Increased cardiac mass
Other causes
Myocarditis
Marfan syndrome
Mitral valve prolapse
Dysrhythmia
Aortic stenosis
Wolff–Parkinson–White syndrome
Idiopathic long QT syndrome
Arrhythmogenic right ventricular dysplasia
Cocaine use
Anabolic steroid use
Bulimia
Anorexia nervosa
Bronchospasm
Heat-related illness
Coronary artery disease

From Lyznicki JM, Nielsen NH, Schneider JF. Cardiovascular screening of student athletes. *Am Fam Physician* 2000;62:765–774, with permission.

TABLE 2.3. *American Heart Association recommendations for cardiovascular preparticipation physical evaluation*

A national standard is needed for preparticipation medical evaluations, including cardiovascular screening, because of heterogeneity in the design and content of preparticipation screening among states. Some form of cardiovascular preparticipation screening is justifiable and compelling for all high school and college athletes, based on ethical, legal, and medical grounds.

Cardiovascular preparticipation screening, including a history and physical examination, should be mandatory for all athletes and should be performed before participation in organized high school (grades 9 through 12) and college sports.

A complete and careful personal and family history and physical examination designed to identify (or raise suspicion of) those cardiovascular lesions known to cause sudden death or disease progression in young athletes is the best available and most practical approach to screening populations of competitive sports participants, regardless of age.

The examination should be performed by a healthcare provider (preferably a physician) who has the requisite training, medical skills, and background to obtain a detailed cardiovascular history reliably, perform a physical examination, and recognize heart disease.

For high school athletes, screening should occur every 2 years, with an interim history in intervening years.

From Maron BJ, Thompson PD, Puffer JC, et al. Cardiovascular preparticipation screening of competitive athletes [Addendum]. *Circulation* 1998;97:2294, with permission.

methods exist for these conditions and because of their relative rarity, diagnosis is difficult. Despite these challenges, the serious nature of such abnormalities makes cardiovascular screening imperative.

A careful cardiovascular history and physical examination may reveal otherwise subtle abnormalities (Tables 2.3 and 2.4). An athlete with a history of chest pain, palpitations, easy fatigability, or a positive family history may be reluctant to share this information unless he or she is specifically asked (49).

HCM, conduction abnormalities, arrhythmias, or valvular problems may manifest with dizziness, light-headedness, excessive dyspnea, palpitations, or syncope. Chest pain may indicate coronary artery disease or abnormality. Additional studies may be warranted in athletes with a previous disqualification, an abnormal cardiac evaluation (electrocardiogram or echocardiogram), high blood pressure, hypercholesterolemia, or a recent viral illness. A history of cardiac murmur or hypertension should heighten the examiner's suspicion.

Dermatologic History

The dermatologic history focuses on infection, such as tinea, herpes simplex, scabies, lice, molluscum contagiosum, warts, impetigo, furunculosis, and carbunculosis. The risk of transmission is increased in sports in which athletes come into contact with one another or with equipment such as mats or helmets.

Acne or tinea versicolor may be exacerbated in athletes as a result of perspiration or occlusive uniforms or equipment. Eczema also may worsen in athletes because of the frequent wet-to-dry cycles, such as those occurring with swimming or from sweating. Although these conditions do not warrant permanent

TABLE 2.4. *American Heart Association recommendations for cardiovascular history and physical examination*

Cardiovascular history: inquire about and seek parental verification of the following:
  Family history of premature death (sudden or otherwise).
  Family history of heart disease in surviving relatives, significant disability from cardiovascular disease in close relatives younger than 50 years, or specific knowledge of the occurrence of conditions (i.e., hypertrophic cardiomyopathy, long QT syndrome, Marfan syndrome, or clinically important arrhythmias).
  Personal history of heart murmur.
  Personal history of systemic hypertension.
  Personal history of excessive fatigability.
  Personal history of syncope, excessive or progressive shortness of breath (dyspnea), or chest pain or discomfort, particularly if present with exertion.
Physical examination
  Perform precordial auscultation in supine and standing positions to identify, in particular, heart murmurs consistent with dynamic left ventricular outflow obstruction.
  Assess femoral artery pulses to exclude coarctation of the aorta.
    Recognize physical stigmata of Marfan syndrome.
  Assess brachial artery blood pressure in the sitting position.

From Maron BJ, Thompson PD, Puffer JC, et al. Cardiovascular preparticipation screening of competitive athletes. *Circulation* 1996;94:850–856, with permission.

disqualification, temporary restriction from play may be indicated while treatment is instituted.

Neurologic and Head Injury History

A thorough neurologic history helps to identify athletes with prior injury or illness that may put them at risk. The most common condition in many sports is concussion. Other neurologic concerns include seizure disorder, severe headaches, numbness or tingling, pinched nerves, burners or stingers, or transient quadriplegia, all of which necessitate further questioning and focused evaluation.

Athletes with a history of concussion must be questioned carefully, specifically with regard to loss of consciousness, confusion, amnesia, headache, and course of care. Any residual deficits indicating possible postconcussion syndrome necessitate further evaluation by a specialist in sports medicine, neurology, or neurosurgery.

Traumatic nerve injury, such as burners or stingers and pinched nerves, involves compression or stretching of the cervical nerves or brachial plexus. These conditions rarely result in permanent deficits (57). Rather, transient unilateral numbness or tingling, pain, or weakness generally resolves within minutes.

Athletes with repeated burners or stingers, transient quadriplegia, or unresolved deficits should undergo a more thorough workup, including cervical spine radiography or magnetic resonance imaging (MRI), and possible referral.

Heat Illness History

Athletes at risk for heat illness will have had frequent cramping, heat exhaustion, or poor exercise tolerance during hot weather. A history of heat illness is the most important predictor of subsequent risk of recurrence (58,59). Preexercise and postexercise weights may help determine athletes who are at risk.

Medications and supplements may predispose athletes to heat-related disorders. In athletes who use antihistamines or stimulants, discontinuation of their use should be considered during hot and humid seasons. Other athletes at risk include those who are obese or poorly conditioned, especially at the onset of the season.

Although heat-related illness may seem inconsequential compared with other disorders (e.g., cardiac abnormalities), exertional hyperthermia in athletes contributes significantly to nontraumatic deaths of noncardiac origin. Among these deaths, 22% are related to hyperthermia, rhabdomyolysis, and status asthmaticus, all of which are considered preventable illnesses (48).

Pulmonary History

Asthma and exercise-induced asthma put the athlete at risk for impaired performance, respiratory distress, or even death in cases of status asthmaticus. Baseline pulmonary function tests or pulmonary function tests after exercise may be advised. Recommendations for follow-up must be given, and guidelines need to be provided for athletes who are seasonally affected, such as those affected during cold weather or allergy season. If an athlete uses an inhaler, it should be available during practice and competition.

Other lung disease, including a history of pneumonia, trauma, or genetic conditions (e.g., cystic fibrosis), also may put the athlete at risk and thus should be evaluated on an individual basis.

Vision History

Vision history determines the risk of participation, in addition to the current function. Prior injury or operation to the eye, including laser-assisted *in situ* keratomileusis (LASIK) or radial keratotomy, should be well documented. Changes or alterations in vision should also be elicited. An athlete with contacts, glasses, or eye guards should use sport-appropriate frames and lenses that are considered safe for participation (Table 2.5) (60). Vision that cannot be corrected to better than 20/40 in one eye is termed as "functionally one-eyed." Such athletes are at risk for becoming legally blind if injury to the dominant eye occurs. This condition may indicate a history of amblyopia and may limit binocular vision.

Nutrition and Weight History

Responses to questions concerning recent weight gain or loss, body image, or perceived ideal weight can give insight into potentially injurious behavior. A rapid weight gain may signal the use of anabolic steroids. Unrealistic ideal weight goals in wrestlers may lead to dangerous practices. Eating disorders reach epidemic proportions in sports with weight classes (wrestling or rowing) or in those with an emphasis on leanness (running or swimming) or appearance (gymnastics, diving, or figure skating) (19). For eating disorders, the female to male ratio is approximately 10 to 1 (61).

When eating disorders are suspected, consultation with a psychological counselor, dietitian, or nutritionist may be of particular value.

TABLE 2.5. *Sports with high risk of eye injury with appropriate eye protectors*

Sport	Eye protection[a]
Badminton	Sports goggles with polycarbonate lenses
Baseball	Polycarbonate face guard or other certified safe protection attached to helmet for batting and base running; sports goggles with polycarbonate lenses for fielding
Bicycling (LER)	Sturdy street-wear frames with polycarbonate or CR-39 lenses
Boxing	None available
Fencing	Full-face cage
Field hockey (both sexes)	Goalie, full-face mask; all others, sports goggles with polycarbonate lenses
Football	Polycarbonate shield on helmet
Full-contact martial arts	Not allowed
Handball[b]	Sports goggles with polycarbonate lenses
Ice hockey	Helmet and full-face protection
Lacrosse (male)	Helmet and full-face protection required
Lacrosse (female)	Should at least wear sports goggles with polycarbonate lenses; should have option to wear helmet and full-face protection
Racquetball[b]	Sports goggles with polycarbonate lenses
Soccer	Sports goggles with polycarbonate lenses
Softball	Polycarbonate face guard or other certified safe protection attached to helmet for batting and base running; sports goggles with polycarbonate lenses for fielding
Squash[b]	Sports goggles with polycarbonate lenses
Street hockey[c]	Sports goggles with polycarbonate lenses; goalie, full-face cage
Swimming and pool sports	Swim goggles recommended
Tennis, doubles	Sports goggles with polycarbonate lenses
Tennis, singles	Sturdy street-wear frames with polycarbonate lenses
Track and field (LER)	Sturdy street-wear frames with polycarbonate or CR-39 lenses
Water polo	Swim goggles with polycarbonate lenses
Wrestling	None available

[a]Abbreviation: LER, low eye risk.
For sports in which a face mask or helmet with eye protection is worn, functionally one-eyed athletes, and those with previous eye trauma or surgery for whom their ophthalmologists recommend eye protection, sports goggles with polycarbonate lenses also must be worn to ensure protection.
[b]Goggles without lenses are not effective.
[c]A street hockey ball can penetrate into a molded goalie mask and injure an eye.
From American Academy of Pediatrics Committee on Sports Medicine and Fitness and American Academy of Ophthalmology Committee on Eye Safety and Sports Ophthalmology. Protective eyewear for young athletes. *Pediatrics* 1996;98:311–313, with permission.

Female athletes with *female athlete triad* have an eating disorder, amenorrhea, and osteoporosis, as evidenced by menstrual history, stress fracture, medication abuses, and dietary habits (62). These athletes are often highly functional, and they may even be praised for their hard work and dedication. Excessive exercise, manifested by training in addition to regular workouts for a sport, has the outward effect of a lean muscular appearance.

Sports in which size is imperative, such as football, may allow an obese athlete to "slip through the cracks." Obesity contributes to the risk for development of diabetes and heart disease in the long term; in the short term, exertion of a deconditioned athlete may contribute to musculoskeletal or heat injuries.

Even athletes of normal body habitus and eating patterns should be counseled on a healthful diet, including the avoidance of saturated fats and fast foods.

The early establishment of good eating habits will help to maintain healthful lifestyles, even after the age of peak performance athletically.

Psychologic History

The PPE history screening shown in Appendix B asks athletes whether they feel stressed. This question often serves as an excellent way to broach the topic of mental health. Performance can be enhanced and overall health can be improved by addressing psychologic factors. These factors include anxiety, depression, suicidal behavior, anger, a history of abuse, and risky behavior.

A personal history of mental illness should be noted. Any psychoactive medication taken by athletes (e.g., for depression or attention-deficit disorder) must be recorded, and a careful history must be taken. The family history of mental health may be important because conditions such as bipolar disorder or schizophrenia manifest in adolescence and young adulthood.

Drug and Alcohol History

Information on a form signed by parents likely is not accurate. The PPE provides a unique setting for screening and counseling young athletes regarding dangerous practices. This part of the PPE should be performed privately with the athlete. Parents, if they are present, should be asked to wait outside the examining room.

Supplement and Ergogenic Aid History

The goal of supplements and ergogenic aids is to enhance performance. Health food stores are replete with formulations that tout enhanced energy, strength, and muscle building. These generally benign measures can become dangerous when they are used in excess or inappropriately.

Anabolic androgenic steroids are extremely effective ergogenic aids in athletic competition. Side effects include testicular atrophy, gynecomastia, liver damage, increased cholesterol level, acne, hirsutism, menstrual changes, and closure of the growth plates. Anabolic steroids are banned by the NCAA and the United States Olympic Committee (63). When they are taken in the injectable form, additional dangers develop from impurities and needle sharing. Because they are illegal, anabolic steroids are often obtained through the black market or from overseas sources, which may further compromise the safety margin for young athletes who use these products.

Immunization History

A record of immunizations should be obtained to ensure adequate protection. Of note is the fact that adolescents need a tetanus booster 10 years after childhood vaccination. Many adolescents have not had a hepatitis B vaccination, and they should be advised to have this done. Additionally, athletes who have not had chickenpox should be vaccinated because the severity of the illness increases with age. Yearly influenza immunization can be considered on a team, institutional, or individual basis.

Female-Only History

Female history should include the age at menarche, the regularity of cycles, the duration of flow, and a history of pregnancy, sexual activity, and method of contraception. Female athletes also should be reminded to perform regular self-examinations of the breasts. Sexually active athletes should have regular Papanicolaou smears. Any findings of concern from the history should be followed up with the primary provider.

Male-Only History

Male history should also include questions regarding sexual activity. Any injury to the genitals should be noted, and athletes should be reminded to perform testicular self-examination because testicular cancer remains the most common form of cancer in young men.

THE PHYSICAL EXAMINATION

The physical examination emphasizes body systems involving sports participation. It also must focus on conditions elicited in the medical history. Table 2.6

TABLE 2.6. *Standard components of the preparticipation physical evaluation*

Height
Weight
Eyes
Visual acuity (Snellen chart)
Differences in pupil size
Oral cavity
Ears
Nose
Lungs
Cardiovascular system
Blood pressure
Pulses (radial, femoral)
Heart (rate, rhythm, murmurs)
Abdomen
Masses
Tenderness
Organomegaly
Genitalia (males only)
Single or undescended testicle
Testicular mass
Hernia
Skin
Rashes
Lesions
Musculoskeletal system
Contour; range of motion; stability; and symmetry of neck, back, shoulder/arm, elbow/forearm, wrist/hand, hip/thigh, knee, leg/ankle, and foot
Neurologic system

From Smith DM, Kovan JR, Rich BSE, et al. *Preparticipation physical evaluation,* 2nd ed. Minneapolis: Mc-Graw-Hill, 1997, with permission.

lists components of the examination, and Appendix B can serve as an outline for the PPE.

General Appearance

General appearance may indicate a syndrome; for example, excessive height with long arms and digits may be signs of Marfan syndrome. Evidence of depression, general nutrition, and hygiene may also be found.

Height and Weight

Body mass index helps to identify overly thin or obese individuals. This information may lead to discussions about eating disorders or obesity. If an eating disorder or growth disturbance is suspected, the athlete should be referred for further evaluation (15).

Vital Signs and Visual Acuity

Determination of vital signs (pulse and blood pressure) remains an integral part of any physical examination. Abnormal heart rate, rhythm, or blood pressure may be indicators of cardiovascular abnormality. Table 2.7 classifies hypertension by age, height, and sex. Care must be taken to determine vital signs as accurately as possible. Regular calibration of sphygmomanometers, the adequate training of staff, and use of the proper cuff size will provide the most accurate readings possible in most settings.

Any deficits found on visual acuity screening should be referred for formal visual evaluation. With use of a standard Snellen eye chart, vision should be 20/40 or better in each eye, either with or without corrective lenses. Athletes involved in sports that require distance vision and hand–eye coordination will be limited by impaired vision, and the athlete could be in danger without proper correction.

Head, Eyes, Ears, Nose, and Throat

Examination of the eyes focuses on signs of injury or infection. Anisocoria, or unequal size of pupils, should be noted as a baseline, and this is important in the evaluation of future head injury. Oral examination should note ulcers, gingivitis, caries, or enamel abnormalities, which are seen in severe bulimia. Athletes who have braces on the teeth may require a mouth guard to lessen the potential for trauma.

Ears should be evaluated for gross hearing by whispering or doing a finger-rub. Abnormalities of hearing should be referred for formal audiologic testing. The tympanic membrane must be evaluated for abnormalities (e.g., perforation, scarring, or infection). Nasal polyps may be indicators of respiratory or systemic illness. A deviated septum should be referred for correction if it is severe.

Cardiovascular System

The PPE hinges on the cardiovascular system because this is where the most serious problems occur. The examination should include (a) precordial auscultation in the standing and supine positions to identify dynamic left ventricular outflow obstruction, (b) comparison of the femoral artery pulses with the upper extremity pulses to screen for the presence of coarctation, (c) recognition of Marfan syndrome, and (d) brachial blood pressure measurement in the sitting position (47).

Blood pressure should be determined, and, if it is abnormal, another reading should be performed. If, after 10 minutes of rest in the supine position, the

TABLE 2.7. *Blood pressure ranges for boys and girls based on height percentiles*

	Blood pressure (mm Hg) by sex							
	Boys				Girls			
	Systolic		Diastolic		Systolic		Diastolic	
Age (yr)	5% Height	95% Height	5% Height	95% Height	5% Height	95% Height	5% Height	95% Height
6–8	109–111	117–120	72–75	76–80	108–112	114–118	71–74	75–78
9–11	113–116	121–125	76–78	81–83	114–118	120–124	75–78	79–81
12–14	119–124	127–132	79–80	83–85	120–123	126–130	79–81	82–85
15–17	127–132	135–140	81–85	86–89	124–126	131–132	82–83	86

[a]Hypertension was defined as the 95th percentile or more for height, age, and sex, measured on at least three separate occasions.

Modified from Falkner B, Daniels SR, Horan MJ, et al. *Update on the Task Force Report (1987) on high blood pressure in children and adolescents: a working group report from the National High Blood Pressure Education Program.* NIH Publication No. 96-3790. Bethesda, MD: National Institutes of Health, National Heart, Lung, and Blood Institute, 1996:7–8.

blood pressure remains increased, questions should be asked regarding stimulant use, including caffeine, cocaine, nicotine, or ephedrine (49). Elevated blood pressure requires further investigation by the athlete's primary care physician.

Cardiac auscultation in the supine and standing positions yields the most accurate examination. HCM can be detected more easily in the standing position. The presence of normal heart sounds and the volume of these sounds should be assessed. Documentation of murmurs must include quality, timing, and volume. Extra heart sounds, such as S3 and S4, and rubs should be recognized.

Maneuvers, such as Valsalva or deep inspiration, may be helpful for further characterizing murmurs. Timing, duration, volume, intensity, radiation, quality, and relationship to respiration or body position may all give clues to the origin and severity of murmurs. With HCM, squatting increases venous return, and thus the obstruction and intensity of the murmur are decreased. Conversely, the Valsalva maneuver reduces venous return, increasing obstruction and murmur intensity. Aortic stenosis produces the opposite effect, so that squatting increases the intensity of the murmur and the Valsalva maneuver reduces it. Innocent murmurs act similarly to aortic stenosis, but they differ by location, intensity, quality, and radiation.

Murmurs in the pediatric and adolescent population are common, but any systolic murmur rated 3/6 or greater, any diastolic murmur, or a murmur that grows louder with the Valsalva maneuver merits further evaluation before clearance for participation. The cardiac history alone may warrant a cardiology consultation, as should any murmur that is not clearly characterized.

Any arrhythmia should be carefully examined. Generally, irregular beats that resolve on exertion indicate a benign course and a normal heart. Electrocardiography should be considered if any irregularity is found, and a cardiologist should formally evaluate any multifocal premature ventricular contractions, doublets, or triplets.

When structural heart disease is suspected, workup by the primary physician should include the history and physical examination, standard 12-lead electrocardiography, echocardiography, and stress testing. A cardiologist should conduct any further evaluation that is required. The 26th Bethesda Conference guidelines (64) provide primary physicians with recommendations for cardiovascular workup and clearance.

Pulmonary System

Any finding on the lung examination should be evaluated further. Wheezing, diminished breath sounds, or rubs may indicate asthma or other significant respiratory abnormality. Athletes carrying cigarettes or smelling of tobacco should be counseled about the risks and long-term effects of tobacco use.

Abdomen

Examination of the abdomen should include auscultation for bowel sounds and possible bruits and palpation of all four quadrants, looking for tenderness, guarding, rigidity, masses, or organomegaly. Any suspicious findings warrant further evaluation. In particular, clearance for sports participation should be postponed if the liver or spleen is enlarged, pending further evaluation. In female athletes, the uterus also should be palpated externally to determine whether the patient might be pregnant or have tenderness or a mass.

Genitalia

Any lesions on the glans or shaft of the penis should be noted, as should any irregularities of the meatus. Testicles should be examined for tenderness, mass, and nodularity, and the physician should ensure that they are descended. Athletes with a single or an undescended testicle must be counseled on protection and the decision to participate in contact sports. The patient also should be evaluated for the presence of a hernia. Depending on the size and reducibility of the hernia, it may or may not require evaluation or repair before participation.

Recent high-profile cases of testicular cancer among Olympic and collegiate athletes and in well-known Hollywood personalities have heightened the public awareness of testicular cancer. Of all cancer-related deaths of men aged from 18 to 35 years, more are caused by testicular cancer than by any other type. Because testicular cancer is often treatable, early detection is of primary importance. The PPE can serve as an opportunity to educate male athletes on testicular self-examination.

The female athlete should have her primary care physician provide any genitourinary or breast examination that may be necessary because this is beyond the scope of the PPE. If the history indicates the need for pelvic or breast examination, the patient should schedule an appointment with her physician.

Skin

Examination of the skin should be incorporated into the PPE, whether it is office-based or station-based. Acne should be noted, and, if appropriate, a recommendation should be made to follow up with the athlete's primary care physician. Additionally, the presence of eczema, psoriasis, infection, or infestation should be documented. Specifically, the examiner should look for impetigo, furuncles, herpes simplex, molluscum contagiosum, tinea, scabies, and lice. An infection may need to be treated before allowing participation in sports in which close contact may spread the infection among athletes. For example, tinea corporis could be spread among wrestlers.

In some cases, covering the lesion may allow the individual to participate.

Musculoskeletal System

The musculoskeletal examination can be performed as a general screening examination, a more compre-

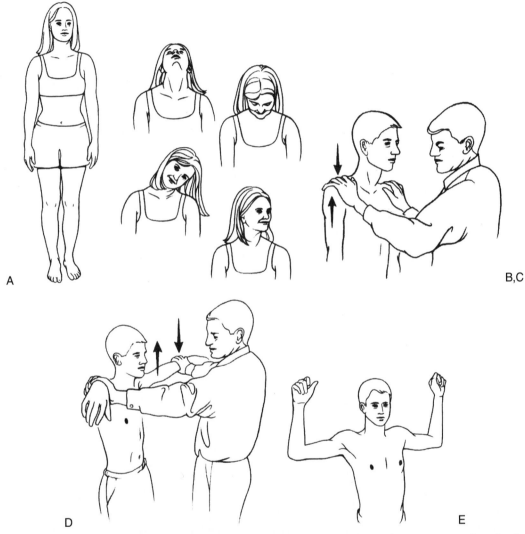

FIG. 2.1. Components of general screening evaluation. Patient performs the maneuvers described. **A:** Stands facing the examiner. Common abnormalities found include asymmetric waist (indicating scoliosis or leg-length discrepancy), swollen joints, and enlargement of acromioclavicular or sternoclavicular joint. Lower extremities are inspected with the quadriceps contracted to evaluate alignment and symmetry. **B:** Extends neck, flexes neck, laterally bends neck, and rotates neck. Diminished mobility, asymmetry, or pain may indicate previous neck injury. **C:** Stands facing examiner and shrugs shoulders against resistance. Atrophy or weakness may indicate nerve injury. **D:** Abducts extended arms and raises them against resistance. Deltoid muscle size and strength should be equal. **E:** Abducts arms with elbows bent to 90 degrees and then raises hands as far as able. Loss of external rotation may indicate prior dislocation. Internal rotation also should be assessed. Range of motion and glenohumeral joint are evaluated. *Continued on next page*

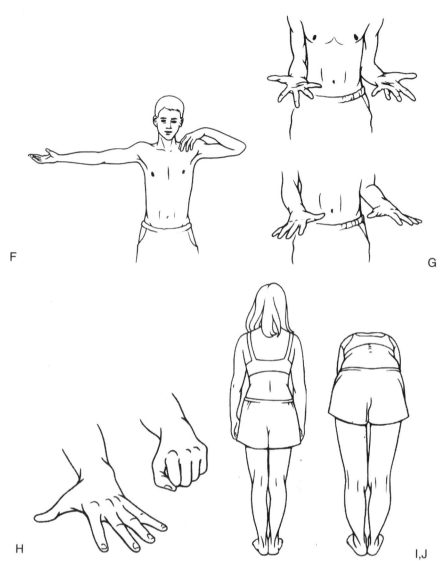

FIG. 2.1. (*Continued*) **F:** Abducts arms with palms up, then completely bends and straightens elbows. Asymmetric movements or loss of flexion or extension may indicate prior elbow injury. **G:** Holds arms at sides with elbows bent at 90 degrees and then achieves full pronation and supination of hands. Inability to do so suggests prior injury to elbow or wrist. **H:** Makes a fist and then opens hand and spreads fingers. Fist should be tight, knuckles symmetric, and fingers straight and without swelling when extended. **I:** Stands erect with back to examiner. Asymmetry of shoulders, prominent rib cage, or asymmetric waist may indicate scoliosis or leg-length discrepancy. Atrophy of musculature may indicate old injury, such as an atrophic calf from ruptured Achilles tendon. Back is extended, with knees straight, to determine pain from spondylolysis or spondylolisthesis. **J:** Bends forward, reaching for toes, with legs straight. Asymmetry indicates possible scoliosis, and twisting to one side may indicate low back pain. Hamstring flexibility also can be assessed.

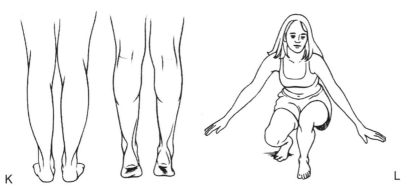

FIG. 2.1. (*Continued*) **K:** Stands on heels and toes. Equal elevation, balance, symmetry, and arch are evaluated. Patient also may be evaluated for ambulating on heels, on toes, and in tandem gait. **L:** Squats and duckwalks. Asymmetry of gait, pain in joints, or imbalance may indicate prior injury. (From Kurowski K, Chandran S. The preparticipation athletic evaluation. *Am Fam Physician* 2000;61:2683–2690,2696–2698, with permission.)

hensive joint-specific evaluation, or a sport-specific examination. History alone can identify 92% of significant musculoskeletal injuries (65). When prior injury or instability is identified through either the history or a general screening examination, a more thorough joint-specific evaluation should be performed, and, if warranted, a referral to a specialist should be given.

The general screening examination is used to evaluate range of motion, gross motor function, and significant injury (Fig. 2.1, A to L) (65). Joint-specific evaluation should be performed when deemed necessary from the history or general screening. Figures 2.2 through 2.9 provide further elaboration of joint-specific testing.

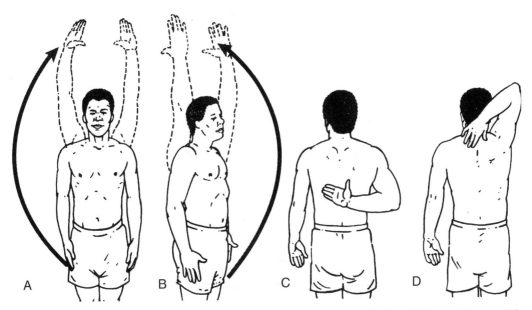

FIG. 2.2. Shoulder range of motion is evaluated in four directions: abduction **(A)**, forward flexion **(B)**, internal rotation **(C)**, and external rotation **(D)**. Asymmetries of the scapular or reach should be noted. (From Smith DM, Kovan JR, Rich BSE, et al. *Preparticipation physical evaluation*, 2nd ed. Minneapolis: McGraw-Hill, 1997, with permission.)

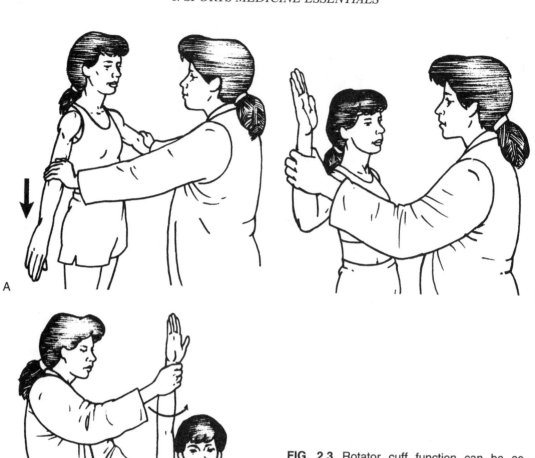

FIG. 2.3. Rotator cuff function can be assessed through several tests, including the empty can test, with isolation of the supraspinatus muscle **(A)**, resistance to internal and external rotation with 90-degree abduction **(B)**, and full abduction with internal rotation to look for impingement **(C)**. (From Smith DM, Kovan JR, Rich BSE, et al. *Preparticipation physical evaluation*, 2nd ed. Minneapolis: McGraw-Hill, 1997, with permission.)

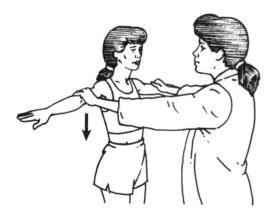

FIG. 2.4. Resisting straight arm abduction and noting symmetry is a test for deltoid strength. (From Smith DM, Kovan JR, Rich BSE, et al. *Preparticipation physical evaluation*, 2nd ed. Minneapolis: McGraw-Hill, 1997, with permission.)

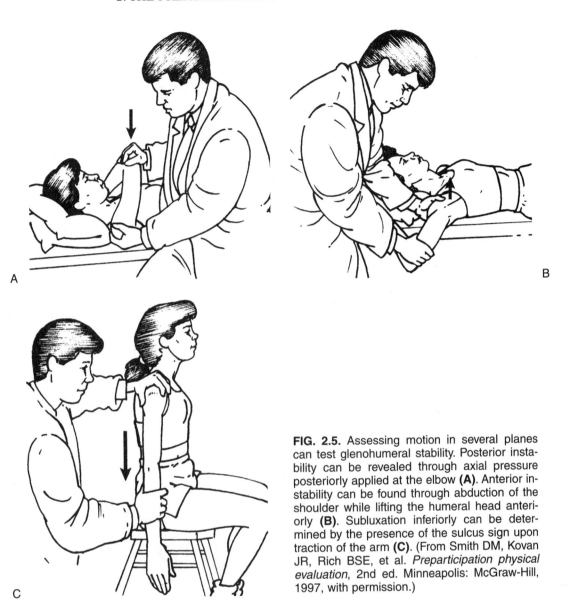

FIG. 2.5. Assessing motion in several planes can test glenohumeral stability. Posterior instability can be revealed through axial pressure posteriorly applied at the elbow **(A)**. Anterior instability can be found through abduction of the shoulder while lifting the humeral head anteriorly **(B)**. Subluxation inferiorly can be determined by the presence of the sulcus sign upon traction of the arm **(C)**. (From Smith DM, Kovan JR, Rich BSE, et al. *Preparticipation physical evaluation*, 2nd ed. Minneapolis: McGraw-Hill, 1997, with permission.)

Sport-specific examinations focus on the athlete's specific sport and specific systems that are more likely to be placed under additional stress. Sport-specific testing includes a general musculoskeletal examination, but it also may incorporate further evaluations for strength, endurance, flexibility, and range of motion. Isokinetic testing and gait or throw analysis may play a role in further testing. These more detailed assessments may help to prevent injury and to improve form and performance, but they are much more costly and time-consuming, and they require a higher level of expertise.

Neurologic System

In the normal asymptomatic athlete, the musculoskeletal screening evaluation also provides a limited degree of neurologic testing. When the history so indicates, further examination should be performed. For example, an athlete with a history of stingers, burners, or concussion should have a more complete examination, including testing of the deep tendon reflexes, strength, cranial nerves, and cerebellar and cognitive function. Any impairment noted should be evaluated further before clearance.

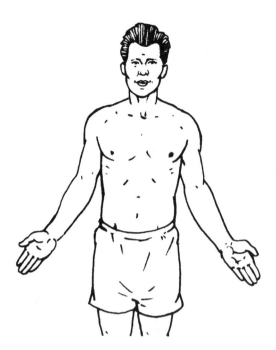

FIG. 2.6. Excessive or insufficient valgus may indicate instability or prior injury. The normal angle of the elbow with palms forward is 15-degree valgus. (From Smith DM, Kovan JR, Rich BSE, et al. *Preparticipation physical evaluation*, 2nd ed. Minneapolis: McGraw-Hill, 1997, with permission.)

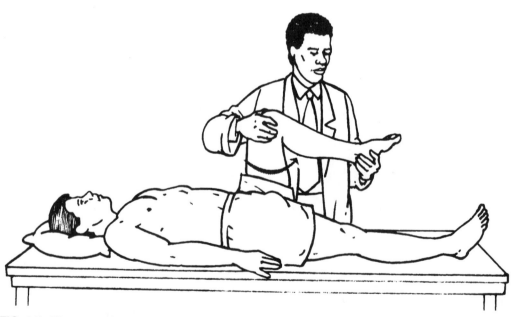

FIG. 2.7. Hip range of motion, evaluated with athlete in supine position. With knee flexed to 90 degrees, hip rotation should equal 60 degrees, with symmetric components of internal and external rotation. (From Smith DM, Kovan JR, Rich BSE, et al. *Preparticipation physical evaluation*, 2nd ed. Minneapolis: McGraw-Hill, 1997, with permission.)

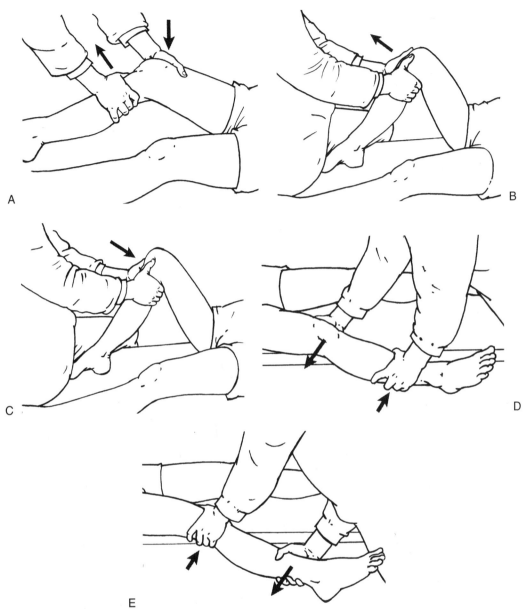

FIG. 2.8. Knee stability can be assessed with several tests. The Lachman test **(A)**, to assess the anterior cruciate ligament, is performed with the knee at 20 degrees and muscles relaxed. The femur is stabilized with one hand, and the other hand rocks the tibia anteriorly; a solid end point is sought. The anterior drawer test **(B)** and posterior drawer test **(C)** are used to test for insufficiency of the anterior and posterior cruciate ligaments. This is accomplished with the knee at 90 degrees and by pulling or pushing the tibia with foot placement fixed. The tibial plateau should be palpated for excessive movement. Excessive movement and lack of end point reveal possible ligamentous injury. Sag of the tibia, compared with the unaffected knee, may indicate a posterior cruciate ligament rupture. Varus **(D)** and valgus **(E)** stresses of the knee test for instability or injury of the medial and lateral collateral ligaments. The knee should be examined at full extension and at 20 degrees. Comparison must be made because normal laxity is highly variable. (From Smith DM, Kovan JR, Rich BSE, et al. *Preparticipation physical evaluation*, 2nd ed. Minneapolis: McGraw-Hill, 1997, with permission.)

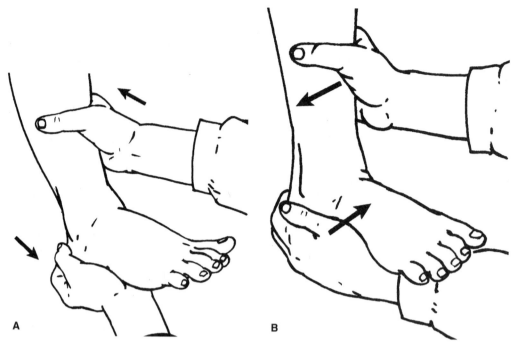

FIG. 2.9. The ankle can be assessed with the anterior drawer test by pulling on the heel, while pushing against the distal tibia **(A)**. The talar tilt test involves inverting the ankle by pushing against the medial tibia and the lateral calcaneus **(B)** to determine whether excessive movement of the foot is occurring medially compared to the contralateral side. (From Smith DM, Kovan JR, Rich BSE, et al. *Preparticipation physical evaluation*, 2nd ed. Minneapolis: McGraw-Hill, 1997, with permission.)

CLASSIFICATION OF SPORTS

Sports can be classified by the level of contact (Table 2.8) or the intensity (Table 2.9). Athletes should be evaluated on an individual basis, and the intended sport and any abnormalities on the history or physical examination should be taken into account.

CLEARANCE FOR PARTICIPATION

The fulcrum for the PPE is the determination of clearance. This can be categorized as (a) unrestricted, (b) dependent on further evaluation or rehabilitation, and (c) not cleared for any sport or for a specific sport.

Determination for clearance for a particular sport should be based on overall risk. Sports are stratified by level of contact or collision and by degree of strenuousness (Tables 2.8 and 2.9) (66). Strenuousness becomes important in athletes who have cardiovascular or pulmonary disease. Static activity produces increased pressure load, whereas dynamic activity strains the left ventricle through a volume load (67).

The American Academy of Pediatrics (AAP) has created guidelines for specific conditions and recommendations for clearance (Table 2.10) (66). Clearance should always be determined on an individual basis, and the specific sport, its contact potential, and level of strenuousness should be considered (66).

When station-based PPE is used, clearance should be determined at the final station by a physician well versed in the specific condition in question, the current recommendations for clearance, and the demands of the desired sport. Follow-up should then be recommended as he or she deems necessary.

Final recommendations for follow-up and clearance determination should be made clear to the athlete and, if the athlete is a minor, to the parents. Once permission has been received from the athlete or parents, this information should be shared with coaches and school officials, with any restrictions and recom-

TABLE 2.8. *Classification of sports by contact*

Contact/collision	Limited contact	Noncontact
Basketball	Baseball	Archery
Boxing[a]	Bicycling	Badminton
Diving	Cheerleading	Body building
Field hockey	Canoeing/kayaking (white water)	Bowling
Football, tackle	Fencing	Canoeing/kayaking (flat water)
Ice hockey[b]	Field events	Crew/rowing
Lacrosse	High jump	Curling
Martial arts	Pole vault	Dancing[d]
Rodeo	Floor hockey	Ballet
Rugby	Football, flag	Jazz
Ski jumping	Gymnastics	Modern
Soccer	Handball	Field events
Team handball	Horseback riding	Discus
Water polo	Racquetball	Javelin
Wrestling	Skateboarding	Shot put
	Skating	Golf
	Ice	Orienteering[e]
	In-line	Power lifting
	Roller	Race walking
	Skiing	Riflery
	Cross-country	Rope jumping
	Downhill	Running
	Water	Sailing
	Snowboarding[c]	Scuba diving
	Softball	Swimming
	Squash	Table tennis
	Ultimate frisbee	Tennis
	Volleyball	Track
	Windsurfing/surfing	Weight lifting

[a]Participation not recommended by the American Academy of Pediatrics. The American Academy of Family Physicians, American Medical Society for Sports Medicine, American Orthopaedic Society for Sports Medicine, and American Osteopathic Academy of Sports Medicine take no stand against boxing.
[b]The American Academy of Pediatrics recommends limiting the amount of body checking allowed for hockey players 15 yr or younger to reduce injuries.
[c]Snowboarding has been added since the previous statement was published.
[d]Dancing has been further classified into ballet, jazz, and modern since the previous statement was published.
[e]A race (contest) in which competitors use a map and compass to find their way through unfamiliar territory.
From American Academy of Pediatrics. Medical conditions affecting sports participation. *Pediatrics* 2001;107:1205–1209, with permission.

mendations for follow-up or rehabilitation clearly outlined. This communication can be accomplished through the use of a clearance form, such as the one shown in Appendix C, which is separate from the history and physical form. This approach ensures the confidentiality of the medical record and yet makes the recommendations and clearance status available to the appropriate individuals.

Acute Illness (Including Infectious Mononucleosis)

The AAP recommends that athletes not participate while they are ill with fever or diarrhea. The inherent risks include dehydration, overheating, and the risk of injury during a viral infection, such as splenic rupture from a collision when one is ill with infectious mononucleosis. Another rare, but serious, complication of viral illness can be myocarditis (68). Clearance is rarely denied on the basis of acute illness, as the PPE generally predates participation; but, if the examination is just prior to participation, clearance should be postponed, pending the appropriate follow-up.

Cardiac Abnormalities

Certain cardiac conditions may be worsened by strenuous activity or may be related to an increased risk of sudden death. Clearance should be given only with

TABLE 2.9. *Classification of sports by strenuousness*

High-to-moderate intensity			Low intensity
High-to-moderate dynamic and static demands	High-to-moderate dynamic and low static demands	High-to-moderate static and low dynamic demands	Low dynamic and low static demands
Boxing[a]	Badminton	Archery	Bowling
Crew/rowing	Baseball	Auto racing	Cricket
Cross-country skiing	Basketball	Diving	Curling
Cycling	Field hockey	Field events (throwing)	Golf
Downhill skiing	Lacrosse	Gymnastics	Riflery
Fencing	Orienteering	Horseback riding (jumping)	
Football	Race walking	Karate or judo	
Ice hockey	Racquetball	Motorcycling	
Rugby	Soccer	Rodeo	
Running (sprint)	Squash	Sailing	
Speed skating	Swimming	Ski jumping	
Water polo	Table tennis	Water skiing	
Wrestling	Tennis	Weight lifting	
	Volleyball		

[a]Participation not recommended by the American Academy of Pediatrics. The American Academy of Family Physicians, American Medical Society for Sports Medicine, American Orthopaedic Society for Sports Medicine, and American Osteopathic Academy of Sports Medicine take no stand against boxing.
From American Academy of Pediatrics. Medical conditions affecting sports participation. *Pediatrics* 2001;107:1205–1209, with permission.

TABLE 2.10. *Medical conditions and sports participation*[a]

Condition	May participate
Atlantoaxial instability (instability of the joint between C-1 and C-2) Explanation: Athlete needs evaluation to assess risk of spinal cord injury during sports participation.	Qualified yes
Bleeding disorder Explanation: Athlete needs evaluation.	Qualified yes
Cardiovascular disease	
Carditis (inflammation of the heart) Explanation: Carditis may result in sudden death with exertion.	No
Hypertension (high blood pressure) Explanation: Those with significant essential (unexplained) hypertension should avoid weight and power lifting, body building, and strength training. Those with secondary hypertension (hypertension caused by a previously identified disease) or severe essential hypertension need evaluation. The National High Blood Pressure Education Working Group defined significant and severe hypertension.	Qualified yes
Congenital heart disease (structural heart defects present at birth) Explanation: Those with mild forms may participate fully; those with moderate or severe forms or those who have undergone surgery need evaluation.[b]	Qualified yes
Dysrhythmia (irregular heart rhythm)	Qualified yes
Mitral valve prolapse (abnormal heart valve) Explanation: Those with symptoms (chest pain, syncope, dizziness, shortness of breath, or other symptoms of possible dysrhythmia) or evidence of mitral regurgitation (leaking) on physical examination need evaluation. All others may participate fully.	Qualified yes
Heart murmur Explanation: If murmur is innocent (does not indicate heart disease), full participation is permitted. Otherwise, the athlete needs evaluation (see "Congenital heart disease" and "Mitral valve prolapse" above).	Qualified yes
Cerebral palsy Explanation: Athlete needs evaluation.	Qualified yes
Diabetes mellitus[c] Explanation: All sports can be played with proper attention to diet, blood glucose concentration, hydration, and insulin therapy. Blood glucose concentration should be monitored every 30 min during continuous exercise and 15 min after completion of exercise.	Yes

TABLE 2.10. *Continued*

Condition	May participate
Diarrhea[d]	Qualified no
Explanation: Unless disease is mild, no participation is permitted because diarrhea may increase the risk of dehydration and heat illness. See "Fever" below.	
Eating disorders	
Anorexia nervosa, bulimia nervosa	Qualified yes
Explanation: These patients need both medical and psychiatric assessment before participation.	
Eyes	
Functionally one-eyed athlete, loss of an eye, detached retina, previous eye surgery, or serious eye injury	Qualified yes
Explanation: A functionally one-eyed athlete has a best corrected visual acuity of less than 20/40 in eye with worse acuity. These athletes would suffer significant disability if the better eye were seriously injured, as would those with loss of an eye. Some athletes who previously have undergone eye surgery or who have had a serious eye injury may have an increased risk of injury because of weakened eye tissue. Availability of eye guards approved by the American Society for Testing Materials and other protective equipment may allow participation in most sports, but this must be judged on an individual basis.	
Fever[d]	No
Explanation: Fever can increase cardiopulmonary effort, reduce maximum exercise capacity, make heat illness more likely, and increase orthostatic hypotension during exercise. Fever may rarely accompany myocarditis or other infections that may make exercise dangerous.	
History of heat illness	Qualified yes
Explanation: Because of the increased likelihood of recurrence, athlete needs individual assessment to determine the presence of predisposing conditions and to arrange a prevention strategy.	
Hepatitis	Yes
Explanation: Because of the apparent minimal risk to others, all sports may be played as the athlete's state of health allows. In all athletes, skin lesions should be covered properly, and athletic personnel should use universal precautions when handling blood or body fluids with visible blood.	
Human immunodeficiency virus infection[d]	Yes
Explanation: Because of the apparent minimal risk to others, all sports may be played that the athlete's state of health allows. In all athletes, skin lesions should be properly covered, and athletic personnel should use universal precautions when handling blood or body fluids with visible blood.	
Kidney: absence of one	Qualified yes
Explanation: Athlete needs individual assessment for contact/collision and limited-contact sports.	
Liver, enlarged	Qualified yes
Explanation: If the liver is acutely enlarged, participation should be avoided because of risk of rupture. If the liver is chronically enlarged, individual assessment is needed before contact/collision or limited-contact sports are played.	
Malignant neoplasm	Qualified yes
Explanation: Athlete needs individual assessment.	
Musculoskeletal disorders	Qualified yes
Explanation: Athlete needs individual assessment.	
Neurologic disorders	
History of serious head or spine trauma, severe or repeated concussions, or craniotomy	Qualified yes
Explanation: Athlete needs individual assessment for contact/collision or limited-contact sports and also for noncontact sports, if deficits in judgment or cognition are present. Recent research supports a conservative approach to management of concussion.	
Seizure disorder, well controlled	Yes
Explanation: Risk of seizure during participation is minimal.	
Seizure disorder, poorly controlled	Qualified yes
Explanation: Athlete needs individual assessment for contact/collision or limited-contact sports. The following noncontact sports should be avoided: archery, riflery, swimming, weight or power lifting, strength training, or sports involving heights. In these sports, occurrence of a seizure may be a risk to self or others.	

Continued on next page

TABLE 2.10. *Continued*

Condition	May participate
Obesity	Qualified yes
Explanation: Because of the risk of heat illness, obese persons need careful acclimatization and hydration.	
Organ transplant recipient	Qualified yes
Explanation: Athlete needs individual assessment.	
Ovary: absence of one	Yes
Explanation: Risk of severe injury to the remaining ovary is minimal.	
Respiratory	
Pulmonary compromise, including cystic fibrosis	Qualified yes
Explanation: Athlete needs individual assessment, but generally, all sports may be played if oxygenation remains satisfactory during a graded exercise test. Patients with cystic fibrosis need acclimatization and good hydration to reduce the risk of heat illness.	
Asthma	Yes
Explanation: With proper medication and education, only athletes with the most severe asthma will have to modify their participation.	
Acute upper respiratory infection	Qualified yes
Explanation: Upper respiratory obstruction may affect pulmonary function. Athlete needs individual assessment for all but mild disease. See "Fever" above.	
Sickle cell disease	Qualified yes
Explanation: Athlete needs individual assessment. In general, if the status of the illness permits, all but high-exertion and contact/collision sports may be played. Overheating, dehydration, and chilling must be avoided.	
Sickle cell trait	Yes
Explanation: Individuals with sickle cell trait are unlikely to have an increased risk of sudden death or other medical problems during athletic participation, except under the most extreme conditions of heat, humidity, and possibly increased altitude. These individuals, like all athletes, should be carefully conditioned, acclimatized, and hydrated to reduce any possible risk.	
Skin disorders (boils, herpes simplex, impetigo, scabies, molluscum contagiosum)	Qualified yes
Explanation: While the patient is contagious, participation in gymnastics with mats, martial arts, wrestling, or other contact/collision or limited-contact sports is not allowed. Herpes simplex virus probably is not transmitted via mats.	
Spleen, enlarged[d]	Qualified yes
Explanation: A patient with an acutely enlarged spleen should avoid all sports because of the risk of rupture. Those with a chronically enlarged spleen need individual assessment before playing contact/collision or limited-contact sports.	
Testicle, undescended or absence of one	Yes
Explanation: Certain sports may require a protective cup.	

[a]This table is designed for both medical and nonmedical personnel. In the "Explanation" section below, "needs evaluation" means that a physician with appropriate knowledge and experience should assess the safety of a given sport for an athlete with the listed medical condition. Unless otherwise noted, this is because of the variability of the severity of the disease, the risk of injury among the specific sports, or both.

[b]Mild, moderate, and severe congenital heart disease are defined in 26th Bethesda Conference, January 6–7, 1994. Recommendations for determining eligibility for competition in athletes with cardiovascular abnormalities. *Med Sci Sports Exerc* 1994;26:S246–S253.

[c]Well controlled.

[d]The American Academy of Pediatrics recommendation as indicated.

Modified from American Academy of Pediatrics. Medical conditions affecting sports participation. *Pediatrics* 2001;107:1205–1209, with permission.

adherence to the 26th Bethesda Conference (64), which gives recommendations for athletes with congenital heart disease, ischemic heart disease, arrhythmias, hypertension, valvular disorders, and cardiomyopathy. Any remaining questions should be referred to a cardiologist for the final determination of participation level. Specific recommendations from the Bethesda guide-lines for hypertension, benign murmurs, mitral valve prolapse, HCM, and arrhythmia are summarized below.

Hypertension

Athletes with mild to moderate hypertension and no end-organ damage may participate in all levels of competition. They should continue to receive treatment and should be followed closely. Athletes with severe hypertension should be treated and must attain controlled blood pressure on follow-up before any clearance is given.

Benign Murmurs

As was discussed previously, innocent murmurs are often found in young athletes, and clearance may be given. Any systolic murmur of grade 3/6 or greater, any diastolic murmur, or a murmur that increases in volume with the Valsalva maneuver should be evaluated further.

Mitral Valve Prolapse

Mitral valve prolapse (MVP) precludes participation only if one of the following is present: (a) a history of arrhythmia with syncope, (b) a family history of sudden death that is believed to be MVP-related, (c) a history of embolic event, (d) arrhythmia exacerbated by exercise, or (e) moderate to severe mitral regurgitation. Consideration on an individual basis may be made for participation in a low-intensity sport if one of the above conditions applies.

Hypertrophic Cardiomyopathy

Athletes with confirmed HCM should not be given clearance for athletic participation, with the possible exception of low-intensity sports. This restriction is justified because of the risk for sudden cardiac death (69,70). Some researchers have proposed that the poor prognosis of HCM may be exaggerated because of a selection bias in studies from tertiary centers (71). Several of the following factors have been identified as contributing to morbidity and mortality of HCM: (a) advanced symptoms at time of diagnosis, (b) atrial fibrillation, (c) basal outflow obstruction, and (d) marked left ventricular hypertrophy (71). Referral to a cardiologist is appropriate, and he or she may assist the primary care physician with questions about clearance.

Arrhythmias

Recommendations for specific arrhythmias are outlined in the 26th Bethesda Conference guidelines (64).

Skin Disorders

Infectious conditions of the skin, which were previously discussed, may prevent participation in some

contact sports and in sports in which mats are used, such as wrestling and gymnastics. Some conditions may be adequately covered to permit participation. As a general rule, however, infectious skin disorders should be treated before the participation in a sport is resumed.

Eye Injuries

The potential for eye injury exists in many sports, and precautions must be taken in order to keep the risk to a minimum. Athletes who are functionally one-eyed with vision in the affected eye correctable to less than 20/40 or who have had eye trauma or surgery should wear protective eyewear. Eye protectors should be worn by all athletes in some sports, such as hockey. Table 2.5 provides recommendations by sport.

If unresolved questions are present or if the athlete has a history of significant eye injury or operation, an ophthalmologist should be consulted for eye clearance and recommendation. The athlete, parents, coaches, and trainers must be aware of the risks and potential consequences. For example, a functionally one-eyed athlete who sustains injury to the "good" eye may be unable to obtain a driver's license.

Heat Illness

Heat illness is often recurrent, and thus a possible cause should be determined. Causes include obesity, medications, dehydration, or febrile illness. Prevention should be emphasized. Any history of heat stroke or rhabdomyolysis should be evaluated further before clearance is granted. Clearance may be given to an athlete who is at risk for heat-related illness only after establishing that the athlete and parents have a clear understanding of the risks. Alternatively, restriction may be appropriate for practices and competitions when environmental conditions involve extremes in temperature and humidity.

Inguinal Hernia or Testicular Disorders

Athletes with an inguinal hernia may participate in any sport. Consultation with a general surgeon, however, is appropriate. Any symptomatic hernia should be repaired prior to practice or competition because physical activity may exacerbate the symptoms.

Athletes with an undescended testicle should be referred for further evaluation because the condition is associated with a higher risk for testicular cancer. Hydroceles and varicoceles should be assessed on an individual basis. Clearance may be given, but, similar

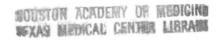

to symptomatic inguinal hernias, if the hydrocele or varicocele is symptomatic, referral should be made.

Gynecologic Disorders or Pregnancy

In general, athletes with menstrual disorders may participate, even while the medical evaluation is proceeding. For young athletes with amenorrhea, close observation for signs and symptoms of eating disorders or osteoporosis is necessary. If pregnancy is suspected, clearance should be contingent on a negative pregnancy test, and/or referral should be made to the athlete's physician.

Pulmonary Disorders or Asthma

Exercise-induced asthma remains the most common respiratory problem encountered in the PPE. This disorder alone should not prevent participation, but adequate evaluation and treatment must be initiated. Pulmonary function testing can aid in confirming the diagnosis. Treatment goals should focus on preventing and treating exacerbations of respiratory compromise. The examiner should emphasize the proper use and availability of medication and the benefits of a peak flowmeter.

More serious respiratory abnormalities, such as cystic fibrosis or pulmonary hypertension, should be referred for more complete testing and monitoring.

Neurologic Disorders

History of neurologic injuries or disorders requires a thorough assessment of the potential risk of long-term morbidity that could result from practice or competition. In particular, a history of concussion, burners, stingers, and convulsion may affect clearance.

Concussion remains the leading serious head injury in contact and collision sports. As many as 250,000 such injuries occur each year in football alone (72). Concussion can be defined as a traumatically induced alteration in mental status (73). Although no clear-cut consensus exists on concussion classification (74,75) and the cumulative effects elude investigators (76,77), many guidelines on classification and management can help physicians in determining risk and clearance (72,73,78–80).

Every athlete with a history of concussion should be evaluated on an individual basis. Some of the concern for concussions comes from second impact syndrome, which can occur with minor head trauma after a concussion. Ensuing cerebral edema can result in significant morbidity or death (73,81,82).

If an athlete who has sustained a concussion presents with any prolonged signs or symptoms of post-concussion syndrome, such as headache, confusion, dizziness, irritability, or impaired memory, he or she should be referred to a neurologist for further testing before participation (83). Conversely, an athlete who has had a history of concussion and who presents free of neurologic impairment for a significant time should be allowed to compete.

Athletes who have sustained brachial plexus or nerve root injuries, which are commonly referred to as burners and stingers, can participate if their neurologic examination is normal and if they are currently asymptomatic. Recurrent injury or persistent symptoms should be cause for concern, and cervical spine films may be obtained to look for instability or degeneration. Additional imaging studies may be indicated if signs and symptoms are frequently recurring, more severe, or persistent.

Any athlete with a history of transient quadriplegia requires further evaluation and consideration for referral. When significant structural abnormalities are detected, they should be considered a contraindication to contact and collision sports (84–86).

Clearance for participation in sports for athletes with seizure disorders should be considered on an individual basis. If the seizure disorder is adequately controlled, the affected athletes may participate. Participation in contact sports requires close monitoring. When seizures are poorly controlled, clearance may be given for noncontact sports that involve little risk to the athlete or others. More comprehensive clearance should be withheld until adequate control is achieved. Consultation with a neurologist should be considered in any athlete with a history of convulsion, in order to optimize therapy and delineate the risks.

Musculoskeletal Disorders

Musculoskeletal disorders lead to the majority of sports restrictions (4). The most common injuries that result in restriction involve the knee and ankle (45). Without proper rehabilitation, knee and ankle injuries have a high risk of reinjury (87). Examining physicians should assess the impact of the previous injury on safe participation. Injuries that do not affect performance in a sport may not require restriction (e.g., a wrist injury in a cross-country runner). Rehabilitation plays a major role in the determination of clearance, and it may be an appropriate condition for clearance.

In athletes with chronic musculoskeletal injuries or acute injuries considered safe for participation, comfort and stability may be achieved through bracing, taping, or padding. Proper fitting is essential, as a poorly fitting brace may actually increase the risk of further injury. When the appropriateness of clearance becomes uncertain, referring the athlete to a specialist for further recommendations and treatment plans is suitable.

Sprains, Subluxations, and Dislocations

Any history of sprain, subluxation, or dislocation must be fully evaluated before the physician gives any athlete clearance to participate in practice or competition. Specifically, examiners should look for decreased range of motion, effusion or swelling, diminished strength (less than 80% to 90% of the corresponding uninjured joint), symptomatic ligamentous instability, or functional limitation. An example of functional limitation is the inability to sidecut after a rehabilitation regimen.

Restriction may be placed until a specialist further evaluates the athlete or until the problem resolves with rehabilitation. Normal function may be achieved with bracing or taping in certain situations.

Muscle Strains or Contusions

Strains and contusions also should be evaluated for range of motion, strength, and functional ability. Any limitations on activity should be thoroughly considered on the basis of safe participation in the particular activity in which the athlete is involved. Appropriate measures should be instituted to assure the full rehabilitation of all previous injuries.

Overuse Injuries

Overuse injuries generally result from repetitive microtrauma. Such injuries begin with pain and inflammation and, with continued insult, may progress to tears or fractures. Disability may result if these injuries develop into chronic lesions. Common examples of this pattern of injury include stress fracture, Achilles tendonitis, plantar fasciitis, patellofemoral pain syndrome, lateral epicondyle tendinopathy, impingement syndrome, and rotator cuff injury. Considerations similar to those for sprains or strains must be made for clearance, treatment, and rehabilitation of overuse injuries.

Fractures

Clearance for athletes with fractures should be made on an individual basis. Factors for consideration include location, classification, risk of reinjury, and potential risk to others during treatment. Participation with a playing cast may be considered if the risk for exacerbating the injury or injuring others with the cast is negligible. The examiner must be aware of any regulations for participation with a protective device and should refer the athlete to a specialist if he or she is unsure of the regulations. If the physician is unsure of the risk of the injury worsening during participation, referral is also warranted.

Developmental Conditions

Abnormalities of the spine, such as spondylolysis, spondylolisthesis, or scoliosis, generally require evaluation beyond the scope of the PPE. Athletes should follow up with their primary care physician or sports medicine specialist with any concerns found on the PPE. Physical findings, symptoms, and radiographic abnormalities contribute to the need for further evaluation or restriction. Spondylolisthesis can progress and may warrant radiographic follow-up. In broad terms, athletes with spinal deformities may participate, but they should be educated on avoiding activities that may contribute to a worsening of their condition.

Other developmental conditions include apophysitis of the tibial tuberosity (Osgood–Schlatter disease), calcaneus (Sever disease), ischium, and ilium, which generally do not limit clearance. Rather, athletes may be limited by symptoms of pain with activity. The approach to these conditions is similar to that for overuse injuries. As with other musculoskeletal disorders, any ambiguity with regard to clearance might benefit from referral to a sports medicine specialist.

Communicable Diseases

HIV and other blood-borne pathogens, including hepatitis B, C, and D, complicate issues for participation in athletics. Athletes and providers should be aware of methods of transmission and should make efforts to minimize these risks. Athletes with these illnesses also carry higher risks to themselves with participation. One of the greatest impediments to participation by infected athletes may be a public misconception and fear.

HIV is transmitted through sexual contact, parenteral exposure to blood and blood products, contamination of infected blood into open wounds or mucous membranes, and perinatal exposure. The virus is present in urine, tears, saliva, sweat, vomitus, and respiratory droplets; however, only its presence in blood poses a recognized risk in sports. In sports, the risk of transmission has been estimated at less than one case per 1 million games (88).

The hepatitis viruses are spread in a manner similar to that of HIV. Hepatitis B virus (HBV) is present at a concentration of 100 million per milliliter; in comparison, the concentration is a few hundred or a few thousand for HIV (89,90). Despite this difference in concentration, only one suspected case of each has been related to athletic participation (91,92).

Hepatitis C virus (HCV) represents 20% to 50% of all cases of viral hepatitis in the United States (93). Hepatitis D virus (HDV) depends on concomitant HBV infection. Neither HCV nor HDV has contributed to an increased risk of spread from athletic participation.

Participation of an athlete with HIV is a complex issue. Initially, the health of the infected athlete should be fully evaluated. HIV is a chronic disease that eventually leads to immunosuppression and acquired immunodeficiency syndrome (AIDS). However, with proper care, infected persons can maintain good health for many years. The athlete should be on an approved medication regimen and should receive follow-up care with an HIV specialist. The presence of HIV does not preclude an asymptomatic athlete from participation (94); in fact, moderate physical activity has even been shown to be beneficial to HIV-infected persons (95).

Athletes with HBV, HCV, or HDV should be monitored for manifestations of active disease, such as pain, anorexia, fatigue, fever, or malaise. Participation depends on the status of the illness, but asymptomatic athletes may participate in their sport of choice with proper monitoring and guidance by an experienced physician.

With all blood-borne pathogens, universal precautions must be taken to minimize the risk to other athletes, trainers, coaches, and physicians. Open wounds must be covered during participation. Transmission during practice or competition is extremely rare, but, with proper education and techniques, this low risk can be further reduced. Confidentiality must be strictly maintained; however, some states require reporting of blood-borne illnesses. Physicians should be aware of their state's requirements and should inform athletes accordingly. In addition to the illness being treated, recommendations for counseling may prove beneficial for dealing with the psychosocial implications of the illness. Developments in understanding and treatment occur frequently with HIV and viral hepatitis, and providers must keep abreast of these. Referral should be made when appropriate to ensure proper management and education.

A more complete overview of HIV and other blood-borne pathogens as related to athletics is provided in the Joint Position Statement by the American Medical Society for Sports Medicine and the American Orthopaedic Society for Sports Medicine (94).

Single Organ

Whenever an athlete with a single paired organ participates, an inherent risk is present. Injury to the remaining organ could result in catastrophic impairment. Perhaps of most concern is the spector of dialysis and premature death may follow injury to a single kidney. These risks must be made absolutely clear to athletes before participation so that they can make informed decisions. When a single kidney is abnormal, such as in polycystic kidney disease, athletes should be restricted from contact and collision sports.

Injury to a remaining eye could lead to blindness or functional blindness if corrected vision is less than 20/40. Athletes with a single functional eye should be evaluated by an ophthalmologist before participation (38). Such athletes may participate in sports that do not involve projectiles and that easily allow the use of protective eyewear. Contraindicated sports include martial arts, wrestling, and boxing.

Injury to a remaining testicle may result in infertility. Athletes who want to participate in athletics must understand this risk. If a contact or collision sport is being played, a protective cup should be used. The risk of orchiectomy from scrotal injury is low, and recommendations for clearance remain controversial (96). Providers must be aware that a single testicle on examination may indicate an undescended testicle, and the athlete should therefore be informed of the increased risk for testicular cancer.

Genetic Syndromes

Genetic syndromes may increase an athlete's risk. One such common genetic condition is sickle cell disease and trait. Approximately 8% of African-Americans carry the sickle cell trait, as do about 0.8% of nonblacks. With sickle cell trait, less than half of a patient's hemoglobin is affected, and affected patients have no associated anemia. Generally, athletes with the trait have no restrictions (97,98).

Under the extremes of training (e.g., altitude, heat, or humidity), an increased risk for rhabdomyolysis may be observed, with a potential for renal failure and death in carriers of the sickle cell trait (99,100). These athletes must be properly educated about this risk and the methods for reducing risk, including conditioning, acclimatization, and hydration.

Athletes with actual sickle cell disease should be evaluated on an individual basis. With exertion, these athletes become prone to sickling and crises attendant to hypoxemia and acidosis. Therefore, such athletes should be counseled to participate in low-intensity sports. With avoidance of temperature extremes and dehydration, athletes with the disease may participate in all but contact or collision and high-exertion sports, with the understanding that they may have more frequent pain crises as intensity increases.

The myriad of genetic syndromes must be considered on an individual basis. If any question remains with regard to clearance or if the examiner is not sufficiently versed in the syndrome, consultation should be sought.

Disability

Disabled athletes have the same thrill for competition and drive for excellence as athletes without disabilities. Within their sphere, disabled athletes can achieve elite levels and face the same hazards and challenges. The difference is that disabled athletes can face additional challenges, often with sports-relevant impediments.

The Paralympic Games allow physically disabled athletes to excel. Media exposure has ensured their growth in popularity and skill development. Each of these athletes has a unique story of overcoming adversity.

The Special Olympics provide another arena for disabled athletes. The most common disabilities of these athletes are Down syndrome, cerebral palsy, seizure disorders, and developmental problems (101). Thousands of these special athletes compete yearly in a broad range of sports. They require a PPE every year before participation because they have a higher incidence of sports-significant abnormalities—39% compared with 1% to 3% in the general high school population (6,102). Sport-significant disabilities include diminished visual acuity, clonus, spasticity, scoliosis, heart murmur or congenital cardiac abnormality, seizure disorder, and, particularly among athletes with Down syndrome, atlantoaxial instability and patellar instability. Although these disabilities increase risk, they do not obviate athletic participation.

When a disability (e.g., atlantoaxial instability with gymnastics or a seizure disorder with skiing) creates excessive risk, clearance may not be offered for a particular sport. Emphasis should be made, however, on offering alternative sports that are safer for the athlete or others. With disabilities often comes heightened risk, and parents, guardians, and athletes must be made aware of these risks.

Providers must become acquainted with the special concerns and needs of athletes with various disabilities and should be versed in standards for ensuring safe athletic participation. The requirements of sponsor organizations, such as the Special Olympics, should also be familiar to these examining physicians. Disabled athletes should be encouraged to participate in sports, rather than being left out as the exception to the rule. As with any athlete, sports participation can contribute to the overall health and well being of disabled athletes.

WHEN SHOULD THE ATHLETE BE REFERRED TO A CONSULTANT?

Referral to a consultant should be considered whenever a serious health concern arises, either through history or physical examination. When risks from participation cannot be adequately delineated, consultation should be similarly considered. Providers should also refer athletes to primary care physicians for issues of health maintenance or lifestyle concerns. Some concerns may be effectively addressed by the primary care physician; this approach makes the follow-up more cohesive and allows continuity of care.

MEDICAL-LEGAL CONCERNS

High-profile cases illustrate that some athletes choose to participate against medical advice. The Rehabilitation Act of 1973 and the Americans With Disabilities Act of 1990 provide legal precedent for such decisions (103a). Athletes generally seek a second opinion for clearance, but, even when specialty consultants cannot provide clearance, athletes may still seek to participate.

When athletes seek to participate against medical advice, the athlete and others involved, including parents, coaches, and trainers, must be made aware of the attendant risks of such a decision. The athlete then can make an informed decision, and appropriate documentation regarding this situation should be made. In such circumstances, athletes and parents should sign a risk release, documenting the informed decision and absolving the physician, coaches, and sponsoring institution or school from liability (103b). Despite a signed waiver, the examining physician should be aware that validity can vary among states and that the physician may not truly be protected from lawsuits (104). Whenever a question remains, legal counsel should be obtained.

Another, more insidious legal concern with the PPE involves allegations of sexual abuse or harassment (105). The station-based examination may pose a heightened risk for such problems because the athlete generally does not know the examiner. This unfamiliarity can be allayed by the inclusion of a third person in the room or simply by explaining the full extent of the examination before performing it. Consistency will serve the examiner well. Performing the same examination on all athletes prevents differences on comparison between athletes. Proper attire also can help to standardize and facilitate examination; male athletes can wear shorts and female athletes, shorts with a tank top. Female breast and genital examinations should be done in a more appropriate setting or circumstance. Such standardization in routine can prevent misunderstandings or uncomfortable situations.

Volunteers may assume the same legal risks as paid examiners. Some states provide volunteer examiners with protection under Good Samaritan statutes (103c), but this status is lost if the examiner accepts payment in any form.

CONCLUSION

The PPE serves as a tool to encourage safe athletic participation, and its emphasis is on identifying and averting the causes of exercise-related sudden death. Although the PPE should not be mistaken as a substitute for a health maintenance examination, it remains an excellent opportunity to make a difference in the lives of athletes. This can be achieved by developing a rapport with the athlete and then providing information and guidance on issues ranging from lifestyle to injury prevention and conditioning. Some of the greatest risks to young athletes are the same as those faced by all young people—suicide, alcohol and drug use, sexually transmitted diseases, and unwanted pregnancy. These risks should be addressed as time and setting permit. Properly planned and executed, the PPE can contribute to the overall well being of the athlete, in both the short term and over a lifetime.

REFERENCES

1. Goldberg B, Saraniti A, Witman P, et al. Preparticipation sports assessment—an objective evaluation. *Pediatrics* 1980;66:736–745.
2. Risser WL, Hoffman HM, Bellah GG Jr. Frequency of preparticipation sports examinations in secondary school athletes: are the University Interscholastic League guidelines appropriate? *Tex Med* 1985;81:35–39.
3. Cavanaugh RM Jr, Miller ML, Henneberger PK. The preparticipation athletic examination of adolescents: a missed opportunity? *Curr Probl Pediatr* 1997;27:109–120.
4. Smith J, Laskowski ER. The preparticipation physical examination: Mayo Clinic experience with 2,739 examinations. *Mayo Clin Proc* 1998;73:419–429.
5. Linder CW, DuRant RH, Seklecki RM, et al. Preparticipation health screening of young athletes. Results of 1,268 examinations. *Am J Sports Med* 1981;9:187–193.
6. Thompson TR, Andrish JT, Bergfeld JA. A prospective study of preparticipation sports examinations of 2,670 young athletes: method and results. *Cleve Clin Q* 1982;49:225–233.
7. Tennant FS Jr, Sorenson K, Day CM. Benefits of preparticipation sports examinations. *J Fam Pract* 1981;13:287–288.
8. Magnes SA, Henderson JM, Hunter SC. What conditions limit sports participation? Experience with 10,540 athletes. *The Physician and Sports Medicine* 1992;20:143–160.
9. McKeag DB. Preparticipation screening of the potential athlete. *Clin Sports Med* 1989;8:373–397.
10. Carek PJ, Futrell M. Athletes' view of the preparticipation physical examination. Attitudes toward certain health screening questions. *Arch Fam Med* 1999;8:307–312.
11. DuRant RH, Pendergrast RA, Seymore C, et al. Findings from the preparticipation athletic examination and athletic injuries. *Am J Dis Child* 1992;146:85–91.
12. McKeag DB. Preseason physical examination for the prevention of sports injuries. *Sports Med* 1985;2:413–431.
13. Kibler WB, Chandler TJ, Uhl T, et al. A musculoskeletal approach to the preparticipation physical examination. Preventing injury and improving performance. *Am J Sports Med* 1989;17:525–531.
14. Kibler WB, Chandler TJ. Sport specific screening and testing. In: Renström PAFH, ed. *Sports injuries: basic principles of prevention and care*. Oxford: Blackwell Science, 1993.
15. Smith DM, Kovan JR, Rich BSE, et al. *Preparticipation physical evaluation*, 2nd ed. Minneapolis: McGraw-Hill, 1997.
16. Laure P. High-level athletes' impressions of their preparticipation sports examination [Letter]. *J Sports Med Phys Fitness* 1996;36:291–292.
17. Bratton RL, Agerter DC. Preparticipation sports examinations. Efficient risk assessment in children and adolescents. *Postgrad Med* 1995;98:123–132.
18. Smith DM, Lombardo JA, Robinson JB. The preparticipation evaluation. *Prim Care* 1991;18:777–807.
19. Tanner SM. Preparticipation examination targeted for the female athlete. *Clin Sports Med* 1994;13:337–353.
20. Johnson MD, Kibler WB, Smith DS. Keys to successful preparticipation exams. *The Physician and Sports Medicine* 1993;21:109–126.
21. Tanji JL. The preparticipation physical examination for sports. *Am Fam Physician* 1990;42:397–402.
22. Group on Science and Technology, American Medical Association. Athletic preparticipation examinations for adolescents. Report of the Board of Trustees. *Arch Pediatr Adolesc Med* 1994;148:93–98.
23. Feinstein RA, Soileau EJ, Daniel WA. A national survey of preparticipation physical examination requirements. *The Physician and Sports Medicine* 1988;16:51–59.
24. Earle MV, ed. *1998–1999 NCAA sports medicine*

handbook, 11th ed. Overland Park, KS: National Collegiate Athletic Association, 1998.

25. Smith NJ, ed. *Sports medicine: health care for young athletes*. Evanston, IL: American Academy of Pediatrics, 1983.

26. Lombardo JA, Robinson JB, Smith DM, et al. *Preparticipation physical evaluation*, 1st ed. Leawood, KS: American Academy of Family Physicians, American Academy of Pediatrics, American Medical Society for Sports Medicine, American Orthopaedic Society for Sports Medicine, American Osteopathic Academy of Sports Medicine, 1992.

27. Dodge WF, West EF, Smith EH, et al. Proteinuria and hematuria in schoolchildren: epidemiology and early natural history. *J Pediatr* 1976;88:327–347.

28. Peggs JF, Reinhardt RW, O'Brien JM. Proteinuria in adolescent sports physical examinations. *J Fam Pract* 1986;22:80–81.

29. Taylor WC III, Lombardo JA. Preparticipation screening of college athletes: value of the complete blood cell count. *The Physician and Sports Medicine* 1990; 18:106–118.

30. Vehaskari VM, Rapola J. Isolated proteinuria: analysis of a school-age population. *J Pediatr* 1982;101: 661–668.

31. Ades PA. Preventing sudden death: cardiovascular screening of young athletes. *The Physician and Sports Medicine* 1992;20:75–89.

32. Epstein SE, Maron BJ. Sudden death and the competitive athlete: perspectives on preparticipation screening studies. *J Am Coll Cardiol* 1986;7:220–230.

33. Feinstein RA, Colvin E, Oh MK. Echocardiographic screening as part of a preparticipation examination. *Clin J Sport Med* 1993;3:149–152.

34. Lewis JF, Maron BJ, Diggs JA, et al. Preparticipation echocardiographic screening for cardiovascular disease in a large, predominantly black population of collegiate athletes. *Am J Cardiol* 1989;64:1029–1033.

35. Maron BJ, Bodison SA, Wesley YE, et al. Results of screening a large group of intercollegiate competitive athletes for cardiovascular disease. *J Am Coll Cardiol* 1987;10:1214–1221.

36. Rupp NT, Brudno DS, Guill MF. The value of screening for risk of exercise-induced asthma in high school athletes. *Ann Allergy* 1993;70:339–342.

37. Rupp NT, Guill MF, Brudno DS. Unrecognized exercise-induced bronchospasm in adolescent athletes. *Am J Dis Child* 1992;146:941–944.

38. Weidenbener EJ, Krauss MD, Waller BF, et al. Incorporation of screening echocardiography in the preparticipation exam. *Clin J Sport Med* 1995;5:86–89.

39. Rice SG, Bierman CW, Shapiro GG, et al. Identification of exercise-induced asthma among intercollegiate athletes. *Ann Allergy* 1985;55:790–793.

40. Shield S, Wang-Dohlman A. Incidence of exercise-induced bronchospasm (EIB) in high school football players [Abstract]. *J Allergy Clin Immunol* 1991;87: 166.

41. Voy RO. The U.S. Olympic Committee experience with exercise-induced bronchospasm, 1984. *Med Sci Sports Exerc* 1986;18:328–330.

42. Feinstein RA, LaRussa J, Wang-Dohlman A, et al. Screening adolescent athletes for exercise-induced asthma. *Clin J Sport Med* 1996;6:119–123.

43. Mitten MJ. HIV-positive athletes. When medicine meets the law. *The Physician and Sports Medicine* 1994;22:63–68.

44. Krowchuk DP. The preparticipation athletic examination: a closer look. *Pediatr Ann* 1997;26:37–49.

45. Grafe MW, Paul GR, Foster TE. The preparticipation sports examination for high school and college athletes. *Clin Sports Med* 1997;16:569–591.

46. Maron BJ, Gohman TE, Aeppli D. Prevalence of sudden cardiac death during competitive sports activities in Minnesota high school athletes. *J Am Coll Cardiol* 1998;32:1881–1884.

47. Maron BJ, Thompson PD, Puffer JC, et al. Cardiovascular preparticipation screening of competitive athletes [Addendum]. *Circulation* 1998;97:2294.

48. Van Camp SP, Bloor CM, Mueller FO, et al. Nontraumatic sports death in high school and college athletes. *Med Sci Sports Exerc* 1995;27:641–647.

49. Lyznicki JM, Nielsen NH, Schneider JF. Cardiovascular screening of student athletes. *Am Fam Physician* 2000;62:765–774.

50. Liberthson RR. Sudden death from cardiac causes in children and young adults. *N Engl J Med* 1996;334: 1039–1044.

51. Maron BJ, Shirani J, Poliac LC, et al. Sudden death in young competitive athletes. Clinical, demographic, and pathological profiles. *JAMA* 1996;276:199–204.

52. Williams RA, ed. *The athlete and heart disease: diagnosis, evaluation & management*. Philadelphia: Lippincott Williams & Wilkins, 1999.

53. Basilico FC. Cardiovascular disease in athletes. *Am J Sports Med* 1999;27:108–121.

54. Futterman LG, Myerburg R. Sudden death in athletes: an update. *Sports Med* 1998;26:335–350.

55. Luckstead EF. Cardiovascular evaluation of the young athlete. *Adolesc Med* 1998;9:441–455.

56. Franklin BA, Fletcher GF, Gordon NF, et al. Cardiovascular evaluation of the athlete. Issues regarding performance, screening and sudden cardiac death. *Sports Med* 1997;24:97–119.

57. Sallis RE, Jones K, Knopp W. Burners: offensive strategy for an underreported injury. *The Physician and Sports Medicine* 1992;20:47–55.

58. Epstein Y. Heat intolerance: predisposing factor or residual injury? *Med Sci Sports Exerc* 1990;22:29–35.

59. Epstein Y, Shapiro Y, Brill S. Role of surface area-to-mass ratio and work efficiency in heat intolerance. *J Appl Physiol* 1983;54:831–836.

60. American Academy of Pediatrics Committee on Sports Medicine and Fitness and American Academy of Ophthalmology Committee on Eye Safety and Sports Ophthalmology. Protective eyewear for young athletes. *Pediatrics* 1996;98:311–313.

61. Squire DL. Eating disorders. In: Mellion MB, ed. *Sports medicine secrets*, 2nd ed. Philadelphia: Hanley & Belfus, 1999:139–144.

62. Hobart JA, Smucker DR. The female athlete triad. *Am Fam Physician* 2000;61:3357–3364.

63. Ferenchick GS, Adelman S. Myocardial infarction associated with anabolic steroid use in a previously healthy 37-year-old weight lifter. *Am Heart J* 1992; 124:507–508.

64. 26th Bethesda Conference. Recommendations for determining eligibility for competition in athletes with cardiovascular abnormalities. January 6-7, 1994. *J Am Coll Cardiol* 1994;24:845–899.

65. Gomez JE, Landry GL, Bernhardt DT. Critical evaluation of the 2-minute orthopedic screening examination. *Am J Dis Child* 1993;147:1109–1113.

66. American Academy of Pediatrics Committee on Sports Medicine and Fitness. Medical conditions affecting sports participation. *Pediatrics* 1994;94:757–760.

67. Mitchell JH, Haskell WL, Raven PB. Classification of sports. *Med Sci Sports Exerc* 1994;26:S242–S245.

68. Rich BS. Sudden death screening. *Med Clin North Am* 1994;78:267–288.

69. Van Camp SP. Sudden death in athletes. In: Grana WA, Lombardo JA, eds. *Advances in sports medicine and fitness.* Chicago: Year Book Medical Publishers, 1988: 121–142.

70. Corrado D, Basso C, Schiavon M, et al. Screening for hypertrophic cardiomyopathy in young athletes. *N Engl J Med* 1998;339:364–369.

71. Maron BJ, Casey SA, Poliac LC, et al. Clinical course of hypertrophic cardiomyopathy in a regional United States cohort. *JAMA* 1999;281:650–655.

72. Cantu RC. Guidelines for return to contact sports after a cerebral concussion. *The Physician and Sports Medicine* 1986;14:75–83.

73. Kelly JP, Nichols JS, Filley CM, et al. Concussion in sports. Guidelines for the prevention of catastrophic outcome. *JAMA* 1991;266:2867–2869.

74. Office of Continuing Medical Educaton, UCLA School of Medicine. Multiple concussion guidelines provoke controversy. *Sports Med Digest* 1995;17:1–2.

75. Office of Continuing Medical Education, UCLA School of Medicine. Tough call: when is it safe to return to play after concussion? *Sports Med Digest* 1995;17:1,3,5–6.

76. McCrory P, Maddocks D, Dicker G. Multiple concussive brain injury: lack of evidence for cumulative damage in a pilot study [Abstract]. *Med Sci Sports Exerc* 1995;[Suppl 27]:S168.

77. Office of CME, UCLA School of Medicine. Can repeated mild concussions cause long-term damage to the brain? *Sports Med Digest* 1995;17:6.

78. Gennarelli TA. Cerebral concussion and diffuse brain injuries. In: Torg JS, ed. *Athletic injuries to the head, neck, and face,* 2nd ed. St. Louis: Mosby-Year Book, 1991: 270–282.

79. Nelson WE, Jane JA, Gieck JH. Minor head injury in sports: a new system of classification and management. *The Physician and Sports Medicine* 1984;12: 103–107.

80. Colorado Medical Society. *Guidelines for the management of concussion in sports [Revised].* Denver: Colorado Medical Society, 1991.

81. Saunders RL, Harbaugh RE. The second impact in catastrophic contact-sports head trauma. *JAMA* 1984; 252:538–539.

82. Cantu RC, Voy R. Second impact syndrome: a risk in any contact sport. *The Physician and Sports Medicine* 1995;23:27–34.

83. Mittenberg W, Burton DB. A survey of treatments for post-concussion syndrome. *Brain Inj* 1994;8:429–437.

84. Torg JS. Management guidelines for athletic injuries to the cervical spine. *Clin Sports Med* 1987;6:53–60.

85. Torg JS, Pavlov H, Genuario SE, et al. Neurapraxia of the cervical spinal cord with transient quadriplegia. *J Bone Joint Surg Am* 1986;68:1354–1370.

86. Torg JS, Glasgow SG. Criteria for return to contact activities following cervical spine injury. *Clin J Sports Med* 1991;1:12–26.

87. Abbott HG, Kress JB. Preconditioning in the prevention of knee injuries. *Arch Phys Med Rehabil* 1969; 50:326–333.

88. Goldsmith MF. When sports and HIV share the bill, smart money goes on common sense [News]. *JAMA* 1992;267:1311–1314.

89. Guidelines for prevention of transmission of human immunodeficiency virus and hepatitis B virus to health-care and public-safety workers. *Morb Mortal Wkly Rep* 1989;38:1–37.

90. Ho DD, Moudgil T, Alam M. Quantitation of human immunodeficiency virus type 1 in the blood of infected persons. *N Engl J Med* 1989;321:1621–1625.

91. Brown LS, Drotman P. What is the risk of HIV infection in athletic competition [Abstract]? *International Conference on AIDS* 1993;9:734.

92. Kashiwagi S, Hayashi J, Ikematsu H, et al. An outbreak of hepatitis B in members of a high school sumo wrestling club. *JAMA* 1982;248:213–214.

93. Dolan PJ, Skibba RM, Hagan RC, et al. Hepatitis C: prevention and treatment. *Am Fam Physician* 1991;43: 1347–1350, 1355–1360.

94. The American Medical Society for Sports Medicine (AMSSM) and the American Academy of Sports Medicine (AASM). Human immunodeficiency virus and other blood-borne pathogens in sports. *Clin J Sport Med* 1995;5:199–204.

95. Calabrese LH, LaPerriere A. Human immunodeficiency virus infection, exercise and athletics. *Sports Med* 1993;15:6–13.

96. Dorsen PJ. Should athletes with one eye, kidney, or testicle play contact sports? *The Physician and Sports Medicine* 1986;14:130–138.

97. Eichner ER. Sickle cell trait, exercise, and altitude. *The Physician and Sports Medicine* 1986;14:144–157.

98. American Academy of Pediatrics Committee on Sports Medicine. Recommendations for participation in competitive sports. *Pediatrics* 1988;81:737–739.

99. Ramirez A, Hartley LH, Rhodes D, et al. Morphological features of red blood cells in subjects with sickle cell trait: changes during exercise. *Arch Intern Med* 1976;136:1064–1066.

100. Eichner ER. Sickle cell trait, heroic exercise, and fatal collapse. *The Physician and Sports Medicine* 1993;21: 51–61.

101. Tanji JL. The preparticipation exam: special concerns for the Special Olympics. *The Physician and Sports Medicine* 1991;19:61–68.

102. McCormick DP, Ivey FM Jr, Gold DM, et al. The preparticipation sports examination in Special Olympics athletes. *Tex Med* 1988;84:39–43.

103. Gallup EM. *Law and the team physician.* Champaign, IL: Human Kinetics, 1995:77,80–81[a];45[b];76–77 [c].

104. Herbert DL. Prospective releases: will their use protect sports medicine physicians from suit? *Sports Medicine Standard and Malpractice Reporter* 1994;6:33,35–36.

105. Herbert DL. Professional considerations related to the conduct of preparticipation examinations. *Sports Medicine Standard and Malpractice Reporter* 1994;6:49, 51–52.

3

Growth and Maturation

Applications to Children and Adolescents in Sports

Robert M. Malina

Participation in sports is an important aspect of the lives of children and adolescents, many of whom have had their first experiences in organized sports by 5 to 8 years of age. The number of participants in organized sports increases during childhood, but it subsequently declines during the transition into and in early adolescence (i.e., after 12 to13 years of age); however, the ages of declining participation vary with specific sports (1). The decline in participation is related to several factors, but three related factors are especially significant. First, interests change during the transition into adolescence, so that participation in organized sport does not have the primacy that it once had in childhood. Second, at these ages, many sports become more selective and specialized, and they tend to focus on the more talented children, and, in turn, eliminate many youths. Third, many communities and schools do not have organized sport programs for the less talented, or general, populations of youths. The decline in youth sports participation after 12 to 13 years of age parallels the declining rates of participation in physical activities in general across adolescence (2–4).

Participation in sports is a major context for physical activity among children and adolescents. Middle school youth actively involved in organized sports have a greater estimated total daily energy expenditure and higher energy expenditure in moderate-to-vigorous physical activity than those who are not involved in sport (5). Regular physical activity, including training for sports, is often assumed to be important for supporting normal growth and maturation, but precisely how much activity is needed is not known. Because of questions raised by parents and, indeed, often by the medical community, a need is seen for the critical evaluation of evidence dealing with the potential influence of regular training for sports on indicators of growth and maturity and of related issues in organized sports for children and adolescents.

Young athletes in many sports have size, physique, and functional characteristics that are similar to adult athletes in respective sports (6–8). This appears to emphasize an important role for growth and maturation, and perhaps constitutional factors, in the processes through which children and adolescents are selected for or excluded from many sports. Therefore, appreciating variation in the growth and maturity characteristics of participants in specific sports is important.

This chapter has four objectives. First, the expected changes in growth and maturity during childhood and adolescence are summarized. Second, trends in the growth and maturity status of young athletes in a variety of sports are highlighted. Third, the potential role of training for sports as a factor influencing growth and maturation is discussed. Finally, several current issues related to children and adolescents in sports are considered.

GROWTH, MATURATION, AND DEVELOPMENT

As children and adolescents progress from birth to adulthood, they experience the following three interacting processes: growth, maturation, and development. Although these terms are often treated as having the same meaning, they refer to three distinct entities in the daily lives of children and adolescents during approximately the first two decades of life.

Growth

Growth refers to the increase in the size of the body as a whole and to that of its parts. Thus, as children grow, they become taller and heavier, they increase in lean and fat tissues, their organs increase in size, and so on. Heart volume and mass follow a growth pattern similar to that of body weight, while the lungs and lung functions grow proportionally to height. Different parts of the body grow at different rates and different times, resulting in changes in body proportions. The legs grow faster than the trunk during childhood; hence, the child becomes relatively longer-legged for his or her height.

Maturation

Maturation refers to progress towards maturity—that is, the biologically mature state. Maturation is a process, whereas maturity is a state. All tissues, organs, and systems of the body mature. Maturity and maturation should be viewed in the following two contexts: timing and tempo. Timing refers to when specific maturational events occur (e.g., age at the beginning of changes in breast morphology in girls, the age at the appearance of pubic hair in boys and girls, or the age at peak height velocity or maximum growth during the adolescent growth spurt). Tempo refers to the rate at which maturation progresses (e.g., how quickly or slowly the youngster passes through the adolescent growth spurt or from the initial changes to the mature state of breast morphology). Timing and tempo are highly individual characteristics, and thus they vary considerably.

Development

Development refers to the acquisition of behavioral competence—the learning of appropriate behaviors expected by society. As children experience life at home, school, and church and participate in sports, recreation, and other community activities, they develop cognitively, socially, emotionally, morally, and so on. They are learning to behave in a culturally appropriate manner. Motor development, an important aspect of behavioral competence, is related to sports. Proficiency in motor skills and in sports-specific skills is central to performance, and it is related to body size and maturity. Although used here in the context of behavioral competence, the term development is also used in the context of biologic maturation (e.g., breast, pubic hair, or genital development).

Interactions

The three processes of growth, maturation and development occur at the same time and thus interact with each other. They cooperate to influence the child's self-concept, self-esteem, body image, and perceived competence. Parents, teachers, coaches, and other adults who work with children and adolescents should be aware of these interactions. Pediatricians are in an ideal position to educate adults about their actual or potential importance. How a youngster copes with sexual maturation or the adolescent growth spurt may influence his or her behavior, including peer relationships and sports-related behavior and performance. A mismatch between the demands of sport and those of normal growth and maturation may be a source of stress among young athletes that may potentially influence their behavior and performance.

GROWTH IN BODY SIZE AND COMPOSITION

Height and weight are the two body dimensions used most often to monitor the growth of children and adolescents. With age, children are expected to become taller and heavier. Size attained at a given age (status) and rate of growth (progress) are usually monitored relative to growth charts, which are the reference for the comparison of the height and weight of individuals or samples of children and adolescents. Revised charts for height, weight, and body mass index (BMI) (see below) for American children from birth to 20 years of age were recently made available (see Appendix D) (9). The charts, based on nationally representative samples of American children and adolescents, replace the earlier international charts (10).

Height and weight increase gradually during childhood. Approximately by the age of 9 to 10 years in girls and 11 to 12 years in boys, the rate of growth in height begins to increase, thus marking the beginning of the adolescent growth spurt. The rate of growth increases until it reaches a peak, known as the peak height velocity (PHV) or maximum rate of growth in height, during the adolescent spurt. The rate of growth then gradually decreases, and the growth in height eventually stops. Girls, on average, start their growth spurts, reach PHV, and stop growing about 2 years earlier than boys. Nevertheless, the age at which the growth spurt starts, PHV is reached, and growth stops are highly variable among individuals. Most other body dimensions follow a growth pattern similar to that for height and weight. Malina and Bouchard (11) and Malina et al. (12) provide a comprehensive discussion of growth-related and maturity-related changes in body size, specific dimensions and tissues, body composition, and a variety of functional parameters.

The growth spurt in body weight begins slightly later than that of height. Body weight is a composite measure of many tissues, but it is often viewed in terms of lean (fat-free) mass and fat components. The following formula is used:

Body weight = fat-free mass (FFM) + fat mass (FM)

Two major components of FFM are skeletal muscle and bone mineral. FFM has a growth pattern analogous to that of body weight and shows a well defined adolescent spurt. FM increases more gradually during childhood and adolescence. General guidelines for expected changes in height, weight, and body composition are summarized in Table 3.1.

Height and weight are frequently used in the form of BMI, or as weight divided by height squared (kg/m^2). After an increase in infancy, BMI declines through early childhood. It reaches its lowest point at about 5 to 6 years of age and then increases with age through

TABLE 3.1. *Guidelines for expected changes in height, weight, and body composition*

Preadolescence or prepuberty (about 6 to 10 yr of age)
Children are expected to grow (i.e., increase in weight and height). Although much variation is seen among individuals, children gain, on average, about 5 to 8 cm (2 to 3 in) per year and about 2 to 3 kg (5 to 7 lb) per year between 6 and 10 yr of age. As adolescence and puberty begin, growth rates increase, first in height and then in weight.
Adolescence and puberty
Adolescence is characterized by the growth spurt and sexual maturation. It is a time of considerable variation in event occurrence and rate.
The following highlights general trends that characterize the growth spurt:
• Girls: begins around 9 to 10 yr
         reaches maximum around 12 yr
         rate slows after 12 yr, but growth continues
         to about 16 to 18 yr
• Boys: begins around 11 to 12 yr
         reaches maximum around 14 yr
         rate slows after 14 yr, but growth continues
         to about 18 to 20 years
• Growth in height continues into the early 20s in some girls and boys
• Considerable variation among individuals in
         Timing: when the adolescent spurt occurs
         Tempo: rate of progress through the spurt
• Body weight, fat-free mass (FFM), and muscle mass also show adolescent spurts; they occur, on average, several months after the maximum rate of growth in height
• During the interval of maximum growth in height (about 11 to 13 yr in girls and 13 to 15 yr in boys), girls gain about 7 kg (15 lb) in FFM, while boys gain double this value (14 kg [31 lb]); girls gain a bit more fat mass than boys during the interval of the growth spurt, 3 kg (6 lb) vs. 1.5 kg (3 lb)
• In a sense, during the growth spurt, "First you stretch them and then you fill them out!"

Adapted from Malina RM. Bouchard C. *Growth, maturation, and physical activity.* Champaign, IL: Human Kinetics, 1991; and Malina RM, Bouchard C, Bar-Or O. *Growth, maturation, and physical activity,* 2nd ed. Champaign, IL: Human Kinetics (*in press*), with permission.

childhood and adolescence into adulthood. Sex differences in BMI are small during childhood, they rise during adolescence, and they persist into adulthood. The rise in BMI after its low point at about 5 to 6 years of age has been labeled the "adiposity rebound." Children who have an early "rebound" have been suggested to have an increased probability of being overweight in late adolescence and young adulthood.

An elevated BMI is generally accepted as an indicator of adiposity or fatness in public health and nutritional surveys. An international reference for the definitions of "overweight" and "obesity" during childhood and adolescence has recently been developed (13). These internationally recommended age-specific and sex-specific cutoff points of BMI for defining overweight and obesity between 2 and 18 years of age are based on pooled data from representative cross-sectional growth surveys performed in Brazil, Great Britain, Hong Kong, the Netherlands, Singapore, and the United States. In establishing cutoff points, a BMI of 25.0 kg per m^2 at 18 years of age was considered overweight, and a BMI of 30.0 kg per m^2 at 18 years of age was considered obese. The curves, in a process known as retrofitting, were then mathematically fit to the pooled BMI data from 2 years of age onward so that they passed through a BMI of 25 kg per m^2 and 30 kg per m^2 at 18 years of age. The values at each half-year from 2 to 18 years of age are the respective cutoff points for being overweight and obese.

The interpretation of BMI in childhood, adolescence, and young adulthood as an indicator of fatness requires care. Elevated BMI is not necessarily indicative of fatness during childhood and adolescence. Although BMI is reasonably well correlated with total body fat and the percentage of fat in heterogeneous samples, it is also related to FFM in children and adolescents. Associations between BMI and fatness indicate a wide range of variability; children with the same BMI can differ considerably in their percentage of fat and total FFM, thus emphasizing the need for care and sensitivity in the use and interpretation of BMI as an indicator of fatness in individual children and adolescents.

BIOLOGIC MATURITY

The term maturity usually refers to the level or extent to which a child or adolescent has progressed to the mature state. It is an operational concept because the process cannot be observed or measured directly. Individuals vary in their attained level of maturity at a point in time (maturity status at a given age), in timing (when maturational events occur), and in tempo (rate of maturation).

Commonly used indicators of biologic maturity are the skeleton, the secondary sex characteristics, and the timing of maximal growth during adolescence. Detailed descriptions of methods of assessment and interrelationships among maturity indicators are presented in Malina and Bouchard (11) and Malina et al. (12).

Skeletal Maturity

The skeleton is an ideal indicator of maturity because its maturation spans the entire period of growth. The bones of the hand and wrist provide the primary basis for assessing skeletal maturity. Other areas of the skeleton can be used (e.g., the knee, foot, and ankle), but the hand–wrist area is most widely used in growth studies. Methods for the assessment of skeletal maturity of the hand and wrist include the Greulich–Pyle, Tanner–Whitehouse, and Fels. The Greulich–Pyle and Tanner–Whitehouse methods are widely used in pediatric clinics and in growth studies. The Fels method has been more recently developed, and it is gradually finding a wider use in these settings.

Methods of skeletal maturity assessment are similar in principle. A hand–wrist radiograph must be matched to a set of criteria. The criteria for making assessments and the procedures used to construct a scale of skeletal maturity from which skeletal ages are assigned vary among the methods. The reference samples upon which each is based also differ.

Skeletal age (SA), sometimes referred to as bone age, corresponds to the level of skeletal maturity attained by a child, relative to the reference sample for each method. It is expressed relative to a child's chronological age (CA). SA may be simply compared to CA. For example, a child may have a CA of 10.5 years and an SA of 12.3 years. The child has attained the skeletal maturity equivalent to that of a child of 12.3 years and therefore is advanced in skeletal maturity status for his or her CA. SA may also be expressed as the difference between SA and CA (i.e., SA minus CA). Thus, in the example given above, the SA could be expressed by the following: 12.3 − 10.5 = +1.8 years. At times, SA is simply divided by CA to yield a relative SA. A relative SA above 1.0 indicates advancement, and a relative SA below 1.0 indicates delay in skeletal maturation.

Assessment of SA is basically a method for estimating the level of skeletal maturity that a child has attained at a given point in time relative to reference data for healthy children. The three commonly used methods for assessing skeletal maturity and deriving SA each have strengths and limitations; the SA derived with each method is not equivalent.

Sexual Maturity

Assessment of sexual maturation is based upon secondary sex characteristics—breasts and menarche in girls, penis and testes in boys, and pubic hair in both sexes. The utility of these characteristics is obviously limited to the pubertal or adolescent phase of growth and maturation.

Secondary sex characteristics are outward indicators of the level of sexual maturity at a point in time. The development of secondary sex characteristics is ordinarily summarized as composite five-stage or six-stage scales for each characteristic. The most commonly used criteria are the stages for pubic hair, breasts, and male genitalia (described by Tanner [14]), which are based, in part, upon the criteria of earlier studies (e.g., Reynolds and Wines [15,16]). They are illustrated in Figs. 3.1 through 3.4. Stage 1 indicates

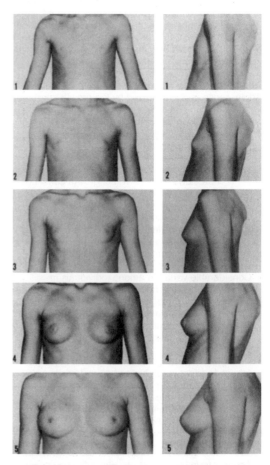

FIG. 3.1. Stages of breast development. (From Tanner JM. *Growth at adolescence*, 2nd ed. Oxford: Blackwell Science, 1962, with permission.)

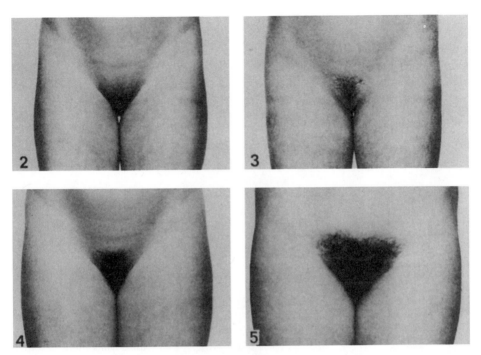

FIG. 3.2. Stages of female pubic hair development. (From Tanner JM. *Growth and adolescence*, 2nd ed. Oxford: Blackwell Science, 1962, with permission.)

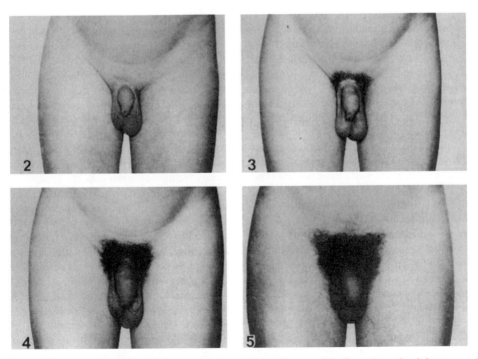

FIG. 3.3. Stages of male pubic hair development. (From Tanner JM. *Growth and adolescence*, 2nd ed. Oxford: Blackwell Science, 1962, with permission.)

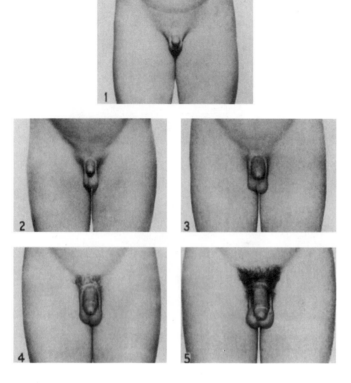

FIG. 3.4. Stages of male genital development. (From Tanner JM. *Growth and adolescence*, 2nd ed. Oxford: Blackwell Science, 1962, with permission.)

the prepubertal state of development, which is the absence of development of each characteristic. Stage 2 indicates the initial overt changes in each characteristic—the initial elevation of the breasts in girls, the initial enlargement of the genitals in boys, and the initial appearance of pubic hair in both sexes. Stages 3 and 4 indicate the continued maturation of each characteristic, and they are somewhat more difficult to evaluate. Stage 5 indicates the adult or mature state of development for each characteristic. Some scales for pubic hair include stage 6, which marks the expansion of pubic hair upward in the midline of the abdomen in about 80% of males and laterally, and to a lesser extent upward, in about 10% of females (17).

Ratings of stages of sexual maturity are usually made by direct observation at clinical examination. Because of the difficulty of direct assessment in nonmedical settings, self-assessments by youth are increasingly used. Youngsters are asked to rate their stage of sexual maturity relative to the photographs of Tanner (14) or van Wieringen et al. (17) or relative to schematic drawings of the respective stages. Good quality photographs of the stages with simplified descriptions should be used; the quality of schematic drawings varies among studies using self-assessment.

Limited data on the concordance of self-ratings of youth and those of experienced assessors exist. Correlations between self-ratings and physician ratings of the breasts, genitals, and pubic hair are moderate to high, ranging from 0.59 to 0.92 (18); but some data suggest a tendency for youngsters to overestimate early stages and to underestimate later stages (19).

The stages are superimposed onto the ongoing process of maturation, which is not necessarily continuous in its tempo. Progress in sexual maturation appears continuous when data are grouped and reported in terms of average trends. However, considerable variability is found among individuals. Some may show a relatively long period of minimal change that is followed by rapid change in a specific characteristic, whereas others may show seemingly continuous progress. Alternatively, pubic hair and breasts in girls or pubic hair and genitalia in boys may show uneven progress or may demonstrate a different tempo. Although the stages are somewhat arbitrary and they have limitations, they are a convenient way to facilitate observation of the maturity of secondary sex characteristics during puberty.

Pediatric and sports medicine literature commonly refer to the assessment of secondary sex characteristics as "Tanner staging." This is erroneous. Secondary sex characteristics are assessed using the criteria of Tanner; they are not "Tanner stages." The stages of pubertal development are specific to the breasts, genitals and pubic hair, respectively. For example, genital stage 3 (G 3) is not equivalent to pubic hair stage 3 (PH 3) in boys; breast stage 3 (B 3) is not equivalent to PH 3 in girls; G 3 in boys is not equivalent to B 3 in girls; and PH 3 in boys is not equivalent to PH 3 in girls. Taking the average of breast and pubic hair stages to characterize the level of sexual maturity of a girl or group of girls or the average of genital and pubic hair stages to summarize the level of sexual maturity of a boy or group of boys is also incorrect. Furthermore, individuals should not be assessed or data should not be reported as "puberty stage 2" or "Tanner stage 3" without specifying the particular secondary sex characteristic to which the designation is referring. Specific stages of each indicator should be noted (e.g., G 4 or PH 3).

Although prepubertal children (B 1, G 1, PH 1) are often assumed to be a homogeneous group that does not vary in maturity status, they do, in fact, vary in skeletal maturity; this range of variation can be considerable. Stages 2 through 4 of the respective characteristics indicate the pubertal or pubescent state, whereas stage 5 indicates maturity or the mature state, respectively, for each secondary sex characteristic. General guidelines for normal variation in sexual maturity during puberty are outlined in Table 3.2.

Age at Menarche

Menarche refers to the first menstrual period, and the age at which menarche occurs is the most commonly reported maturity indicator of female puberty. It, however, is a late event in the sequence of pubertal changes. Menarche has significant value judgments associated with its attainment in many cultures, and the psychologic importance of menarche in the development of girls has no counterpart in the sexual maturation process of boys. Age at menarche is also a common focus in discussions of training with young female athletes.

Age at menarche can be estimated in three ways. In longitudinal studies (the prospective method), the girl or her mother is interviewed, on each occasion, about whether menarche has or has not occurred; if it has occurred, the interviewees are asked to provide the date of occurrence. Girls are ordinarily examined at 3-month or 6-month intervals so that an accurate estimate of when menarche occurred can be made. Sample sizes in prospective studies are generally small, so the range of variability may be limited.

The status quo method provides a sample or population estimate. It is a statistical method based on probits that requires a large sample of girls who range in age from 9 to 17 years. The following two pieces of information are needed: the exact age of each girl and whether or not she has attained menarche. Probits for each percentage are then plotted for each chronologi-

---

TABLE 3.2. *Guidelines for normal variation in sexual maturation*

Girls
- The first physically apparent sign of sexual maturation in girls is the initial enlargement of the breasts. It occurs, on average, at about 10 yr of age, but it may occur before 9 yr in about 10% of girls and not until after 12 yr in another 10%.
- Initial enlargement of the breasts is, on average, followed by the appearance of pubic hair, but variation is found among girls.
- Maturity of the breasts and pubic hair occurs, on average, between 14 and 15 yr of age, but it may occur as early as 12 to 13 yr in some girls and not until 16 to 17 yr in others.
- Progress from initial to mature breast and pubic hair development is highly variable among girls. Some girls may pass through the process in 2 yr, while others may take 5 yr or more.
- Menarche is a rather late event of puberty. It occurs, on average, near 13 yr of age in many samples of European girls, about 1 yr after peak height velocity, and a bit earlier in North American girls.

Boys
- Initial enlargement of the genitals (testes and penis) marks the first physically apparent sign of sexual maturation in boys. It occurs, on average, at about 11 yr of age, but it may occur around 9 yr in about 10% of boys and not until after 13 yr in another 10% of boys.
- Pubic hair usually appears after initial enlargement of the genitals, but variation is observed among boys.
- Maturity of the genitals and pubic hair occurs, on average, at about 15 yr of age, but it may occur as early as 13 yr and after 18 yr in some boys.
- Progress from initial appearance to maturity of the genitals and pubic hair is highly variable among boys. Some boys may pass through the process in 2 yr, while others may take about 5 yr or more.

Adapted from Malina RM, Bouchard C. *Growth, maturation, and physical activity.* Champaign, IL: Human Kinetics, 1991; and Malina RM, Bouchard C, Bar-Or O. *Growth, maturation, and physical activity,* 2nd ed. Champaign, IL: Human Kinetics (*in press*), with permission.

cal age group, and a straight line is fitted to the points, and the point at which 50% of the girls attained menarche is estimated. This is the estimated median age at menarche for the sample. The method provides a standard deviation and confidence intervals. The estimated median age applies only to the population and does not apply to individual girls.

The retrospective method is limited to samples of postmenarcheal adolescents and adult women. The subjects are asked to recall, as accurately as possible, when menarche occurred. If the interview is done at close intervals, as in longitudinal studies, the method is quite accurate. However, if it is done with older girls or adult women, it has an error component. The method relies on the individual's memory and thus includes the potential for error associated with accuracy of recall. As a rule, the longer the interval between the occurrence of menarche and the age at which the individual is asked to recall the event, the lower the accuracy is. Nevertheless, most teenagers and women can recall this landmark within a range of about 3 to 6 months.

The retrospective method has limited utility with samples that include girls who have not yet attained menarche. The mean will be biased toward a younger age by the inclusion of girls who have attained menarche and the exclusion of girls who have not yet attained menarche. The retrospective method is often used with older adolescents and adult women. Data for athletes are based largely on the retrospective method.

Age at Peak Height Velocity

If longitudinal data for height that span the adolescent years are available, the resulting growth curve has several parameters that provide useful information about the adolescent growth spurt. The two primary parameters are take-off (initiation of the spurt) and PHV (maximum rate of growth during the spurt). Age at PHV is an indicator of somatic maturity. This maturity indicator is obviously limited to adolescence, and it requires longitudinal data for its estimation.

Interrelationships Among Maturity Indicators

The following two issues are important regarding indicators of skeletal, sexual, and somatic maturity in children and adolescents: relationships among the indicators and the consistency of maturity ratings over time. The issue of interrelationships is complex because only skeletal maturity spans the prepubertal and pubertal years, whereas secondary sex characteristics and age at PHV are limited to puberty.

A general maturity factor that discriminates among individuals who are early, average ("on time"), or late in the timing of maturity appears to exist. However, variation among indicators is seen so that no one system (sexual, skeletal, or somatic) provides a complete description of the timing and tempo of maturity of an individual boy or girl during adolescence. Some evidence suggests that the tempo of prepubertal growth and maturity may be somewhat independent of pubertal events, but skeletal maturity is the primary indicator for the prepubertal years.

GROWTH AND MATURITY STATUS OF YOUNG ATHLETES

In order to evaluate the potential influence of training for sports on growth and maturation, one must be familiar with the selective or exclusive nature of many sports and with the growth and maturity characteristics of young athletes in a variety of sports. Some sports selectively choose or exclude youths on the basis of body size during childhood. A primary example in this context is artistic gymnastics, which often attempts to identify potential athletes at 5 to 6 years of age (20). Body size plays a more important role in other sports later in childhood and during the transition into adolescence. At this time, size is closely related to individual differences in the timing and tempo of the adolescent growth spurt and sexual maturation. This section summarizes current information on trends in height and weight, as well as the biologic maturity status of young athletes in a several of sports.

Size Attainment

Average heights of athletes in different sports are expressed relative to percentiles (P) of United States growth charts in Tables 3.3 and 3.4 for boys and girls, respectively. For example, male athletes in many sports have heights that, on average, fluctuate just above and below the reference medians; this is indicated in the table as ±P50. If average heights are consistently above the median, this is indicated as >P50; and, if average heights of athletes in a sport are consistently below the median, this is indicated as <P50.

Athletes of both sexes and in most sports have, on average, heights that equal or exceed the reference medians. Gymnastics is the only sport that consistently presents a profile of short height in both sexes. Average heights for most samples of gymnasts are near P10. Figure skaters of both sexes also present with shorter heights, on average, although the data are

TABLE 3.3. *Heights and weights of young male athletes relative to percentiles[a] of United States reference data[b]*

Sport	Height	Weight
Basketball	P50 to >P90	P50 to >P90
Soccer	±P50	±P50
Ice hockey	±P50	P50
Distance runs	±P50	≤P50
Sprints	≥P50	≥P50
Swimming	P50 to P90	>P50 to P75
Diving	<P50	≤P50
Gymnastics	≤P10 to P25	≤P10 to P25
Tennis	±P50	≥P50
Figure skating	P10 to P25	P10 to P25
Ballet	<P50	P10 to P50

[a]Abbreviation: P, percentiles.
[b]United States reference data from Hamill PVV, Drizd TA, Johnson CL, et al. *NCHS growth curves for children, birth–18 years.* PHS 78-1650. Washington, D.C.: United States Government Printing Office; 1977.
Adapted from Malina RM. Physical growth and biological maturation of young athletes. *Exerc Sport Sci Rev* 1994;22:389–433; and Malina RM. Growth and maturation of young athletes: is training for sport a factor? In: Chan KM, Micheli LJ, eds. *Sports and children.* Hong Kong: Williams & Wilkins Asia Pacific, 1998:133–161, with permission.

TABLE 3.4. *Heights and weights of young female athletes relative to percentiles[a] of United States reference data[b]*

Sport	Height	Weight
Basketball	P75 to >P90	P50 to P75
Volleyball	P75	P50 to P75
Soccer	P50	P50
Distance runs	≥P50	<P50
Sprints	≥P50	≤P50
Swimming	P50 to P90	P50 to P75
Diving	≤P50	P50
Gymnastics	≤P10 to <P50	P10 to <P50
Tennis	>P50	±P50
Figure skating	P10 to <P50	P10 to <P50
Ballet	≤P50	P10 to <P50

[a]Abbreviation: P, percentiles.
[b]United States reference data from Hamill PVV, Drizd TA, Johnson CL, et al. *NCHS growth curves for children, birth–18 years.* PHS 78-1650. Washington, D.C.: United States Government Printing Office, 1977.
Adapted from Malina RM. Physical growth and biological maturation of young athletes. *Exerc Sport Sci Rev* 1994;22:389–433; and Malina RM. Growth and maturation of young athletes: is training for sport a factor? In: Chan KM, Micheli LJ, eds. *Sports and children.* Hong Kong: Williams & Wilkins Asia Pacific, 1998:133–161, with permission.

less extensive than for gymnasts. These trends are based on group means. Given the range of normal variation among individuals and the variation associated with individual differences in pubertal timing and tempo, individual exceptions to the trends suggested in the tables are observed.

Body weight presents a similar pattern. Young athletes in most sports tend to have body weights that, on average, equal or exceed the reference medians. Gymnasts, figure skaters, and ballet dancers of both sexes, however, consistently show lighter body weights. Gymnasts and figure skaters have appropriate weight-for-height, while ballet dancers generally display low weight-for-height. A similar trend of low weight for height is suggested for female distance runners.

Body Composition of Young Athletes

Child and adolescent athletes have less relative fatness (percentage body fat) than nonathletes of the same age and sex. Male athletes and nonathletes both show a decline in percentage body fat during adolescence, but athletes generally have less relative fatness. Female athletes also have a lower percentage body fat than nonathletes, especially during adolescence, and the differences between female athletes and nonathletes appear to be greater than the corresponding differences in males. Relative fatness in female athletes does not increase much with age during adolescence, but it does in nonathletes (12). As expected, variations among athletes and among athletes in different sports are observed.

Maturity Status of Male Athletes

With few exceptions, male athletes in a variety of sports tend to be average (on time) or advanced (early) in biologic maturity (8,21). Other than gymnasts, who show, on average, SA that lags behind CA, a lack of late maturing boys who are successful in sports during early adolescence and mid-adolescence (about 12 to 15 years) is observed. In some sports, advanced maturity is more apparent in adolescence. For example, among youth soccer and ice hockey players, a broad range of skeletal maturity is represented among participants from 10 to 12 years of age (i.e., boys with delayed [late], "on time" [average], and advanced [early] SA are almost equally represented). However, among players 13 to 16 years of age, late maturing boys (SA behind CA by more than 1 year) are minimally represented. Thus, with advancing CA and experience and the tendency for the sports to become more selective or exclusive, boys advanced in biologic maturity are more common among elite adolescent players in soccer and ice hockey (22). This may reflect selection or exclusion (self, coach, sport system, or some combination), differential success of boys advanced in maturity, the changing nature of the games (more physical contact may be permitted in older age groups with an advantage for larger, stronger, or more mature boys), or some combination of these factors.

In contrast, late maturing boys are often successful in some sports (e.g., track and basketball) in later adolescence (16 to 18 years) (23). This is associated with catch-up in biologic maturity and late adolescent growth. All youths eventually reach maturity, and maturity-associated differences in body size are reduced, and they thus have less significance for performance in late adolescent boys.

Maturity Status of Female Athletes

Most discussions of biologic maturity of female athletes focus on the age at menarche. Mean ages at menarche in North American and European girls vary, in general, between 12.5 and 13.5 years, but the age range within which menarche may normally occur is 9 through 17 years. Menarche is a late event during puberty, and it occurs, on average, about 1 year after PHV.

Later mean ages at menarche are often reported in athletes in many, but not all, sports (21,24–26). When the distribution of recalled ages at menarche are considered in large samples of athletes and nonathletes of the same CA and from similar social backgrounds, considerable overlap between the samples is seen. The distribution for athletes is simply shifted to the right, or to later ages, by about 1 year or so. Both early and late maturing athletes and nonathletes are observed, but more later maturing athletes than nonathletes are found.

Information on the age at menarche in adolescent athletes (i.e., teenage athletes) is rather limited. Reliable information is derived from longitudinal studies and status quo surveys. Use of the retrospective method with adolescent athletes excludes those who have not yet attained menarche and thus biases the mean age for the sample. Presently available data from status quo and longitudinal studies of adolescent athletes are summarized in Table 3.5. If an average of 13.0 years and a standard deviation of 1.0 year is accepted for North American and European girls, about 95% of girls will attain menarche between 11.0 and 15.0 years. Most samples of adolescent athletes have mean ages at menarche within the range of normal variation. However,

TABLE 3.5. *Ages at menarche (years) in samples of adolescent athletes in prospective and status quo studies[a]*

Prospective studies	
Gymnastics	
Poland	15.1 ± 0.9
Switzerland	14.5 ± 1.2
Sweden	14.5 ± 1.4
United Kingdom[b]	14.3 ± 1.4
Swimming, United Kingdom	13.3 ± 1.1
Tennis, United Kingdom	13.2 ± 1.4
Track, Poland	12.3 ± 1.1
Rowing, Poland	12.7 ± 0.9
Elite ballet, United States	15.4 ± 1.9
Status quo studies	
Gymnastics	
world[c]	15.6 ± 2.1
Hungarian	15.0 ± 0.6
Figure skating, United States, Canada	14.2 ± 0.5
Swimming, age group, United States	13.1 ± 1.1
Swimming, age group, United States	12.7 ± 1.1
Diving, Junior Olympic, United States	13.6 ± 1.1
Ballet, Yugoslavia	13.6
Ballet, Yugoslavia	14.1
Track, Hungary	12.6
Soccer, age group, United States	12.9 ± 1.1
Several team sports, Hungary	12.7

[a]Prospective data report means, while status quo data report medians.

[b]Among British athletes, 13% had not yet attained menarche; therefore, the estimated mean ages will be somewhat later. Small numbers of Swiss and Swedish gymnasts and ballet dancers also had not reached menarche at the time of the respective studies.

[c]This sample is from the 1987 world championships in Rotterdam. It did not include girls under 13 yr of age; therefore, the estimate may be biased toward an older age.

References for specific studies, with the exception of figure skaters, from Malina RM. Growth and maturation of young athletes: is training for sport a factor? In: Chan KM, Micheli LJ, eds. *Sports and children.* Hong Kong: Williams & Wilkins Asia Pacific, 1998:133–161, with permission. Figure skating data from Vadocz EA, Siegel SR, Malina RM. Age at menarche in competitive figure skaters: variation by level and discipline. *J Sports Sci* 2002;20:93–100, with permission.

ever, several samples of gymnasts and ballet dancers have mean ages at menarche older than 15.0 years. Both of these activities have extremely selective criteria that tend to favor the late maturing girls.

Sample sizes in studies of adolescent athletes are generally small, and studies in which the athletes are followed from prepuberty through puberty are often limited to small select samples. A potentially confounding issue in such studies is selective dropout. Do earlier maturing girls selectively drop out of gymnastics or figure skating? Or, do sports like gymnastics, figure skating, and ballet systematically select late maturing girls or systematically eliminate early maturing girls?

REGULAR TRAINING FOR SPORTS AND GROWTH AND MATURATION

In the past decade or so, concern has been expressed on a more or less regular basis about the potential negative influences of intensive training for sports on growth (i.e., the size attained and maturation—the timing and tempo of progress to the mature state, especially in young female athletes). One suggestion is, for example, that intensive training during childhood and adolescence may stunt growth and delay the sexual maturation of girls (27,28). On the other hand, the potential negative influences of training for sports on the growth and maturation of boys is only marginally expressed, usually in the context of young wrestlers who may drastically modify their diets to meet specific body mass criteria for the sport.

What Is Training?

Training refers to the systematic specialized practice for a specific sport or sport discipline for most of the year. It also may refer to specific short-term experimental programs. Physical activity is not the same as regular training. Training programs are ordinarily specific (e.g., endurance running, strength training, or sport skill training), and they vary in intensity and duration. Training is often quantified as hours per week. However, what is important is the duration and intensity of specific activities performed during this time. Training in gymnastics and figure skating includes stretching, light weights, choreography, and formal instruction by coaches, in addition to numerous repetitions of specific stunts and routines. Soccer training includes stretching, endurance-related and strength-related activities, skill instruction and drills, and game situations. Thus, not all "training" time is spent in intensive physical activity. The quantification and specification of training programs by sport needs closer attention in order to evaluate the potential effects on growth and maturity. The subsequent discussion of training as a potential influence on growth and maturation is derived from several earlier reviews (20,21,25,29).

Training and Growth in Height and Weight

Sport participation and training for sport have no apparent effect on growth in height and the rate of growth in height in healthy, adequately nourished children and adolescents. The heights of young athletes probably reflect the size demands of specific sports. The smaller size of athletes in gymnastics and figure skating is evident long before systematic training was initiated. Athletes in these two sports also have parents who are shorter than average, suggesting a familial contribution to their smaller size. Both sports also tend to favor shorter participants selectively.

Short-term longitudinal studies of athletes in several sports indicate rates of growth in height that are well within the range of normally expected variation among children and adolescents.

In contrast to height, body weight can be influenced by regular training for sport, which results in changes in body composition. Training is associated with a decrease in fatness in both sexes and occasionally with an increase in FFM, especially in boys. Changes in fatness depend on continued regular activity or training (or caloric restriction, which often occurs in sports like gymnastics, ballet, figure skating, and diving in girls and wrestling in boys) for their maintenance. When training is significantly reduced, fatness tends to accumulate. Separating the specific effects of training on FFM from the expected changes that occur with normal growth and sexual maturation during adolescence is difficult. This is especially so in boys who almost double their estimated FFM during adolescence.

Training and Specific Tissues

Bone, skeletal muscle, and adipose tissues are the three primary components of body composition. The skeleton is the framework of the body and the main reservoir of minerals. Skeletal muscle is the major work-producing and oxygen-consuming tissue, while adipose tissue represents energy in stored form.

Bone

Regular physical activity and training during childhood and adolescence are associated with increased bone mineral content and mass. The beneficial effects are more apparent in weight-bearing (e.g., running, soccer, or gymnastics) than non–weight-bearing (e.g., swimming) activities. Of particular importance to physical activity and the integrity of skeletal tissue is the observation that bone mineral levels established during childhood and adolescence may be an important determinant of bone mineral status in adulthood.

In contrast to the positive influence of physical activity and training on bone mineralization, excessive training associated with changes in the menstrual cycle in some, but not all, postmenarcheal adolescent athletes may potentially be associated with the loss of bone mineral if the alterations in menstrual function persist for some time. This is labeled the "female athlete triad," which consists of altered menstrual function, disordered eating, and the loss of bone mineral. Most of the data dealing with this issue are derived from adult athletes who have been intensively training in their given sport, quite often distance running, for a long period of time. One should note, however, that variation in menstrual cycles after menarche among adolescent girls is the rule rather than the exception. Menstrual cycles ordinarily take about 2 to 3 years to become "regular." Hence, some "irregularity" may be common in adolescent athletes.

Skeletal Muscle

Information on skeletal muscle tissue is derived largely from short-term specific training studies of small samples. Muscular hypertrophy is associated with heavy-resistance exercise programs, such as weight or strength training in adolescent boys, and does not occur, or may occur to a much lesser extent, in preadolescent boys and girls and in other forms of training.

No strong evidence that exists suggests that fiber type distribution in children and adolescents can be changed as a result of training. Limited data for adolescent boys suggest that regular endurance training has the potential to modify the activities of oxidative enzymes, whereas regular sprint training has the potential to modify the activities of glycolytic enzymes. However, after the cessation of the specific training programs, enzyme levels return to pretraining values, indicating the following important feature of training studies: physiologic changes in response to short-term programs are not permanent, and they depend upon regular training for their maintenance. An important question that remains is, "how much training is needed to maintain beneficial changes?"

Adipose Tissue

In studies of children and adolescents, subcutaneous fat is most often measured in the form of skinfold thickness. Regularly active young athletes generally have thinner skinfold thicknesses when compared to reference samples, but individual skinfolds change differentially with age, (e.g., skinfolds on the extremities but not those on the trunk generally decline during adolescence in boys). As was noted earlier, data for percentage body fat indicate similar trends—lower fatness in young athletes of both sexes than in nonath-

letes. As with skeletal muscle enzymes, regular training is necessary to maintain these beneficial effects. When training stops, fatness increases. Just how much training or activity is essential to modify skinfold thickness or to maintain lower levels of fatness in growing children and adolescents is not known.

Training and Biologic Maturation

The timing and tempo of biologic maturation are highly individual characteristics. This individuality, which has a significant genotypic component, needs to be considered in evaluating potentially positive or negative influences attributed to regular training for sports.

Skeletal Maturity

Regular training for sport does not influence the skeletal maturity of the hand and wrist. Short-term longitudinal studies of male and female athletes in several sports and of nonathletes indicate similar gains in SA and CA.

Somatic Maturity

Regular training for sports does not influence the age at PHV and the rate of growth in height during the spurt in boys and girls. The suggestion that intensive training may delay the timing of the growth spurt and stunt the growth spurt in female gymnasts has been made (30). The data upon which this conclusion is based are not sufficiently longitudinal to warrant such a conclusion, and many potentially confounding factors, especially the rigorous selection criteria for gymnastics, the marginal diets, and so on, were not considered. Female gymnasts, as a group, show the growth and maturity characteristics of short normal, slow maturing children with short parents (20).

Sexual Maturity

Longitudinal data on the sexual maturation of either girls or boys who are regularly active in and/or training for sports are not extensive. The limited longitudinal data indicate no effect of regular physical activity or training on either the timing and progress of breast and pubic hair development in girls or genital and pubic hair development in boys.

Discussions of the potential influence of training on sexual maturity focus most often on later average ages at menarche that, as noted earlier, are often observed in athletes in many, but not in all, sports. Training for sports is commonly indicated as the factor that is responsible for later ages at menarche among athletes, with the inference that training "delays" this late pubertal landmark. Unfortunately, studies of athletes do not consider factors that are known to influence menarche. Diet is an obvious factor, and athletes in sports with characteristically late ages at menarche (gymnastics and ballet) often demonstrate energy intakes that are consistently lower than their energy expenditures (i.e., a chronic energy deficit). A familial tendency for later maturity in athletes is also found. Mothers of ballet dancers, gymnasts, figure skaters, and athletes in several other sports attain menarche later than mothers of nonathletes, and sisters of athletes also attain menarche later than average (31,32). The number of siblings in a family is also related to the age at menarche in both nonathletes and athletes (33). The complexity of factors related to the timing of menarche is highlighted in the conclusions of two comprehensive discussions of exercise and reproductive health of adolescent girls and women. The first states that "although menarche occurs later in athletes than in nonathletes, it has yet to be shown that exercise delays menarche in anyone" (Loucks et al., S288 [34]), and the second concludes that "the general consensus is that while menarche occurs later in athletes than in nonathletes, the relationship is not causal and is confounded by other factors" (Clapp and Little, 2–3 [35]).

The literature on training and menarche is confused in part by altered menstrual function, which is common in athletes. Menarche refers only to the first menstrual period. Cessation of menstrual cycles after menarche has occurred (secondary amenorrhea) or infrequent cycles (oligomenorrhea) are different issues that are beyond the scope of this discussion (25). However, in the context of normal puberty, menstrual cycles immediately following menarche tend to be anovulatory, and they are often irregular (12). The development of more or less regular menstrual cycles takes place over the several years after menarche. Hence, some of the menstrual irregularities observed in adolescent athletes may, in fact, reflect the normal process of sexual maturation involved in the establishment of regular menstrual cycles.

Overview of the Potential Influence of Regular Training

Intensive training for sports does not appear to have a negative influence on growth and maturity. In adequately nourished children and adolescents, growth in height and biologic maturity is under genotypic regulation (12). Regular training for sport has the potential to

influence body composition favorably by increasing bone mineral and skeletal muscle and by decreasing fatness. In the few athletes who may present problems related to growth and maturity, factors other than training must be more closely evaluated before attributing the observations to regular training for the sport (21). In many cases of short stature, the shortness has a familial component (i.e., short parents tend to have short children). Shortness may also be related to late maturity, which may also be familial. Linearity of build is associated with later maturation in both sexes, and some sports select for this characteristic of physique.

In some sports, the growth and maturity of young athletes may be compromised by chronically marginal or poor nutritional status and occasionally by disordered eating. Dietary practices associated with an emphasis on thinness, an optimal weight for performance, or specific weight categories for competition may possibly influence growth and maturity, especially if they involve energy deficits for prolonged periods. Disordered eating behaviors are related factors in these contexts. The energetic demands of intensive training may also compete with the energy and nutrient requirements of the growth and maturational processes in rapidly growing children and adolescents. Psychologic and emotional stresses associated with training and competition are additional concerns, especially the high levels of stress associated with coach–athlete or parent–athlete interactions. Thus, if intensive training for sport influences growth and maturity, it most likely interacts with, or is confounded by, other factors so that a specific effect of training *per se* may be impossible to extract.

When one allows for the wide range of individual variation in normal growth and maturity (12) and responsiveness to training (36), why would all children and adolescents be expected to respond to training in a similar manner? Rather, can clinicians identify the young athlete who might be at risk for potentially compromised growth and maturation? If so, how can the sports environment be modified to eliminate the risk? A unique feature of the sport environment of young athletes is its adult control, which is provided by coaches, parents, sport administrators, judges, and other officials. Presumably, these adults have the health, safety, and best interests of child and adolescent athletes at heart!

ISSUES IN SPORTS RELATED TO GROWTH AND MATURITY

Participation in sports has associated risks. The concerns regarding compromised growth and maturity have already been discussed. The risks of injury and psychologic stress are two other major concerns. A related issue in organized sports is the use of maturity matching to equalize competition and reduce the risk of injury.

Risk of Injury

Risk of injury is real in sports and in many other activities of childhood and adolescence. The injury-related literature in youth sports often focuses on risk factors related to the young athlete (internal) and to the sports environment (external) (37–40). Needless to say, interactions between the athlete and the sports environment are important considerations in the risk of injury.

Data on the prevalence and incidence of injuries in child and adolescent athletes are limited by the lack of suitable exposure data for practices and competitions to enable rates to be estimated accurately. The definition of an injury, which varies considerably among studies, is a confounding factor. The National Athletic Trainers Association conducted a high school injury surveillance project for the academic years of 1995 through 1997. The study permitted comparison of five sports in males and five in females, as well as that of similar (baseball and softball) or the same (e.g., basketball, soccer) sports in males and females. All injuries were reported by certified athletic trainers, a unique feature of this study (41,42). Corresponding data for youth sports, especially at the local level, are extremely limited. Injury data for youth athletes below the high school level are often limited to those who present to clinics and emergency rooms or to those who are included in insurance company statistics. Individuals who are injured but who are not presented to medical and/or insurance personnel are not represented in the statistical base. Such surveys, thus, probably underestimate the true incidence of injuries in youth sports, since many minor injuries likely are unreported or self treated.

Potential risk factors related to the young athlete include a variety of characteristics that are related to size, physique, maturity status, and performance and/or physical fitness. These factors, of course, may change with age, and they are interrelated as follows: (a) physique (i.e., the child may not have the body build suitable for a specific sport); (b) problems in structural alignment; (c) lack of flexibility; (d) lack of muscular strength or strength imbalance; (e) marginal and/or poor skill development; (f) behavioral factors, including risk taking and an inability to cope with stress; (g) injury history, specifically inadequate re-

habilitation from a prior injury; (h) the adolescent growth spurt, including individual differences in timing and tempo, strength imbalance, reduction in flexibility, and adolescent awkwardness; and (i) maturity-associated variation, such as maturity mismatches in size and strength and/or late maturation.

Discussions of internal risk factors are generally descriptive and speculative. The specific contributions of risk factors related to young participants with injuries sustained in sports activities are not known with certainty.

What about the growth spurt places the adolescent athlete at risk? The association between the increased prevalence of injuries and the adolescent growth spurt has been long recognized (43–47). The use of the term association must be emphasized. No existing prospective or longitudinal data specifically relate the occurrence of injuries to the parameters of the adolescent growth spurt. Youths who present to a clinic with an injury are ordinarily seen only on this occasion. Estimating where a youngster is in his or her growth spurt based on one observation is virtually impossible. If secondary sex characteristics are assessed, they provide only an estimate of sexual maturity and do not indicate where a youth is in the course of his or her growth spurt. In this context, for example, the suggestion that a boy in "Tanner stage 3" is experiencing maximal growth during adolescence and that this places him at risk for injury has been made in the following:

> During the Tanner Stage III (maximum height velocity), significant risk is present because of decreased strength at the epiphyses. During this growth spurt, decreased flexibility and strength also add potential factors for injury (Stanitski, 690 [40]).

The limited utility of the term *Tanner stages* was discussed earlier. These refer to stages of pubic hair and/or genital development in boys; thus, the two are not interchangeable. Tanner stage 3 does not refer to age at PHV or to the maximum velocity of growth in height during the growth spurt. The same applies to stages of pubic hair and breast development in girls.

The range of variation among individuals in the timing and sequence of the events of sexual maturation and adolescent growth spurt should be noted. Age at PHV can only be estimated from longitudinal data that span the duration of the adolescent growth spurt in height; thus, estimating PHV from a single observation is not possible. Although most boys are in PH 3 and G 4 at the time of PHV, all five pubic hair stages and stages G 2 through G 5 can be represented at PHV. Similarly, most girls are in breast and pubic hair stages 2 and 3 at the time of PHV, but all five breast stages and stages 1 through 4 of pubic hair can be represented among girls at PHV (12). Because of this variability, inferences about the rate of growth from the stage of puberty have limited accuracy, and they must be interpreted with caution.

Longitudinal data on bone mineral accrual during the adolescent growth spurt indicate that the peak velocity of growth in bone mineral content occurs after the peak velocity of growth in height by more than 1 year, on average (48). The lag in bone mineral accrual relative to linear growth may suggest a period of skeletal "fragility," which might contribute to the increased occurrence of injuries, both in sports and nonsports activities, during the adolescent spurt. This, however, should be verified with more specific observations on the growth, maturity, and perhaps even the body composition of young athletes.

Other changes during the adolescent growth spurt also need consideration. Loss of flexibility, for example, is indicated as a risk factor. Flexibility is joint specific, and it is a highly individual characteristic. Girls, on average, are more flexible than boys, and the range of motion of some joints increases during puberty, which contrasts to the general suggestion that flexibility decreases. Loss of flexibility in athletes during adolescence may be sport specific (e.g., shoulder and back flexibility in tennis players or the loss of quadriceps flexibility in soccer players) (49). Although flexibility and strength (both static and explosive) are not related, an imbalance between strength and flexibility has been suggested to lead to abnormal movement mechanics, which, in turn, may be a risk factor for injury.

Peak gains in muscular strength and power occur, on average, after PHV and closer in time to the peak velocity of body weight. Does this contribute to the strength imbalance described in some adolescent athletes? The role of "adolescent awkwardness," which is often attributed to rapid growth (50), also needs consideration in the context of injuries.

Maturity-associated variations in body size, strength, power, and other performance characteristics are magnified in adolescence, especially during early and mid-adolescence (i.e., about 9 to16 years of age). An important question is, "How do maturity mismatches in size, strength, and power factor into injuries and to what extent?" Unfortunately, the maturity status of youth sport participants has not been systematically related to injury. Sexual maturity status was evaluated as a factor related to injury in a North Carolina study of high school football injuries

(51). The criterion for maturity was a composite score based on the testicular volume and stages of pubic and axillary hair at the start of the season. Within single-year age groups at 13, 14, and 15 years, the injured players were slightly less mature. Differences between mean composite scores were 0.6, 0.2, and 0.3, respectively. Among older players, the differences in maturity were small and inconsistent. Most boys are either sexually mature or are approaching maturity by these ages, so one would expect to see less variation in maturity status among older players. The results of this football study, however, should be tempered with caution because, in general, the players had advanced maturity status compared to nonplayers and the range of maturity scores among players was less than in nonplayers. The results also indicate the need for a more sensitive index of maturity. Stages of puberty are limited; in this study, they simply indicate the youth's current status and not when he entered a stage or how long he had been in that stage. Nevertheless, the study of Violette (51) is one of the few to consider biologic maturity in the context of football injuries.

Three studies on injuries among soccer players considered biologic maturity. Vidalin (52) described 11 youth soccer players from 12.2 to 15.7 years of age who were injured during a season. Nine of the 11 injured players had a SA that was considered to be late maturing; the other two players were average or "on time" in skeletal maturity. Using grip strength and height as an indicator of maturity, Backous et al. (53) reported more injuries in a summer camp for soccer among boys who were classified as "tall and weak" ("skeletally mature but muscularly weak") than among those who were perceived as "tall and strong" ("mature") or "short and weak" ("immature"). The reader should note, however, that biologic maturity was not assessed. The authors assumed that height was directly related to the stage of development of secondary sex characteristics. This assumption does not allow for individual differences in timing and tempo and for genotypic differences in height. Furthermore, weight-for-height relationships were not considered in the analysis. In a study of elite young British athletes, on the other hand, no differences were observed in the incidence of injury among male soccer players in different stages of puberty. With the exception of a slightly higher incidence of injury in male tennis players who were advanced in pubertal status, the incidence of injury was not related to pubertal status in male swimmers and gymnasts (54,55).

Corresponding data that relates maturity status to injury among female athletes are extremely limited. No association was found between pubertal stage and the incidence of injury among swimmers in the study of young British athletes, but, in tennis players and gymnasts, an association was seen between the later stages of puberty and the incidence of injury. The association was significant only in gymnasts (54,55). By contrast, in another study, elite gymnasts in stages B 2 and B 3 were apparently more at risk for injury than were prepubertal (B 1) and postmenarcheal gymnasts (56).

Results of presently available studies of maturity status and risk of injury in young athletes are limited. A need exists for systematic study of variations in maturity status and in size, strength, and power associated with individual differences in maturity as potential risk factors for injury in sport. Advanced maturity is associated with larger body size and greater muscular strength and power in adolescent boys. The corresponding differences among girls of contrasting maturity status are not as large.

Growing Pains

"Growing" or limb pains that cannot be traced to bone, muscle, or joint disorders or to trauma are common in the pediatric age group, with an incidence of 4.2% to 36%. This condition, which is poorly understood and whose etiology is unknown, is unrelated to physical growth. Growing pains are typically observed from 3 to 5 years of age and from the ages of 8 to 12, although they can occur at any time in infancy and adulthood. They are self-limiting, and they generally affect females more often than they do males. The pain is usually deep or intermittent, and it occurs in the muscles of both the thighs and the calves and sometimes behind the knees and in the groin. It rarely affects the arms. The pain, which can resemble cramps or creeping sensations or can manifest as restless legs, typically occurs at the end of the day or at night, and it may arouse the child from sleep. It usually lasts for 3 months, with symptom-free intervals of days, weeks, or even months. The physical examination, laboratory data, and radiographs are all normal. Children with growing pains exhibit the same growth velocities as children without growing pains. The differential diagnosis should include serious disorders, such as infection, malignancy, and arthritis. Specific differential diagnoses include osteoid osteoma, intermittent nocturnal leg cramps, somatization disorders, benign hypermobility syndrome, and patella femoral pain syndrome. Because the condition is benign and self-limiting, a moderate exercise program with emotional support is appropriate.

Psychologic Stress

Discussions of potential psychologic risks in sports for children and youth are usually set in the context of competitive stress. Stress may be accentuated in individual sports (e.g., gymnastics, figure skating, diving, and distance running) in which athletes compete and perform as individuals. An additional factor in aesthetic sports is the presence of adults in the capacity as officials who evaluate the performances. In contrast, team sports involve a greater number of participants interacting at one time. The larger number of athletes and the highly interactive nature of activities in team sports tend to diffuse responsibility so that the performance of an individual athlete may be less conspicuous and performance evaluation may be less of a threat. In other words, team sports have the buffer of team members, which may alleviate some of the stress associated with performance, errors, and losing.

The potential consequences of competitive stress and, more specifically, the negative outcomes associated with it include low self-esteem, elevated anxiety, aggressive behavior, a possibly increased risk for injury, and "burnout". The latter term, which is commonly used in the context of high performance sports, refers to withdrawal from the sport in response to chronic stress that is associated with the demands of training and competition. Signs of chronic stress include behavioral alterations, such as agitation, sleep disturbances, and a loss of interest in practice and in the sport itself. Other manifestations include depression, a lack of energy, skin rashes, nausea, and frequent illness (57). Unfortunately, data on the prevalence or incidence of such conditions among elite young athletes or among youth sports participants are not available; a good deal of information is anecdotal, and it often is limited to individual sports, such as tennis and swimming.

Many factors are involved in competitive stress and burnout. Two especially important factors are negative performance evaluations and inconsistent feedback from coaches and officials. Negative evaluations are usually critical, rather than supportive, while inconsistent feedback often translates into mixed messages for the young athlete. Other contributing factors are the athlete's perception of not being able to meet the expectations imposed by self and/or others (e.g., coaches and parents), a training environment that is not supportive, and the stress of intensive competition *per se*. Overprotection by coaches, trainers, parents, and sport officials is an additional factor. This tends to limit the exposure of young athletes to new situations and, in turn, denies the athletes opportunities for developing coping mechanisms. These sport-related stresses are superimposed on and interact with the normal stresses of adolescence (i.e., school, peer pressures, social relationships [boyfriends and girlfriends], economic independence, and so on).

Growing, maturing, and developing young athletes also have the need to be a child or adolescent. All too often, some young athletes find themselves in the microcosm of a sport that is organized and operated by and for the satisfaction of adults. Thus, the fact that a factor in stress and burnout may be the conflicting demands between the sport and the universal tasks of childhood and adolescence (growth, maturation, and development) should come as no surprise.

Equalizing Competition by Maturity Matching

The issue of maturity matching in youth sports is ordinarily set in the context of the following two related issues: (a) grouping children for a sport by ability, grade, or maturity status and (b) "playing up" or "moving up" (i.e., children moving up a grade to participate). Moving up may occur in some small communities that may not have enough children to constitute a team, or it may take place because an individual is skilled and he or she wants to play at a higher level of competition. These are legitimate problems for which a simple solution is not available. They occur most often among middle school children who are from 11 to 15 years of age. Malina and Beunen (58) present a more detailed discussion of issues in maturity matching.

Size, strength, and skill mismatches are common in many youth sports despite the efforts to group participants for competition by age and skill. Matching participants by body size and biologic maturity is often suggested as a means for equalizing competition to reduce the risk of injury and to increase the chance for success.

Matching in youth sports is largely done on the basis of CA and sex and, to some extent, the level of skill. Body size (most often body weight) and biologic maturity (almost exclusively sexual maturity) are used less often. As has been noted earlier, skill, strength, size, and maturity are interrelated. Sex differences in pubertal timing and in size, strength, and skill, which become especially apparent at about 10 to 14 years of age, are also important.

Participants in youth sports are ordinarily grouped on the basis of CA. Two-year CA categories are often used. Limited numbers of participants in some programs, especially in smaller communities, may result in broader CA categories that can span up to 4 years. Although 2 years appears to be a relatively narrow range, considerable variation in size, strength, and skill is found among children of the same CA during the initial stages of the transition into puberty (i.e., about 9 to 11 years of age in girls and 10 to 12 years in boys). This emphasizes the need for narrower CA categories for youth sports at this time.

An issue related to age grouping deals with cutoff dates for a season. The selection of the cutoff point for age is somewhat arbitrary, and a youngster's fate in sport may be dictated by the calendar. Little League baseball, for example, has a CA limit of 12 years as of August 1 of the current season (i.e., the boy has not reached his thirteenth birthday by August 1). Boys born on August 1 and 2, 1988, would thus be classified differently. The boy born on August 1 is classified as a 13-year-old and is considered too old for Little League because he is 13 years as of August 1, 2001, while the boy born on August 2 plays as a 12-year-old. The latter is an "old" 12-year-old boy, while the former is a "young" 13-year-old boy. This problem is a concern in many organized youth sports.

The level of skill and previous experience in a sport may be considered in the matching process. Many programs have several competitive levels that are aligned on the basis of proficiency in the skill demands of the sport. The initial assessment of skill can be an issue. Assessment of skill levels should be done by individuals who are not involved in coaching in the respective leagues and whose own children are not involved. Children should then be assigned to a team, and the team should then receive a coach. Player drafts, lotteries, player recruitment, and so on often create extreme competitiveness and, at times, ill will, among coaches and parents.

Matching participants for sport by body size, independent of CA and biologic maturity, can be misleading given their interrelationships. As youngsters enter puberty, variability in height and weight within a CA group is magnified. Matching by size, especially body weight, is common in football. The potential for injury associated with size mismatches in sports that feature body contact on a regular basis (e.g., football, ice hockey and soccer) should be of concern. The strength and impact force disparities between large and small boys can be considerable.

The most commonly used indicators of biologic maturity for purposes of maturity matching are secondary sex characteristics. Which specific indicators of sexual maturity should be used in matching? The stages of secondary sex characteristics are not equivalent within each sex and between the sexes. Corresponding stages of breast and pubic hair in girls and the stages of genital and pubic hair in boys are generally related, so either can be used within each sex; but only one characteristic or the other should be used.

How should a change in maturity status during the course of a season be handled? For example, Little League baseball teams in the South are selected in March, and the season starts in April and continues into July. Pee Wee hockey teams are selected in the early fall, and the season continues through the winter into spring. That some early and rapidly maturing boys will pass through one or more stages of sexual maturity and perhaps will experience their growth spurt during the course of the season is entirely possible. The relatively small size differences associated with variations in maturity status may now be magnified. Thus, should matching be an ongoing process during the season? This obviously is not practical.

Children are ordinarily grouped for sports on the basis of CA. This presents a significant problem, even when the sexual maturity status of the participants is considered. How should variation in maturity status within a given CA group be handled?

Among girls, menarcheal status is often used as a criterion for classification. Girls are classified as premenarcheal or postmenarcheal. Within an age group, postmenarcheal girls are taller, heavier, and stronger than premenarcheal girls, and the differences are more apparent at younger adolescent ages. The 12-year-old postmenarcheal girl is, on average, about 9 cm (3.5 in.) taller and 10 kg (22 lb) heavier than the 12-year-old premenarcheal girl. The differences are only slightly less at older ages (e.g., 14 years) when postmenarcheal girls are, on average, about 5 cm (2.0 in.) taller and 8 kg (17.5 lb) heavier than premenarcheal girls of the same age.

In moving up from middle school to high school sports, the criterion may be menarcheal status independent of CA. A young postmenarcheal girl may move up to play with older girls. However, older postmenarcheal girls are, on average, taller and heavier than younger postmenarcheal girls. The differences between mean heights and weights of 12- and 14-year-old postmenarcheal girls, for example, reach about 5 cm (2 in.) and 4.0 kg (9 lb), respectively. Older postmenarcheal girls are also, on average, stronger than younger postmenarcheal girls.

Although matching may equalize competition and reduce the risk of injury, it generally does not take into consideration individual differences in behaviors (e.g., social, emotional, and cognitive). A child's level of behavioral development does not necessarily pro-

ceed in concert with his or her physical growth and maturity. A late maturing, 13-year-old boy may resent participating with 11-year-old boys of similar maturity status. Similarly, an early maturing, 11-year-old girl may not want to participate with equally mature, but older and more experienced, 13-year-old girls. Matching may thus have potential behavioral consequences that can influence the self-concept and self-esteem of the athlete.

Younger, early maturing boys may be threatened by having to participate and to compete with chronologically older boys of the same maturity status. Conversely, older boys may not want to participate with younger boys of the same maturity status, due largely to social concerns (e.g., the individual may receive less recognition when he successfully competes against less mature individuals).

The peer group is a major force during middle childhood and early adolescence, and the team is a significant peer group. Although children and youth have several peer groups, matching by size, skill, and maturity status often alters peer group structure and, in turn, may influence social relationships and development.

Most discussions of maturity matching and equating for sports competition focus on youth. However, reversing the question is also appropriate—how can sports be modified to meet the characteristics and needs of their youthful participants? How can the tasks and rules of a sport be adjusted to meet the changing needs of growing, maturing, and developing youth? Eliminating body checking in youth ice hockey, for example, significantly reduces the number of injuries. Reducing the size of the playing area and the duration of contests are other examples of modifying sports, such as baseball, football and soccer, to meet the characteristics of children and youths. Other modifications should also be considered (e.g., reducing the height of the basket to improve the possibility for success in basketball, perhaps granting a point if a child's shot hits the rim in basketball, or enlarging the goal in soccer). Undoubtedly, other possibilities abound, and those involved with youth sports programs should be encouraged to consider seriously how sports can be matched to the needs and characteristics of children and adolescents. On the other hand, the demands of sports (e.g., artistic gymnastics and figure skating) have seemingly been altered by administrators, judges, and coaches so that "women's" competitions at elite levels in these sports have essentially become competitions among "prepubertal girls." Suggestions that the rigors of training girls for elite gymnastics and figure skating border on child abuse have even been voiced.

SUMMARY

Young athletes of both sexes in most sports have, on average, heights and weights that equal or exceed reference values for the general population of children and adolescents. Gymnasts and figure skaters of both sexes present shorter heights, on average, but have appropriate weight-for-height values. Female distance runners tend to have low weight-for-height. Intensive training for sports has no negative effects on growth in height and biologic maturity (SA, secondary sex characteristics, or adolescent growth spurt). In adequately nourished children and adolescents, growth in height and biologic maturity is largely genotypically mediated. In the extremely small number of young athletes who may present to a clinic with problems related to growth and maturation, factors other than physical training must be more closely scrutinized. On the other hand, regular training for sports has the potential to influence body composition favorably by contributing to an increase in bone mineral and skeletal muscle and a reduction in fatness.

Involvement in sports has the potential to provide both positive and negative experiences and outcomes for children and adolescents. The line between benefits and risks may be quite fine, and optimizing the risk to benefit ratio for child and adolescent participants in sports is important. Coaches, parents, and the medical community need to be aware of potential benefits and risks, and they must also be good stewards of the sports experiences of children and adolescents.

REFERENCES

1. Malina RM, Clark MA, eds. *Youth sports in the 21st century: organized sport in the lives of children and adolescents*. Monterey, CA: Exercise Science Publishing, 2002.
2. Malina RM. Physical activity and fitness of children and youth: questions and implications. *Med Exerc Nutr Health* 1995;4:123–135.
3. Malina RM. Physical activity and fitness: pathways from childhood to adulthood. *Am J Hum Biol* 2001;13: 162–172.
4. Sallis JF. Age-related decline in physical activity: a synthesis of human and animal studies. *Med Sci Sports Exerc* 2000;32:1598–1600.
5. Katzmarzyk PT, Malina RM. Contributions of organized sports participation to estimated daily energy expenditure in youth. *Pediatr Exerc Sci* 1998;10:378–386.
6. Carter JEL. Somatotypes of children in sports. In: Malina RM, ed. Young athletes: biological, psychological, and educational perspectives. Champaign, IL: Human Kinetics, 1988:153–165.
7. Geithner CA, Malina RM. Somatotypes of junior Olympic divers. In: Malina RM, Gabriel JL, eds. *U.S. diving 1993 sport science seminar proceedings*. Indianapolis, IN: United States Diving, 1993:36–40.
8. Malina RM. Physical growth and biological maturation of young athletes. *Exerc Sport Sci Rev* 1994;22: 389–433.
9. Kuczmarski RJ, Ogden CL, Grummer-Strawn LM, et al. *CDC growth charts: United States*. Advance Data from Vital and Health Statistics, no 314. Hyattsville, MD: National Center for Health Statistics, 2000.
10. Hamill PVV, Drizd TA, Johnson CL, et al. *NCHS growth curves for children, birth—18 years. United States*. Publication no. (PHS) 78-1650. Washington, D.C.: United States Government Printing Office, 1977.
11. Malina RM, Bouchard C. *Growth, maturation, and physical activity*. Champaign, IL: Human Kinetics, 1991.
12. Malina RM, Bouchard C, Bar-Or O. *Growth, maturation, and physical activity*, 2nd ed. Champaign, IL: Human Kinetics, *(in press)*.
13. Cole TJ, Bellizzi MC, Flegal KM, et al. Establishing a standard definition for child overweight and obesity worldwide: international survey. *Br Med J* 2000;320:1240–1243.
14. Tanner JM. *Growth at adolescence*, 2nd ed. Oxford: Blackwell Science, 1962.
15. Reynolds EL, Wines JV. Individual differences in physical changes associated with adolescence in girls. *Am J Dis Child* 1948;75:329–350.
16. Reynolds EL, Wines JV. Physical changes associated with adolescence in boys. *Am J Dis Child* 1951;82: 529–547.
17. van Wieringen JC, Wafelbakker F, Verbrugge HP, et al. *Growth diagrams 1965 Netherlands*. Groningen: Wolters-Noordhoof Publishing, 1971.
18. Matsudo SMM, Matsudo VKR. Self-assessment and physician assessment of sexual maturation in Brazilian boys and girls: concordance and reproducibility. *Am J Hum Biol* 1994;6:451–455.
19. Schlossberger NM, Turner RA, Irwin CE. Validity of self-report of pubertal maturation in early adolescents. *J Adolesc Health* 1992;13:109–113.
20. Malina RM. Growth and maturation of elite female gymnasts: is training a factor? In: Johnston FE, Zemel B, Eveleth PB, eds. *Human growth in context*. London: Smith-Gordon, 1999:291–301.
21. Malina RM. Growth and maturation of young athletes: is training for sport a factor? In: Chan KM, Micheli LJ, eds. *Sports and children*. Hong Kong: Williams & Wilkins Asia Pacific, 1998:133–161.
22. Malina RM, Peña-Reyes ME, Eisenmann JC, et al. Height, mass and skeletal maturity of elite Portuguese soccer players ages 11–16 years. *J Sports Sci* 2000;18: 685–693.
23. Malina RM, Beunen G, Wellens R, et al. Skeletal maturity and body size of teenage Belgian track and·field athletes. *Ann Hum Biol* 1986;13:331–339.
24. Malina RM. Menarche in athletes: a synthesis and hypothesis. *Ann Hum Biol* 1983;10:1–24.
25. Malina RM. Physical activity, sport, social status and Darwinian fitness. In: Strickland SS, Shetty PS, eds. *Human biology and social inequality*. Cambridge: Cambridge University Press, 1998:165–192.
26. Beunen G, Malina RM. Growth and biological maturation: relevance to athletic performance. In: Bar-Or O, eds. *The child and adolescent athlete*. Oxford: Blackwell Science, 1996:3–24.
27. American Medical Association and American Dietetic

Association. *Targets for adolescent health: nutrition and physical fitness.* Chicago: American Medical Association, 1991.

28. Tofler IR, Stryer BK, Micheli LJ, et al. Physical and emotional problems of elite female gymnasts. *N Engl J Med* 1996;335:281–283.

29. Malina RM. Growth and maturation: do regular physical activity and training for sport have a significant influence? In: Armstrong N, van Mechelen W, eds. *Oxford textbook of paediatric exercise science and medicine.* Oxford: Oxford University Press, 2000:95–106.

30. Theintz AGE, Howald H, Weiss U, et al. Evidence for a reduction of growth potential in adolescent female gymnasts. *J Pediatr* 1993;122:306–313.

31. Malina RM, Ryan RC, Bonci CM. Age at menarche in athletes and their mothers and sisters. *Ann Hum Biol* 1994;21:417–422.

32. Vadocz EA, Siegel SR, Malina RM. Age at menarche in competitive figure skaters: variation by level and discipline. *J Sports Sci* 2002;20:93–100.

33. Malina RM, Katzmarzyk PT, Bonci CM, et al. Family size and age at menarche in athletes. *Med Sci Sports Exerc* 1997;29:99–106.

34. Loucks AB, Vaitukaitis J, Cameron JL, et al. The reproductive system and exercise in women. *Med Sci Sports Exerc* 1992;24:S288–S293.

35. Clapp JF, Little KD. The interaction between regular exercise and selected aspects of women's health. *Am J Obstet Gynecol* 1995;173:2–9.

36. Bouchard C, Malina RM, Perusse L. *Genetics of fitness and physical performance.* Champaign, IL: Human Kinetics, 1997.

37. Caine DJ, Lindner K. Preventing injury to young athletes. I. Predisposing factors. *Canadian Association for Health, Physical Education and Recreation Journal* 1990;56:30–35.

38. Micheli LJ. Overuse injuries in children's sports: the growth factor. *Orthop Clin North Am* 1983;14:337–360.

39. Micheli LJ. Preventing youth sports injuries. *Journal of Physical Education. Recreation and Dance* 1985;56: 52–54.

40. Stanitski CL. Management of sports injuries in children and adolescents. *Orthop Clin North Am* 1988;19: 689–697.

41. Powell JW, Barber-Foss KD. Injury patterns in selected high school sports: a review of the 1995–1997 seasons. *Journal of Athletic Training* 1999;34:277–284.

42. Powell JW, Barber-Foss KD. Sex-related injury patterns among selected high school sports. *Am J Sports Med* 2000;28:385–391.

43. Dameron TB, Reibel DB. Fractures involving the proximal humeral epiphyseal plate. *J Bone Joint Surg* 1969; 51A:289–297.

44. Peterson CA, Peterson HA. Analysis of the incidence of injuries to the epiphyseal growth plate. *J Trauma* 1972; 12:275–281.

45. Burkhart SS, Peterson HA. Fractures of the proximal tibial epiphysis. *J Bone Joint Surg* 1979;61A:996–1002.

46. Bailey DA, Wedge JH, McCulloch RG, et al. Epidemiology of fractures of the distal end of the radius in children as associated with growth. *J Bone Joint Surg* 1989; 71A:1225–1231.

47. Blimkie CJR, Lefevre J, Beunen GP, et al. Fractures, physical activity, and growth velocity in adolescent Belgian boys. *Med Sci Sports Exerc* 1993;25:801–808.

48. Iuliano-Burns S, Mirwald RL, Bailey DA. The timing and magnitude of peak height velocity and peak tissue velocities for early, average and late maturing boys and girls. *Am J Hum Biol* 2001;13:1–8.

49. Kibler WB, Chandler TJ. Musculoskeletal adaptations and injuries associated with intense participation in youth sports. In: Cahill BR, Pearl AJ, eds. *Intensive participation in children's sports.* Champaign, IL: Human Kinetics, 1993:203–216.

50. Beunen G, Malina RM. Growth and physical performance relative to the timing of the adolescent spurt. *Exerc Sports Sci Rev* 1988;16:503–540.

51. Violette RW. *An epidemiologic investigation of junior high school football injury and its relationship to certain physical and maturational characteristics of the players* [dissertation]. Chapel Hill, NC: University of North Carolina; 1976.

52. Vidalin H. Football. Traumatismes et age osseux. Estude prospective de 11 cas. *Medicin du Sport* 1988;62: 195–197.

53. Backous DD, Friedl KE, Smith NJ, et al. Soccer injuries and their relation to physical maturity. *Am J Dis Child* 1988;142:839–842.

54. Sports Council. *TOYA and sports injuries.* London: The Sports Council, 1992.

55. Baxter-Jones A, Maffulli N, Helms P. Low injury rates in elite athletes. *Arch Dis Child* 1993;68:130–132.

56. Caine D, Cochrane B, Caine C, et al. An epidemiologic investigation of injuries affecting young competitive female gymnasts. *Am J Sports Med* 1989;17:811–820.

57. Weinberg RS, Gould D. *Foundations of sport and exercise psychology*, 2nd ed.. Champaign, IL: Human Kinetics, 1999.

58. Malina RM, Beunen G. Matching opponents in youth sports. In: Bar-Or O, ed. *The child and adolescent athlete.* Oxford: Blackwell Science, 1996:202–213.

4

Sports Nutrition

Kim Edward LeBlanc

The period of most rapid growth of the human body occurs during childhood and adolescence. This has a marked effect on the nutritional requirements of these individuals. Additional nutritional demands are placed by physical and sports activities. These additional requirements have a significant impact on decisions regarding choices, particularly in the caloric content, in the diet of these athletes. With the added stress of training, the primary care physician is challenged to ensure that dietary intake is appropriately balanced between sport and maturation. Attention to this detail is essential to avoid any impairment of growth and development that might occur as a result of poor nutritional intake.

ENERGY REQUIREMENTS

Regardless of age, the caloric requirements of the body will be increased with physical activity. As a consequence, additional calories that will compensate for athletic activities must be consumed on a daily basis. As a general rule of thumb, the daily caloric requirement is highest during the first year of life (80 to 120 kcal per kg per day). After this first year, the caloric requirements decrease by approximately 10 kcal per kg per day every 3 years, as Table 4.1 depicts (1). These requirements allow normal growth and development. As was noted above, these amounts will be inadequate during periods of physical activity. The estimated average requirement for physical activity is 15 to 25 kcal per kg per day (2).

Most athletes will need an additional 500 to 1,500 calories per day to cover these additional activities (2). The current recommended daily allowance (RDA) for calories for children 7 to 10 years of age is 2,000 calories (3). The RDA for males between the ages of 15 and 18 years old is 3,000 calories per day, while females in that age range require 2,200 calories per day (2).

The reader should bear in mind that the above RDAs are those for normal daily activities. This amount should be sufficient for growth and development. However, additional calories must be consumed for sporting activities. For example, current information indicates that the moderately active teenager, whether male or female, will require between 1,500 and 3,000 additional calories to cover his or her energy requirements (1,4).

As children and adolescents generally eat poorly, athletes in this age group should be encouraged to consume three meals a day. One should be as well balanced as possible, containing food from all major food groups. In addition, they should be allowed to have healthy nutrient-dense snacks.

Although following caloric consumption accurately is difficult, some attempt should be made to verify that growth and development will not be impeded by inadequate intake. One useful method is plotting the athlete's growth pattern, while comparing his or her weight-for-height to previously established standards. This allows a fairly accurate assessment of whether or not these athletes are consuming enough calories to support their growth and development.

TABLE 4.1. *Daily caloric requirements for various ages*

Age (yr)	Requirements (kcal/kg/d)
2–4	70–110
5–7	60–100
8–10	50–90
11–13	40–80
14–16	30–70
17–20	25–30

MACRONUTRIENT REQUIREMENTS

Macronutrients refer to the major components of the diet—carbohydrates, proteins, and fats. Whether the child or adolescent is an athlete or not, the nutritional needs are the same. The difference is that the exercising individual should pay particular attention to the intake of calories provided by these macronutrients. With increasing levels of activity, the number of calories that are ingested should be increased as well. This is also true for fluid intake on a daily basis.

Usually, the exercising person begins to consume more food as a compensatory mechanism to keep up with caloric expenditure. However, in this population of patients, monitoring the type of calories that are ingested to be certain that they are healthy choices is prudent.

Carbohydrates

Once exercise commences, most of the energy that is released to support the activity comes from carbohydrates. Carbohydrates are the most important source of fuel for the exercising muscle, especially at high levels of exercise intensity. Therefore, the ability to engage in physical activity is crucially dependent on the ingestion of adequate carbohydrates.

In the older child and adolescent, carbohydrates should make up approximately 55% to 60% of caloric intake, which is similar to the balance recommended for adults. For the adolescent who is engaged in prolonged activity, these daily intake amounts may need to be increased by an additional 5% to 10% to maintain adequate glycogen stores in the skeletal muscle and liver.

Following exercise, the athlete should begin to replenish the glycogen stores. Research has indicated that this restoration should begin as soon after the event as is feasible. The first 2 hours following the completion of exercise appears to be the period of most rapid reabsorption of ingested carbohydrates. Some authors recommend that 1.0 to 1.5 g of carbohydrates per kg of body weight be consumed immediately following exercise in an effort to replenish the depleted reserves (5). This should be modified according to the athlete's individual ability to consume these amounts. The replenishment should continue throughout each day to ensure the presence of adequate glycogen stores. No noticeable difference is found when these carbohydrates are consumed in either the liquid or solid form.

Many carbohydrate replacement drinks can be found on the market today. These may be of benefit mainly for their ability to replace glycogen stores rapidly without outpacing the stomach's ability to receive large amounts of this macronutrient. These drinks may also be utilized during a sporting event in an attempt to delay glycogen depletion and, hence, the onset of fatigue. By using carbohydrate supplementation in this manner, endurance performance may be enhanced. However, these drinks should contain no more than an 8% concentration of the carbohydrate.

Fluid with a concentration exceeding 8% may cause a delay in gastric emptying.

Finally, with regard to carbohydrate replacement, one should remember that the ingestion of large amounts of fructose whether in a liquid or solid form can result in gastrointestinal difficulties, such as cramping, bloating, and diarrhea. However, the use of some fructose in carbohydrate supplements is recommended because it appears to be more effective than glucose in restoring liver glycogen (5).

Dietary sources of carbohydrates include starches, vegetables, fruits, cereals, milk, and syrups. The ingested carbohydrates should be complex (e.g., potato), and an active attempt should be made to avoid simple sugars, such as table sugar.

Proteins

Proteins function in the body primarily in the growth and repair of tissue. Accordingly, in the younger individual, this an extremely important macronutrient. The child or adolescent athlete must be certain that, in addition to consuming an adequate supply of protein to allow normal growth and development, he or she also eats enough to compensate for the repair of tissues that are microscopically damaged during the training process. During times of rapid growth, such as infancy and younger childhood, protein demands are higher than they are for adults per unit of body mass (Table 4.2) (3). In this table, one should also note that females above the age of 14 years typically require less protein in their diets than do their male counterparts.

Generally speaking, protein should make up 10% to 15% of the total calories in the diet. Strength training and muscle building athletes typically wish to increase their protein intake in hope of increasing muscle mass and bulk. However, they must be reminded that simply increasing protein intake in the diet does not result in muscle hypertrophy. Resistance exercise

TABLE 4.2. *Protein recommended daily allowances*

Category	Age (yr)	Protein (g/d)	Protein (g/kg)
Children	4–6	24	1.2
	7–10	28	1.0
Males	11–14	45	1.0
	15–18	59	0.9
Females	11–14	46	1.0
	15–18	44	0.8

is required to stimulate protein synthesis in the muscle and, consequently, hypertrophy. In adult body builders and weight training athletes, an increased protein intake does seem beneficial. However, this has not been demonstrated in the nonadult population. In fact, consuming excess protein increases the work of the liver and kidneys for deamination and excretion, respectively. Furthermore, any extra protein calories that are not consumed will be converted into fat and stored.

Finally, although the common feeling among high school athletes, particularly football players, is that consuming amino acids will help in building muscle or in hormone excretion or will enhance exercise performance, no supporting data can be found for this assumption (6). The excess amino acids are simply excreted.

Dietary sources of protein would include eggs, milk, fish, meat, poultry, legumes, cheese, cereals, and nuts.

Fats

Fats are the storage form of energy in the body. These macronutrients are highly efficient in their ability to store energy. They also serve as vehicles for the fat-soluble vitamins A, D, E, and K. Additionally, they afford palatability to many foods, making them tasty and quite appealing (one of the reasons that Americans overeat this particular nutrient). As the intensity of exercise increases, so does the relative utilization of carbohydrates. However, as the duration of exercise increases, particularly beyond 15 minutes, the relative utilization of fat increases. Fats within the bloodstream, as well as intramuscular triglycerides, are important sources of energy during prolonged exercise. Therefore, adipose tissue should be considered a fuel reserve of maximal proportion.

On the other hand, the utilization of fat as a form of energy does not occur readily. In addition, the untrained individual is poorly adapted for using this energy source in a timely fashion. Consequently, glycogen remains the preferred source of fuel during exercise in almost all circumstances.

Important dietary sources of fat include milk, cheese, egg yolk, meat, nuts, and vegetable oils. However, the usual diet of an older child or adolescent contains an excessive amount of fat calories. The intake of the normal teenage diet consists of many fast foods and snacks that contain excessive fat (e.g., candy bars, potato chips, and cookies).

Although athletes need to consume adequate amounts of fats in their daily diet, excess fat intake should still be avoided. No more than 30% of the daily caloric intake should consist of fats.

Every attempt should be made to avoid the intake of excessive amounts of fat, whether or not the person is an athlete. Excess fat intake contributes to the obesity among American youth, as well as being detrimental to athletic performance. Estimates from the United States Department of Agriculture indicate that fat makes up 40% to 50% of calories in the average American diet. This is considerably more than the recommended intake of less than 30% of daily caloric consumption. Saturated fats are particularly undesirable. The recommendation is that saturated fat make up no more than 10% of the total calories consumed. These measures help minimize cardiovascular risk in youths, as well as in adults.

MICRONUTRIENT REQUIREMENTS

Vitamins

Vitamins are essential organic compounds that are required by all cells in the body. These substances are present in minute quantities within each cell. They are necessary for their individual or interrelated roles in various, highly specific metabolic functions. As a consequence, vitamins are crucial for normal cellular metabolism to ensure normal growth, development, and function.

Although they are highly important to normal bodily functioning, vitamins do not supply energy or serve as compounds that are substrates for building other compounds. Their importance lies in their ability to function as catalysts for a variety of cellular metabolic activities unique to each particular vitamin.

Although vitamin deficiency is a known cause of suboptimal athletic capabilities, no convincing data exists to suggest that supplementation in otherwise healthy athletes with a normal vitamin status will enhance performance. Athletes rarely are subject to any deficiency state because of the normal increase in dietary consumption that occurs with physical activity (7). As daily caloric consumption increases, the logical result would be an increase in daily vitamin consumption as well. Most athletes consume quantities far in excess of the RDA for any particular vitamin. In actuality, research indicates that only the following four vitamins demonstrate declines in their levels with exercise due to increased metabolism: ascorbic acid, pyridoxine, thiamin, and riboflavin. However, they are normally replaced by the aforementioned increase in dietary intake. Table 4.3 provides a listing of the current RDA of vitamins for children and adoles-

TABLE 4.3. *Recommended daily allowances for vitamins and minerals*

Age (yr)	Fat-soluble vitamins					Water-soluble vitamins						Minerals				
	A (µg)	D (µg)	E (mg)	K (µg)	C (mg)	Thiamine (mg)	Riboflavin (mg)	Niacin (mg)	B_6 (mg)	Folate (µg)	B_{12} (µg)	Calcium (mg)	Phosphorus (mg)	Magnesium (mg)	Iron (mg)	Zinc (mg)
7–10 (M,F)	700	10	7	30	45	1.0	1.2	13	1.4	100	1.4	800	800	170	10	10
11–14 (M)	1,000	10	10	45	50	1.3	1.5	17	1.7	150	2.0	1,200	1,200	270	12	15
15–18 (M)	1,000	10	10	65	60	1.5	1.8	20	2.0	200	2.0	1,200	1,200	400	12	15
11–14 (F)	800	10	8	45	50	1.1	1.3	15	1.4	150	2.0	1,200	1,200	280	15	12
15–18 (F)	800	10	8	55	60	1.1	1.3	15	1.5	180	2.0	1,200	1,200	300	15	12

Abbreviations: F, female; M, male.

cents (3). These recommendations are the same for both the sedentary and the physically active individual.

One of the difficulties in conveying the message that no data or convincing research support the enhancement of athletic performance via vitamin supplementation is the frequent advertisements to the contrary. Scattered throughout all forms of media presentations are testimonials and claims made by famous athletes or coaches to suggest that the use of a particular supplement will improve athletic ability. None of these statements is supported by legitimate scientific investigations. However, as a result of these claims, vitamin supplementation is a multibillion dollar a year industry. Certainly, no athlete should attempt to supplement a poor diet with vitamins.

Minerals

Minerals are inorganic compounds, and at least 31 such substances have been identified in the body. Twenty-four of them are considered essential for life. The minerals may be divided into two groups: macrominerals and microminerals. Macrominerals are required in amounts greater than 100 mg per day, while the microminerals are necessary in daily amounts less than 100 mg. Macrominerals are made up of the following elements, which are listed in descending order of quantity within the body: calcium, phosphorus, potassium, sulfur, sodium, chlorine, and magnesium. Microminerals are considered trace minerals and consist of the following (also listed according to decreasing bodily concentrations): iron, fluoride, zinc, copper, silicon, vanadium, tin, nickel, selenium, manganese, iodine, molybdenum, chromium, and cobalt.

As was noted above, vitamins may activate certain chemical processes without being incorporated into the products of the reaction. However, minerals often are fundamental to the structures that they help produce. Generally speaking, minerals have three major responsibilities within the body. First, they may become part of enzymes and hormones that control cellular activity and that also play a regulatory role in cellular metabolism. Second, they play an integral role in acid–base regulation, muscular contractility, cardiac rhythm, and nerve conduction. Third, some provide structure for bones and teeth.

Although many minerals exist, this discussion centers on the most commonly deficient minerals—calcium, magnesium, and iron. These minerals are important in all individuals, but they are especially important in the growing athletic population in which they attain an even higher significance. For example, weaker bones may result if calcium intake is inadequate, or decreased performance may be noted due to iron deficiency anemia. Adults take for granted the fact that these young athletes will eat properly. However, this frequently is not the case. Any physician caring for these individuals should be aware of the possibilities of inadequate intakes of calcium, magnesium, and iron.

Calcium

Calcium is important to mention in any topic related to children and other growing populations. Available data indicate that more than 50% of American children do not consume the RDA of calcium. They also suggest that children may require more than the RDA to maximize bone formation (8,9). When individuals are engaging in sporting activities, optimal bone health undoubtedly is extremely important. Every effort should be made to ensure that these children consume adequate quantities of calcium-rich foods.

Although childhood is an important time for bone growth, the most critical time for bone mass development occurs during the adolescent years. Generally speaking, athletes do exhibit higher bone density than their sedentary counterparts due to mechanical loading; however, sufficient calcium must be ingested to maximize this process. No data suggests that calcium ingestion enhances athletic performance. However, calcium intake should be stressed to all children and particularly to adolescents. Calcium accumulation in bone will markedly decline after the third decade. Therefore, to avoid the onset of osteoporosis, calcium intake must minimally coincide with the current RDA for each particular age group (Table 4.3). If the child is between 7 and 10 years of age, the RDA is 800 mg per day. The RDA for the individual between the ages of 11 and 18 years is 1,200 mg per day, regardless of gender.

The most important source of calcium in the diet is dairy products. Other good sources include calcium-fortified foods (e.g., orange juice), canned fish, and green leafy vegetables (e.g., broccoli).

If calcium supplements are ingested, the athlete should be mindful of the timing of the ingestion. The recommendation is that these supplements be ingested in divided doses (e.g., 500 mg or less) between meals to enhance their absorption. However, calcium carbonate requires stomach acid for optimal absorption, and therefore, it should be ingested with meals. Excess consumption of certain food products (e.g., coffee, alcohol, meat, and salt) may impair absorption as well, while vitamin D facilitates its uptake.

The two most common forms of calcium that are recommended for supplementation are calcium citrate and calcium carbonate. One should also note that the calcium content of milk is the same whether the milk is whole, fat free, 1%, or 2% (300 mg per 8-ounce glass). Therefore, as long as one of these forms of milk is ingested, the calcium availability is the same.

One important role of calcium relates to exercise-induced amenorrhea in adolescent females. Exercise-induced amenorrhea may be seen in any sport, but it is most commonly observed in certain athletic arenas, such as ballet dancing and gymnastics. Regular menses must be established in these athletes because of the known incidence of decreased bone density and increased stress fractures in the amenorrheic female. This is followed by the development of premature osteoporosis. Furthermore, some of the bone loss may be irreversible if the amenorrhea is allowed to continue beyond 2 to 3 years (9).

Magnesium

Although calcium is perhaps the most discussed mineral, the role that magnesium plays in many of the processes that occur with physical activity is often not appreciated. Magnesium is extremely important for both physiologic and biochemical effects within the exercising body. It plays an important role in the conduction of nerve impulses and muscle contraction via its function in maintaining electrical potentials at the membranes of muscles and nerves. It also serves as an essential cofactor in certain enzymes that are involved with carbohydrate metabolism. This role is important in the formation of glycogen in the liver and muscle from glucose in the bloodstream. Magnesium also plays a role in the breakdown of fatty acids, glucose, and amino acids and in the synthesis of protein.

The status of magnesium in the body may be affected by physical activity. Strenuous exercise has been shown to have the ability to lower magnesium concentrations in the athlete (10). Furthermore, a small loss may occur in sweat (11). The reasons for these are not clear, and these declines have been documented in adults only. A few case reports highlight the beneficial effect of magnesium supplementation in adult athletes who chronically experience muscle cramps or spasms. Therefore, how this relates to the child and/or adolescent has not yet been determined. Furthermore, no data indicating that supplementation

will provide any benefit in the normal individual exists. Magnesium supplementation should not be automatically incorporated into the athlete's diet. Instead, blood levels of magnesium should be determined prior to the initiation of supplementation. Magnesium may interact with other minerals and interfere with absorption. In particular, this interaction has been noted with calcium. Magnesium and calcium are antagonistic as an excess of magnesium has the potential to impair bone mineralization, which could have profound consequences, especially in the young female athlete.

Currently, the RDA for magnesium is 170 mg per day for children between the ages of 7 and 10 years. In males, the RDA is 270 mg and 400 mg per day for those between the ages of 11 to 14 and 15 to 18 years, respectively. In females, the RDA is 280 mg and 300 mg per day for those between the ages of 11 to 14 and 15 to 18 years, respectively (Table 4.3). These amounts should be obtained from dietary sources. The food sources of magnesium include legumes, meat, vegetables, whole-grain products (e.g., cereal), sunflower seeds, and popcorn. If a plant source is used, boiling the item may result in a loss of 50% of the magnesium content.

Iron

Although no research specifically indicates that iron supplementation is beneficial to athletic performance in a normal individual, low iron stores will result in a decline in exercise capacity. Iron plays a critical role in the body, whether one is sedentary or physically active. However, it is even more significant if one is trying to perform at an optimal level.

Iron is important as a result of its association with the protein globin and its ability to form hemoglobin. Hemoglobin is located in red blood cells, and it enables the oxygen-carrying capabilities of these cells. In addition, iron is found in myoglobin, which is similar to hemoglobin; myoglobin functions in the storage and transport of oxygen within the muscle cells. A third function of iron is observed in the mitochondria. The iron located in mitochondria enables the functional capability of a series of specialized enzymes called cytochromes. Simply stated, cytochromes allow the transmission of energy within the mitochondria via the ability of iron to transfer electrons. This transfer of electrons results in the generation of energy for cellular function, and it provides power for all forms of biologic work.

Iron is stored in the spleen, liver, and bone marrow. The iron stored within the liver and spleen is referred to as hemosiderin, while that stored in the bone marrow is referred to as ferritin. These sites serve as reservoirs for iron when inadequate intake or iron depletion via blood loss occurs. The serum level of ferritin is highly correlated to the amount of iron stored in the body. This is important because athletes often have an expanded plasma volume. As a consequence, their hemoglobin and/or hematocrit concentration may be factitiously low, resulting in so-called "sports anemia." If actual anemia is a possibility, the clinician should obtain a serum ferritin level. A level below 12 μg per L is a reliable indicator of storage iron depletion, which is the first stage of iron deficiency.

Iron deficiency anemia in the child athlete, whether male or female, and the male adolescent athlete is most likely the result of inadequate dietary intake of iron. Although blood loss is an unlikely etiology of iron deficiency anemia in these individuals, it should be investigated and ruled out.

Iron deficiency anemia in the female adolescent is a different matter. Menstruating females have a higher potential for the development of iron deficiency anemia on two fronts. First, adolescents typically do not consume a nutritionally sound diet. This results in an inadequate daily intake of iron. Second, menstruating females have a certain amount of blood loss every month. This combination of events makes females prone to the development of iron deficiency anemia.

Once iron deficiency anemia develops, the athlete may complain of a decline in exercise performance. One of the earliest complaints may be undue fatigue during a normal workout. These athletes should begin dietary iron replacement and should receive instruction on proper dietary management. Excess dietary intake of iron does not result in improved performance and may have toxic side effects. Therefore, children and adolescents and their parents should be made aware of this potential for chronic toxicity with excess ingestion.

The intestine will increase its absorption of iron during times of increased need. However, the source and bioavailability of iron are vital in the prevention and/or correction of anemia. This must be taken into account when deciding the makeup of a diet. Iron obtained from animal sources is much better absorbed by an order of 10% to 35%. In contrast, iron obtained from plant sources is only absorbed in the range of 2% to 20%. Giving these facts to athletes is particularly important for athletes who are vegetarians. The consumption of red meat along with grains and vegetables enhances the overall absorption of iron. Additionally, the ingestion of vitamin C improves the absorption of iron.

The RDA of iron for children from the ages of 7 to 10 years is 10 mg per day. The current RDA for males aged 11 to 14 and 15 to 18 years is 12 mg per day. As was explained above, that the RDA for adolescent females is higher is not surprising. Females aged from 11 to 14 and those between 15 to 18 years have an RDA of 15 mg per day (Table 4.3). Good dietary sources of iron include meat (e.g., fish, poultry, and beef), liver, egg yolk, legumes, whole grains, and green vegetables. Additional sources might include nuts, tomatoes, and potatoes. Cooking with an iron skillet also adds some iron into the diet.

FLUIDS

During all forms of exercise, fluids are lost. These fluids must be monitored and replaced to avoid the unpleasant and potentially devastating consequences of dehydration. Although an exercising child's response may appear to be physiologically similar to that of an adult, some distinct differences exist. Children are at a considerable disadvantage when they exercise in extremes of cold or heat.

Children do not tolerate the extremes of temperature as well as adults. They are not as able to dissipate heat loss via sweating due to their lower sweating rate, and they are less able to transfer heat produced as a result of exercise from muscles to skin. Furthermore, children have excess heat loss in the cold and excess heat gain in extreme heat when compared to an adult, due to their greater relative surface area. Moreover, children at any given level of metabolism have a lower cardiac output, which diminishes their ability to transfer heat from their core to their periphery. Additionally, children take longer to acclimatize to changes in weather conditions than do adults.

These differences mean that the fluid needs of children must be frequently assessed and replaced to avoid dehydration. Guidelines have been devised and position statements have been put forth by both the American College of Sports Medicine and the American Academy of Pediatrics (12,13). They indicate that the children should be observed and should be strongly encouraged to drink at least 4 to 6 ounces of fluid in every 20 to 30 minutes of exercise (12–14). Adolescent athletes should be encouraged to consume 8 to 12 ounces of fluid every 20 to 30 minutes during exercise (12–14). The fluid should be in the form of cold water or a flavored beverage, and the child or adolescent should drink even if he or she does not feel thirsty.

One method of monitoring fluid status is by weighing the athlete. Thirst is a poorly developed mechanism for monitoring hydration in humans, and the sensation should not be relied upon to determine fluid needs. No more than a 2% decrease in body weight should be allowed. In the younger athlete, this should be limited even further to a no more than a 1% decrease (12,13). Performance begins to decline at these levels, and they could rapidly lead to unfavorable circumstances, both in terms of the sporting activity and of the potential for dehydration. The maintenance of plasma volume should be stressed as the primary aim of fluid replacement. Maintaining a normovolemic state ensures that both sweating and circulation continue at the most favorable levels.

The best replacement fluid is water for events lasting less than 1 hour; it should preferably be consumed cool (50° to 55°F), as this speeds gastric emptying (12). For events that last longer than 1 hour, the addition of carbohydrate to the fluid replacement beverage is advantageous. The ingestion of carbohydrates in these situations will maintain blood glucose concentration, as well as enhance carbohydrate utilization (12). Moreover, sport drinks may offer some advantage in the maintenance of plasma volume by increasing the gastrointestinal absorption of fluid or maintaining the electrolyte concentrations for those events lasting longer than 1 hour (12).

Moreover, children and adolescents may more readily consume adequate fluids when a sport drink is provided, due to its pleasant taste. Therefore, in this age group of athletes, the major advantage of sport drinks may lie in their ability to encourage rehydration in these athletes when compared to the consumption of plain water.

Certain precautions are mandated when suggesting replacement fluids to this population of athletes. Drinks that have a high carbohydrate (i.e., sugar) concentration (>10%), such as carbonated beverages and/or undiluted fruit juice, may cause gastric discomfort and a delay in gastric emptying. Therefore, the amount of carbohydrates that should be added to the water should contain no more than a 5% to 8% concentration of glucose polymer (12). This conveys the advantage of carbohydrate replacement, while avoiding any of the adverse effects of an excessive concentration. Caffeine is a known diuretic, and thus, it should be avoided in any replacement drinks. The ingestion of caffeine may be inadvertent, and it may go unrecognized, as many youths consume large amounts of caffeinated soft drinks. Additionally, not only do these drinks foster excess caffeine intake, but they also make poor substitutes for proper fluid replacement drinks and represent even further lapses in proper nutrition. Finally, the use of salt tablets should

not be permitted. Salt tablets cause fluid to be drawn into the intestinal lumen at the expense of the intravascular space, resulting in more rapid dehydration. The normal diet should easily replace any electrolytes that are lost during exercise in both children and adolescents alike.

PRECOMPETITION AND POSTCOMPETITION MEALS

Athletes often request information about what should be eaten before or after a competitive event. However, athletes, parents, and coaches must understand that this is not as important as the content of the dietary intake in the days or weeks prior to the event. Attention should be drawn to the daily intake to maintain adequate stores of energy for growth, repair, and physical activity.

Preevent meals are of paramount importance for providing the fuel necessary for muscles to engage in both training and competition. Foods that are chosen should not be new to the normal dietary routine of the athlete. Meals should be consumed approximately 2 to 3 hours before the activity, and they should consist of foods that are both enjoyable to and well tolerated by the athlete. These foods should be low in fat but high in carbohydrates, with low to moderate amounts of protein. Some type of fluid (at least 8 ounces) should also be ingested with the meal, preferably in the form of water or fruit juice while avoiding caffeine and carbonated beverages.

Children should shun foods that are typically considered snack foods, such as candy, honey, or highly sugared items. The simple sugars (carbohydrates) in these foods are not a source of quick energy, and they may, in fact, precipitate hypoglycemia in susceptible individuals. The optimal foods are complex carbohydrates (e.g., bread, pasta, and rice). These will not delay gastric transit time, and they will allow a stable blood sugar during the competition or practice. One to 2 hours before the event, a low fiber fresh fruit and/or fruit juice or an appropriate sport drink may be consumed, if desired.

If the child or adolescent athlete does not want to eat, no effort should be made to force dietary consumption. Some athletes become too nervous prior to competition to eat, and thus, they should avoid eating at this time. If possible, liquids in the form of juice or sports drinks should be encouraged.

Postevent meal guidelines are virtually identical to the preevent recommendations. Fluids should be encouraged to replace lost amounts. Complex carbohydrates should be permitted, as this assists the body in replenishing glycogen stores and begins preparing it for future practice and competition. The best time to "refuel" is within the first 2 hours following the sporting event, as the body then takes up these fuel sources more readily. However, replacement should continue on an ongoing daily basis. Parents should be discouraged from offering snack foods to their athletes, particularly those that contain simple sugars and are of little nutritional value.

CONCLUSION

Society has made participation in athletics an important part of growing up. Children begin to participate in sports at an early age, and many of them continue well into their teens and beyond. Many benefits accompany participation in sports, including social interaction, family togetherness, and the development of motor skills.

All too often, one of the most important elements—sound nutritional practices—of sports participation is lost. Children and adolescents are nearly overwhelmed by advertisements that promote improper dietary practices.

Attention to growth and development should be of prime importance. Although similarities exist among children, adolescents, and adults, many differences are found. These differences must be recognized, and they should influence dietary recommendations.

Certainly, even the best nutritional intake will not create a champion. However, poor nutritional practices will undoubtedly weaken an individual's potential to become one.

REFERENCES

1. Curran JS, Barness LA. Nutrition. In: Behrman RE, Kliegman RM, Jenson HB, eds. *Nelson textbook of pediatrics*, 16th ed. Philadelphia: WB Saunders, 2000: 141.
2. Harvey JS. Nutritional management of the adolescent athlete. *Clin Sports Med* 1984;3:671–678.
3. Food and Nutrition Board, National Research Council. *Recommended daily allowances*, 10th ed. Washington: National Academy Press, 1989.
4. Loosli AR, Benson J. Nutritional intake of adolescent athletes. *Pediatr Clin North Am* 1990;37:1143–1152.
5. Ivy JL. Role of carbohydrate in physical activity. *Clin Sports Med* 1999;18:469–484.
6. McKardle WD, Katch FI, Katch VL, eds. *Sports & exercise nutrition*. Philadelphia: Lippincott Williams & Wilkins, 1999.
7. Johnson WA, Landry GL. Nutritional supplements: fact or fiction? *Adolesc Med* 1998;9:501–513.
8. Kennedy E, Goldberg J. What are American children eating? Implications for public policy. *Nutr Rev* 1995; 53:111–126.
9. Wolman RL. ABC of sports medicine. Osteoporosis and exercise. *BMJ* 1994;309:400–403.
10. Rowe WJ. Extraordinary unremitting endurance exercise and permanent injury to normal heart. *Lancet* 1992; 340:712–714.
11. McDonald R, Keen CL. Iron, zinc, and magnesium nutrition and athletic performance. *Sports Med* 1988;5: 171–184.
12. American College of Sports Medicine Position Stand. Exercise and fluid replacement. *Med Sci Sports Exerc* 1996;28:i–vii.
13. American Academy of Pediatrics. Climatic heat stress and the exercising child and adolescent. *Pediatrics* 2000;106:158–159.
14. Squire D. Heat illness: fluid and electrolyte issues for pediatric and adolescent athletes. *Pediatr Clin North Am* 1990;37:1085–1089.

5

Ergogenic Aids

Bernard A. Griesemer

The use of pharmacologic ergogenic aids in sports has become increasingly common in the last decades of the twentieth century, and this pattern is expected to continue in the twenty-first century. Exact trends in usage are difficult to determine due to the wide differences in the use of ergogenic drugs according to the particular sport, the variation of use by player position in team sports, and the level of competition. Exact trends in usage are also difficult to determine because of the variation in consistency and duration of use in each individual athlete. The reliability of data that is obtained from athletes who self-report the use of these substances is hard to confirm by laboratory testing. This may be a significant variable, especially in younger athletes, where patterns of use are currently being investigated.

In spite of the limitations inherent in research studies involving the use of ergogenic drugs in young athletes, both primary care physicians and clinical researchers have noted an increase in the use of these products in younger athletes in recent years. In general, an existing trend also seems to indicate that the use of these products is increasing in individuals who are not engaging in athletic competition (1). In both young male and female patients, these substances are often used purely for cosmetic physique enhancement. In addition, the increased use of ergogenic pharmacologic aids has been noted in young female athletes who are seeking to enhance their athletic performance. Factors that contribute to this pattern of increased use have been the subject of discussion in the sports medicine community. As competition becomes more intense in both young male and young female athletes, a concurrent increase in the attempts by these young athletes to enhance their performance by pharmacologic methods is observed. Similarly, pressure to achieve a cosmetic "athletic" body image has increased in peer groups and in the media.

Concern over the widespread availability of ergogenic drugs in the retail market has also extended to the pediatric-aged athlete. Many products banned at the collegiate or Olympic level are easily purchased by minors at convenience stores, supermarkets, and nutrition centers in shopping malls. Young athletes are also constantly encountering paid advertisements in both the print and electronic media that, while securing multimillion dollar sales figures for these products, fail to present balanced information. Warnings regarding the potential side effects of these products are either absent, are minimized, or are couched in legalistic jargon that far exceeds the reading and comprehension levels of the younger athlete.

Advertisers seldom include information on the limited potential for incremental gain in performance enhancement that a young athlete will achieve with these products. The potential gain in performance should be related to the gains in performance that can be achieved more effectively by close attention to an adequate baseline nutrition plan, fluid balance, training and conditioning, and skill development. The perception of many young athletes, which is often reinforced by sports celebrity testimonials and endorsements, is that significant performance enhancement can be achieved at their age range and level of competition simply through better biochemistry.

Scientifically controlled studies of consistent, reproducible ergogenic effects in the pediatric-aged athlete are virtually nonexistent for many of these products. Data will undoubtedly remain difficult to obtain in this age range for many reasons.

First, inconsistency in product content appears to be a significant variable when research protocols attempt to determine the extent to which these products produce an incremental gain in athletic performance. The possible impact of this variable on the data may be significant regardless of the age and level of competition. Product content variability becomes increasingly significant in younger and smaller athletes who are competing at elite levels and in study protocols where the incremental gain being measured involves narrow margins of performance measurement.

A second major limitation facing research centers engaged in studies that are attempting to determine the true degree of performance enhancement that pharmacologic ergogenic aids cause in young athletes is the scrutiny of institutional review boards. These institutional review boards are justifiably severe in their inspection of research projects involving minors where the long-term safety of a nonessential non-life-saving intervention or product is the focus of the study. Finally, the legal complexity of using minors in medical research studies is well established.

The adverse effects of these products are equally difficult to quantify; they are generally encountered as anecdotal case reports. Research studies that statistically delineate the significant incidence of a particular side effect of a particular drug or category of ergogenic drugs in the pediatric-aged athlete are almost uniformly unavailable. Prospective controlled studies that seek to confirm or to disprove a causal relationship between a product and an adverse effect operate under the same restrictions mentioned in studying potentially desirable effects.

Primary care physicians should be cognizant of the limitations that the lack of statistical data places on this discussion of the effects and side effects of ergogenic aids in the pediatric-aged athlete.

Because of changes in the legal definitions and regulations of products used in sports for performance enhancement, the legal and ethical ramifications of this topic have become increasingly complicated. Substances may be prohibited on the basis of legal definition of the product, level of play, and specific sport, as well as on the basis of their chemical structure, effects, and side effects. Products with similar ergogenic properties may range from being classified as controlled substances to nonprescription medications to "nutriceuticals" to food supplements. In the United States, many of these products are under the legal umbrella of the 1994 Dietary Supplement and Education Act. The following discussion will hopefully place performance-enhancing substances in perspective for the primary care physician who is caring for physically active young patients.

The term *ergogenic* derives from two Greek words, meaning "to make work." In athletic competition, the expression *ergogenic substances* is most commonly used to refer to a broad group of chemicals that are taken either orally or parenterally to improve performance in physical competition. Training techniques, adjustments in diet and fluid intake, the use of a wide variety of strength and conditioning programs and equipment, and psychologic training methods can all be regarded as ergogenic aids; these, however, are outside of the scope of this discussion.

Determining which ergogenic substances and ergogenic aids constitute ethical attempts to improve performance in competition is a topic of ongoing discussion among competitors and their organizations regarding fair play in their respective sport. Physicians have the following additional historic ethical standard that applies to performance enhancement: "First, do no harm." This mandate dates back to the time of one of the early forms of formal organized competition, the ancient Olympics. The earliest records of the Olympics also contain references to athletes who were under scrutiny because of their use of ergogenic drugs.

Another term that is frequently used to describe the use of performance-enhancing substances in sports is *doping*. The expression doping is derived from a word used to describe a mixture of substances used by the Kaffir tribesmen in South Africa at the time of the Boer Wars. *Stacking* and *cycling* are two terms used frequently by competitors to describe the common practice of using multiple substances at a time (stacking) and rotating substances either to enhance the desired effects or to minimize the adverse effects (cycling). Keeping pace with the ever-changing street vernacular of drug use in sports is a constant challenge. A particular athlete in one area of the world may use the same term for an entirely different drug, doping technique, or ergogenic effect than an athlete from a different region does. When the clinician is confronted in a clinical situation with an athlete's use of an unfamiliar term, querying the young athlete as to the details of the product or technique being used and their understanding of the definition of the term, product, or technique is always advisable.

The categories of ergogenic substances that are most often encountered by primary care physicians are as follows:

1. Anabolic–androgenic steroids
   a. Prescription/controlled substances
   b. Dietary supplement precursors
2. Stimulants
   a. Prescription and nonprescription drugs
   b. Dietary supplements
3. Blood doping
   a. Autologous transfusions
   b. Erythropoietin (EPO)
   c. Plasma expanders and related products
4. Specific drugs and masking agents
   a. Polypeptide hormones

  b. Beta blockers and beta agonists
  c. Diuretics
  d. Alcohol
 5. Dietary supplements
  a. Protein and nucleic acid supplements
  b. Vitamins and minerals

ANABOLIC–ANDROGENIC STEROIDS

Research studies published in the medical literature have reported the use and abuse of anabolic–androgenic drugs in athletic competition for approximately 50 years. Documentation of their use at the high school and collegiate level has been published in the medical literature for approximately 25 years. Over that period of time, no clear trend indicates that the use of these substances is increasing at these ages. (1a). Documentation of the use of these substances at the middle school level has occurred only recently (2).

Anabolic–androgenic steroids are drugs that are either taken orally or are injected. They can also be classified according to their biochemical structure, and Table 5.1 lists these with brief examples of each group.

These chemicals are *anabolic* in that they increase protein synthesis in skeletal muscle. Furthermore, substantial evidence demonstrates that these drugs also have an ergogenic effect in athletic training and competition because they help block the catabolic effect that physical exercise has on human skeletal muscle. Achieving the ergogenic effect, or an increase in both muscle size and muscle strength, requires that the drugs be used in conjunction with adequate caloric intake and a progressive strength training program. The incremental value of these drugs over the base effect of caloric intake and training varies sig-

nificantly from one individual to another. Research confirming that anabolic–androgenic steroids increase muscle strength is a relatively recent finding (3). Previously, the data were not clear as to the extent that strength was truly enhanced above baseline training techniques.

Currently, no definitive evidence proves that these drugs significantly enhance aerobic capability in young athletes.

The degree to which these drugs truly enhance sports performance appears to vary greatly, depending on the sport in question. Athletes participating in sports where brief explosive power is a factor tend to see more of an ergogenic benefit than in those athletic events where this type of activity is less of a competitive advantage.

When presenting the desirable effects of anabolic–androgenic drugs (e.g., increased muscle strength and size and possible increase in performance, depending on the sport), the physician must also provide the athlete with information regarding the undesirable effects of these drugs.

One significant "side effect" is the fact that the use of anabolic–androgenic steroids is considered unethical by most, if not all, sports organizations and governing bodies. Direct detection of these substances and their metabolites is now becoming possible. An alternate method of detection has frequently been used as a basis for sanctions in elite sports. The drug testing agency responsible for the integrity of the competition will often develop a profile of a particular athlete to detect alterations in the testosterone to epitestosterone (T to E) ratio. Athletes may attempt to circumvent the T to E ratio by taking epitestosterone in order to increase the denominator of the ratio. Many doping control agen-

TABLE 5.1. *Anabolic androgenic steroid classification*

Form	Chemical structure	Specific steroids
Oral	17-α-methyl derivatives	Methyltestosterone
		Fluoxymesterone
		Methandrostenolone
		Oxandrolone
		Oxymetholone
		Stanazolol
	17-α-ethyl derivatives	Ethyestrenol
	1-methyl derivatives	Methenolone
Injectable	19-nortestosterone esters	Nandrolone
	Testosterone esters	Testosterone proprionate
	Testosterone cypionate	Depotestosterone
Dietary supplement precursors	—	Dehydroepiandrosterone
	—	Androstenediol
	—	Androstenedione

cies now limit the level of epitestosterone that is allowed in an individual athlete.

In addition to sanctions imposed by sports governing bodies, severe legal penalties are incorporated into United States federal law. The Anabolic Steroid Act of 1990 placed anabolic androgenic steroids under the Controlled Substances regulations as Class III drug (3a). The possession, use, and distribution of a Schedule III Controlled Substance, without appropriate medical indication, a correct written prescription, dispensing, record keeping, and inventory control, is a Class C felony. Furthermore, many states have additional penalties or harsh sentencing guidelines if these products are detected on or within 1,000 feet of a school or university (4). In recent years, the use of anabolic–androgenic precursors has increasingly come to the attention of primary care physicians. Dehydroepiandrosterone, androstenedione, and androstenediol (DHEA) are dietary supplements that are commonly sold in retail outlets and through the Internet or catalog sales throughout the United States. These supplements are nonprescription anabolic–androgenic drugs that are loosely regulated under the Dietary Supplement and Health Education Act of 1994. Product content variability, manufacturer discretion in labeling, and limited controlled studies as to their efficacy and side effects make evaluation of many drugs in this legal category difficult. Products are designated as dietary supplements in the United States if they are taken orally, if they are nonprescription, and if they are not designated as pharmaceuticals by the Food and Drug Administration (FDA). The classification of a particular drug as a dietary supplement rather than as a prescription medication may be determined more by political expediency than by the biochemistry of the drug in question.

Anabolic steroid precursors have been documented to increase testosterone levels in healthy subjects for 1 to 2 hours following ingestion (5). Although they have not been tested in young subjects in controlled situations, the concern is that, if the ingested amounts are sufficient to achieve effects on muscle strength and muscle mass, then these same doses will be sufficient enough to be associated with the same adverse effects as those of pharmaceutical grade anabolic–androgenic steroids.

Serious medical adverse effects of anabolic–androgenic steroids are often classified according to the organ systems that are affected. In addition, any drug used to enhance performance that is given parenterally involves a risk of hepatitis B, hepatitis C, and human immunodeficiency virus (HIV) transmission.

The organ system that the general public most commonly associates with anabolic–androgenic misadventures is the hepatobiliary system. Cholestatic jaundice is one of the more common and reversible side effects of use of these chemicals. Likewise, elevations in serum transaminase levels appear to be a transient finding in most athletes, especially in athletes who use these products inconsistently and for short periods of time. Other side effects of these chemicals are more likely to be irreversible. Liver tumors, both benign and malignant, have been reported in athletes using steroids. Peliosis hepatis, a condition marked by blood-filled cysts in the liver, is an adverse result that has been associated with fatalities in athletes due to the traumatic rupture of the cysts.

The association of hypertrophic changes in the myocardium with the use of anabolic–androgenic steroids is unclear in the clinical setting, although case reports have raised concerns among sports medicine physicians (6). *In vitro* studies in animal models have increased these levels of concern (7). More significant for the primary care physician is the knowledge that these substances have adverse effects on parameters associated with atherosclerotic heart disease, specifically elevation in blood pressure, reduction of high-density lipoprotein levels, an increase in total cholesterol, and an increase in fibrinogenesis. Whether prolonged use of these products in the pediatric-aged population is associated with increased risk of these adverse effects, compared to the risk in the adult-aged athlete, is unknown.

This class of drugs also adversely affects the genitourinary system. In women, clitoral hypertrophy is irreversible. In men, testicular atrophy, oligospermia, abnormal sperm morphology, prostatic hypertrophy, and a possible increased risk of prostatic cancer are all reported adverse effects of anabolic–androgenic steroids. Whether young male athletes who use anabolic–androgenic steroids or their precursors are at increased risk for testicular cancer, which is one of the most common forms of cancer in the young adult male population, is unknown at the present time. As with the hepatobiliary system, whether the risk of side effects on the genitourinary system is increased when adding the variable of age or stage of pubertal development is unknown.

The degree to which anabolic–androgenic steroids increases the risk for birth defects in the offspring of male and female athletes who abuse these substances is unknown. In males, the documented abnormalities of sperm morphology are of obvious concern to physicians who focus on issues related to reproductive health. In the "underground" literature, athletes are admonished to avoid these products if they are interested in procreating. Birth defects in the offspring of former East German female athletes are alleged to have been caused by prolonged exposure to anabolic–androgenic steroids. Multiple reports of serious neuromuscular, neurologic, and musculoskeletal birth defects are under ongoing investigation (8).

Side effects on the integumentary system in both male and female athletes include male pattern baldness, hirsutism, and acne. When compared to older athletes, younger athletes may be at risk for an increased severity of acne and a subsequent increased risk of long-term complications due to scarring. Acne may also be more refractive to therapeutic interventions when it is caused by or aggravated by the use of anabolic–androgenic steroids. Primary care physicians and dermatologists who manage a patient's acne with isotretinoin routinely provide close monitoring of alterations in liver enzyme profiles or those in the lipid profiles in these patients. The potential risks of developing these two adverse effects of isotretinoin and the severity of the adverse alterations of these parameters theoretically are likely to be compounded by the similar adverse effects of anabolic–androgenic steroids on these systems. Recent concerns regarding the risk of depression and suicide with the use of isotretinoin are the subject of ongoing investigations. In a young athlete who is using isotretinoin and who is also using anabolic–androgenic drugs or precursors, additional concerns regarding the risk of depression and/or suicide may be valid, based on the adverse psychologic effects of these compounds.

In young female athletes, another potentially undesirable side effect of this class of ergogenic drugs is hirsutism. The degree to which excessive hair growth is noted and the degree to which it is reversible appear to vary significantly from one female athlete to the next.

In women, permanent thickening of the vocal cords can occur, regardless of pubertal stage, as a result of anabolic–androgenic drug use. Premature deepening of the voice in the physically immature male athlete would also be expected as a result of accelerated pubertal maturation. Whether an increased risk of vocal polyps or of other permanent dysmorphic changes exists for the younger athlete, when compared to the adult who is using these products, is unknown. The degree to which morphologic changes of the vocal cords may partially resolve varies greatly from one athlete to the next.

Adverse psychologic effects are widely reported. Excessive aggression, both during and outside of athletic events, is consistently documented in the literature. This increase in aggression may be a significant contributing factor for enhancing athletic performance because it contributes to increased intensity and duration of training sessions. Similarly, a decreased perception of fatigue during training and competition may be a significant ergogenic aid. Many athletes, both male and female, report significant increases in libido.

Depression, especially in the withdrawal phases of cycling these drugs, and psychosis are documented in the medical literature. Some researchers have argued that these drugs meet the criteria for classification as addictive substances on the basis of their psychologic effects (9). As was stated earlier, young athletes may be at an increased risk for depression and suicide if use of these compounds is coincident with other drug use, whether prescription or otherwise, or if they have a history of preexisting personal or family history of depression.

Permanent premature closure of the epiphyseal growth plate in young athletes who are physically and skeletally immature is an adverse effect of steroids that is specific for this group. Arrested height growth is a significant documented side effect in young patients who are taking anabolic–androgenic steroids for therapeutic indications (e.g., Fanconi anemia) (10). As has been previously mentioned, if a young athlete is taking sufficient quantities of these products to achieve changes in muscle mass and strength and these are enough to achieve changes in the androgenic distribution of body fat and lean muscle mass, then the assumption that the young athlete is receiving a dose that will lead to accelerated pubertal development is reasonable. Premature closure of the epiphyseal growth plate, decelerating linear growth, and a subsequent reduction in ultimate adult height are all consequences of accelerated pubertal development. The effect of smaller doses of anabolic–androgenic steroids with regard to smaller incremental decreases in ultimate height in young athletes have yet to be studied.

In older athletes, the musculoskeletal system is adversely affected by changes in tendons and the muscle–tendon juncture, which leads to an increase risk of rupture (11). Primary care physicians are well aware of the increased risk of both major trauma and overuse injuries to this anatomic area in the young athlete. Relative to the adult population, the risk of injury, the severity of injury, the speed and degree of healing following injury, and the response to rehabilitative interventions in the young athlete who is abusing anabolic–androgenic steroids will require further investigation.

Athletes who use anabolic–androgenic steroids have an increased risk for infection due to the reduction in circulating immunoglobulins. Risk also appears to be increased for certain autoimmune diseases (12). The degree to which younger athletes display an increased risk for these complications and the degree to which these effects are reversible or irreversible in younger athletes will also require further study. Alterations in the immune status of a young athlete who is abusing these compounds is also a factor in ongoing discussions regarding the risk of testicular and hepatobiliary cancer.

In summary, the use of anabolic–androgenic drugs in both athletic and nonathletic populations has been documented for many decades. Adolescents are as likely to use these products for cosmetic physique enhancement as they are to use them for sports performance enhancement. The medical literature has documented the use of these drugs in an increasingly younger population, extending at least to the middle school age range (2). In the prepubertal age range, the young athlete is at a greater risk for the significant side effects of these products than the older, more physically mature, population is. Specifically, the skeletally immature athlete is at risk for adverse consequences on linear growth, secondary to accelerated pubertal development and epiphyseal growth plate closure. Whether younger athletes are at relatively higher risks for the commonly recognized adverse effects of these drugs (e.g., hepatic, dermatologic, and musculoskeletal) is difficult to determine from the existing medical literature. Prospective controlled studies of the effects and side effects of this category of ergogenic drugs are difficult to perform because of ethical constraints involving medical research in minors for products that lack significant medical indications for use.

STIMULANTS

Athletes are often unaware that one of the most commonly used categories of ergogenic drugs is stimulants, a group of drugs that includes caffeine.

Young athletes commonly consume coffee, soft drinks, and foods and use nonprescription drugs that contain caffeine (Table 5.2). At elite levels of competition, caffeine concentrations are tested, and those that exceed certain levels (12 μg/mL in urine for Olympic competition) are prohibited. Caffeine is a xanthine compound that, arguably, is the most widely used stimulant in both athletic and nonathletic populations. The ergogenic effect of caffeine is derived from a combination of central nervous system (CNS) stimulation, a decreased perception of fatigue, improved skeletal muscle contractility, and the increased metabolism of free fatty acids. The ergogenic effect of caffeine in ath-

TABLE 5.2. *Caffeine content of various substances*

Product	Amount/dose	Equivalence in urine within 2 to 3 hr
Coffees and Teas		
Decaffeinated coffee	2.0–3.0 mg	0.03–0.04 mcg/mL
1 cup regular coffee	100.0 mg	1.50 mcg/mL
5 oz instant tea	28.0 mg	0.42 mcg/mL
5 oz brewed tea	20.0–110.0 mg	0.30–1.60 mcg/mL
Soda		
12 oz Coca-Cola, Diet Coke	45.6 mg	0.68 mcg/mL
12 oz Tab	46.8 mg	0.70 mcg/mL
12 oz Dr. Pepper	39.6 mg	0.59 mcg/mL
12 oz Pepsi, Pepsi Light	36.0 mg	0.54 mcg/mL
12 oz Mountain Dew	55.0 mg	0.85 mcg/mL
12 oz Jolt Cola	90.0 mg	1.35 mcg/mL
12 oz Red Bull	115.0 mg	1.73 mcg/mL
Chocolate		
1 oz milk chocolate	6.0 mg	0.08 mcg/mL
1 oz bittersweet chocolate	20.0 mg	0.30 mcg/mL
1 oz baking chocolate	26.0 mg	0.40 mcg/mL
Over-the-counter drugs		
1 No Doz	100.0 mg	1.50 mcg/mL
1 Vivarin	200.0 mg	3.00 mcg/mL
1 Anacin	32.0 mg	0.48 mcg/mL
1 Excedrin	65.0 mg	0.97 mcg/mL
1 Midol	32.4 mg	0.48 mcg/mL

From *Athletic drug reference '99.* Fuentes R, Rosenberg J, eds.

letic competition is more likely to be noted in competitive events lasting longer than 30 minutes.

The principal adverse effect of caffeine that results in performance degradation in young athletes occurs as a result of the diuretic properties of this chemical. Dehydration whether from caffeine or from any other cause diminishes muscle strength and endurance. Caffeine also directly increases the risk of heat-related illness, especially in susceptible individuals. Primary care physicians who care for young athletes are aware that all young athletes, especially those who are female, overweight, poorly trained, and/or inadequately acclimatized, are considered susceptible individuals. The use of excessive amounts of caffeine in these subsets of young athletes may seriously compound the risk of heat-related illness. In the United States, dietary supplements that contain large doses of caffeine, ephedra, and related compounds are marketed and used extensively in the young athlete population. Primary care physicians need to recognize that young men and women who are participating in sports, especially those that are weight-categorized or weight-sensitive, may have a significantly increased risk of heat stress and heat stroke if they combine the risk factors listed above (e.g., overweight, undertrained) with the high-risk ambient heat and humidity conditions and if they are concomitantly using products that contain caffeine, ephedra, and/or related compounds.

An additional adverse effect is that increased tremulousness, subsequent to ingestion of products containing caffeine, may adversely affect an individual's performance in sports that require fine motor precision.

Many herbal products and dietary supplements contain caffeine in relatively large concentrations in comparison to the levels found in soft drinks, coffee, and over-the-counter products used to combat fatigue. One herbal product that primary care physicians may encounter is guarana, a South American herb that contains up to 5% caffeine by weight. Primary care physicians should counsel their young athletic patients about the limited benefit and the potential for serious side effects from products that contain large amounts of caffeine.

Nicotine, especially when it is used as snuff (i.e., smokeless tobacco), is reported by athletes to have a mild stimulant effect; it is commonly used in sports at levels ranging from middle school to the professional level of competition. Whether nicotine truly has ergogenic properties in young athletes is difficult to document. However, the significant side effects of products containing nicotine on the cardiovascular

and pulmonary system are well established. The relative risk of oral, laryngeal, and esophageal cancer appears to be related to the delivery system used by the athlete (e.g., snuff, chewing tobacco, and/or cigarettes). Technically, nicotine is a stimulant in an herb, namely tobacco.

Other dietary supplements and herbal medications may have performance-enhancing components that are also considered stimulants. The most common stimulant in this group is ephedrine. This chemical is derived from plants in the genus *Ephedra*. Herbal teas, gingko biloba, ginseng, and other dietary supplements that contain ephedrine or ephedrine-like compounds are often used to reduce fatigue, to enhance mental alertness, and to increase metabolic rates in weight reduction scenarios. Nonprescription medications, in which ephedrine is the single component or one of multiple drugs combined in one product, are also available to athletes. The widespread use of ephedrine and pseudoephedrine, in a wide variety of products ranging from dietary aids to decongestants, may pose a problem for the primary care physician who is assisting in the care of athletes competing at elite levels. The gymnastic competition at the Sydney Olympics in September 2000 provided an unfortunate example of a young pediatric-aged athlete who was severely sanctioned because of her use of a product containing ephedrine. Allegedly, her team physician inadvertently administered the product to her when she was being treated for flu-like symptoms. At this elite level of competition, the presence of the substance in an athlete's system during competition is prohibited. Who gave the athlete the banned substance, whether the use was intentional or unintentional, whether the use was medically indicated or not, and whether the athlete knew about the product are not mitigating circumstances to the international governing bodies.

The beneficial effects of increased energy and/or a decreased perception of fatigue of ephedrine and ephedrine-like products on endurance and strength vary significantly in individual young athletes. The potential enhancement in sports performance is offset by the detrimental side effects of dehydration, heat intolerance, and decreased fine motor coordination. Potentially lethal episodes of hyperthermia, cardiac arrhythmia, and hypertensive crises have been documented in the medical literature.

A drug with properties similar to ephedrine and pseudoephedrine is phenylpropanolamine. This stimulant is also a banned drug at the elite Olympic level of competition. As with ephedrine, this product historically has been found in a wide variety of products that were used in clinical settings to treat upper respiratory tract infections, especially in the pediatric age group. Phenylpropanolamine was also the main ingredient in many nonprescription products that were used as appetite suppressants in attempts to cause or to facilitate weight loss. This chemical is becoming increasingly difficult to obtain because of recent concerns expressed by the United States FDA. A recent study in men and women from 18 to 49 years of age suggests that this chemical is a significant risk factor for hemorrhagic stroke in women (13).

The most potent drug in the stimulant category is amphetamine. Currently, law enforcement officials are facing a growing epidemic of home-based methamphetamine production laboratories as is often reported in the popular press. The proliferation of production facilities has markedly increased the availability of these illicit products and, consequently, has increased the possibility that a primary care physician may encounter these compounds in young athletes.

Amphetamines are rapidly absorbed by oral and parenteral routes of administration, and approximately 60% of the dose is excreted rapidly in the urine. Detection in an athletes' urine specimen is increasingly difficult after 48 hours. Many athletes use additional drugs as masking agents to alkalinize their urine specimens, in an attempt to both evade detection and to prolong or increase the amount of amphetamine in the circulation. In competitive events that are drug tested, increasingly sensitive methods used to detect amphetamine metabolites have effectively reduced the ability of alkalinizing agents to mask amphetamine use in athletic competition.

The ergogenic effects of amphetamine and its related substances are the result of multiple actions of these compounds. Amphetamines and amphetamine-like compounds increase cardiac output, boost the speed of fatty acid metabolism, and augment glycogenolysis. All of these factors serve to increase energy availability for athletic competition. In addition, these compounds have significant effects on the CNS. The primary effects on the CNS include a decreased perception of fatigue, increased mental alertness, and increased aggression. Many adult athletes also report a significant improvement in coordination and reaction time; however, the degree to which these are enhanced in younger athletes is unknown.

Primary side effects for athletes include cardiac arrhythmias, especially tachyarrhythmias, and an increased risk of heat-related illness. Even in competitive scenarios where ambient temperature and humidity conditions do not place an athlete at high risk for heat-related illness, the presence of amphetamine and amphetamine-like substances in the athlete's system is more likely to result in hyperthermia. Especially in endurance events, the excessive load that these compounds place on an athlete's metabolic pathways may lead to significant reductions in performance. Mental agitation, confusion, and insomnia are also side effects of these compounds that can have adverse effects on performance.

This category of ergogenic drugs also includes prescription medications that are used to treat attention deficit disorder and/or hyperactivity. At elite levels of competition, use of these controlled substances is prohibited. Primary care physicians are likely to encounter athletes who use these medications on a daily maintenance basis for the appropriate management of correctly diagnosed disorders. The primary care physician is especially likely to encounter these medications in competitive scenarios such as the Special Olympics. The combination of high-risk ambient temperature and humidity; a physically challenged athlete, especially one with spinal cord compromise; and the concurrent use of these drugs poses an extremely high risk for serious heat-related illness. Close attention to fluid and electrolyte intake, equipment modification, and an adjustment of medication dosage are appropriate. Close monitoring of the athlete's status for signs and symptoms of heat-related illness during competition is critical.

For physicians to prescribe these medications to athletes who do not meet the attention deficit disorder diagnostic criteria recently established by the American Academy of Pediatrics (14) and the current *Diagnostic and statistical manual of mental disorders*, fourth edition (DSM-IV) is inappropriate (15). If an athlete's condition meets specific diagnostic criteria and it is also a true limiting factor in athletic competition that requires close attention to the execution of play strategy, then using these compounds in athletic competition may be both appropriate and ethical. The fine ethical line between the appropriate use of medications for attention deficit disorder during competition and the abuse of these medications in order to enhance performance is an appropriate topic of discussion between a primary care physician and patient.

BLOOD DOPING

In endurance sports, especially at the elite level of competition, a primary care physician may encounter athletes who resort to blood doping to enhance athletic performance. The majority of cases of blood doping in athletic competition have utilized one of the following three techniques: autologous blood transfusion, synthetic EPO, and new compounds that are often referred to as synthetic hemoglobin. All of these techniques seek to enhance athletic performance by making more oxygen available at the muscle tissue level during physical activity. The increased efficiency in oxygen-carrying capability secondarily decreases cardiac output and energy consumption per unit of work. Other training techniques also achieve these effects. Strength and conditioning alone will increase an athlete's hemoglobin concentration and the efficiency of oxygen transport. Training at higher altitudes will further improve the level of hemoglobin in the athlete. These performance enhancements, secondary to appropriate and ethical training and conditioning regimens, are also noted in younger athletes. The term *blood doping* is used when an athlete resorts to the unethical manipulation of the hematocrit and hemoglobin in an effort to improve athletic performance in endurance events.

Unless a primary care physician is providing care for a young athlete who is competing in an elite event, the physician is less likely to encounter an athlete who is utilizing autologous blood transfusion as a method of enhancing performance. In this form of doping, an athlete's own packed cells are harvested at least 6 weeks prior to a competitive event in order to allow enough time for the red blood cell (RBC) supply to recover endogenously prior to the event. Within days of the competitive event, the harvested cells are then transfused back to the athlete in an attempt to shift the hematocrit and hemoglobin above the training baseline. Because the maximum concentration of blood in packed cells is usually in the range of 55%, it is unlikely that a young athlete will achieve hematocrits in excess of 60% with the use of this technique. The elevation in the hematocrit level resulting from an autologous transfusion persists for approximately 1 week before it begins to return to baseline. The detection of autologous blood transfusions in athletic competition is possible by performing studies on RBC age in samples with suspiciously high hematocrits.

In contrast, EPO may be seen more frequently at the elite level of endurance sports. Unlike autologous transfusions, the use of which seldom results in a hematocrit above 55%, repeated EPO injections commonly move the hematocrit above 60%. EPO is a glycoprotein that is produced endogenously by the kidney. Multiple factors influence the production of this chemical via a negative feedback system that affects the kidneys. Negative feedback mechanisms appear to be extremely limited at the RBC production level

in the bone marrow, and therefore RBC concentrations will continue to increase in response to ongoing exogenous EPO administration. Recombinant DNA technology has resulted in widely available synthetic EPO that is virtually indistinguishable from the natural product. Detection of exogenous EPO and its metabolites has only recently become possible, and the processes that are involved in the detection of exogenous EPO will need significant refinement over the next decade.

Primary care physicians are also less likely to encounter the use of the newer transfusion products in younger athletes. The degree to which plasma expanders and other products that carry oxygen enhance athletic performance requires ongoing study. At the elite Olympic level, compounds that artificially carry oxygen and products that are classified as plasma expanders are prohibited.

All of these blood doping techniques are associated with potentially lethal complications from hyperviscosity. Younger athletes are physiologically at higher risk for dehydration with exercise, and they are also at higher risk for heat-related illness than is the adult population. Because of these factors, younger athletes who are manipulating their athletic performance by blood doping are theoretically at greater risk for developing hyperviscosity than are their adult counterparts. Endurance athletes of all ages who have artificially elevated their hematocrits beyond 60% and who are competing in high temperature and high humidity conditions are at extreme risk for the potentially lethal complications of hyperviscosity syndrome.

POLYPEPTIDE HORMONES

Recombinant DNA technology has made another polypeptide compound more readily available to athletes of all ages, and, consequently, primary care physicians may encounter this compound at all levels of competition. Human growth hormone (HGH), a polypeptide hormone, is endogenously produced in the anterior lobe of the pituitary gland. Its production and release are regulated, in part, by HGH releasing factor. In humans, HGH acts primarily on the liver and skeletal muscle to increase the production of somatomedin (insulin-like growth factor). Primary care physicians who have experience in the diagnostic procedures that are used to detect a clinical deficiency in young patients are familiar with the drugs that are utilized to test the integrity of a patient's HGH production and release. Unfortunately, athletes are also aware of these same clinical protocols. L-Dopa, propranolol, vasopressin, clonidine, 5-hydroxytyrpta-mine, caffeine, and drugs that induce hypoglycemia (e.g., insulin) are all used by athletes who are attempting to stimulate endogenous HGH production. Additionally, many recent herbal and dietary supplement products have been promoted as sources of exogenous somatomedin or of HGH releasing factor. The effects of these products on athletic performance is questionable, especially in young athletes.

HGH is used by prepubertal athletes to accelerate linear growth, to increase body weight, and to enhance muscle mass. In skeletally mature athletes, this synthetic product is useful only in attempts to increase body weight and muscle mass. The degree to which HGH truly increases muscle strength is currently being investigated. Limited research evidence in adult subjects indicates that this compound also has a positive effect on $\dot{V}_{O_2}$ max.

The adverse effects of exogenous HGH in the physiologically mature young athlete are identical to the aberrations seen in pathologic states in which HGH is produced in excess, specifically clinical acromegaly. Coarse facial features, acne, and cardiovascular complications are noted in both the clinical condition and in athletes who misuse HGH. Untreated, clinical acromegaly has been reported have a fatality rate of 50% by the age of 50 years.

Similar to synthetic EPO, HGH that is produced with recombinant DNA technology is indistinguishable from the naturally occurring form. Emerging technology may facilitate the detection of HGH in athletic competition in the near future. Many physicians who care for athletes who participate at the elite level of sports have expressed concerns that use of HGH may be more pervasive than is commonly suspected.

Adrenocorticotropic hormone (ACTH) and human chorionic gonadotropin (hCG) are two additional polypeptide hormones that are used to enhance body weight and muscle mass. The effect of these compounds on body weight and muscle mass occurs secondary to their influence on endogenous testosterone production in the adrenal gland (ACTH) and the testes (hCG). The efficacy of this category of drugs as ergogenic aids is difficult to determine, and it appears to vary significantly from one athlete to another and from one sport to another. In addition to possible long-term adverse health effects, side effects, such as alterations in glucose metabolism, may adversely affect performance. Whether younger athletes are at a higher risk for complications from inappropriate use of ACTH and hCG than is the adult population requires additional study.

BETA BLOCKERS

Beta blockers, such as propranolol, are considered performance-enhancing substances—and, as such, are banned—in specific sports (e.g., shooting, archery) in which a lower heart rate and improved fine motor control offer a competitive advantage. As was mentioned previously, certain drugs in this category (e.g., propranolol) are also used in attempts to induce production of endogenous HGH. The clinical indications for beta agonist use in younger athletes are significantly more limited than in the past. Alternative medical treatment regimens for chronic migraine headaches, asthma, arrhythmias, and hypertension in younger patients have reduced the need for, and the potential for conflict resulting from the use of, these medications in younger athletes.

The beta agonists that are used to control asthma are an extremely common category of medications used by young athletes. These oral, parenteral, or inhaled medications (e.g., albuterol) are common interventions used as rescue medications for acute exacerbations of asthma. Whether a certain drug is allowable in competitive events may vary according to the route of administration, the provision of a medical clearance prior to competition, the level of competition, or the specific sport in question. Primary care physicians who care for young athletes who have asthma and who are competing at elite levels of sports should be aware of the restrictions that are placed on the use of these medications by national and international governing bodies. One beta agonist used in veterinary medicine, clenbuterol, has been used by athletes because of its anabolic effect, and it is a considered a banned substance. Conventional inhaled beta agonists have limited effect on skeletal muscle. Beyond correcting the adverse effects of reactive airway disease, these products also have limited ergogenic effects on athletic performance. Antiinflammatory medications, both steroidal and nonsteroidal, that are used as maintenance medications for the control of asthma are generally allowable in athletic competition. In the case of antiinflammatory steroids, sports governing organizations may restrict the use of these steroidal preparations to inhaled preparations of these products only.

DIURETICS

Primary care physicians also need to be aware of the fact that many commonly used diuretics are prohibited by sports governing bodies. Unfortunately, popular press reports indicate that the use of diuretics has apparently increased in youth sports over the past decade. Controlled studies investigating the incidence of use of these products is limited; however, public exposure of the abuses of diuretics in weight-sensitive youth sports has prompted increased levels of concern among primary care physicians and their supporting organizations (16). Athletes may also use diuretics in a drug stacking scenario in an attempt to evade detection of other ergogenic drugs in a urine specimen. Excessive weight loss resulting from diuretics or other techniques is highly likely to result in decreased athletic performance in young athletes. Similar to the side effects of medications in the stimulant category, diuretics place a young athlete at a much higher risk for heat-related illness, compared to that of the physically mature athlete.

ALCOHOL

Surveys of behavior in young people in the United States, such as the National Youth Risk Behavior Survey of the Centers for Disease Control and Prevention, continue to provide documentation that alcohol is the most widely used and abused drug. The positive or negative ergogenic effects of ethanol are directly related to its serum concentration at the time of athletic practice or competition.

With a low dose of ethanol in the bloodstream, some athletes may achieve a lessening of fine motor tremulousness. As with beta blockers, this would be a positive ergogenic effect in shooting sports. Alcohol is a banned substance in these sports, and breath analysis is utilized in drug testing scenarios to monitor compliance. Other than acting as a suboptimal source of calories for energy, alcohol has few other positive ergogenic effects on athletic performance.

At higher doses of alcohol in the bloodstream, the adverse effects on coordination, balance, judgment, and reaction time impair athletic performance and substantially increase the risk of injury in young athletes. Adverse effects on the cardiorespiratory system cause a negative ergogenic effect, especially in endurance events. Specific athletes and competitive scenarios may have additional risks. The diuretic effects of ethanol increase the risk of heat-related illness in situations where ambient conditions already place a young athlete at risk for occurrence. Alcohol also markedly increases the risk for hypothermia if the young athlete endures a prolonged exposure to cold temperatures.

Young athletes who are exercising at high altitude and who have consumed alcohol are more likely to experience a quicker onset of altitude-related difficulties, and they also suffer from adverse symptoms that are more severe than those of their alcohol-free counterparts. Similarly, young SCUBA (self-contained underwater breathing apparatus) divers who consume alcohol are at higher risk for the complications of nitrogen saturation and for potentially fatal errors in judgment.

Besides ethanol, glycerol is another alcohol that is used in athletic competition. Athletes have used this chemical to increase the absorption of water from the gastrointestinal tract and to decrease urinary excretion in an effort to improve hydration prior to athletic competition, especially in endurance events. The safety and efficacy of glycerol supplementation as an ergogenic aid in young athletes is highly questionable.

DIETARY SUPPLEMENTS

The manipulation of the components of an athlete's diet in an attempt to enhance performance has a lengthy history in athletic competition.

Managing fluid intake correctly and adjusting dietary caloric balance to enhance performance in competitive events are definitely valuable and effective ergogenic aids. Primary care physicians commonly encounter questions regarding the effectiveness of increasing intake above the baseline recommendations.

In almost all categories of dietary supplements, product variability and inaccurate labeling are ongoing problems for research efforts that attempt to validate claims regarding performance enhancement scientifically.

The most common food groups that are supplemented are protein, amino acids, and nucleic acids. The baseline intake of protein is 0.8 to 1.0 g per kg per day. Adequate protein intake for most athletes can be achieved by maintaining approximately 15% of the daily caloric intake as protein. Supplementing the diet with an additional 0.5 to 1.0 g per kg per day of protein may enhance muscle mass during rigorous training schedules, but a total intake beyond 2 g per kg per day has not been shown to be a consistent ergogenic aid. Excessive protein intake (>2 g per kg per day) may result in performance degradation due to dehydration. All protein and amino acid supplements may cause gastrointestinal upset, and they can aggravate runner's diarrhea, causing a subsequent worsening of dehydration. Prolonged use of a diet or a dietary supplement that contains excessive amounts of protein may result in renal system damage.

Determining whether supplementation of amino acids is effective as an ergogenic aid in the young athlete is also difficult. The human body cannot synthesize nine of the amino acids required for optimal health and exercise capability. These essential amino acids are present in adequate amounts in a properly balanced diet. Supplementation with individual essential amino acids or combinations with these chemicals is unlikely to provide significant performance enhancement in a young athlete, when compared to an adequately balanced diet.

Lysine is the essential amino acids on which athletes have historically focused. Anecdotal claims that lysine enhances HGH production and that, subsequently, it leads to an increase in muscle mass have been made. However, no consistent data support the use of lysine supplementation in young athletes as a significant factor in enhancing performance. Arginine and ornithine, two nonessential amino acids that the human body is capable of synthesizing from other amino acid components, are also are promoted as ways for stimulating endogenous growth hormone production and secretion. As with lysine, research has failed to show any significant positive effect in young athletes.

Altering muscle fatigue or the perception of muscle fatigue has been the goal of some athletes who supplement their diets with additional amino acids. Aspartic acid, another nonessential amino acid, has been suggested as a means for reducing muscle fatigue peripherally. Tyrosine and choline supplementation have been studied with regard to their effect on dopamine and acetylcholine levels and the consequent effect on central muscle fatigue. Research studies are not conclusive as to whether a significant ergogenic effect can be achieved for all sports, but supplemental choline may improve muscle function in certain situations (e.g., swimming), in addition to reducing the perception of fatigue.

Glutamine, another nonessential amino acid, is often used in an attempt to reduce the degree of metabolic acidosis associated with strenuous exercise and to ameliorate the free radical damage to cells that is associated with strenuous exercise. Improvement in anabolic metabolism, increased resistance to infection, and decreased fatigue are all anecdotally reported effects of glutamine supplementation. The exact impact that glutamine has on these components of exercise physiology is unclear at the present time.

Branched chain amino acids (i.e., isoleucine, leucine, and valine) are used in an attempt to affect tryptophan levels in the brain, and, like tyrosine and choline, they may affect central muscle fatigue in endurance sports. The positive ergogenic effects of these chemicals, if they are present to any degree, appear to be limited to endurance sports; they have not

been extensively studied in young athletes. A metabolite of leucine, β-hydroxy-β-methylbutyrate, has also been studied to determine if its supplementation will increase muscle strength and lean body mass. Definitive studies, especially in younger athletes, to delineate the safety and efficacy of this supplement have yet to be performed.

L-Carnitine, a derivative of the amino acids lysine and methionine, has been used as an ergogenic supplement in an effort to improve the efficiency of fatty acid metabolism and to preserve muscle glycogen stores during exercise. However, studies have failed to demonstrate improved athletic performance with carnitine supplementation.

Nucleic acid supplementation has recently become one of the most closely watched and most widely promoted ergogenic supplements. Methyl guanidine acetic acid, commonly referred to as creatine, has been studied since the early nineteenth century; however, it came into prominence in sports at the end of the twentieth century. In recent years, the use of creatine in high school and middle school athletes has increased substantially. The exact number of individuals in the pediatric population that consistently uses creatine in an attempt to increase lean muscle mass and improve athletic performance is unknown.

Creatine in a young athlete's daily diet is obtained from adequate amounts of meat and fish. After the monohydrate form of the chemical is transported to the muscle cell membrane, it is pumped into the cell and is trapped by phosphorylation. The phosphorylated creatine found in dietary supplements is impermeable to muscle cell membrane. Intracellular creatine is used by the skeletal muscle cell to resynthesize adenosine triphosphate (ATP), and it is an integral component of muscle energy production and the maintenance of intracellular hydrogen ion homeostasis.

Usually, athletes will load their skeletal muscle system by taking 20 g of creatine daily for 5 days, and then they attempt to maintain creatine stores by taking 2 g per day. Doses in excess of 2 g per day have not been shown to confer significant advantages in maintaining intramuscular creatine stores. Excessive amounts of creatine in the young athlete's diet may increase the risk of dehydration and muscle cramps and, consequently, may result in performance degradation.

In research studies, the maximum performance enhancement that has been attributed to creatine supplementation has been in the range of 5% to 7%. Performance enhancement above the levels that would be attributed to training and conditioning alone has been noted in, and is probably limited to, sports where short bursts of anaerobic activity are a competitive advantage. Performance degradation has been noted in sports where endurance is a key factor. Most published researchers echo a caution issued by the National Institutes of Health (17), that pointed out that the long-term effects of creatine supplementation in healthy and diseased states is unknown. The extensive use of products containing creatine has prompted extensive review of both the effects and the side effects of this supplement (18–20). Recent concern regarding the accuracy of labeling and the quality control of product content have caused concern in sports governing bodies, primary care organizations, and secondary school associations.

VITAMINS

Almost all vitamins have been extensively studied with regard to their ergogenic properties. Most often the research has centered on improving the function of the immune system or reducing free radical damage by increasing the amounts of antioxidants present in the body. Most studies confirm that a well balanced diet will serve to meet or exceed the daily requirements for vitamins adequately, even in a competitive athlete. In the absence of a vitamin deficiency or disease state, vitamin supplementation is unlikely to improve athletic performance.

The antioxidant vitamins that are commonly used by athletes are ascorbic acid, α-tocopherol, and retinoic acid. Athletes often use β-carotene supplementation, a precursor to retinoic acid, in an attempt to increase the levels of that particular vitamin. Whether supplementation of these chemicals provides any incremental benefit to athletic performance or the health of the athlete, when compared to an adequately balanced diet, is unclear. Excessive doses of these chemicals are associated with gastrointestinal disturbance, renal calculi (ascorbic acid), liver damage (retinoic acid), and an increased risk of skeletal fractures (retinoic acid).

Primary care physicians may encounter products containing other chemicals that are not classified as vitamins but that, nonetheless, are used by athletes for their antioxidant characteristics. Coenzyme Q, glutathione, γ-oryzanol, and octacosanol may be used individually or in combinations with antioxidant vitamins. The efficacy of these products, especially in younger athletes, is questionable, whether used individually or in combination with other drugs and supplements.

B-complex vitamins are commonly employed as ergogenic aids because of their importance in multi-ple metabolic pathways. Pyridoxine and its related compounds are often promoted to athletes for their purported ability to improve multiple parameters that theoretically influence athletic performance, such as the prevention of anemia and improvement in the efficiency of energy production. As with many of the products discussed in this section, the determination of whether any significant performance improvement results in young athletes with these supplements is difficult. However, additional supplementation of these compounds appears to be unnecessary for athletic performance unless the young athlete has an inborn metabolic error or a nutritional deficiency state that affects a particular vitamin or related compound. Vitamin preparations are also plagued with wide variation in product content and inconsistencies in labeling.

MINERALS

Mineral supplementation as a component of a regimen attempting to enhance athletic performance has focused primarily on chromium and iron. Attempts to improve glucose metabolism by increasing the dietary intake of chromium have revolved around the role of chromium as a cofactor for insulin. Chromium supplementation is most commonly employed using chromium picolinate in an effort to improve the relatively poor absorption of chromium in oral preparations. Chromium picolinate is promoted in athletic circles for its supposed anabolic-like effect on lean muscle mass and its positive effect on muscle energy metabolism. Controlled studies in subjects that have included late adolescent and young adult age ranges have shown that supplementation with this compound failed to provide any incremental gain over routine training protocols in the athletes' body composition or athletic performance (21). As with most supplementation, an adequately balanced diet will provide appropriate amounts of chromium for an athlete. Vanadyl and boron are two other trace elements that athletes utilize either individually or in combination with chromium. Research studies have failed to document any significant improvement in sports performance with the addition of these two chemicals.

Similarly, supplementation with iron has not been shown to enhance performance, except when it is used to correct an iron-deficient state. Recently, increasing attention has been given to chronic iron overload conditions. Individual young athletes may be at higher risk for complications of iron supplementation if they are genetically predisposed to abnormalities in iron storage. As before, routine intake from a well balanced diet should provide the young athlete with adequate amounts of iron for optimal athletic performance. Young female athletes who experience excessive iron loss with menstruation may, however, require appropriate oral iron supplementation.

Many other drugs, herbal derivatives, and dietary supplements have been used in athletes in an attempt to enhance performance. While including all of the products in this discussion is impossible, several examples are worth noting because of the likelihood that a primary care physician may encounter their usage in a young athlete.

Sodium bicarbonate is often taken orally in an attempt to increase the hydrogen ion buffering capability during athletic competition and thus to improve athletic performance by reducing the signs and symptoms of muscle fatigue. Exercise physiologists confirm that athletes, including young athletes, tend to develop metabolic acidosis during practice and competition, relative to the resting state. The degree to which oral sodium bicarbonate, either prior to or during practice or competition, alters this parameter is unclear. Excessive amounts of sodium bicarbonate are likely to be required in order to affect blood pH significantly. These large loads of sodium are likely to have significant adverse effects on the gastrointestinal tract, and they require the concomitant intake of large volumes of water to reduce the risk of dehydration. Primary care physicians who care for elite young athletes may also encounter a young athlete who is attempting to mask the use of other illicit ergogenic drugs via the ingestion of sodium bicarbonate or other alkalinizing agents.

Significant controversy has occurred in the past decade as to whether marijuana and other products that contain δ-9 tetrahydrocannabinol (THC) are appropriately classified as ergogenic drugs.

From the standpoint of exercise physiology, THC increases cardiac output in athletes; however, its ability to increase performance is unclear. Adverse effects on judgment, memory, coordination, and reaction time all serve to decrease athletic performance in competitive scenarios. In 1996 at the Nagano Winter Olympics, the controversy over the ergogenic effects of THC in skiing and snowboarding events garnered a large amount of international media coverage. In competitive events that require elements of risk taking and physical flexibility, the "release of inhibition" may confer a competitive advantage. The International Olympic Committee subsequently listed products containing THC as banned substances. Likewise, narcotic analgesics and related substances were also banned at elite levels of competition, even though

they have little or no positive effect on the parameters of exercise physiology that would usually result in performance enhancement.

Products derived from Asian ginseng root are also becoming increasingly popular among athletes and nonathletes. Multiple components of ginseng products have both negative and positive biologic activity with regard to athletic performance. The 17-β-hydroxy components in ginseng are being utilized for their CNS stimulation properties. However, other components of ginseng may have CNS depression activity. In younger athletes, incremental performance enhancement, above the improvement seen with training and conditioning alone, is unlikely. Higher doses and prolonged use of these products may result in significant adverse effects on fluid and electrolyte imbalance, hemolysis, and hypertension. Wide variation in product content and the accuracy of labeling is also a major concern in product lines that promote ginseng use.

Another Asian herb that has recently been the focus of concern because of its increasing use among younger athletes is tribulus. Tribestan, a compound that is found in the oriental plant *Tribulus terrester*, is marketed to young athletes as a method of increasing endogenous testosterone. It is often included in multiple component products with DHEA and androstenedione and/or androstenediol in an effort to augment the anabolic effect of those compounds. At the present time, products that are labeled as containing tribulus appear to be ineffective in enhancing athletic performance in young athletes. Likewise, the safety of this product in large amounts or for prolonged periods of use is unknown in the pediatric age range.

Bee pollen, echinacea, garlic, and many other food products are being utilized in athletic circles and are being promoted to young athletes as ergogenic aids. The efficacy and safety of large amounts of these foods in the diet is questionable. To the degree in which they are substituted for adequate amounts of properly balanced nutrients in the diet of a young and growing athlete, they are likely to be detrimental to athletic performance.

SUMMARY

The list of chemicals, drugs, herbal preparations, supplements, and dietary manipulations is constantly changing, and, as such, it is a constant challenge for the primary care physician. Limited scientific data exist to support the theory that any of these products provides significant performance enhancement in young athletes over and above the gains seen from the routine growth and maturation associated with puberty, adequate nutrition and fluid intake, and appropriate training and conditioning. Unfortunately, the safety of these products may remain difficult to determine for many years. Whether younger, physiologically immature athletes are at a higher risk for complications from many of these products than the adult population is will require even further and more in-depth evaluation.

Similar to many adult athletes, young athletes are often looking for the magic pill or exotic shortcut to provide an edge in competition or a quick alternative to the hard work and repetitive practice that fosters skills development. In general, one statement regarding the use of the ergogenic substance tricks that are used by many young athletes in attempts to enhance performance is reliably accurate. When primary care physicians have the opportunity to discuss this topic with young athletes under their care, the following statement may be a valuable beginning point in the discussion: *if you don't get the basics down, the tricks don't work; if you do get the basics down, the tricks are of little incremental value.* Young athletes are more likely to enhance their performance in competitive athletics significantly by focusing most of their efforts on ergogenic aids that have been proven to have the most substantial positive effects on physical activity. These effective ergogenic aids are close attention to dietary caloric balance, adequate fluid consumption, skills development appropriate for the sport, and appropriate strength and conditioning regimens.

REFERENCES

1. Terney R, McClain L. The use of anabolic steroids in high school students. *Am J Dis Child* 1990;144:99–103.
1a. Rogol A, Yesalis C. Anabolic-androgenic steroids and the adolescent. *Pediatr Ann* 1992;21:175–188.
2. Faigenbaum A, Zaichkowsky L, Gardner D, et al. Anabolic steroid use by male and female middle school students. *Pediatrics* 1998;101:E6–E10.
3. Bhasin S, Storer T, Berman N, et al. The effects of supraphysiologic doses of testosterone on muscle size and strength in normal men. *N Engl J Med* 1996;335: 1–8.
3a. *Anabolic Steroids Act of 1990.* Public Law 101–644. Washington, D.C.: United States Government Printing Office, 1990.
4. State of Missouri. *Revised Statutes*. 195.211–195.214.
5. Leder B, Longcope C, Catlin D, et al. Oral androstenedione administration and serum testosterone concentrations in young men. *JAMA* 2000;283:779–782.
6. Mochizuki R, Richter K. Cardiomyopathy and cerebrovascular accident associated with anabolic-androgenic steroid use. *Physician and Sports Medicine* 1988;16:109–114.
7. Melchert R, Herron T, Welder A. The effect of anabolic-androgenic steroids on primary myocardial cell cultures. *Med Sci Sports Exerc* 1992;24:206–212.
8. Ungerleider S. *Faust's gold.* New York: St. Martin's Press, 2001.
9. Brower K. Evidence for physical and psychological dependence on anabolic-androgenic steroids in eight weight lifters. *Am J Psychiatry* 1990;147:510–512.
10. Bourguignon JP. Linear growth as a function of age at onset of puberty and sex steroid dosage: therapeutic implications. *Endocr Rev* 1988;9:467–488.
11. Laseter J, Russell J. Anabolic steroid-induced tendon pathology: a review of the literature. *Med Sci Sports Exerc* 1991;23:1–3.
12. Clabrese L, Kleiner S, Barna B. The effects of anabolic steroids and strength training on the human immune response. *Med Sci Sports Exerc* 1989;21:386–392.
13. Kernan W, Viscoli C, Brass L, et al. Phenylpropanolamine and the risk of hemorrhagic stroke. *N Engl J Med* 2000;343:1826–1832.
14. American Academy of Pediatrics. Clinical practice guideline: diagnosis and evaluation of the child with attention-deficit/hyperactivity disorder. *Pediatrics* 2000; 105:1158–1170.
15. American Psychiatric Association. *Diagnostic and statistical manual of mental disorders*, 4th ed. Washington, D.C.: American Psychiatric Association, 1994.
16. Jurik P. Weight factor: parents examine why kids must slim down. *Chicago Tribune* 1995 Sept 10:A1,A8.
17. Office of the Director, National Institutes of Health. *Dietary supplements for physically active people*. Washington, D.C.: United States Government Printing Office, 1996.
18. Terjung RL, Clarkson P, Eichner ER, et al. American College of Sports Medicine roundtable. The physiological and health effects of oral creatine supplementation. *Med Sci Sports Exerc* 2000;32:706–717.
19. Juhn M, Tarnopolsky M. Oral creatine supplementation and athletic performance: a critical review. *Clin J Sports Med* 1998;8:286–297.
20. Juhn M, Tarnopolsky M. Potential side effects of oral creatine supplementation: a critical review. *Clin J Sports Med* 1998;8:298–304.
21. Walker L, Bemben M, Bemben D, et al. Chromium picolinate effects on body composition and muscular performance in wrestlers. *Med Sci Sports Exerc* 1998;30: 1730–1737.

6

Strength Training and Endurance Training for the Young Athlete

Paul R. Stricker and Jaci L. VanHeest

The number of young people involved in sports continues to increase. The benefits of exercise should continually be stressed for increasing fitness and self esteem, reducing risk factors for cardiovascular disease, and helping combat the nationwide problem of obesity. Despite the ongoing problem of obesity, literally millions of youths participate in some sort of exercise, whether it is in physical education class, during recess play, or as part of organized team sports. Not long ago, youth involvement in sports such as long distance running, triathlons, or weight lifting, was unheard of, yet now training and competing in such events has become more commonplace. In addition, more opportunities for kids to participate are available. Because of the intense and the more focused training in which these young athletes are participating, the rise of overuse injuries is significant, and physicians are seeing more of these injuries in the pediatric population. Approaching children and young adolescents as unique "structures" who are different from their adult counterparts is necessary in order to help diagnose, treat, and educate these athletes, their parents, and coaches. This chapter focuses on the issues of strength and conditioning in the pediatric and adolescent population. Pediatric strength training in this chapter refers to children in the earliest states of sexual maturation (Tanner stages 1 and 2), which would include girls less than the age of 11 years and boys less than 13 years of age.

STRENGTH TRAINING

Training with weights used to be a relative nonissue for the pediatric age group because the thinking was that weights would not enhance strength due to the lack of testosterone necessary for increasing strength and muscle mass (1). Much concern was expressed over the fear of significant injury to the growth plate and resulting stunted growth. Moreover, rarely were children involved in such focused partici-

pation that they required additional strength training. With the rise of specialization in a specific sport at earlier ages, the issue of strength training to enhance a sport program is being raised more frequently. Recent investigations have provided support for the idea that preadolescents can gain strength with adequate weight training programs (2,3). Information regarding the appropriateness of strength training and the potential results of training with weights will help provide better guidance for the young athlete.

Sports performance is determined by a myriad of variables. Genetics, environment, and opportunity all provide forces that can help or hinder an athlete's development. Two youngsters can be the same age yet differ markedly in physical size, as well as ability. Intrinsic factors that contribute to differing levels of ability include flexibility, coordination, balance control, reaction time, visual maturity, body composition, motivation, self-esteem, muscle strength and endurance, and cardiorespiratory efficiency. Thus, increasing strength clearly is only one aspect of performance, and it should not be the main focus of the training regimen.

Many of the earlier fears regarding weight training stemmed from a lack of knowledge and assumed negative outcomes. Those fears are now being overcome with research studies that provide valuable information showing that young people can gain strength in a safe manner. However, this information should not become a blanket approval of a strength program for any young athlete who asks to participate. Important factors must be considered, such as the age of the athlete, the level of development, his or her maturity and desire, the level of sport skill proficiency he or she has already attained, the risks versus the benefits, and the reason why the strength program is being pursued.

Stories of training programs of prominent college and professional athletes can mislead a young athlete. He or she often believes that, if a professional is capable of a particular feat, then he or she must do the same thing, even though the child is much younger and less developed. This expectation is not only unrealistic, but it is also dangerous because these strength training programs would be quite different. The age is also important because the development of sports skills is a process of acquisition that follows a sequential course (4). Just as a baby follows a sequence of rolling over, sitting, and pulling up in developing major motor skills, a child develops sports skills in a similar sequential pattern. As is usual for developmental processes, children go through the pattern at different rates, but the order is generally consistent. Since training with weights involves issues of balance and coordination, a program involving weights should not be started until these milestones have been reached. Postural and balance skills usually mature and become automatic by age 7. Other skills also mature quite rapidly during the 6-year to 9-year age group. Running improves to adult levels usually by the age of 8; fundamental skills, such as throwing, progress to more transitional skills, such as throwing for accuracy; and visual maturity provides the child with a better ability to track moving objects and judge velocity. From the ages of 10 to 12 years, more marked attainment of complex skills develops, attention becomes more selective and focused, and increasing mental maturity allows for more complex and rapid decision making, as well as the integration of information from multiple sources. All of these factors can coalesce to result in marked improvement in ability and an increased interest in participation in sports activities.

The maturity of the young athlete, both physically and emotionally, helps in making the determination about whether the athlete has required desire and discipline for adding a strength training program to their sport activity. Additionally, the desire must stem from the participant, and not just that of the parents or coaches. If the child has the desire, then he or she must also be able to listen to instruction and to accept coaching. Usually, older children and young adolescents that have already specialized in a certain sport for a few years will be at a stage in which a strength program may be appropriate for them.

A certain level of sport skill proficiency must already have been attained in order for a strength program to be appropriate. If someone is just starting to learn a sport, working to become stronger without having the skills to compete in the sport does not make sense. Gaining strength is done to enhance skills that already exist.

Without a doubt, training with weights involves risks for injury. The benefits of increased strength, potentially enhanced performance, and potentially reduced injuries may outweigh the risks of serious injury if the program is performed under strict supervision and with adequate technique (5).

Determining the reason for which a strength program is being pursued is crucial. Often the pressure to do so is coming from an outside source (i.e., one other than the child athlete), such as the parents or coaches. But even more significant is the role of pressure from peers and the media.

An increasing number of youths want to strength train simply because of the aesthetic standard of the beautiful bodies that are featured in magazines, movies, and television. Reports regarding the use of anabolic steroids in high school and junior high populations show that the reasons for their use may have nothing to do with sports participation; instead, they are often used only to enhance looks (6). Simply getting more in shape and toned can be a healthy activity for a youngster who is not otherwise involved in sports, but, in this instance, development, maturity, and desire should again play a role in the decision to approve or to withhold approval of a program for such an individual. However, the clinician must remember that all factors must be taken into consideration. Even though a young athlete may be the right age and he or she spends significant time in sports, these factors do not mean that he or she is necessarily ready for a strength training program or for that level of participation, even if it could be considered appropriate.

As with any exercise program, the potential benefits should exceed the risks. Many potential risks are accepted as part of weight training among youth, and they range from overuse tendonitis and muscle strains to acute fractures and serious injuries (7). The young, rapidly growing skeleton contains the growth plate, or physis, which is the weakest link of the entire musculoskeletal chain. This "fault-line" of cartilage and maturing bone cells is weaker than the surrounding bone, and it can fail with certain shearing and rotational forces. During the prepubertal and pubertal phases of growth, the strength of the muscle–tendon unit is often greater than that of the physeal areas, and it can even cause avulsion fractures of the attachment sites, or apophyses, until these areas fuse with skeletal maturity.

The potential for injury is high (8–10), and injuries that have been reported include fractures, avulsion fractures, spondylolysis, cartilage tears, ligament sprains, muscle strains, disk herniations, shoulder separations and dislocations, ankle fractures, wrist dislocations, and even cardiac rupture. Certainly, this litany of injuries should stimulate the practitioner to use caution when giving advice concerning strength training and to assign a high priority to correct technique and strict supervision.

The Consumer Product Safety Commission's National Electronic Injury Surveillance System uses data reported from selected emergency departments about injuries due to exercise equipment (9). These injuries almost always occur on home gym equipment or school equipment in unsupervised settings. The lack of supervision allows dangerous situations, such as competitive lifts, the use of improper technique, attempts to lift excessive weight, and inadequate spotting, to occur. Unfortunately, fatal accidents have happened. Some preadolescents and early adolescents have sustained serious injuries with Olympic and power lifting techniques, so the American Academy of Pediatrics recommends that these more ballistic and heavy types of lifting be postponed until skeletal maturity has been reached (11). Skeletal maturity does not always correlate to chronological age, and using sexual maturity scales, such as pubertal staging according to the Tanner method, can be helpful in this regard (see Chapter 2). Even though strength training can cause injuries, the incidence of injuries from training with weights is reported to be less than that associated with sports such as football, wrestling, and gymnastics (8).

Reducing the risk of injury is paramount to the big picture of youth strength training. Requiring a preparticipation physical examination can aid in recognizing the athlete's level of physical and emotional maturity, assessing the level of conditioning, and examining the areas of potential injury or previous injury. Individuals with uncontrolled hypertension and uncontrolled seizure disorders should not be allowed to participate in strength training (see Chapter 2). The importance of technique and strict supervision must be emphasized, and the athlete should be educated to avoid competitive or maximum lifts, to exhale during exertion, to avoid hyperventilation, and to use lower weights with higher repetitions (Table 6.1). The American Orthopaedic Society for Sports Medicine provides guidelines for prepubescent weight training (12).

Although most types of weight equipment can be used to gain strength, important general factors that might influence the risk for injury should be taken into consideration. Weight machines can be easier to use, and they do not require significant balance control. However, these machines are usually built for individuals of adult-size, and, thus, the weight increments are too large. Conversely, free weights require mature balance and coordination skills, as well as adequate spotters, yet these have the ability to be made more sports specific by mimicking certain movements, as well as to start light and to add weight in small increments.

As was stated previously, many of the earlier concerns regarding strength training prior to puberty centered around the risk of injury and the fear of negative effects on growth. Many of the early studies were poorly controlled, they used weights that were too light to have an effect, and the protocols used were not long enough to elicit a response. Fortunately, over

TABLE 6.1. *Risks and recommendations for strength training*

Risks	Recommendations
Starting a strength training program too young	Not appropriate to start until balance and postural maturity attained: about age 7 to 8 yr.
Performing a strength training program at home on home gym equipment/weights	Too dangerous to be unsupervised and using poor technique. (Deaths have been reported on home equipment.)
Doing maximum lifts or competing with friends while working out	Too dangerous for young skeleton. High risk for sprains, strains, or more serious injury. These should not occur until child has gone through puberty.
Lifting weights for appearance	Will not get large muscles until child has hormones associated with puberty.
Holding breath during lifting or hyperventilating before a lift	Too much risk for syncope. Child should exhale during the lift and should not hyperventilate prior to lift.
Losing form while lifting	Risk for injury. Use less weight to allow for better form and technique.
Doing a strength training program to increase speed or athletic performance	One part of overall training. Evidence shows good ability to get stronger, but consistent evidence is lacking to show that increasing strength in prepubertal subjects increases performance.
Doing a strength training program to make up for deficits in sports performance	Must also have good conditioning and good proficiency at sport skills before starting a strength training program.
Using heavier weights to get stronger	Youth strength training should employ light weights with higher repetitions. Strength increases due to neurologic recruitment; heavier weights only add risk for injury.

the past 20 years, research in this area has improved and has provided valuable information that has calmed these fears.

Good prospective controlled studies consistently support the ability to gain statistically significant strength, with little risk of injury, if good technique and strict supervision are maintained (2,3,8,13–22). Injuries reported in the literature have been rare and minor, and they have resolved quickly (15). No reported cases of physeal injury and stunted growth have been found. Many of these research projects have performed bone scintigraphy and have found no evidence of skeletal injury.

Of notable interest is the fact that injuries were more frequent and more severe among the control groups in recess play than in the strength training groups (8,23). Even more surprising is the other health benefits that have appeared among various studies, although many of the benefits have not been consistent enough to draw conclusions from the results. Promising benefits that have been found with strength training programs include increased flexibility and improved coordination (16), increased aerobic capacity (17), decreased serum lipids (24,25), and increased bone density (9,26).

The main focus of investigation, however, has been directed at discovering whether strength gains among these prepubescent subjects are genuine. The obvious hesitation for recommending training with weights at young ages stems from the lack of hormones available in individuals of these ages for increasing strength. Most of the original research in this area did not support gains in strength; but this research did not include matched controls, it did not control for the effects of learning, it used loads that were too light to produce changes in strength, and it was too short in duration. With the advent of more scientifically correct research, the vast majority of recent studies support statistically significant gains in strength in youngsters in the earliest stages of sexual maturity. Although they make smaller absolute gains than their adolescent and adult counterparts, these children appear to make the same or larger percentage gains in strength during a training program with weights (9,21,22,27–30).

Various prospective matched, controlled studies that have been performed have used Tanner stage 1 and/or stage 2 boys and girls and have involved multiple modes of training and different durations. Results consistently showed significant gains in strength in untrained children, compared to those in matched controls in recess play. Average gains of 30% to 40% have been observed (9). The modes of training included the range of isometric, isotonic, and isokinetic resistance, with durations of 8 to 12 weeks and even up to 9 months. Both boys and girls attained significant gains in strength (31).

Recent metaanalyses (2,3) note several studies with positive results, and more have certainly been reported since then. The fact that, with adequate intensity, volume, and duration, increases in strength can occur is now evident. The effectiveness of the training program seems to depend more on the intensity, rather than the mode, of training or its duration, although programs that are less than 8 weeks in duration do not consistently produce gains in strength.

Obviously, strength gains in developmentally immature youths happen with structured strength training programs; yet they do not have the pubertal hormones that normally account for such increases in strength, and the strength gains are more than would occur simply from growth alone. Any act that is performed repetitively usually becomes easier, and a similar effect occurs in a strength program. In this regard, a small portion of the gains in strength could be attributed to motor learning and improvements in coordination. However, even when the effects of learning are controlled for by evoked twitch responses (14), the gains in strength are still greater.

Another possible contribution could come from morphologic changes, such as increases in muscle size or hypertrophy. Computerized tomography scans in some studies have shown that, even with 20 weeks of strength training, no evidence of muscle hypertrophy could be found to accompany the significant gains in strength (14). Although reports of increased muscle size do exist (32), the vast majority of studies (those that are longer than 8 weeks in duration) have not shown evidence of muscle hypertrophy that would account for this increased strength.

Benchmark studies (14,18) have revealed that increases in strength in these young athletes occur due to a neurologic phenomenon whereby increases in motor unit recruitment contribute to increased strength. Increases in motor unit activation around 12% and electromyogram amplitude by about 17% are significant in the strength training groups. Thus, neurologic changes of the increased recruitment of muscle fiber activation are large contributors to the increased strength without muscle hypertrophy.

Of noteworthy interest is the fact that the bulk of the studies have used prepubescent school children and their classmates as controls. Investigations using highly trained young athletes are extremely limited and are virtually nonexistent at this time. One such effort studied prepubescent boy and girl swimmers in a strength training program, in comparison to teammates who did not strength train; the gain in strength was approximately 10% (33). Despite the fact that this is a significant gain, this result is one of the lowest reported, thus raising the question of the effect of sports activity on the neurologic recruitment of muscle fibers. Whether these youngsters have already maximized the recruitment effect, thus producing less of an impact from actual strength training, remains open to more thorough investigation.

Substantial support for the ability of preadolescents to gain strength before the onset of puberty now exists. Some evidence supports the hypothesis that a stronger muscle-tendon unit protects the adolescent athlete from injury (34,35). However, long-term prospective studies are still required, and many variables would need to be controlled. Therefore, at this point, the idea that strength training could have a similar protective effect in preadolescents is only speculation. Mixed results with regard to the effect of strength training on actual performance have also been reported (20,33,36–38).

Studies have shown additional benefits from strength training, such as increased flexibility, coordination, and aerobic capacity, as well as a decrease in serum lipids. No detrimental effect on growth or blood pressure has been seen. As more investigations are performed and these potential benefits are consistently found, more support for strength training programs is seen.

If a young boy or girl is involved in sports activities and desires to start a strength training program, certain minimal criteria should be met. The desire should come from the individual, not just the parents or coach. The young boy or girl should have the maturity to accept coaching and instruction and should be disciplined enough to stick with the program. A moderate level of proficiency in the skills of the particular sport should already have been achieved. The strength training program should not be the center of focus, nor should it be a substitute for general aerobic fitness development; it should, however, be one component of a well-balanced and varied exercise program. The program should be general, with appropriately sport-specific techniques. Most importantly, strict technique should be demonstrated, and extremely close supervision must be available.

Strength training should be approached with caution, respect, and the knowledge that it has the potential to have positive benefits with relatively little risk of injury or detriment to stature and blood pressure, if it is conducted appropriately and is supervised. How-

ever, simply because research supports the ability to gain strength does not mean that a cavalier recommendation should be made for all kids to lift weights. When a child starts depends on his or her attainment of good balance, as well as of coordination skills. A strength training program should not be the main objective, but it should complement a youth sports program. If approached in this manner, then it can contribute to the overall beneficial effects of exercise activity in children.

ENDURANCE TRAINING

Aerobic endurance is the foundation of performing physical work. Aerobic metabolism or aerobic pathways generate energy from fuels within the body, such as carbohydrates, fats, and proteins, while using oxygen in the process. The aerobic pathways can produce energy for extended periods of time (large capacity) when the intensity of exercise is low. Maximal aerobic power (represented by $\dot{V}_{O_2}$ max), or endurance capacity, is the ability to take in, transport, and utilize oxygen. Maximal aerobic power has traditionally been described as a marker of endurance performance capacity and cardiovascular fitness. Changes in endurance capacity have been studied in normal children and adolescents, as well as in child and adolescent athletes. The following section describes the normal development of aerobic power and the alterations in endurance capacity with endurance training.

Endurance capacity is influenced by a number of factors, such as genetic endowment, developmental rate, body composition, and habitual physical activity. Maximal aerobic power is achieved through a rather complex series of reactions within the human body that involves the lungs, heart, circulatory system, and skeletal muscle. Maximal oxygen consumption is used to represent aerobic power. Maximal oxygen consumption ($\dot{V}_{O_2}$ max) is the sum of cardiac output (heart rate times stroke volume) times the arteriovenous (AV) O_2 difference. Endurance performance is highly related to the $\dot{V}_{O_2}$ max possessed by the athlete and the percentage of $\dot{V}_{O_2}$ max that can be maintained over long periods of physical work.

Many studies have attempted to identify the biologic determinants of maximal oxygen consumption. Various factors have been described, such as improved stoke volume (i.e., increased preload, increased blood pressure, reduced resting heart rate, increased cardiac contractility, and decreased afterload) and improved AV O_2 oxygen difference (i.e., increased hemoglobin mass, capillary density, myoglobin concentration, and cellular aerobic enzyme activity) (39–41). Most of these alterations have been reported as changes in autonomic nervous control (42). These changes result in reduced submaximal sympathetic tone and increased plasma volume (42). To date, the triggers for these changes are unknown.

When evaluating aerobic capacity, the values can be expressed in either absolute terms (L per minute) or relative terms (mL per kg per minute). Cross-sectional data support a progressive increase in absolute $\dot{V}O_2$ max, with increasing age in healthy untrained children (43–46). Further study indicates a 200 mL per minute increase, up to the age of 12 years, for both boys and girls (47,48). Following puberty, a gender difference becomes clearly evident. The increase seen in young girls plateaus, while that of boys continue to rise. By the age of 16 years, a 50% difference between the genders is observed (43,49). Regardless of gender or age, a large variability of 10% to 20% in maximal aerobic power is seen (42). These differences in children and adolescents are due to differences in the development of many components of $\dot{V}O_2$ Relative $\dot{V}O_2$ max in boys between the ages of 6 and 16 years remains relatively stable (approximately 50 mL per kg per minute). However, the values for young girls decline during the same period (age 8 = 50 mL per kg per minute; age 12 = 45 mL per kg per minute; age 16 = 40 mL per kg per minute) (50–52). The difference that is observed in young women is due primarily to the alterations in body composition that occur during this time period, with an increase in body fat relative to lean tissue.

Training has been shown to improve maximal oxygen consumption by approximately 15% to 20% in previously untrained adults (53). That children should also improve their aerobic capacity with training also seems logical. However, the question that must be answered is whether young children are miniature adults in terms of aerobic power. Furthermore, one could suggest that children might actually possess an enhanced capacity for growth in this area, compared to adults. They may be more capable of adapting many of the factors that control maximal oxygen consumption and may to adjust a larger extent. Finally, the temporal pattern of adaptation in children and adolescents is important. Are any differences in the adaptation process observed in prepubescent as compared to postpubescent youngsters? Many studies have been performed to evaluate these concepts in both boys and girls.

Early studies showed that children had little improvement (<10%) in $\dot{V}O_2$ max relative to body weight (54–58). The studies evaluated boys and girls from the ages of 8 to 15 years who were involved in training programs for between 7 weeks and 22 months. The children and adolescents trained, using various techniques (e.g., long slow distance training, interval training sets and games), 2 to 4 times per week (5,58–60). These researchers and others have suggested that the low response in aerobic power was associated with the training stimulus. Further evaluation of these studies indicated that the training stimulus was much smaller than that which is typically used in adult studies.

When specific training program criteria were used, improvements were seen in maximal oxygen consumption in both children and adolescents in several studies (39,54,58,61,62). The criteria utilized included (a) aerobic activity stimulus, such as swimming, running, or other activities; (b) training 3 to 5 times per week; and (c) heart rate that was 60% to 90% of the maximal heart rate (63). The children ranged from 7 to 15 years of age. Total training duration for the various studies ranged from 6 weeks to 32 months. The average increases in maximal oxygen consumption were approximately 10% (range 7% to 26%) (54,58,64–66). Clearly, an appropriate stimulus must be applied to children and adolescents for significant improvements in aerobic power to occur. Furthermore, many of these studies indicated that the improvements in aerobic power were similar to those observed in adults.

Both absolute and relative $\dot{V}O_2$ max can be improved with aerobic training in children and adolescents. However, the trainability of the aerobic system is less in children and adolescents than it is in adults. Determining whether child athletes already possess an enhanced endurance capacity compared to their normal age-matched counterparts is important.

Researchers have sought to determine the plasticity of endurance capacity in both child and adolescent endurance-trained athletes. Several studies have evaluated young runners and swimmers from the ages of 9 to 15 years. The studies, which included both male and female children, assessed maximal oxygen consumption. Relative $\dot{V}O_2$ max ranged from 55.4 to 65.9 mL per kg per minute in boys and 52.2 to 61.0 mL per kg per minute in girls. Several research studies have been performed on male and female endurance athletes in the ages of 15 to 19 years. Young male runners exhibited $\dot{V}O_2$ max values ranging from 66.4 to 74.6 mL per kg per minute (42,67–70). Endurance-trained young females had values ranging from 62.2 to 66.1 mL per kg per minute (67,68,70).

Although young athletes appear to have increased aerobic capacities, one must understand the temporal pattern of endurance adaptations. Do young athletes merely follow the normal pattern of aerobic power expansion annually, or is the growth of their aerobic abilities unique in some way? One speculation has focused on the influence of puberty in the plasticity of endurance capacity in young athletes training for endurance events. Studies evaluating child athletes prior to puberty remain unclear. One study assessing male swimmers showed that $\dot{V}O_2$ max increased progressively during each state of puberty and that it was independent of age, height, and weight. This trend did not occur in the females in the study. A review of prepubescent studies shows that some studies report increases, while others show no change in maximal aerobic power (71–75). In contrast, research evaluating postpubescent youths is more conclusive. Relative $\dot{V}O_2$ max is enhanced with athletic training during the teen years (70,76–78).

Endurance training is clearly important in the development of both normal children and young athletes. However, a discussion of the potential risks of endurance training in children and adolescents is crucial (Table 6.2). Primary concerns related to endurance training are issues of overtraining (i.e., too much stimulus) and early specialization.

Overtraining or maladaptation to training is common in competitive adult athletes (79–82). Unfortunately, this is also seen in child athletes. Training adaptation occurs along a continuum. Appropriate training load results in adaptations in the bodily systems, whereas too much training stimulus overloads the body and results in maladaptation. Negative consequences can be seen on many systems, including the endocrine, neuromuscular, cardiovascular, and immune systems. Additionally, psychologic changes do occur that also result in negative performance outcomes.

Physiologic alterations cross many bodily systems. The body responds to training by activating the hypothalamic–pituitary–adrenal axis. Cortisol is one hormone that affects many body functions. Elevations in basal cortisol are commonly associated with training and overtraining (9,80,81). Negative adaptations in cardiac function are often expressed through an increase in the resting heart rate (80,81). Gastrointestinal disturbances that include increased motility, flatulence, and nausea have also been reported by athletes who negatively responding to training (81). Muscle-related issues, such as chronic muscle soreness, are classic signs of overtraining; and these are often associated with elevations in skeletal muscle damage markers, including creatine phosphokinase, total protein, and urea (81,82). Finally, immune function is typically compromised, as poor healing and increased illness demonstrate (80,81).

Alterations in bodily function create a physiologic environment that is not optimized for peak performance. Reductions in performance outcomes are often evident in young athletes who maladapt to training. They show signs of intolerance to training, coupled with prolonged recovery time (81). In addition, coordination is compromised, resulting in poor technique,

TABLE 6.2. *Risks and recommendations for endurance training*

Risks	Recommendations
Increases in training loads to adult levels to increase endurance in children (the concept of training children as if they are small adults, when they are not).	A "ceiling" for the amount that $\dot{V}O_2$ max can increase prior to puberty appears to exist. $\dot{V}O_2$ max can be increased with training stimulus in children, but the trainability of the child's aerobic system is less than that in adults.
Significantly increasing training before puberty to improve performance	How much difference this can make is unclear. $\dot{V}O_2$ max can be more clearly enhanced by increased training during the postpuberty years.
Overtraining: increased risks of negative consequences on muscle/tendon, hormone, heart, immune, and psychologic systems	Reduce training loads as necessary. Balance training volume; it should be different for level of development (prepuberty vs. postpuberty), regardless of chronological age.
Nutritional restriction	If volume of food is a problem, use concentrated caloric sources. Watch for disordered eating patterns and emphasize the need for calories to optimize performance.
Staleness and plateau of performance	Make sure athlete is not overtrained, underrested, or lacking adequate calories.
Using adult heart rate parameters for training	Children actually require higher heart rates to gain improvements in endurance capacity.
Sport specialization too early	Maintain a good mix of exposure to different sports. This will maximize many different skills before complete specialization.

which can be critical in sports like swimming or running. Maximal work output is also suppressed in overtrained young endurance athletes. Overall, training capacities, as well as recovery abilities, are reduced. The young athlete is unable to adapt to the training stimulus. Reductions in training load must be used to allow recovery to occur, but complete rest must also be considered for these young endurance athletes.

Early sport specialization has grown in popularity over the past decade. Children often train year round for sports, and they train at levels that could be considered elite. Many factors influence this phenomenon, including the media exposure of young athletes, an increased focus on scholarships, and Olympic development programs that identify youngsters quite early in their development. The American Academy of Pediatrics study on sport specialization (83) suggested that, regardless of the factors that may influence children and parents, potential negative issues must be considered when an athlete is specializing early. Two of these areas that must be considered are musculoskeletal injury and nutritional issues.

Bone loading is important in the normal growth of this tissue. Assuming that repetitive stresses on long bones may impact the epiphysis, resulting in delayed growth or fracture at this point in the bone, seems logical. Researchers are continuing to evaluate this concept in prepubescent children. To date, research supporting an increased incidence of epiphyseal injuries in the long bones of athletes in weight-bearing sports remains unclear. Growth in child athletes, both in total size and in the rate of growth, is similar to that for nonathletes (84). Clearly, however, investigation in this critical area must continue to strive to reduce risks for children participating in endurance sports. Physicians should evaluate young athletes for overuse injuries (e.g., tendonitis, stress fractures, shin splints) on a regular basis as a measure of assessment.

Nutritional considerations should address both macronutrient (carbohydrate, fat, and protein) and micronutrient (iron and calcium) needs when assessing a young athlete (see Chapter 4). Child athletes should consume a variety of foods from each food category of the food pyramid. In addition, the ingestion of ample total calories is important to normal growth and development. Caloric intake must support normal growth and development, as well as the additional energy needs of sport activity. For young athletes, especially girls, controlling the amount and variety of foods that are consumed is not uncommon. Caution must be taken to avoid creating environments that support the development of disordered eating habits among these young athletes.

Two specific minerals, iron and calcium, are important in the growing years. Iron is important in oxygen transport, aerobic metabolism, and mental functioning (83). Support is found for the potential for additional losses of iron through various means from chronic endurance training. The requirement for iron is 10 mg per day in young children and 12 to 15 mg per day in adolescents, compared to 10 to 15 mg per day in adults (85). The consumption of foods high in iron, such as red meat, spinach, liver, and other dark green vegetables, is crucial to ensure ample iron in the diet. If the diet is not rich in these foods, suggesting a multivitamin for these developing athletes might be prudent in order to fulfill the requirements for iron.

Relative calcium requirements for children are also greater than for adults. Calcium is critical in the formation of bone, as well as in appropriate skeletal muscle function. Inadequate calcium intake is common in young athletes because of reduced diary intakes (83). The requirement for calcium is 800 mg per day for children and 1,200 mg per day for adolescents and adults (85). Dairy products, as well as almonds, apricots, pears, raisins, and leafy green vegetables, are good sources of calcium.

Overtraining and overuse injuries are often reported in young athletes. However, research evaluating the impact of excessive endurance training on prepubescent children and adolescents is limited. The safety of young endurance athletes should be a primary concern for parents, coaches, and physicians. A proactive approach is the most successful in preventing negative physical outcomes in these developing endurance athletes. Anecdotal evidence supports the notion that the prevention of problems results in the maximization of performance potential in adulthood.

Endurance training in young children and adolescents balances between presenting an appropriate training stimulus and preventing it from becoming so large that it overloads the youngster inappropriately. Separate training parameters should be applied to prepubescent children and postpubescent adolescents. Although the principles of training (i.e., progressive overload, individualization, and specialization) should be applied to both groups, the volume of training is different. The following two criteria are similar: training should occur 3 to 5 times per week and heart rate should reach 60% to 90% of maximal heart rate. These two parameters have been shown to produce increases in aerobic power or endurance capacity.

Prepubescent children should be exposed to general aerobic activity. Children should participate in running, swimming, cycling, and sport games to increase endurance capacity. In doing so, children should respond to training stimuli by meeting specific criteria as described above. Of importance is noting the fact that traditional adult formulas underestimate the appropriate target heart rate stimulus for children. Therefore, children require higher heart rates to gain improvements in endurance capacity. Endurance training during prepubescent and early puberty periods allows the enhancement of overall technical skills associated with endurance events (e.g., running, swimming, and cycling). Aerobic workloads provide increased economical performances of technique, based on the natural maturation of neuromuscular processes, as well as of motor centers in the brain.

Continuous training is one technique that can be used to develop endurance capacity in prepubescent athletes. Young athletes can improve aerobic metabolic processes with work intensity in the range of 50% to 60% $\dot{V}_{O_2}$ max (i.e., a heart rate of approximately 150 to 170 beats per minute in children from the ages of 8 to 12 years) (40,41). Interval training is also effective with this age group. Maximal oxygen consumption can be increased in 9-year-old to 12-year-old children by incorporating serialized exercise of 7 to 19 minutes, at an intensity of 70% to 80% $\dot{V}_{O_2}$ max (approximate heart rate of 170 to 180 beats per minute) (40,41). One caution the clinician should note is that the adaptive capacity of prepubertal children to work of this type and intensity is limited; therefore, the volume of work in this category must be restricted.

Postpubescent youngsters can acquire aerobic potential with the use of a wide range of cyclic exercises. Endurance capacity will expand severalfold during puberty and following puberty. Endurance athletes can begin to increase the volume of training (total distance) at this point, which then results in increased performance aerobically, both in training and in competition.

Training programs for young endurance athletes are varied. Scientific literature that proves one training protocol is more advantageous than another is not available. Most coaches attempt to use their experience and best judgment in developing training programs that effectively overload the child, without placing too large a demand on their bodies. One model from the sport of swimming can be used as an illustration. The reader should note that boys and girls are separated, based on age, due to a delay in the maturation of young boys compared to young girls.

Girls aged from 7 to 9 years and boys aged between 8 and 10 years enter the structured swimming program. The program focuses on technical skills and aerobic activities. Swimmers participate 3 to 6 times per week with a gradual progressive increase in swimming load. The swimmers swim only three times per week initially, and, over a period of 1 year, they progress to a level of six times per week. Natural progression of the training load results.

Girls aged from 9 to 10 years and boys 10 to 11 years of age are then progressed into a second stage of training. This stage places a greater focus on the aerobic development of the young athlete, in addition to a further development of technical proficiency in swimming strokes. This stage lasts for 3 to 4 years. Annual training distances range from 1,200 to 1,400 km for girls and from 1,000 to 1,200 km for boys. Training is focused on aerobic work, in which 60% to 65% of the total training volume is designed to load the aerobic metabolic pathways.

Depending on the pace at which the young athlete progresses, he or she may pass into the third stage of training. This stage begins between 12 and 14 years in girls and 13 to 15 years in boys. Initiation of this stage is dependent upon the rate of biologic or sexual maturation of the youngster. This stage typically is designed to last for 3 to 4 years. When the swimmer reaches the Tanner stage 3 of physical development, he or she is viewed as having the capacity to increase training loads rapidly. Up to this point, the focus has primarily been on aerobic work that results in enhanced performance in both long and short distances. In this stage, however, total swimming volume may reach 1,600 to 1,700 km. The work is designed to stress metabolic capacities to allow interplay between the aerobic and anaerobic systems. Typically, less than 25% of the overall volume is strictly aerobic in nature. This training program must be viewed merely as one example in a large number of possibilities. The training of both prepubescent and postpubescent athletes must follow the principles of training. Monitoring training adaptations regularly and involving medical personnel when any signs of overuse or overtraining are evident are essential components.

In summary, the plasticity of the aerobic system in children is reduced prior to puberty compared to that of adults. Studies do support improvements in maximal oxygen consumption, but one must realize that methodologic problems are found with many of these studies. Cross-sectional and longitudinal training studies of child endurance athletes report a reduced improvement in maximal aerobic power until puberty is initiated. Adolescent athletes increase $\dot{V}_{O_2}$ max readily with training. Normal adolescents can improve aerobic capacity by 20% to 25% with training. Prepubescent children, however, show improvements of approximately 10%. Endurance training programs must be designed appropriately for children at the various stages of puberty. Training the aerobic systems is appropriate, but the goals of improvement must be realistic for prepubertal boys and girls. Following puberty, rapid gains that plateau and/or decrease with increasing age are typical.

Training young children to become champion endurance athletes is a challenge. Care must be taken to construct training programs carefully so that they optimally load the aerobic metabolic system without overloading its capacities. If the load is too high, the youngster will show signs of overtraining and/or overuse. Loading the athlete less than desired will result in poor adaptation and performances that are subcaliber. Additional research is necessary to elucidate further the factors that impact the development of aerobic power and endurance capacity in young athletes. In addition, applied research is needed to decipher optimal training protocols for both prepubescent and postpubescent endurance athletes.

REFERENCES

1. American Academy of Pediatrics. Weight training and weight lifting: information for the pediatrician. *The Physician and Sports Medicine* 1983;11:157–161.
2. Falk B, Tenenbaum G. The effectiveness of resistance training in children: a meta-analysis. *Sports Med* 1996; 22:176–186.
3. Payne V, Morrow J, Johnson L, et al. Resistance training in children and youth: a meta-analysis. *Res Q Exerc Sport* 1997;68:80–89.
4. Brant C, Haubenstricker J, Seefeldt V. Age changes in motor skills during childhood and adolescence. *Exerc Sport Sci Rev* 1984;12:467–520.
5. Rowland T. Effects of training on a child's body. In: Sullivan JA, Anderson SJ, eds. *Care of the young athlete*. Rosemont, IL: American Academy of Orthopaedic Surgeons and American Academy of Pediatrics, 2000: 57–63.
6. Faigenbaum A, Zaichkowsky L, Gardner D, et al. Anabolic steroid use by male and female middle school students. *Pediatrics* 1998;101:E6–E10.
7. Brady T, Cahill B, Bodnar L. Weight training related injuries in the high school athlete. *Am J Sports Med* 1982; 10:1–5.
8. Risser W. Weight training injuries in children and adolescents. *Am Fam Phys* 1991;44:2104–2110.
9. Faigenbaum A. Strength training for children and adolescents. *Clin Sports Med* 2000;19:593–619.
10. Tanner S. Weighing the risks. *The Physician and Sports Medicine* 1993;21:105–110.
11. American Academy of Pediatrics. Strength training, weight and power lifting, and bodybuilding by children and adolescents. *Pediatrics* 1990;86:801–803.
12. American Orthopaedic Society for Sports Medicine. *Proceedings of the Conference on Strength Training and the Prepubescent*. Chicago: American Orthopaedic Society for Sports Medicine, 1988.
13. Blimkie C. Resistance training during preadolescence. *Sports Med* 1993;15:389–407.
14. Ramsay J, Blimkie C, Smith K, et al. Strength training effects in prepubescent boys. *Med Sci Sports Exerc* 1990;2:605–614.
15. Rians C, Weltman A, Cahill B, et al. Strength training for prepubescent males: is it safe? *Am J Sports Med* 1987;15:483–489.
16. Sewall L, Micheli L. Strength training for children. *J Pediatr Orthop* 1986;6:143–146.
17. Weltman A, Janney C, Rians C, et al. Effects of hydraulic resistance strength training in pre-pubertal males. *Med Sci Sports Exerc* 1986;18:629–638.
18. Ozmun J, Mikesky A, Surburg P. Neuromuscular adaptations during prepubescent strength training. *Med Sci Sports Exerc* 1991;[Suppl 23]:31.
19. Lillegard W. Strength training in children. *Sports Med Prim Care* 1995:S5–S8.
20. Lillegard W, Brown E, Wilson D, et al. Efficacy of strength training in prepubescent to early postpubescent males and females: effects of gender and maturity. *Pediatr Rehabil* 1997;1:147–157.
21. Pfeiffer R, Francis R. Effects of strength training on muscle development in prepubescent, pubescent, and postpubescent males. *The Physician and Sports Medicine* 1986;14:134–143.
22. Nielsen B, Nielsen K, Behrendt-Hansen M, et al. Training of "functional muscular strength" in girls 7-19 years old. In: Berg K, Eriksson B, eds. *Children and exercise IX*. Baltimore: University Park Press, 1980:69–77.
23. Mazur L, Yetman R, Risser W. Weight training injuries. *Sports Med* 1993;16:57–63.
24. Fripp R, Hodgson J. Effect of resistive training on plasma lipid and lipoprotein levels in male adolescents. *J Pediatr* 1987;111:926–931.
25. Weltman A, Janney C, Rians C, et al. Effects of hydraulic resistance strength training on serum lipid levels in prepubertal boys. *Am J Dis Child* 1987;141:777–780.
26. Morris F, Naughton G, Gibbs J, et al. Prospective ten month exercise intervention in premenarcheal girls: positive effects on bone and lean mass. *J Bone Miner Res* 1997;12:1453–1462.
27. Westcott W. Female response to weight lifting. *J Phys Educ* 1979;77:31–33.
28. Sailors M, Berg K. Comparison of responses to weight training in pubescent boys and men. *J Sports Med Phys Fitness* 1987;27:30–37.
29. Sale D. Strength training in children. In: Gisolfi G, Lamb D, eds. *Perspectives in exercise science and sports medicine*. Indianapolis: Benchmark Press, 1989: 165–216.
30. Vrijens F. Muscle strength development in the pre-and post-pubescent age. *Medicine and Sport* 1978;11: 152–158.
31. Blimkie C. Age- and sex-associated variation in strength during childhood. Anthropometric, morphologic, neurological, biomechanical, endocrinologic, genetic, and physical activity correlates. In: Gisolfi C, Lamb D, eds. *Perspectives in exercise science and sports medicine*. Indianapolis: Benchmark Press, 1989.
32. Fukunga T, Funato K, Ikegawa S. The effects of resistance training on muscle area and strength in prepubescent age. *Ann Physiol Anthropol* 1992;11:357–364.
33. Blanksby B, Gregor J. Anthropometric, strength, and physiological changes in male and female swimmers with progressive resistance training. *Aust J Sport Sci* 1981;1:3–6.

34. Cahill B, Griffith E. Effect of preseason conditioning on the incidence and severity of high school football knee injuries. *Am J Sports Med* 1978;6:180–184.

35. Hejna A, Rosenberg A, Buturusis D, et al. The prevention of sports injuries in high school students through strength training. *National Strength and Conditioning Association Jounal* 1982;4:28–31.

36. Williams D. The effect of weight training on performance in selected motor activities for preadolescent males. *J Appl Sport Sci Res* 1991;5:170.

37. Faigenbaum A, Zaichkowsky L, Westcott W, et al. The effects of a twice per week strength training program on children. *Pediatr Exerc Sci* 1993;5:339–346.

38. Ford H, Puckett J. Comparative effects of prescribed weight training and basketball programs on basketball skill test scores of ninth grade boys. *Percept Mot Skills* 1983;56:23–26.

39. Eriksson BO, Koch G. Effect of physical training on hemodynamic response during maximal and submaximal exercise. *Acta Physiol Scand* 1973;87:27–39.

40. Koch G. Muscle blood flow in prepubertal boys. Effect of growth combined with intensive physical training. In: Borms J, Hebbelink M, eds. *Medicine and sport*. Basel: Karger, 1978:34–46.

41. Eriksson B, Gollnick P, Saltin B. Muscle metabolism and enzyme activities after training in boys 11-13 years old. *Acta Physiol Scand* 1973;87:485–497.

42. Lehmann M, Keul J, Korstein-Reck U. The influence of graduated treadmill exercise on plasma catecholamines, aerobic and anaerobic capacity in boys and adults. *Eur J Appl Physiol* 1981;47:301–311.

43. Krahenbuhl G, Skinner J, Kohrt W. Developmental aspects of maximal aerobic power in children. *Exerc Sport Sci Rev* 1985;13:503–538.

44. Malina R, Bouchard C. *Growth, maturation, and physical activity*. Champaign, IL: Human Kinetics, 1991.

45. Andersen K, Seliger V, Rutenfranz J, et al. Physical performance capacity of children in Norway. *Eur J Appl Physiol* 1974;33:177–195.

46. Rutenfranz F, Andersen K, Seliger V, et al. Maximum aerobic power and body composition during the pubertal growth period: similarities and differences between children of two European countries. *Eur J Pediatr* 1981;136:123–133.

47. Mirwald R, Bailey D. *Maximal aerobic power. A longitudinal analysis*. London, Ontario: Sport Dynamics, 1986.

48. Binkhorst R, de Jong-va de Ker M, Vissers A. Growth and aerobic power of boys aged 11-19 years. In: Ilmarinen J, Valimaki I, eds. *Children and sport*. Heidelberg: Springfield, 1984:99–105.

49. Bar-Or O. *Pediatric sports medicine for the practitioner*. New York: Springer-Verlag New York, 1983.

50. American Alliance for Health, Physical Education, Recreation and Dance. *Youth fitness testing manual*. Washington, D.C.: American Alliance for Health, Physical Education, Recreation and Dance, 1980.

51. Cumming G, Everatt D, Hastman L. Bruce treadmill test in children: normal values in a clinic population. *Am J Cardiol* 1978;41:69–75.

52. Astrand P. *Experimental studies of physical working capacity in relationship to sex and age*. Copenhagen: Munksgaard, 1952.

53. Saltin B, Hartley L, Kilbom A, et al. Physical training in sedentary middle-aged and older men. II. Oxygen uptake, heart rate, and blood lactate concentrations at sub-maximal and maximal exercise. *Scand J Clin Lab Invest* 1969;24:323–334.

54. Ekblom B. Effect of physical training on oxygen transport systems in man. *Acta Physiol Scand Suppl* 1969;328:5–45.

55. Bar-Or O, Zwiren L. Physiological effects of frequency and content variation of physical education classes and of endurance conditioning on 9 to 10-year-old girls and boys. In: Bar-Or O, ed. *Pediatric work physiology IV*. Nantanya, Israel: Wingate Institute, 1973:190–208.

56. Mocellin R, Wasmund U. Investigations on the influence of a running training program on the cardiovascular and motor performance capacity in 53 boys and girls of a second and third primary school class. In: Bar-Or O, ed. *Pediatric work physiology IV*. Natanya, Israel: Wingate Institute, 1973:279–288.

57. Stewart K, Gutin B. Effects of physical training on cardiorespiratory fitness in children. *Res Q* 1976;47:110–120.

58. Lussier L, Buskirk E. Effects of an endurance training regimen on assessment of work capacity in prepubertal children. *Ann N Y Acad Sci* 1977;30:734–747.

59. Yoshida T, Ishiko I, Muraoka I. Effect of endurance training on cardiorespiratory function of 5-year-old-children. *Int J Sports Med* 1980;1:91–94.

60. Benedict G, Vaccaro P, Hatfield B. Physiological effects of an eight week precision jump program in children. *American Corrective Therapy Journal* 1985;5:108–111.

61. Brown C, Harrower J, Deeter M. The effects of cross country running on preadolescent girls. *Med Sci Sports Exerc* 1972;4:1–5.

62. Shasby G, Hagerman F. The effects of conditioning on cardiorespiratory function in adolescent boys. *J Sports Med* 1975;3:97–107.

63. Rowland T. Aerobic response to endurance training in prepubescent children: a critical analysis. *Med Sci Sports Exerc* 1985;17:493–497.

64. Gilliam T, Freedson P. Effects of a 12-week school physical fitness program on peak VO2, body composition, and blood lipids in 7 to 9 year old children. *Int J Sports Med* 1980;1:73–78.

65. Vaccaro P, Clarke D. Cardiorespiratory alteration in 9 to 11 year old children following a season of competitive swimming. *Med Sci Sports Exerc* 1978;10:204–207.

66. Massicotte D, MacNab R. Cardiorespiratory adaptations to training at specified intensities in children. *Med Sci Sports Exerc* 1979;11:172–176.

67. VanHuss W, Evans S, Kurowski T, et al. Physiologic characteristics of male and female age-group runners. In: Brown E, Branta C, eds. *Competitive sports for children and youth*. Champaign, IL: Human Kinetics, 1988:143–158.

68. Nudel D, Hassett I, Gurain A, et al. Young long distance runners: physiologic characteristics. *Clin Pediatr* 1989;28:500–505.

69. Rowland T, Varzeas M, Walsh C. Aerobic responses to walking training in sedentary adolescents. *J Adolesc Health* 1991;12:30–34.

70. Baxter-Jones A, Goldstein H, Helms P. The development of aerobic power in young athletes. *J Appl Physiol* 1993;75:1160–1167.

71. Kobayashi K, Kitamura K, Miura M, et al. Aerobic power as related to body growth and training in Japanese boys: a longitudinal study. *J Appl Physiol* 1978;44:666–672.

72. Mirwald R, Bailey D, Cameron N, et al. Longitudinal

comparison of aerobic power in active and inactive boys aged 7 to 17 years. *Ann Hum Biol* 1981;8:404–414.

73. Weber G, Kartodihardjo W, Skissouras V. Growth and physical training with reference to heredity. *J Appl Physiol* 1976;40:211–215.

74. Eisenmann P, Golding L. Comparison of effects of training on VO₂ max in girls and young women. *Med Sci Sports Exerc* 1975;7:136–138.

75. Savage M, Petratis M, Thomson W, et al. Exercise training effects on serum lipids of prepubescent boys and adult men. *Med Sci Sports Exerc* 1986;18:197–204.

76. Rusko H. Development of aerobic power in relation to age and training in cross-country skiers. *Med Sci Sports Exerc* 1992;24:1040–1047.

77. Murase Y, Kobayashi K, Kamei S, et al. Longitudinal study of aerobic power in superior junior athletes. *Med Sci Sports Exerc* 1981;13:180–184.

78. Miyashita M, Miura M, Murase Y, et al. Running performance from the viewpoint of aerobic power. In: Folinsbee L, ed. *Environmental stress: individual human adaptations.* New York: Academic Press, 1978:183–193.

79. Uusitalo A. Hormonal responses to endurance training and overtraining in female athletes. *Clin J Sport Med* 1988;8:178–186.

80. Urhausen A. Blood hormones as markers of training stress and overtraining. *Sports Med* 1995;20:251–276.

81. Stone M, Keith R, Kearney J, et al. Overtraining: a review of the signs, symptoms and possible causes. *J Appl Sports Sci Res* 1991;5:35–50.

82. Rowbottom D, Keast D, Morto A. The emerging role of glutamine as an indicator of exercise stress and overtraining. *Sports Med* 1996;21:80–97.

83. American Academy of Pediatrics, Committee on Sports Medicine and Fitness. Intensive training and sports specialization in young athletes. *Pediatrics* 2000;106: 154–157.

84. Malina R. Physical growth and biological maturation of young athletes. *Exerc Sports Sci Rev* 1994;22: 389–434.

85. National Research Council, National Academy of Sciences. *Recommended dietary allowances,* 10th ed. Washington: National Academy Press, 1989.

7

Environmental Conditions and Youth Sports

Robert C. Gambrell

Children and adolescents exercising in extreme temperatures are at risk for a variety of environmental injuries. Morphologic and physiologic differences between children and adults place children at increased risk of injury when exercising in extreme environments. This chapter focuses on the effects and problems that may occur when children exercise in extreme heat or cold. Knowledge about the potential environmental dangers children face when exercising will prepare physicians for the diagnosis, treatment, and prevention of such problems.

HEAT-RELATED ILLNESS AND HYPERTHERMIA

Children exercising in hot environments are vulnerable to minor heat-related illnesses, as well as to severe hyperthermic syndromes that may become life threatening. Heat-related illnesses arise in response to physiologic adaptations that occur in individuals who are exercising in hot environments. Hyperthermic syndromes, heat exhaustion, and heat stroke occur when normal physiologic mechanisms for heat dissipation are overwhelmed, and they become inadequate to maintain the core body temperature (CBT) at normal levels. Children and adults alike are susceptible to heat injuries, but children do not adapt to increased heat stress, as well as adults do (1). Children have a larger surface area to body mass ratio than adults, which leads to a greater heat gain from the environment; and they produce more heat per mass unit from metabolic processes than adults (2). Children also have a lower sweating capacity than adults (1), limiting their ability to dissipate heat, which serves as the primary method of heat loss in hot environments. An understanding of the physiologic mechanisms involved in thermoregulation is necessary to explain how individuals may become hyperthermic and how heat injuries may be avoided.

Pathophysiology

Thermoregulation is maintained through a complex set of mechanisms that attempt to maintain the CBT at 37°C (98.6°F). Heat is generated, absorbed, and lost in the exercising child from both endogenous and exogenous sources. Endogenous heat comes from exercising muscles and cellular metabolism. Exogenous heat comes from the environment. Children lose heat by conduction, convection, radiation, and evaporation. At rest, when the environmental temperature is below body temperature, thermoregulation is maintained primarily by the convection of heat to the skin and the radiation of heat to the environment, with an additional small contribution from evaporation of moisture from the lungs (3). As heat production increases with exercise, sweating provides additional heat loss through evaporation. When the environmental temperature exceeds the body temperature, athletes rely almost entirely on evaporative heat loss to regulate body temperature (3,4).

Athletes exercising in hot environments put extreme demands on their thermoregulatory mechanisms. The key components of thermoregulation are the cardiovascular and integumentary systems. Compromise of either of these systems places an exercising child at risk for heat injury. When one takes this into consideration, one realizes that individual, medical, and environmental factors may all increase the risk for heat illness or injury.

As was previously mentioned, children are at increased risk for heat illnesses due to a larger surface area to body mass ratio and lower sweating capacity than adults. Additional individual and medical factors that place individuals at risk for heat illness include obesity, dehydration, a low degree of physical fitness, recent febrile or gastrointestinal illness, cardiovascular disease, sweat gland dysfunction, drugs, alcohol, a past history of heat stroke, sunburn, midday overeating, heat-retaining clothing, and inadequate acclimatization (4–7). Medications may also increase an individual's risk for heat illness. Antihistamines, anticholinergics, phenothiazines, and benztropine mesylate decrease sweat production. Sedatives and haloperidol decrease thirst recognition. Thyroid hormones and amphetamines increase heat production (4,5,6,8).

Environmental heat stress is the major risk factor for developing heat illness. Temperature, relative humidity, wind, and the degree of cloud cover combine to determine the actual environmental heat stress and how hot one actually feels. The wet bulb globe temperature (WBGT) index is a temperature/humidity/radiation index that is used to measure environmental heat stress. The risk for heat illness increases with increasing environmental heat stress, and it can reach a point at which it can overwhelm any individual's thermoregulatory mechanisms, thus becoming a tremendous risk for exercising individuals (Fig. 7.1) (9).

Heat acclimatization is one of the key components of an athlete's ability to exercise in a hot environment. Acclimatization occurs through repeated exposures, over 1 to 2 weeks, to a hot environment, which leads to improved heat-dissipating mechanisms. Physiologic changes that occur with acclimatization include increased cardiac output, extracellular fluid volume expansion, increased sweat volume, and decreased sweat sodium concentration (4,10–12). Acclimatiza-

tion allows athletes to experience a smaller rise in rectal temperature at any given workload in the heat, which enhances performance and decreases the risk for experiencing a heat-related illness (4,9). Cardiovascular fitness has also been shown to decrease the risk for hyperthermia in athletes, independent of the effects of acclimatization (5,12).

Dehydration is thought to be a major factor in the development of heat exhaustion, and it places the athlete at risk for exertional heat stroke. Performance is impaired with as little as a 2% reduction in circulating volume, and progressive dehydration is believed to cause hyperthermia in proportion to the fluid deficit (13). Adequate fluid consumption before and during exercise in a hot environment can reduce the risk of heat illness (9).

Heat-related Illnesses

Minor heat-related illnesses are generally benign and self-limited, and they are easily treated by removing the individual from the hot environment and rehydrating the athlete. *Heat cramps* usually affect the large, heavily worked muscles in the legs and abdomen, although they may affect any muscle group. Heat cramps result from excessive electrolyte loss in sweating, and they may occur even in highly acclima-

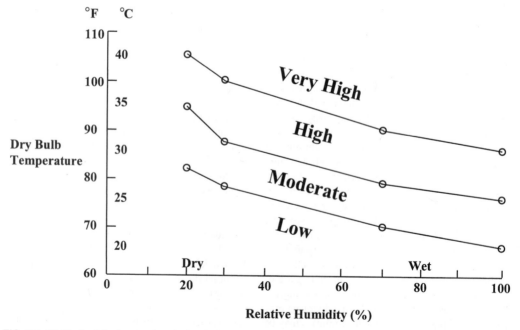

FIG. 7.1. Wet bulb globe temperature index. (Modified from American College of Sports Medicine. Position stand: heat and cold illnesses during distance running. *Med Sci Sports Exerc* 1996;28:i–x, with permission.)

tized individuals. Treatment of heat cramps involves rest, massage, and replacing electrolytes, especially sodium. *Heat edema* is benign swelling of the extremities that often occurs in poorly acclimatized individuals who are exposed to hot environments. The swelling results from peripheral vasodilatation in response to aldosterone-mediated sodium retention (4). Treatment of heat edema includes elevation of the extremities and acclimatization. Diuretics are not needed, and, in fact, they should be avoided in the treatment of heat edema. *Heat syncope* occurs from the same mechanisms as heat edema, but peripheral vasodilatation is severe enough to cause orthostatic hypotension and loss of consciousness. The treatment of heat syncope includes hydration, removing the individual from the hot environment, and rest. Sitting or lying down may prevent syncope if lightheadedness or weakness is experienced.

Hyperthermia

Heat exhaustion and heat stroke represent a spectrum of hyperthermic syndromes. Heat exhaustion is defined as the inability to continue exercise in the heat, and it has no known chronic harmful effects. Heat stroke occurs when the body temperature is elevated to a level that causes damage to body tissues, oftentimes affecting multiple organ systems. Elevated body temperatures of 40°C (104°F) or higher can quickly lead to irreversible neurologic damage, and prolonged or extreme periods of temperature elevation may lead to widespread tissue damage with multisystem organ failure. At the initial presentation, differentiating between heat exhaustion and heat stroke is extremely difficult, with the primary clinical sign of heat stroke being central nervous system (CNS) dysfunction. CBT above 40°C (104°F) is typically used to diagnose heat stroke, but temperatures above 40.6°C (105.1°F) have been recorded following a race in conscious adult runners who suffered no ill effects (9). Additionally, CBTs below 40°C (104°F) have been recorded in individuals with exertional heat stroke. This may reflect either the body's early attempts at cooling before a core temperature was obtained or individual susceptibility to hyperthermia. Heat stroke is divided into two categories, classic heat stroke and exertional heat stroke. CBT in excess of 40°C (104°F), mental status changes, and anhydrosis are the hallmarks of classic heat stroke. Classic heat stroke predominantly affects the elderly or debilitated individual who becomes overwhelmed by environmental heat stress; this may be seen with summertime heat waves and confinement in a poorly ventilated dwelling. Exertional heat stroke, by contrast, is

associated with initial profuse sweating, and it usually occurs in healthy young active individuals, such as the pediatric athlete.

Heat exhaustion occurs when the cardiovascular system is overwhelmed in its attempt to maintain the competing demands of exercise and thermoregulation. Heat exhaustion is the most common heat-related illness among athletes, and it occurs from excessive sweating in a hot environment, leading to dehydration and decreased cardiac output. (5) Common symptoms include weakness, headache, tachycardia, dizziness, nausea, vomiting, diarrhea, hypotension, goose flesh, and irritability. Symptoms may appear abruptly because athletes frequently maintain high levels of performance up until the moment they collapse. Major neurologic impairment is absent, which helps to distinguish heat exhaustion from exertional heat stroke. CBT rises, but it usually remains below 40°C (104°F). Heat syncope or heat cramps may accompany heat exhaustion. The treatment for heat exhaustion includes rest, cooling, and rehydration. Oral electrolyte solutions are preferred for rehydration if the patient is conscious and is able to tolerate them. Intravenous administration of 5% dextrose in 0.9% (normal) saline solution is frequently used as it expedites recovery. Most young athletes recover quickly.

Exertional heat stroke should be considered in any child exhibiting neurologic symptoms while exercising in a hot environment. Exertional heat stroke is an emergency that necessitates rapid cooling. The severity of heat stroke is related to the length of time before cooling measures are instituted and the degree of hyperthermia. Symptoms of exertional heat stroke include the same symptoms as heat exhaustion, plus neurologic symptoms, such as headache, confusion, agitation, seizures, stupor, or coma. An accurate CBT is necessary for the diagnosis and treatment of exertional heat stroke. CBT should always be measured rectally because oral, axillary, and aural temperatures are not reliable measures (4,6). Early mortality from heat stroke is related to CNS injury. Widespread cellular injury may occur in heat stroke, leading to liver injury, rhabdomyalysis, acute renal failure, pulmonary edema, and disseminated intravascular coagulation. Evidence of cellular injury by measurement of serum transaminases, lactate dehydrogenase, creatine phosphokinase, blood urea nitrogen, creatinine, complete blood count, platelets, fibrin split products, prothrombin time, and fibrinogen may aid in making the diagnosis of exertional heat stroke. Poor prognostic indicators for individuals suffering from exertional heat stroke are CBT more than 42.2°C (107.6°F), aspartate aminotransferase (AST, also known as SGOT) greater than 1,000 during the first 24 hours, and coma that lasts for more than 2 hours (5,6).

The first and most important step in the treatment of exertional heat stroke is lowering CBT below 39°C (102°F). The patient should be moved to a cooler location, and active external cooling measures should be instituted immediately. Many active cooling measures have been used successfully to treat exertional heat stroke, including cool or cold water immersion, ice packs, ice water cooling blankets, warm water mist with fanning, and combinations of these measures. Cooling measures should not restrict access to the patient for monitoring and treatment. The fastest cooling rates and the lowest mortality rates have been observed with cool and cold water immersion (9). A number of internal cooling measures (e.g., cardiopulmonary bypass and peritoneal or gastric lavage) have also been used, but they have never been shown to be superior to external active cooling (14). Because of their invasiveness and risks, internal cooling measures should be reserved for cases when external cooling measures fail. CBT should be closely monitored to avoid overcorrection of hyperthermia, which leads to hypothermia.

Prevention of Heat-Related Illness

Heat-related illness is a preventable problem. Prevention begins with identifying athletes who are at risk. The risk for heat-related illness increases with increasing heat stress. Accordingly, the WBGT or heat stress should be monitored, and activities must be modified accordingly; special consideration must be given to children exercising in the heat because of their increased vulnerability (Table 7.1) (4). Preventive measures may include unlimited substitutions, shedding restrictive clothing and equipment, mandatory water breaks, and avoiding extreme efforts in heat. Athletes, parents, and coaches should be aware of the early signs and symptoms of heat illness, including dizziness,

weakness, nausea, headache, cramping, or confusion. The clinician should be aware that any heat-related illness, however minor, among members of an athletic team suggests that others are at risk. Children should be given free access to fluids that should be cooled; these may be flavored to improve their palatability, thus promoting consumption. Recent febrile, respiratory, or diarrheal illness should preclude exercise in heat. Parents and coaches should ensure that children have adequate time for heat acclimatization and that they are in good physical condition before they begin exercising vigorously in the heat. By taking all of these factors into consideration, the goal of preventing heat-related illness and hyperthermia in children can be accomplished.

COLD-RELATED INJURIES

Risk for the development of cold-related injuries occurs in many outdoor and winter sports. In addition to traditional winter sports, a significant risk of hypothermia is associated with water sports, mountaineering, and endurance events. Cold-related injuries may be local, such as frostbite, or systemic, such as hypothermia. Frostbite occurs when fluid crystallizes in the skin and subcutaneous tissues from exposure to subfreezing temperatures, thereby causing cellular damage. Hypothermia occurs when heat loss exceeds heat production, and CBT drops below 36°C (97°F). Frostbite and hypothermia may occur alone or in combination.

Frostbite

Frostbite among athletes during training or competition has been reported, but its exact incidence is unknown (9). Frostbite occurs because of the individual's inability to protect himself or herself from the elements. Frostbite may occur within seconds or after hours of exposure, depending upon the degree of skin

TABLE 7.1. *Guidelines for team activities based on wet bulb globe temperature*

Wet bulb globe temperature	Activity
<65°F (18°C)	Follow regular schedules; allow full access to fluids.
65° to 72°F (18° to 22°C)	Add quarterly fluid breaks; allow free access to fluids.
73° to 82°F (23° to 28°C)	Shorten games or allow unlimited substitutions; add quarterly fluid breaks; allow full access to water.
82° to 85°F (28° to 30°C)	Establish an alternate schedule (in advance) to hold more midday games at earlier and later hours; allow unrestricted substitution at all age levels; shorten game times; add quarterly fluid breaks; allow fluid breaks during play.
>85°F (31°C)	Cancel all exertion and avoid sun exposure at rest.

From Bracker MD. Environmental and thermal injury. *Clin Sports Med* 1992;11:431, with permission.

protection and the severity of cold exposure. Multiple factors contribute to the development of frostbite, but the type and duration of cold contact are the two most important factors in determining the extent of frostbite injury (9,15,16). Frostbite occurs when the body is unable to protect against heat loss. Direct contact with substances, such as metal, that have high thermal conductivity is much more likely to cause frostbite than is contact with wood or fabric. Air is a poor thermal conductor.

Cold ambient temperature alone is not as dangerous as when it is combined with windy conditions. The wind chill index factors the wind speed with the ambient temperature to determine the relative cold stress in the environment (Fig. 7.2) (17). For example, an ambient temperature of 10°F (−12.2°C) with a 30-mile-per-hour wind feels as cold as −33°F (−36.1°C) with no wind. Additional factors that increase the risk for developing frostbite include humidity and skin wetness (15,16).

The clinical appearance of frostbite and severity of symptoms generally parallels the severity of injury. Frostbite usually affects the extremities, nose, or ears. Frostbitten skin may appear white, yellow–white, or mottled blue (9,15,16). Most patients initially complain that the extremity is cold and numb, followed by the appearance of extreme pain and hyperemia upon rewarming. After rewarming, edema appears, followed by blisters and eventually a hard, dry eschar,

depending upon the severity of the injury. In the pre-hospital phase, the injured extremity should be rapidly rewarmed, unless some danger of refreezing exists. Additional details of the treatment are beyond the scope of this chapter, and they can be found elsewhere (15–18). Frostbite should be prevented by the use of proper protective clothing.

Hypothermia

In ambient air temperatures above 28°C (82.5°F), heat produced by basal metabolic processes is adequate to maintain CBT at 37°C (98.6°F). At environmental temperatures below 28°C (82.5°F), the body must produce additional heat to maintain thermoregulation. Consequently, two factors are required for hypothermia to develop, the environmental temperature must be below the CBT, and heat loss must exceed heat production. (6,9) Hypothermia is defined as a CBT below 36°C (97°F). Athletes can develop hypothermia through exposure to cold environmental air, but they are at greater risk from cold-water immersion. In spite of the high physiologic production of heat from muscle activity during sports such as swimming, kayaking, sailing, scuba diving, or rafting, athletes can experience tremendous conductive heat loss to the environment when they are immersed in cold water. Conductive heat losses may increase by five times in wet clothing and twenty-five times in water. (18) En-

Air Temperature in F (C)	Estimated Wind Speed in mph (kph)				
	0 (0)	10 (16)	20 (32)	30 (48)	
30 (-1.1)	30 (-1.1)	16 (-8.9)	4 (-15.6)	-2 (-18.9)	Little Risk
20 (-6.7)	20 (-6.7)	4 (-15.6)	-10 (-23.3)	-18 (-27.8)	
10 (-12.2)	10 (-12.2)	-9 (-22.8)	-25 (-31.7)	-33 (-36.1)	
0 (-17.8)	0 (-17.8)	-24 (-31.1)	-39 (-39.4)	-48 (-44.4)	Increased Risk
-10 (-23.3)	-10 (-23.3)	-33 (-36.1)	-53 (-47.2)	-63 (-52.8)	
-20 (-28.9)	-20 (-28.9)	-46 (-43.3)	-67 (-55)	-79 (-61.7)	Great Risk

FIG. 7.2. Wind chill index. (From Milesko-Pytel D. Helping the frostbitten patient. *Patient Care* 1983;17:90–115, with permission.)

durance athletes, by contrast, may develop hypothermia slowly through convective heat loss, especially when they are running in cold, windy conditions. Runners are especially vulnerable when they become exhausted and slow down at the end of a race, thus reducing the heat production from exercising muscles but continuing to lose heat to the environment rapidly.

Pathophysiology of Hypothermia

As in hyperthermia, hypothermia develops when thermoregulatory mechanisms are overwhelmed and the body is unable to maintain CBT within a narrow range. Factors that decrease heat production or increase heat loss will place individuals at risk for hypothermia. Risk factors for hypothermia include dehydration, fatigue, hypothyroidism, cardiovascular disease, infection, neurologic disease, alcohol or drug use, trauma, burns, and extremes of age (18). Environmental factors that place an individual at risk include cold water immersion, wind chill, and inadequate or wet clothing and/or equipment. Children are at increased risk for hypothermia because of a greater surface area to body mass ratio than adults, which increases the conductive heat loss to the environment (2).

Hypothermia is frequently categorized as mild (CBT of 34°C [93.2°F] to 36°C [96.8°F]), moderate (CBT of 30°C [86°F] to 34°C [93.2°F]), or severe (CBT <30°C [86°F]) (19). The degree of hypothermia generally parallels the severity of symptoms, but some variation may occur. Hypothermia affects the function of all body systems, but it is most apparent in the cardiovascular and neurologic systems. Symptoms of mild hypothermia reflect the body's attempt to increase heat production and to decrease heat loss. Initial signs and symptoms include shivering, tachycardia, peripheral vasoconstriction, tachypnea, cyanosis, dysarthria, ataxia, and amnesia (6,18,19). Peripheral vasoconstriction that occurs with mild hypothermia stimulates cold diuresis in response to the increasing central blood pool. The intravascular volume losses from cold diuresis may be excessive, and they can result in hypovolemic shock during rewarming as constricted peripheral vascular beds dilate. The victim who suffers from a slower onset of hypothermia generally experiences a larger cold diuresis, and thus, he or she is more likely to require larger volumes of fluid during resuscitation (6).

As CBT drops below 32°C (89.6°F), individuals begin to lose the shivering reflex and heat production falls sharply (6,18). Symptoms of moderate hypothermia include worsening cognitive function, hypotension, bradycardia, and cardiac arrhythmias. Worsening cognitive function may prevent the affected individual

from recognizing that he or she is in danger, and seeking warmth oftentimes manifests paradoxically as undressing. Severe hypothermia is associated with the loss of reflexes, stupor or coma, dilated pupils, and ventricular fibrillation. The basal metabolic rate falls by half at a CBT of 28°C (6,18). At this degree of hypothermia, the victim may actually be protected against hypoxic injury, and many cases of recovery from severe hypothermia have been reported (6).

Treatment of Hypothermia

Treatment of hypothermia necessitates early recognition and rapid rewarming, with special attention to fluid replacement. Treatment of severe hypothermia in the field, however, remains controversial. An accurate measurement of CBT is critical in diagnosing and treating hypothermia. Intravenous access and cardiac monitoring should be established quickly. Special care should be taken in the transport of the hypothermic victim to prevent precipitating ventricular fibrillation. Hypothermia increases urine output, causing cold diuresis, which may be significant (6,18). Fluid shifts caused by rewarming may reduce intravascular volume to the point of hypotension and shock. Another potentially fatal complication during rewarming is the CBT afterdrop. Afterdrop is a phenomenon of a continued drop in CBT during early rewarming. Cooling of the core may continue as cold blood from the extremities returns to the heart with early peripheral vasodilatation or as a result of cooling of the relatively warmer central blood pool as it begins to circulate through the cold peripheral tissues.

A variety of cardiac conduction abnormalities may complicate the treatment of hypothermia. In severe hypothermia, the myocardium becomes extremely irritable, to the point that minimal manipulation of the patient may precipitate fatal ventricular arrhythmias. Arrhythmias associated with hypothermia are resistant to treatment while the patient remains cold. The most common electrocardiographic change associated with hypothermia is the Osborne wave (J wave), which is named for the characteristic "J" shape that is formed by the ST segments (6,18). It is typically seen at temperatures below 32°C (89.6°F) and is reported in up to 80% of patients with CBT below 30°C (86°F) (18). Spontaneous ventricular fibrillation and asystole develop at temperatures below 28°C (82.5°F) and resist all forms of defibrillation, including electrical, chemical, and pacing. Rewarming above 28° (82.5°F) to 30°C (86°F) is required before cardioversion may be successful.

Cardiopulmonary resuscitation should be initiated for hypothermic patients with cardiac arrest follow-

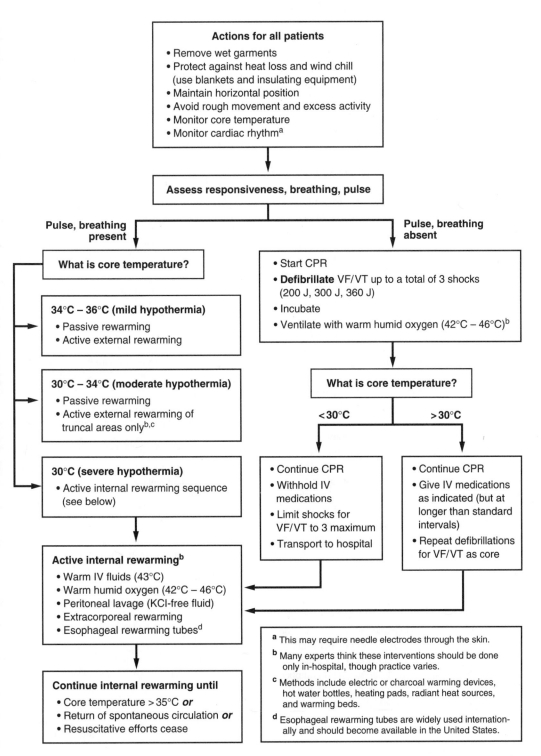

FIG. 7.3. Advanced cardiac life support hypothermia algorithm. Abbreviations: CPR, cardiopulmonary resuscitation; IV, intravenous; VF, ventricular fibrillation; VT, ventricular tachycardia.

ing advanced cardiac life support (19) and pediatric advanced life support (20) guidelines (Fig. 7.3). A commonly held belief is that severely hypothermic patients who appear dead should not be considered dead until the CBT has been returned to near normal and they continue to be unresponsive to resuscitation.

A variety of rewarming strategies exist, and they may be used in combination. Rewarming strategies may be passive or active. Passive rewarming insulates the victim from further heat loss and relies on internal thermogenesis for heat production. Active rewarming applies an extrinsic heat source to the body to increase CBT. Active rewarming measures may be external or internal, depending upon the method used. Passive rewarming is usually initiated in the field to stem the ongoing heat loss by removing wet clothing, drying the victim, and covering the victim with insulating material, such as a space blanket or sleeping bag. Active rewarming must be done with great caution, due to the risks from afterdrop and rewarming hypovolemia, and it is best initiated at an appropriate treatment facility, except under grave or extreme circumstances (6,18).

Active external rewarming techniques include chemical hot packs, which are applied to the groin, axilla, neck, and thorax; warming blankets; radiant heat lamps; and warm water baths. Active external rewarming alone is recommended for the treatment of mild hypothermia, and it should be used in combination with active internal rewarming in severely hypothermic patients (6,18). Active internal rewarming applies heat directly to the victim's core by the use of heated inhalation therapy, heated oral or intravenous fluids, peritoneal lavage, or extracorporeal blood rewarming. The method chosen for rewarming should be based upon the degree of hypothermia, the victim's cardiac status, the available equipment, and the training of the treatment personnel.

SUMMARY

Awareness of the risks associated with exercising in hot or cold environments allows athletes, parents, and coaches to ensure safe participation in recreational and sports activities. Prevention of environmental injuries should be the goal, and this is easily accomplished. Ensuring that athletes are properly dressed and equipped for the climate, well hydrated via access to proper fluids, and closely monitored in potentially dangerous environmental conditions creates a safer environment for participation.

REFERENCES

1. Bar-Or O. Temperature regulation during exercise in children and adolescents. In: Gisolfi C, Lamb DR, eds. *Perspectives in exercise sciences and sports medicine. II. Youth, exercises and sport.* Indianapolis, IN: Benchmark Press, 1989:335–367.
2. Astrand PO. *Experimental studies of physical working capacity in relation to sex and age.* Copenhagen: Munksgaard, 1952.
3. Nadel ER. Temperature regulation and hypothermia during exercise. *Clin Chest Med* 1984;5:13–20.
4. Bracker MD. Environmental and thermal injury. *Clin Sports Med* 1992;11: 419–436.
5. Armstrong LE, Maresh CM. The exertional heat illnesses: a risk of athletic participation. *Med Exerc Nutr Health* 1993;2:125–134.
6. Tom PA, Garmel GM, Auerbach PS. Environment-dependent sports emergencies. *Med Clin North Am* 1994; 78:305–325.
7. Tek D, Olshaker JS. Heat illness. *Emerg Med Clin North Am* 1992;10:299–310.
8. Hubbard RW. An introduction: the role of exercise in the etiology of exertional heatstroke. *Med Sci Sports Exerc* 1990;22:2–5.
9. American College of Sports Medicine. Position stand: heat and cold illnesses during distance running. *Med Sci Sports Exerc* 1996;28:i–x.
10. Armstrong LE, Deluca JP, Hubbard RW. Time course of recovery and heat acclimation ability of prior exertional heatstroke patients. *Med Sci Sports Exerc* 1990;22: 36–48.
11. Armstrong LE, Maresh CM. The induction and decay of heat acclimation in trained athletes. *Sports Med* 1991; 12:303–312.
12. Nielsen B. Heat stress and acclimation. *Ergonomics* 1994;37:49–58.
13. American College of Sports Medicine. Position stand: exercise and fluid replacement. *Med Sci Sports Exerc* 1996;28:i–vii.
14. Harker J, Gibson P. Heat-stroke: a review of rapid cooling techniques. *Intensive Crit Care Nurs* 1995;11: 198–202.
15. Smith DJ, Robson MC, Heggars JP. Frostbite and other cold-induced injuries. In: Auerbach PS, Geehn EC, eds. *Management of wilderness and environmental emergencies,* 2nd ed. St Louis: Mosby, 1989:101–116.
16. Heggars JP, Robson RC, Manavalen K, et al. Experimental and clinical observations on frostbite. *Ann Emerg Med* 1987;16:1056–1062.
17. Milesko-Pytel D. Helping the frostbitten patient. *Patient Care* 1983;17:90–115.
18. Danzl DF, Pozos RS, Hamlet MP. Accidental hypothermia. In: Auerbach PS, ed. *Wilderness medicine: management of wilderness and environmental emergencies,* 3rd ed. St. Louis: Mosby, 1995:51–103.
19. American Heart Association. *Advanced cardiac life support.* Dallas, TX: American Heart Association, 1997.
20. American Heart Association. *PALS provider manual.* Dallas, TX: American Heart Association, 2002.

8

Protective and Supportive Equipment

Richard B. Birrer and Marcia K. Anderson

Protective equipment is often necessary in a variety of sports to protect the athlete from injury and to protect an existing injury from additional trauma. The efficacy of the equipment, however, is limited by the skill, strength, and speed of the athlete, all of which can be augmented by the sense of security imparted by the equipment and the aggression at play (1). The responsibility for the integrity of protective equipment (condition, cleanliness, fit, and use) resides with the certified athletic trainer.

From a liability point of view, a manufacturer's information materials (e.g., brochures and warrantees) should be catalogued for reference in case an injury occurs after the equipment has been purchased. Even when an athlete provides his or her own protective equipment, the responsibilities of the athletic trainer do not change. The athletic trainer still must ensure that the equipment meets safety standards and that it is fitted properly, used appropriately, properly maintained, and cleaned. Athletic trainers and coaches should not allow an athlete to wear any equipment or to alter any equipment that may endanger the individual or other team members.

Injuries secondary to poor technique, inadequate conditioning, the low tolerance of a player to injury, poor quality maintenance or cleanliness of protective equipment, poor technique, poorly matched player levels, a previously injured area that is now vulnerable to reinjury, and an inability to protect an area adequately without restricting motion can be prevented by using the appropriate protective equipment. Table 8.1 lists equipment design factors that are important in mitigating the size and severity of injury. Style, cost, size, comfort, tradition, long-term maintenance costs, and appearance are less significant factors.

MATERIALS

The efficacy of protective equipment is largely determined by the density, thickness, and temperature of the energy-absorbing material. Soft low-density materials (neoprene, foam, gauze padding, Sorbothane, moleskin, and felt) are light and comfortable to wear, but they are ineffective at high impact intensities. Firmer density materials of the same thickness, while they are less comfortable and less cushioned, can absorb more energy by deformation; and therefore, they are the materials of choice for high-impact intensity levels. Examples include casting materials, such as plaster or fiberglass, and high-density materials, such as thermomoldable plastics (e.g., Orthoplast and Thermoplast) (Fig. 8.1). While nonresilient or slow recovery resilient materials offer the best protection to areas subject to occasional or one-time impacts, choosing highly resilient materials that regain their shape after impact in areas subject to repeated trauma may be more appropriate.

Neoprene sleeves provide therapeutic warmth; support for chronic injuries, such as quadriceps or hamstrings tears; and uniform compression. Nylon-coated rubber material is comfortable, it allows full mobility, it provides better absorption of sweat, it causes less skin breakdown, and it supplies the athlete with proprioceptive feedback in the affected area. The impact forces associated with running and walking are

TABLE 8.1. *Equipment design factors that can reduce potential injury*

Increase the impact area.
Transfer or disperse the impact area to another body part.
Limit the relative motion of a body part.
Add mass to the body part to limit deformation and displacement.
Reduce friction between contacting surfaces.
Absorb energy.
Resist the absorption of bacteria, fungus, and viruses.

From Anderson MK, Hall SJ, Martin M. *Sports Injury Management,* 2nd ed. Philadelphia: Lippincott Williams & Wilkins, 2000, with permission.

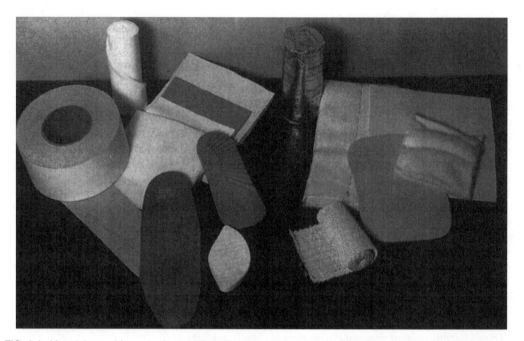

FIG. 8.1. Materials used in protective padding. Examples of low-density material used to cushion low-level impact forces include moleskin, gauze padding, foam materials, neoprene, Sorbothane, and felt **(left)**. Examples of high-density materials, such as thermomoldable plastics and casting materials **(right)**, that can absorb more energy by deformation and thus transfer less stress to an injured area. (From Anderson MK, Hall SJ, Martin M. *Sports injury management*, 2nd ed. Philadelphia: Lippincott Williams & Wilkins, 2000, with permission.)

largely absorbed and dissipated by Sorbothane insoles. Felt (¼ to 1 inch thick) absorbs perspiration but, in doing so, has less of a tendency to move under stress and must oftentimes be replaced daily. Moleskin is useful for friction spots to reduce skin irritation or blisters since its adhesive bonding on one side prevents any movement once it has been applied to the skin. Foam (1/8 to 1 inch thick) ranges in density from a very soft, open-cell foam to a denser, closed-cell foam. Like a sponge in which air passage is possible from cell to cell, open-cell foam absorbs fluids, and it is commonly used to pad bony prominences or to protect the skin under the hard edges of protective equipment or custom-fabricated pads. Because deformation occurs quickly under stress, open-cell foams do not have good shock-absorbing qualities. On the other hand, closed-cell foam, because it does not allow air passage from one cell to another, rebounds and returns to its original shape quickly; and it thus is better for shock absorbance. However, at low levels of impact, it may not be as comfortable as open-cell foam next to the skin.

Layering materials of varying density that combine open- and closed-cell foam in polyurethane or nylon can provide maximal shock absorption. Soft, lower density material placed next to the skin that is covered by increasingly denser, closed-cell material away from the skin absorbs and disperses higher intensity blows. Thus, higher intensity external blows are dispersed by closed-cell material, and soft, lower density material is placed closest to the skin. The entire pad is airtight, preventing quick deformation of the foam, so energy is dissipated over the entire surface of the pad. Such air management pads are frequently used in football for shoulder protection; but they are expensive, and they require extensive maintenance if the nylon covering is torn because air can then pass into the pads, thereby reducing their effectiveness. These liners must be replaced or patched. Nylon prevents the absorption of perspiration or water, thus helping to avoid additional weight and facilitating cleansing with a weak bleach solution. Certain dense foams are thermomoldable, allowing shaping to any body part when heated. They then retain this new shape when cooled. Such pads can be used repeatedly to immobilize a body structure, to absorb shock, and to deflect impact. The pad is secured to the body part with elastic or nonelastic tape.

Hard materials, such as thermoplastics are divided into the two categories of plastic and rubber. Rubber-like materials use a polyisoprene base; they include Ultraform Traditions, Synergy, Orthoplast, and Aquaplast Greenstrip. The plastic group uses a poly-caprolactone base with varying amounts of inorganic elastomer filler and resins to affect the durability, memory, and stiffness of the material. This category tends to conform better than the rubber-type, and it is more appropriate for small splints, such as those applied to the hand. Examples of plastic materials include Orfit, Orthoplast II, Multiform I and II, and Aquaplast Bluestripe.

Most of these materials are heated for 1 minute while lying flat at temperatures between 150°F (65°C) and 180°F (81.4°C). The material is then shaped for 3 to 4 minutes before it returns to a hardened form. Minor changes can be made with a heat gun, but these should never be performed while the splint is on the athlete.

Casting materials, such as plaster or fiberglass, provide the best body part splinting. However, allergic contact dermatitis, rashes, infections, blisters, macerations, burns, and ulcerations can result from extended use. Fiberglass casts with a stockinette or cast padding can limit moisture, but they must be dried, usually with a hair dryer to prevent odor, maceration, and itching. A new Gore-Tex liner that is directly applied to the skin can be used under fiberglass to repel water and permit evaporation, thus allowing sweating, bathing, hydrotherapy, and swimming, without any special drying of the cast or skin. Fiberglass casting material applied over such a liner does not have to be changed as often because it remains more comfortable throughout the immobilization period; however, it is slightly more expensive than traditional casts.

REGULATION AND CERTIFICATION

The use of soft and hard materials to protect the body area is determined by specific rules developed by the National Federation of State High School Associations (NFSHSA) and the National Collegiate Athletic Association (NCAA) (2). Abrasive, unyielding, or hard substances may be used on the hand, wrist, forearm, or elbow, if the substance is covered on all exterior surfaces with no less than ½-inch thick, high-density, closed-cell polyurethane or a material of the same minimum thickness and similar physical properties. The athlete must have a written authorization form signed by a licensed medical physician that indicates the cast or splint is necessary to protect the body part. The onsite referee is responsible for the review of all such forms and the application of such standards prior to the start of the competition. If the referee cannot verify that the material is properly padded according to the guidelines, he or she has the right to eject the player if the athlete uses the cast or splint as a weapon.

The National Operating Committee on Standards for Athletic Equipment (NOCSAE) sets the standards for baseball, football, softball, and lacrosse helmets and masks for the toleration of certain forces when they are applied to different areas of the helmet or mask. Other testing agencies for protective equipment include The American Society for Testing Material (ASTM) and the Hockey Equipment Certification Council (HECC) of the Canadian Standards Association (CSA). These agencies have established material standards for equipment, such as ice hockey helmets and face masks and protective eyewear. In addition, athletic governing bodies, including the NFSHSA, the NCAA, United States Olympic Committee (USOC), and the National Association of Intercollegiate Athletics (NAIA), establish rules for the mandatory use of specific protective equipment and determine rules governing the use of special protective equipment.

HEAD AND FACE

The regular use of properly fitted helmets and facial protective devices, such as ear wear, eyewear, face masks, throat protectors, and mouthguards prevent many significant head and facial injuries (3,4,5). In particular, helmets are required in football, baseball, softball, men's lacrosse, ice hockey, white water sports (kayaking), amateur boxing, snowmobiling, martial arts, and bicycling (6).

Helmets

Football Helmets

Football helmets must be approved by NOCSAE. Helmet face protection must be no less than two bars, according to interscholastic and intercollegiate athletic governing bodies. The single bar does not meet minimum protection standards and should not be allowed on the helmet. Since heat can alter the effectiveness of shock absorption of the liner in some shell materials, the materials compress more easily, and they absorb less shock at higher temperatures. Players must inspect helmets on a daily basis to ensure adequate inflation for the maintenance of proper fit. A warning label on the exterior shell of all new and reconditioned helmets by NOCSAE should be clearly visible. The athletic trainer and coach should continually warn athletes of the risks involved in football and should ensure that the helmet is properly used within the guidelines and rules of the game.

The manufacturer's guidelines should always be followed when fitting a football helmet (Table 8.2). Once it is fitted, however, the helmet should be checked daily for proper fit, which can be altered by the loss of air from cells, hair length, the spread of the face mask, and the deterioration of internal padding. Inspection is performed by inserting a tongue depressor between the pads and face. When the depressor is moved back and forth, a firm resistance should be felt. A well-fitted helmet should not move in one direction when the head moves in another. Finally, the helmet should be checked weekly by the athletic trainer to ensure compliance with safety standards for proper fitting (Table 8.3). All helmets should have the

TABLE 8.2. *Proper fitting of a football helmet*

The player should have a haircut in the style that will be worn during the competitive season; the player should wet his hair to simulate game conditions. Measure the circumference of the head above the ears, using the tape measure supplied by the manufacturer. The suggested helmet size is listed on the reverse side of the tape.

Select the proper sized shell and adjust the front and back sizers and jaw pads for a proper fit.

Inflate the air bladder by holding the bulb with an arch in the hose; to deflate, the hose must be in a straight position.

Ensure that the helmet fits snugly around the player's head and covers the base of the skull but does not impinge the cervical spine when the neck is extended. The ear holes should match up with the external auditory ear canal.

   Check that the four-point chin strap is of equal tension and length on both sides, placing the chin pad an equal distance from each side of the helmet.

   Ensure that the face mask allows for a complete field of vision and that the helmet is one to two finger widths above the eyebrows and extends two finger widths away from the forehead and nose.

   Watch that the helmet does not move when the athlete presses forward on the rear of the helmet and for straight down on the top of the helmet.

   Test that the helmet does not slip when the athlete is asked to "bull" his neck, while the face mask is grasped, pulling left, then right.

From Anderson MK, Hall SJ, Martin M. *Sports Injury Management,* 2nd ed. Philadelphia: Lippincott Williams & Wilkins, 2000, with permission.

TABLE 8.3. *Weekly helmet inspection checklist*

Check proper fit according to manufacturer's guidelines.

Examine the shell for cracks, particularly around the holes. Replace the shell, if any cracks are detected.

Test all mounting rivets, screws, Velcro, and snaps for breakage, sharp edges, and/or looseness. Repair or replace as necessary.

Replace the face mask if bare metal is visible or if it has a broken weld or is grossly misshapen.

Check and replace any parts that are damaged, such as jaw pads, sweatbands, nose snubbers, and chin straps.

Examine the chin strap for proper shape and fit; inspect the hardware to see if it needs replacement.

Inspect shell according to NOCSAE[a] and manufacturer's standards; only approved paints, waxes, decals, or cleaning agents are to be used on any helmet. Severe or delayed reaction to the substances may permanently damage the shell and affect its safety performance.

If air-filled and fluid-filled helmets are used and the team travels to a different altitude, recheck the fit prior to use.

[a]Abbreviation: NOCSAE, National Operating Committee on Standards for Athletic Equipment.

From Anderson MK, Hall SJ, Martin M. *Sports Injury Management,* 2nd ed. Philadelphia: Lippincott Williams & Wilkins, 2000, with permission.

purchase date and tracking number engraved on the inside. The purchase date, reconditioning history, use, and certification seals should be part of a detailed record that is kept on file by the athletic trainer. The athlete should be instructed on proper fit, use, and care of the helmet. A statement that confirms that he or she has read the NOCSAE seal and has been informed of the risk of injury through improper use of the helmet or face mask when striking an opponent should be signed, dated, and kept as part of the player's medical files.

Ice Hockey Helmets

Like football helmets, ice hockey helmets reduce head injuries, but they do not prevent neck injuries due to axial loading. Studies have shown that the risk of spinal cord injury, especially quadriplegia, may be as much as three times greater in hockey than in American football. Headfirst contact with the boards secondary to a push or check from behind, is the major mechanism for this injury. The ASTM and HECC, in conjunction with the CSA, monitor ice hockey helmet standards. Proper fit is achieved when a snug fitting helmet does not move in one direction when the head is turned in the other. The full-face guard may be wire, mesh, or clear polycarbonate.

Batting Helmets

Softball and baseball require batting helmets with NOCSAE certification, and they must have a double earflap design. A thick layer of foam between the primary energy absorber and the head that allows the shell to move slightly and to deform is recommended, as it thus prevents excessive pressure on the cranium from the kinetic energy of missile trauma. The helmet should be snug enough so that it does not move or fall during batting and running the bases.

Other Helmets

Lacrosse helmets are mandatory in the men's game and optional in the women's game, and they are also worn by field hockey goalies. These helmets must meet NOCSAE standards. The helmet, wire face mask, and chin pad are secured with a four-point chin strap. The helmet should not move in one direction when the head moves in another.

An effective bicycle helmet has a plastic or fiberglass rigid shell with a chin strap and an energy-absorbing foam liner (3,7). Mini-shell and no-shell Lycra-covered (expanded polystyrene layer) helmets are lighter, attractive alternatives. Stiffer shells result in better diffusion and resilience to impact. Due to ventilation ports, today's helmets are more lightweight and aerodynamic than ever before, without increasing thermal discomfort to the body or head or any additional impact on core temperature, head skin temperature, thermal sensation, sweat rate, heart rate, and overall perceived exertion. Helmets are rated as American National Standards Institute Z90.4 (minimum for racing), Snell Memorial Foundation B95 (stringent), and ASTM (industry favorite).

A variety of closed-foam helmets have been designed for the martial arts so that not only the head, but also the face and chin, fit snugly. If a plastic or fiberglass head shell is worn, then polycarbonate eyewear is also recommended in all contact forms of the martial arts, as well as competitive tournament situations, even if the styles are considered low or noncontact.

Face Masks

Face masks vary in size and style, and their purpose is to protect and shield the facial region from projectiles. The standards for strength and deflection for football face guards worn at the high school and college levels have been set by NOCSAE. When the face mask is properly fitted, it should extend 1 to 2 finger widths away from the forehead and should allow for the complete field of vision (Table 8.4). No facial protection should be less than two bars, and eye shields made of Plexiglas or polycarbonate can be attached to the face mask as necessary.

Ice hockey face masks are made of steel wire, clear plastic (polycarbonate), or a combination of the two; and they must meet ASTM and HECC standards. Use of full-coverage face masks in amateur ice hockey has greatly reduced facial trauma from penetration of the hockey stick; flying pucks; and collisions with elbows, helmets, sideboards, and the ice. The use of a single chin strap, however, still allows the helmet to ride back on the head when a force is directed to the frontal region, thus exposing the chin to lacerations. The mask stands approximately 1 to 1½ inches away from the nose. If wire mesh is used, the hole should be small enough to prevent penetration by hockey sticks.

Lacrosse face masks must meet NOCSAE standards. The wire mesh mask stands away from the face, but the four-point chin strap has a padded chin region in case the mask is driven back during a collision with another player (Fig. 8.2). Full face masks have been required for youth and high school players since 1975; the Eastern Collegiate Athletic Confer-

TABLE 8.4. *Fitting mouth-formed mouthguards*

Submerge the mouthguard (not the loop strap) in boiling water for 20 to 25 s. Shake off excess water, but do not rinse the mouthguard in cold water as this decreases pliability.

Place the mouthguard directly in the mouth over the upper dental arch. Center the mouthguard with the thumbs, using the loop strap as a guide.

Close the mouth, but do not bring the teeth together or bite down on the mouthguard. Place the tongue on the roof of the mouth and *suck* as hard as possible for 15 to 25 s. The sucking mechanism acts as a vacuum to mold the mouthguard around the teeth and gums.

Rinse the mouthguard in cold water to harden the material. Check the finished product for any significant indentations. If any imperfections or errors are noted, do not reheat the mouthguard as this decreases its effectiveness. Select a new mouthguard and repeat the process.

From Anderson MK, Hall SJ, Martin M. *Sports Injury Management*, 2nd ed. Philadelphia: Lippincott Williams & Wilkins, 2000, with permission.

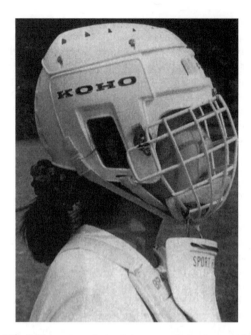

FIG. 8.2. Lacrosse helmet. Lacrosse helmets provide full face and neck protection. (From Anderson MK, Hall SJ, Martin M. *Sports injury management*, 2nd ed. Philadelphia: Lippincott Williams & Wilkins, 2000, with permission.)

ence required usage in 1977 and the NCAA, in 1980. For catchers and home plate umpires in baseball and softball, face masks should fit snugly to the forehead and cheeks, while not impairing vision. Such devices can also be used by players in the field, and they must meet ASTM standards. Men and women's fencing masks have an adjustable spring to prevent the mask from moving during competition.

Eyewear

No interscholastic or intercollegiate sport requires protective eyewear, despite the fact that such injuries are frequent and are almost always preventable (8,9). Goggles, face shields, and spectacles are the three types of protective eye wear (Fig. 8.3). Face shields are usually preferred by athletes wearing contact lenses because less chance exists for a finger or hand to hit the eye. Spectacles or eyeglasses contain the lenses, frame, and side shields that are commonly seen in industrial eye protective wear, and they may be single units or separate. Such lenses should be 3 mm thick and should be made from CR 39 plastic or polycarbonate, both of which can be incorporated with prescription lenses. Only polycarbonate eye protectors and eye frames that meet ASTM and the parallel CSA standards offer enough protection for a sport participant, particularly those playing racquetball, in which the ball reaches 90 miles per hour or 40 m per second. Single-unit face frames without lenses are not recommended. Eye protection is appropriate for soccer, basketball, baseball, football, and cycling.

Athletes with vision in only one eye should wear maximum eye protection during all practices and competitions, after they have been cleared by a physician. The use of a sweatband to keep sweat out of the eye guard may be helpful. Although many athletes wear contact lenses to improve astigmatism and peripheral vision and to avoid clouding during temperature changes, they do not protect against eye injury. Hard contact lenses that cover only the iris of the eye often become dislodged, and they are more frequently associated with irritation from foreign bodies (i.e., corneal abrasions). Foreign matter, particularly dust, may get underneath the lenses and may damage the cornea, or the cornea may be scratched while the in-

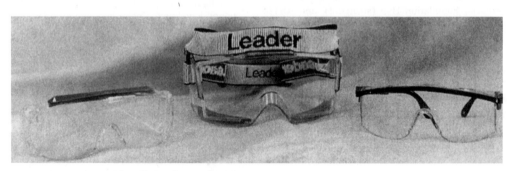

FIG. 8.3. Eye protectors. Protective eyewear should be made from polycarbonate, which is lightweight, scratch-resistant, and impact-resistant, and should meet American Society for Testing Material or Canadian Standards Association standards. (From Anderson MK, Hall SJ, Martin M. *Sports injury management*, 2nd ed. Philadelphia: Lippincott Williams & Wilkins, 2000, with permission.)

dividual is inserting or removing the lens. Soft contact lenses protect the eye from irritation by chlorine and pools, although the wearing of soft lenses while swimming is not recommended despite research that shows that soft lenses adhere to the cornea while in pool water, thus reducing the risk of loss. Further, microorganisms found in pool water, especially *Acanthamoeba*, are responsible for a rare, but serious, keratitis. Wearing goggles and waiting 20 to 30 minutes after leaving the water to remove the contact lenses or using saline drops if the lenses must be removed earlier can achieve protection against this infection. This period of time allows the lens to stop sticking to the cornea. The lenses should then be immediately disinfected.

Ear Protectors

Wrestling, boxing, martial arts, and water polo require specialized ear protection from repeated trauma and friction to the ear that can lead to a permanent deformity called hematoma auris (e.g., cauliflower ear, scrum ear, and wrestler's ear). Proper fit is achieved when the chin strap is snug and the headgear does not move during contact with another player. The protective ear cup should be deep enough so as not to compress the external ear. Ear protection is also essential for target and/or skeet shooting.

Mouthguards

A readily visible intraoral mouthguard is required in all intercollegiate and interscholastic football, field hockey, men's and women's lacrosse, and ice hockey (10). The guard usually attaches to the player's face mask or chin piece by a safety strap. Dental and oral soft tissue injuries and, to a lesser extent, cerebral concussions, temporomandibular joint fractures, and jaw fractures, have been significantly reduced by the use of a properly fitted mouthguard across the upper teeth that absorbs energy, disperses impact, keeps the upper lip away from the incisive edges of the teeth, and cushions contact between the upper and lower teeth. The practice of cutting down mouthguards to cover only the front four teeth voids the manufacturer's warranty because this cannot prevent many dental injuries and it can lead to airway obstruction if the mouthguard becomes dislodged. Thermal set mouth-formed mouthguards are the most frequently used, and they consist of a firm outer shell fit with a softer inner material. When properly fitted, such mouthguards virtually match the efficacy and comfort of a custom-made guard. These mouthguards are

relatively easy to find and inexpensive, and they have a loop strap for attachment to a face mask. The latter has the following two advantages: it prevents individuals from choking on the mouthguard, and it prevents the individual from losing the mouthguard when it is ejected from the mouth. Because such guards often lack full extension into the buccal and labial vestibules, they do not provide adequate protection against oral soft tissue injuries. Finally, the thermoplastic inner material loses its elasticity at mouth temperature, which may cause the protector to loosen. Table 8.4 lists the proper fitting of a thermoplastic mouth-formed mouthguard.

The pressure-formed laminated type of mouth protector is the most effective, but it is also the most expensive; proper fitting requires special training in order to obtain the best results. Vacuum-formed mouthguards are less expensive and are easier to mold. Because of the low heat used in their construction, however, their fit can be compromised by an elastic memory at mouth temperatures, thus making speaking and unrestricted breathing more difficult.

A mouthguard should be thoroughly rinsed with water after each use and should be placed in a plastic mouthguard retainer box to air dry. Periodically, it should be soaked overnight in a weak bleach solution (10 parts water to 1 part bleach).

THROAT AND NECK PROTECTORS

The NCAA requires that catchers in softball and baseball wear a built-in or attachable throat guard on their masks. Those playing field hockey, ice hockey, and lacrosse should also wear fencing masks and helmets to provide anterior neck protection.

Cervical neck rolls and collars (e.g., Cowboy collar, Long Horn neck roll, LaPorta collar) limit motion of the cervical spine, and they are effective in protecting players who have histories of repetitive stingers or burners. However, properly fitted shoulder pads are perhaps the most critical factor in preventing brachial plexus injuries. The collars do not increase the axial load on the cervical spine when the neck is flexed during a tackle.

SHOULDER PROTECTION

The following three types of football shoulder pads are available: flat, cantilevered, and channel. Flat shoulder pads are lightweight, and they provide less protection to the shoulder region but allow more glenohumeral joint motion. Therefore, quarterbacks or receivers who must raise their arms above the head

TABLE 8.5. *Fitting football shoulder pads*

Determine the chest girth measurement at the nipple line or measure the distance between shoulder tips. Select pads that are based on the player's position. Place the pads on the shoulders and tighten all straps and laces. The laces should be pulled together until touching. The straps should have equal tension and should be as tight as functionally tolerable to ensure proper force distribution over the pads. Tension on the straps should prevent no more than two fingers from being inserted under the strap. The entire clavicle should be covered and protected by the pads. If the clavicles can be palpated without moving the pads, refit with a smaller pad.

Anterior view. The laces should be centered over the sternum, with no gap between the two halves. The acromioclavicular joint, clavicles, and pectoral muscles should be fully covered. Caps should cover the upper portion of the arch and entire deltoid muscle.

Posterior view. The entire scapula and trapezius should be covered, with the lower pad arch extending below the inferior angle of the scapula to adequately protect the latissimus dorsi adequately. The laces should be pulled tight and should be centered over the spine.

With the arms abducted, the neck opening should not be uncomfortable or pinch the neck. Finally, inspection should include the shoulder pads, with the helmet and jersey in place, to ensure that no impingement of the cervical region is present.

From Anderson MK, Hall SJ, Martin M. *Sports Injury Management,* 2nd ed. Philadelphia: Lippincott Williams & Wilkins, 2000, with permission.

to throw or to catch a pass favor them. Cantilever pads have a hard plastic bridge over the superior aspect of the shoulder to protect the acromioclavicular (AC) joint. These bridges are lightweight, they distribute impact forces throughout the entire shoulder girdle, and they allow the maximum range of motion at the shoulder. Because of its protective capacity, it is preferred by linemen. The channel system incorporates both types, with impact forces placed entirely on the anterior and posterior aspects of the shoulder. The particular choice of football shoulder pads for an individual should be based on the player's medical history, body type, and playing position. The general steps used in fitting football shoulder pads are outlined in Table 8.5.

ELBOW, FOREARM, WRIST, AND HAND PROTECTION

In high school and collegiate play, no rigid material can be worn at the elbow or below, unless it is cov-

ered on all sides by closed-cell foam padding. A counterforce forearm brace may be worn by certain individuals with lateral epicondylitis to reduce tensile forces in the wrist extensors, particularly the extensor carpi radialis brevis. While some pain relief may be noted on return to play, considerable controversy exists about the effectiveness of counterforce forearm straps. Such straps should not be used for other causes of elbow pain, most especially growth plate problems in children and adolescents. The forearm, wrist, and hand are especially vulnerable to external forces and are often neglected when protective equip-

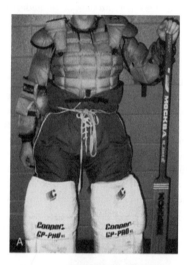

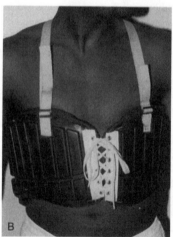

FIG. 8.4. Chest and rib protection. **A:** Several sports require extensive chest protection (e.g., ice hockey). **B:** Rib protectors absorb impact forces caused during tackling. (From Anderson MK, Hall SJ, Martin M. *Sports injury management,* 2nd ed. Philadelphia: Lippincott Williams & Wilkins, 2000, with permission.)

ment is considered. A wide variety of specialized gloves, pads, and splints are available for collision and contact sports (11–14). Newer sports, such as rollerblading, roller hockey, and skateboarding, should include this protection.

RIB, THORAX, AND ABDOMINAL PROTECTION

Catchers in softball and baseball wear full thoracic and abdominal protectors to prevent high-speed blows from a bat or ball. Individuals in fencing, martial arts, and boxing and goalies in many sports wear full thoracic protectors. Quarterbacks and wide receivers in football often wear rib protectors composed of air-inflated, interconnected cylinders whose purpose is to absorb the impact forces caused by tackling (Fig. 8.4).

SPORT BRAS

Despite the fact that sport bras (Fig. 8.5) are designed to prevent excessive vertical and horizontal breast motion during exercise, many women continue to experience sore, tender breasts after exercise. Girls and women with small breasts may not need a special bra. Women with a size C cup or larger need a firm durable supportive bra that has nonslip straps and no irritating seams or fasteners next to the skin. A Lycra/poly/cotton fabric is a popular blend seen in sport bras. In hot weather, an additional outer layer of textured nylon mesh can promote natural cooling of the skin. In sports requiring significant overhead motion, bra straps should stretch to prevent the bra from riding up over the breasts. In activities in which overhead motion is not a significant part of the activity, nonstress straps connected directly to a nonelastic cup are preferable. Women with medium-sized breasts generally prefer compressive bras that bind the breasts to the chest wall.

LUMBAR AND SACRAL PROTECTION

Abdominal binders, weight training belts, and other similar support devices support the abdominal contents, stabilize the trunk, and prevent spinal deformity or injury during heavy lifting. Use of binders or belts significantly increases intraabdominal pressure to reduce compressive forces in the vertebral bodies and lessens the risk of low back strain.

HIP AND BUTTOCK PROTECTION

Special pads that are usually composed of hard polyethylene covered with layers of Ensolite are designed to protect the iliac crest, coccyx, sacrum, and genital region in collision and contact sports. A girdle with special pockets can hold the pads in place effectively. A protective cup placed in the athletic supporter provides the best protection for the male genital region. The female genital region should be similarly protected in activities such as full contact martial arts or high-speed water surfing.

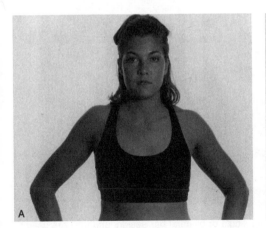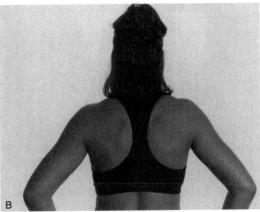

FIG. 8.5. Sport bras. Sport bras made from nonelastic material, with wide shoulder straps and wide bands under the breasts, provide upward support by compressing the breasts against the rib cage. **A:** Anterior view. **B:** Posterior view. (From Anderson MK, Hall SJ, Martin M. *Sports injury management*, 2nd ed. Philadelphia: Lippincott Williams & Wilkins, 2000, with permission.)

THIGH PROTECTION

Girdles with ready-made pockets can be used to prevent injury to the quadriceps area. Thigh pads should be placed over the quadriceps muscle group, approximately 6 to 7 inches proximal to the patella. Genital injury can be avoided by placing the larger flare of an asymmetrical thigh pad on the lateral aspect of the thigh. Neoprene sleeves can provide uniform compression, support for quadriceps or hamstring strains, and therapeutic warmth.

KNEE AND PATELLA PROTECTION

The knee, which is second only to the ankle and foot in incidence of injury, sustains frequent contusions and abrasions during collisions or falls. Frictional injuries also occur to the prepatellar and infrapatellar bursae. The following are the three functional categories of knee braces: functional (FKB), rehabilitative (RKB) and prophylactic (PKB) (Fig. 8.6) (15). FKBs are widely used to protect moderate anterior cruciate ligament (ACL) injuries or in cases of postsurgical ACL repair or reconstruction. RKBs provide absolute immobilization at a selected angle after surgery, permit controlled range of motion through predetermined arcs, and prevent accidental loading in non–weight-bearing patients. PKBs are designed to protect the medial collateral ligament (MCL) by redirecting a lateral valgus force away from the joint itself to more distal points on the tibia and femur.

Two basic styles of ACL or derotational braces are found—hinge–post-shell and hinge–post-strap. Their performance depends on the magnitude of the anterior shear load and the internal torque applied across the tibiofemoral joint, and it may be affected by several factors (Table 8.6). These braces provide protection for individuals with mild to moderate degrees of instability who participate in activities with low or moderate load potential. They do not guarantee increased stability in those sports that require cutting, pivoting, or other quick changes in direction.

The two general types of PKBs include lateral and bilateral bar designs. The American Academy of Orthopedic Surgeons has concluded that the routine use of available PKBs has not been proven effective in reducing either the number or severity of knee injuries and that, in some instances, such use may have been

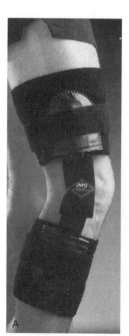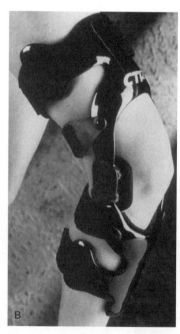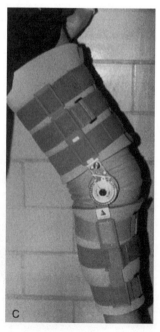

FIG. 8.6. Knee braces. **A:** Prophylactic knee braces may be single or bilateral bar design, and they are used to protect the medial collateral ligament. **B:** Functional knee braces control tibial translation and rotational stress, relative to the femur, and they can provide extension limitations to protect the anterior cruciate ligament. **C:** Rehabilitative braces provide absolute or relative immobilization following surgery. (From Anderson MK, Hall SJ, Martin M. *Sports injury management*, 2nd ed. Philadelphia: Lippincott Williams & Wilkins, 2000, with permission.)

TABLE 8.6. *Factors affecting functional knee braces*

The technique of attachment
The design of the brace:
   Hinge design
   Materials of fabrication
   Geometry of the attachment interface
   Mechanism of attachment
Variables in the attachment interface:
   How the interface molds around the soft-tissue
     contours of the limb
   How much displacement occurs between the rigid
     brace and compliant soft tissues surrounding the
     distal femur and proximal tibia while loads are
     applied across the knee

From Anderson MK, Hall SJ, Martin M. *Sports Injury Management,* 2nd ed. Philadelphia: Lippincott Williams & Wilkins, 2000, with permission.

a contributing factor to the injury. Therefore, clinicians should base decisions on PKB use on the individual needs of the athlete. Finally, decisions to use any of the three major categories of knee braces should rest with the supervising physician or surgeon. Selection should be based on the projected objectives, the cost effectiveness, and the fit needs of the participant, relative to the sport's demands, the durability, and comfort.

Patellar braces are designed to dissipate force, to improve patellar tracking, and to maintain patellar alignment. They relieve anterior knee pain syndrome. An alternative brace for treating patellar pain is the strap worn over the infrapatellar ligament (Fig. 8.7).

LOWER LEG PROTECTION

A wide variety of commercial designs are available to protect the anterior tibia and ankle malleoli. They utilize pads that consist of a hard deflective outer layer and an inner layer of thin foam. Velcro stirrups and straps help stabilize the pad inside the sock.

ANKLE AND FOOT PROTECTION

A large number of commercial ankle braces that can be used to prevent or support a postinjury ankle sprain are available. These braces come in the following three categories: semirigid orthosis, air bladder brace, and lace-up brace (Fig. 8.8). Only inversion and eversion are limited with a semirigid orthosis; a lace-up brace can limit all ankle motions (16). Ankle braces are more effective than adhesive tape in reducing ankle injuries, they are easier for the wearer to apply independently, they provide better comfort and support, they are more cost effective and comfortable to wear, and they do not produce some of the skin ir-

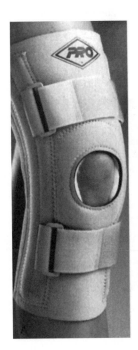
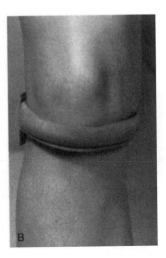

FIG. 8.7. Patellofemoral braces. **A:** A horseshoe-type silicone or felt pad sewn into a sleeve can relieve chronic patella pain. **B:** A strap worn over the infrapatellar ligament may also relieve patellar pain. (From Anderson MK, Hall SJ, Martin M. *Sports injury management,* 2nd ed. Philadelphia: Lippincott Williams & Wilkins, 2000, with permission.)

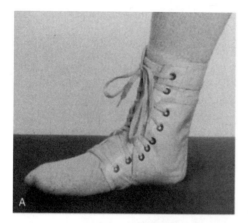

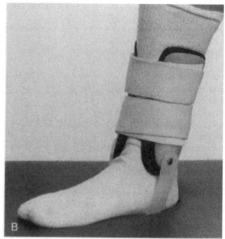

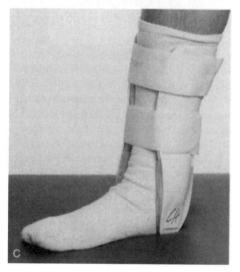

FIG. 8.8. Ankle protectors. Commercial designs include the lace-up brace **(A)**, the semirigid orthrosis **(B)**, and the air bladder brace **(C)**. (From Anderson MK, Hall SJ, Martin M. *Sports injury management*, 2nd ed. Philadelphia: Lippincott Williams & Wilkins, 2000, with permission.)

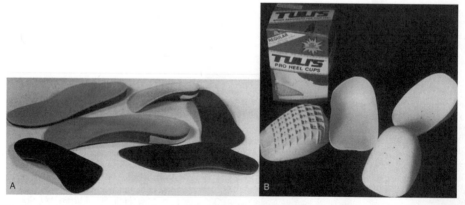

FIG. 8.9. Foot and heel protection. **A:** Semirigid orthotics provide stability and support to the intrinsic structures of the foot. **B:** Heel cups are used to reduce tissue shearing and shock in the calcaneal region. (From Anderson MK, Hall SJ, Martin M. *Sports injury management*, 2nd ed. Philadelphia: Lippincott Williams & Wilkins, 2000, with permission.)

ritations that are associated with adhesive tape. Furthermore, the maximal tensile strength from ankle strapping is lost after 20 minutes or so of exercise.

Innersoles, semirigid orthotics, and rigid orthotics can be successfully used to pad and support fallen arches, medial tibial stress syndrome, pronated feet,

TABLE 8.7. *Factors in the selection and fit of athletic shoes*

Fit shoes toward late afternoon or evening, preferably after a workout, and wear socks typically worn during sport participation.

Fit shoes to the longest toe of the largest foot, providing one thumb's width to the end of the toe box.

The widest part of the shoe should coincide with the widest part of the foot. Eyelets should be at least 1 in. apart, with normal lacing. Women with big or wider feet should consider purchasing boy's and men's shoes.

The sole of the shoe should provide moderate support, but it should not be too rigid. Sole tread typically comes in a horizontal bar (commonly used on asphalt or concrete) or waffle design (used on off-road terrain).

The midsole may be composed of ethylene vinyl acetate (EVA), polyurethane, or, preferably, a combination of the two. EVA provides good cushioning, but it will break down over time. Polyurethane has minimal compressibility and provides good durability and stability.

A thermoplastic heel counter maintains its shape and firmness, even in adverse weather conditions.

Running shoes should position the heel at least 0.5 in. above the outsole to minimize stretch on the Achilles tendon.

While wearing the shoes, approximate athletic skills (walking, running, jumping, and changing directions).

Individuals with specific conditions need special shoes:
Runners with normal feet—more forefoot and toe flexibility.
Overpronation—greater control on the medial side.
Achilles tendinitis—at least 15-mm heel wedge.
Court sports—added side-to-side stability.
High rigid arches—soft midsoles, curved lasts, and low or moderate hindfoot stability.
Normal arches—firm midsole, semicurved lasts, and moderate hindfoot stability.
Flexible low arch—very firm midsole, straight last, and strong hindfoot stability.

After purchasing the shoes, walk in the shoes for 2 to 3 d to allow them to adapt to the feet. Then begin running or practicing in the shoes for about 25% to 30% of the workout. To prevent blisters, gradually extend the length of time the shoes are worn.

Avid runners should replace shoes every 3 mo and recreational runners every 6 mo.

From Anderson MK, Hall SJ, Martin M. *Sports Injury Management,* 2nd ed. Philadelphia: Lippincott Williams & Wilkins, 2000.

and the abnormalities of the forefoot (e.g., bunions, hammertoes, etc.) (Fig. 8.9). While a wide variety of commercial products are available, the cost can be prohibitive; off-the-shelf products often suffice.

Injuries to the lower extremity can be significantly influenced by the selection and fit of footwear. Shoes should adequately cushion impact forces and should guide and support the foot during the stance and final push-off phase of running. Additional heel cushioning should be available in sports that entail repeated heel impact. The length of the shoe should be sufficient to allow all the toes to be fully extended, and a wider toe box should be provided for those individuals with toe abnormalities or bunions. Table 8.7 outlines the key factors for athletic footwear selection and fit. Flat-soled, long cleat, short cleat, or multicleated shoes should be chosen for field sports. Cleats should be properly positioned under the major weight-bearing joints of the foot, and they should not be able to be felt through the sole of the shoe. Only flat-soled, basketball-type turf shoes have low-release coefficients at varying elevated temperatures, and, therefore, these should be chosen for playing on turf when increased temperature is a factor. Adequate forefoot arch and heel support is essential for athletes with arch problems. All athletic footwear selections should be based on the demands of the activity.

REFERENCES

1. Saliba E, Foreman S, Abadie RT Jr. Protective equipment consideration In: Zachezewski JE, Magee DJ, Quillen WS. *Athletic injuries and rehabilitation.* Philadelphia: WB Saunders, 1996.
2. Protective equipment. In: Benson M, ed. *1997–1998 NCAA sports medicine handbook.* Overland Park, KS: The National Collegiate Athletic Association, 1997: 58–83.
3. Cheng TL, Fields CB, Brenner RA, et al. Sports injuries: an important cause of morbidity in urban youth. *Pediatrics* 2000;105:E32.
4. Rice MR, Alvanos L, Kenney B. Snowmobile injuries and deaths in children: a review of national injury data and state legislation. *Pediatrics* 2000;105:615–619.
5. Thompson DC, Nunn ME, Thompson RS, et al. Effectiveness of bicycle safety helmets in preventing serious facial injury. *JAMA* 1996;276:1974–1975.
6. Thompson MJ, Rivara FP. Bicycle-related injuries. *Am Fam Physician* 2001; 63:2007–2014.
7. Shafi S, Gilbert JC, Loghmanee F, et al. Impact of bicycle helmet safety legislation on children admitted to a regional pediatric trauma center. *J Pediatr Surg* 1998; 33:317–321.
8. Knorr HL, Jonas JB. Retinal detachments by squash ball accidents. *Am J. Ophthalmol* 1996;122:260–261.
9. Livingston LA, Forbes SL. Eye injuries in women's lacrosse: strict rule enforcement and mandatory eyewear required. *J Trauma* 1996;40:144–145.
10. Berg R, Berkey DB, Tang JM, et al. Knowledge and at-

titudes of Arizona high-school coaches regarding oral-facial injuries and mouthguard use among athletes. *J Am Dent Assoc* 1998;129:1425–432.

11. Machold W, Kwasny O, Gassler P, et al. Risk of injury through snowboarding. *J Trauma* 2000;48:1109–1114.

12. American Academy of Pediatrics Committee on Injury and Poison Prevention and Committee on Sports Medicine and Fitness. In-line skating injuries in children and adolescents. *Pediatrics* 1998;101:720–722.

13. Schrieber RA, Branche-Dorsey CM, Ryan GW, et al. Risk factors for injuries from in-line skating and the effectiveness of safety gear. *N Engl J Med* 1996;335:1630–1635.

14. Orenstein JB. Injuries and small-wheel skates. *Ann Emerg Med* 1996;27:204–209.

15. Wichman S, Martin DR. Bracing for activity. *The Physician and Sports Medicine* 1996;24:88–94.

16. Gross MT, Clemence LM, Cox BD, et al. Effect of ankle orthoses on functional performance for individuals with recurrent lateral ankle sprains. *J Orthop Sports Phys Ther* 1997;25:245–252.

9

Psychosocial Aspects of Sport Participation

Cora Collette Breuner

Athletic programs are flourishing in the United States, where more children are involved in sports than ever before. Twenty-five million children and adolescents in the United States between the ages of 6 and 16 years participate in a multitude of non–school-sponsored sports programs (1), and an estimated 6 to 7 million high school students are involved in interscholastic athletics (2). Without question, sports participation plays a solidly established role in United States culture. On the positive side, athletic involvement provides a framework for regular physical activity, which helps children develop lifestyle patterns that may follow them into adulthood (3). Competitive experiences on the playing fields may possibly help to prepare youth for parallel situations that may arise as they mature into adulthood. Through sports, children can learn how to cooperate and work as a team. The grace children learn in both winning and losing can be assimilated into all aspects of life.

While participation in sports may produce all positive outcomes for some athletes, the potential negative effects should not be ignored (4). For those children who are involved in higher levels of competitive sport, the average time spent in or preparing for participation is 11 hours per week for an 18-week season (5). This dedication comes at a time when critical developmental tasks must be accomplished, including the promotion of positive self-esteem and effective social interactions. Another potential negative outcome may result from exposure to poor modeling. Wining at all costs or zero tolerance for losing are attitudes that are not suitable for children. Experiential knowledge, in the setting of poor modeling, can potentially negate the benefits obtained from involvement in youth sport.

In this chapter, the pressures of athletic commitment on the mind and the body are examined.

EATING DISORDERS

While the fact that eating disorders exist in young athletes, especially women, is well known, this phenomenon is much more prevalent than was previously thought (6,7). Many woman athletes make concerted efforts to lose weight either by restricting food intake or by binging and purging. This may result from the extreme pressure many athletes face to be competitive in their sport. In the general population of athletes and nonathletes, over 90% who present with the classic signs and symptoms of anorexia and bulimia are female, and greater than 95% of these are white. Most are teenagers when they first demonstrate the disease, and they generally come from middle to upper socioeconomic class families. Many young women feel compelled to diet, which places them at risk for the development of harmful eating habits.

In a study of female collegiate athletes, 32% engaged in at least one form of behavior that characterized an eating disorder, including vomiting, laxative use, excessive weight loss, or the use of diuretics or diet pills. These athletes reported that they had done this daily in the 1 month prior to the survey (8). Among female gymnasts, 62% reported using weight control behaviors at least twice weekly for 3 months or more. The methods used included vomiting (26%), diet pill use (24%), fasting (24%), diuretic use (12%), and laxative use (7%) (8). The athletes had been told repeatedly by coaches that they were too heavy; this may have influenced their progression into eating-disordered behavior (9).

Anorexia nervosa and bulimia nervosa are the most common forms of eating disorders. Anorectics have a distorted body image and an overwhelming fear of becoming obese. They often develop amenorrhea. The challenging aspect of providing care for these individuals is in the denial of abnormality and the angry resistance to intervention.

Bulimics eat episodically, which then leads them to feel guilty and ultimately to purge. Like anorectics, they feel pressure to change their bodies via vomiting or laxative use, and they are governed by the stereotype "thin is beautiful;" bulimics, however, realize that their behavior is abnormal.

Bulimia and anorexia may coexist, as some athletes may restrict food intake prior to an event and may then resort to binging and purging when restricting becomes too difficult.

Athletes with eating disorders are seen in all sports, but sports that are particularly at high risk include gymnastics, diving, dance, figure skating, wrestling, synchronized swimming, cross country skiing, long-distance running, rowing, and martial arts. These sports place a high emphasis on the small petite figure, or they stress meeting weight goals for optimal performance. Tragic outcomes have resulted among both gymnasts and figure skating because of the incessant demands for a perfect appearance in tight costumes (9).

The diagnosis of anorexia or bulimia nervosa can be made with the help of the diagnostic criteria delineated in Tables 9.1 and 9.2 (10). For those athletes who meet the criteria, the diagnosis is straightforward. However, for athletes with abnormal eating behavior, the diagnostic criteria of a full-blown eating disorder may not be met. Disordered eating in the athlete may range from moderate to severe. The moderate form is seen as a restrictive pattern, where the athlete fails to take in the caloric requirements appropriate for meeting the demands of his or her exercise schedules. Severely disordered eating is evident when an athlete is intentionally not taking in minimal calories. In anorexia nervosa, athletes deliberately restrict their foods to vegetarian or low-fat foods, thus severely limiting the

TABLE 9.2. *Diagnostic criteria for bulimia nervosa*

Recurrent episodes of binge eating, characterized by both (a) eating in a discrete period of time (e.g., within any 2 hr period) an amount of food that is definitely larger than most people would eat during a similar period of time and under similar circumstances and (b) a sense of lack of control during the episode (i.e., a feeling that one cannot stop eating or control what or how much one is eating).

Recurrent inappropriate compensatory behavior to prevent weight gain, which may include self-induced vomiting; misuse of laxatives, diuretics, enemas or other medications; fasting; or excessive exercise.

Episodes average at least twice a week for 3 mo.
Self-evaluation unduly influenced by body shape and weight.
Does not occur exclusively during episodes of anorexia nervosa.
Subtypes
  purging
  nonpurging

From American Psychiatric Association. *Diagnostic and statistical manual of mental disorders,* 4th ed. Washington, D.C.: American Psychiatric Association, 1994, with permission.

TABLE 9.1. *Diagnostic criteria for anorexia nervosa*

Refusal to maintain body weight at or above a minimally normal weight for age and height (e.g., weight loss leading to maintenance of body weight less than 85% of that expected or failure to make expected weight gain during a period of growth leading to a body weight less than 85% of that expected).
Intense fear of gaining weight or becoming fat, even when underweight.
Disturbance in the way one's body weight or shape is perceived; undue influence of body weight or shape on self-evaluation; denial of the seriousness of the current low body weight.
In postmenarchal females, amenorrhea, that is, the absence of at least three consecutive menstrual cycles. (A woman is considered to have amenorrhea if her periods occur only following hormone [e.g., estrogen] administration.)
Two subtypes:
  Restricting
  Binge-eating and purging

From American Psychiatric Association. *Diagnostic and statistical manual of mental disorders,* 4th ed. Washington, D.C.: American Psychiatric Association, 1994, with permission.

numbers of acceptable foods. Clearly, research indicates that the majority of female athletes may have some degree of abnormal eating behavior, but, for many of them, the diagnostic criteria may not be met. One must be aware of the fact that those athletes who have abnormal or disordered eating behaviors may progress to an eating disorder. These young athletes are at risk for a number of adverse health consequences.

Risk factors for the development of eating disorders are multifaceted (Table 9.3). In women's sports, the constant pressure for optimum performance for many is weight related. Weight or body fat goals that are implemented over a short period of time can force a young athlete to develop disordered eating habits and distorted body image. The drive to win may become another motivator for the athlete to be thin. Additionally, some have acquired the ability to block distractions, such as pain; and they may extend this to block hunger as well (11). Finally, when an athlete's education is tied to his or her sport (e.g., by a scholarship), he or she may be willing to take risks with his or her body in order to maintain funding.

The sociocultural factors that contribute to the development of disordered eating are perpetuated in a culture where thinness is equated with success, power, beauty, and control. Gender disparity in this disorder is

TABLE 9.3. *Risk factors for developing an eating disorder*

Pressure to be the best.
Heightened awareness of the body.
Perfectionism.
Compulsion and obsession.
Involvement in highly competitive sports: gymnastics, diving, figure skating, dance, synchronized swimming, long-distance running, swimming, cross-country skiing, rowing, judo, weight lifting, and tae kwondo.
Sociocultural factors: desire to be thin, which leads to "power, success, and beauty."
Biologic factors: gender (10:1 are women), imbalances in neurotransmitters.
Psychological factors: family of origin has difficulty dealing with conflict or stress; response to sexual or physical abuse, low self-worth, or lack of identity outside of eating disorder.

quite high, as only 5% to 10% of eating disorder patients are male. However, one must be able to recognize this disorder in male athletes. Male body perceptions can be quite abnormal in sports oriented to meet certain weight goals, such as wrestling. While males may not "diet," they may attempt extreme and excessive weight control behaviors that are medically dangerous.

Imbalances in neurotransmitters have been postulated as causative factors for eating disorders. Serotonin (5-hydroxytryptamine [5-HT]), norepinephrine, and melatonin have all been implicated (12). Appetite is decreased at the medial hypothalamus by higher levels of 5-HT. Lower levels of 5-HT decrease satiety. In patients with anorexia nervosa, the central nervous system precursor of 5-HT, 5-hydroxyindolacetic acid (5-HIAA), tends to be significantly reduced. After recovery, it returns to normal, which suggests that a disturbance of 5-HT activity may predispose certain people who are vulnerable to manifest symptoms of anorexia and bulimia nervosa.

Psychologic factors may be present in young athletes with poor coping skills. Some athletes may have difficulty expressing negative emotions, tolerating negative emotions, or resolving conflict. The families of these athletes may be either completely enmeshed with the child or totally disengaged, both of which may foster the need for the child to perpetuate closeness through thinness or to reengage the attention of the parent who seems too busy to care. Victimization is another important factor in the development of eating disorders. Sexual abuse has been reported among 20% to 35% of people with eating disorders. These etiologies may or may not be common in athletes, but they should be considered (11). Many athletes may

feel overwhelmed when they juggle academic demands, poor sports performance, financial issues, or family concerns. They may be able to deal with stress on the playing field but not that found in their everyday lives. The female athlete especially may find managing her weight, rather than her life, to be easier for her. Other psychologic predisposing factors include low self-esteem and a lack of identity. Anyone whose self-esteem is dictated by performance in some area is inherently exposed to a normal fluctuation of positives and negatives. If a female athlete does not have a solid foundation of positive self-worth, she may "punish herself" by restricting food if she does constantly perform perfectly. The final psychologic factor, lack of identity, may be noted when an athlete is defined by his or her sport. This may lead to a failure to develop in other areas of life. Not surprisingly, as the athlete's career and competence change, he or she may feel that life is nothing without sports. The female athlete who has progressed to bulimia nervosa may present in one of three ways. She may continuously binge and purge on a daily basis, sometimes up to six times per day. The purging may occur in a cyclical pattern during a competition or during hormonal cycles. The episodic presentation may occur sporadically, during a vacation, or while under specific pressure from another commitment. For these athletes, initial food restriction is followed by severe hunger, which leads to eating an amount of food, whether large or small. Afterward, she may "purge," which can occur through vomiting, via laxative and/or diuretic abuse, or by exercise.

An eating disorder can affect the performance of an athlete by a reduction in energy, strength, reaction time, cognitive functions, and speed. The athlete may severely restrict food intake prior to competition, which may precipitate dehydration and induce poor reaction times. The athlete may have electrolyte abnormalities (e.g., hypokalemia), which can cause cardiac arrhythmia and death. Neutropenia and reduced immune function, which decrease the ability to resist infections, can also result. The risk of injury is increased, especially with the abnormal bone densitometry findings that are secondary to the low estrogen state that is often seen in amenorrhea (13).

Screening for eating disorders should occur during the preparticipation physical examination. The potential athlete should fill out a questionnaire that includes a nutritional screen, a question about his or her highest and lowest weight and happiness with body habitus, and a menstrual history (females). Table 9.4 gives examples of questions that may be diagnostic. The nutritional screen ideally includes a 24-hour recall of the number

TABLE 9.4. *SCOFF inventory*

1. Do you feel **S**ick because you feel uncomfortably full?
2. Do you worry that you've lost **C**ontrol over how much you eat?
3. Have you lost **O**ver 6 kg (13 lbs) pounds in a recent 3-mo period?
4. Do you believe yourself to be **F**at when others say you are too thin?
5. Would you say that **F**ood dominates your life?

Two or more affirmative answers have a 100% sensitivity in identifying individuals with bulimia or anorexia nervosa. The false positive rate is 12%.

From Morgan JF, Reid F, Lacey JH. The SCOFF questionnaire: assessment of a new tool for eating disorders. *BMJ* 1999;319:1467–1468, with permission.

of daily meals and snacks eaten and a list of the athlete's "forbidden foods" (those which are avoided).

Although the diagnosis of an eating disorder is primarily clinical, laboratory tests can be ordered to help confirm the diagnosis and also to follow the progression of the disease. Laboratory evaluation includes a complete blood count, urinalysis, electrolytes, calcium, magnesium, phosphorus, and thyroid-stimulating hormone.

The results of many tests depend on the state of hydration of the athlete. Persistently abnormal values should cause the tests to be repeated in order to determine if an underlying organic disease is present.

Leukopenia and thrombocytopenia may occur with starvation. Leukopenia may be due to the increased margination of leukocytes, but is not associated with an increased risk of infection. The hemoglobin is usually normal. Thrombocytopenia may be seen in as many as one-third of those with anorexia.

Glucose levels may be low because of lack of glycogen stores or glucose precursors. Blood urea nitrogen and creatinine are normal, unless the athlete is dehydrated. If the athlete is vomiting or taking laxatives, the electrolyte levels may be abnormal. In those who vomit, hypokalemic hypochloremic metabolic alkalosis is found. Acidosis may be associated with laxative use (14).

If menses are absent or abnormal, tests of follicle stimulating hormone and luteinizing hormone are required. A pregnancy test should also be obtained. If amenorrhea has been prolonged (greater than 1 year), a bone densitometry evaluation is warranted. An electrocardiogram should be obtained in all athletes suspected of having an eating disorder. Electrocardiographic findings associated with eating disorders include bradycardia (less than or equal to 60 beats per minute), low volt-

age, low or inverted T waves, and prolonged QT interval (14). Of note, reviewing all prescribed and nonprescribed medications taken by an athlete suffering from an eating disorder is crucial. Some may cause dysrhythmias in athletes with prolonged QT interval.

Serum protein and albumin are generally normal; however, pre-albumin levels may be low. Liver function tests are normal, as is the bilirubin level. Cholesterol may be elevated because of low cholesterol or binding globulin or from cholesterol breakdown resulting from depressed triiodothyronine (T3) levels (14). When a complete lipid profile is obtained, most of the cholesterol will be high-density lipoprotein (HDL).

The approach to evaluation and treatment requires the use of a multidisciplinary team consisting of health care professionals knowledgeable in the treatment of eating disorders.

Sometimes activity must be restricted to allow the athlete to return to a healthy weight. The coach and trainer need to be aware of the restrictions. They can provide gentle assurance to the athlete about the return to full activity when he or she is healthy.

The criteria for hospitalization include weight loss to below 30% of normal, altered mental status, hypotension or dehydration, electrolyte abnormalities, or the failure of outpatient treatment. Proper preparation for inpatient treatment is imperative. Hospitalization should never be considered punitive. Rather, it should be considered a more intensive from of treatment. The goals of hospitalization should be to provide more involved planning and eating of healthy meals, the improvement of the individual's physiologic and metabolic status, enhanced communication skills, and the development of a different coping strategy. Intense behavior modification can also occur in the hospital. Athletes may need to learn *"how to eat"* and how to express emotions in other ways besides a refusal to eat.

The prognosis for patients with eating disorders is generally favorable, provided that a multidisciplinary team manages the patient. The healthcare provider should be aware that treatment may last anywhere in the range of 6 months to 2 years. Success rates with an experienced team may be 70% to 85%. Unfortunately, even with exceptional care, 15% to 25% of these individuals may persist in abnormal eating behaviors and may do poorly. Affective or personality disorders and osteoporosis may develop. The mortality rate may be 5% from suicide, cardiovascular collapse or arrest, sepsis, and gastric or intestinal perforation (15).

Stressing that prevention is the absolute first step when dealing with eating disorders is key. Figure 9.1 delineates a conceptual model of unhealthy coping mechanisms used by the athlete with disordered eat-

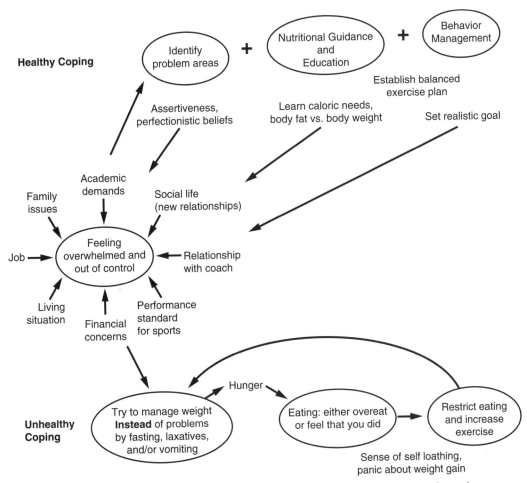

FIG. 9.1. Conceptual model of the athlete with disordered eating, delineating unhealthy coping mechanisms used by the athlete and illustrating the therapeutic process utilized in the acquisition of healthy coping skills. (From Priscilla Wright, with permission.)

ing, as well as the therapeutic process used in the development of healthy coping skills.

Women with female athlete triad have an eating disorder, amenorrhea, and osteoporosis. Elite gymnasts have higher rates of developing this disorder, and they should be screened earlier than athletes in other sports (16). They should be managed in the same manner as patients with an eating disorder. The use of hormones for preventing osteoporosis is controversial. The use of an oral contraceptive is indicated in the sexually active athlete with female athlete triad.

The male athlete is not immune to the pressures of competition, and he can also develop disordered eating

that progresses to an eating disorder. Men are more likely to present with involvement in sports that require weight control, such as wrestling, diving, or biking. The age at which men present is slightly older than that for women. Men also may be more likely to purge at presentation, as dieting may not be as acceptable.

Coaches, training staff, athletes, and parents should be aware of the risks and warning signals for eating disorders that are noted in Table 9.5. Prevention of eating disorders begins in the home, in schools, and on playing fields. All of those involved with children must be aware of the subtle messages that are being sent to children about their appearance and about how

TABLE 9.5. *Risks and warning signals of an eating disorder*

Preoccupation with food, calories, and weight
Repeated concerns about feeling fat, even when weight is average or below average
Increasing criticism of one's body
Eating large meals and then disappearing or taking trips to the bathroom
Stealing food or secretly eating food
Bloodshot eyes, especially after trips to the bathroom
Vomitus or odor of vomit in bathroom
Laxative use
Periods of excessive calorie restriction
Mood swings
Continuous drinking of diet soda or water
Refusal to eat in front of teammates (e.g., on road trips)
Swollen parotid glands at the angle of the jaw, giving a chipmunk-like appearance
Appearing preoccupied with the eating of others
Expression of self-deprecating thoughts following eating
Compulsive excessive exercise that is not part of the athlete's training regimen
Wearing baggy or layered clothing
Wide fluctuations in weight over short periods of time

best to promote healthy eating habits and self-confidence before disordered eating habits become an ingrained part of the athlete's daily routine.

MOTIVATION FOR PARTICIPATION

Why do children play sports? Most do it to have a good time, to develop something they can do well, and to be with friends or to make new friends. In one survey, 8,000 youths were asked to rank their reasons for sport participation in order of importance (17). The results were separated into important motivators for nonschool and school sports. In order of importance, girls in nonschool sports participated to have fun, to stay in shape, to get exercise, to "do something I am good at," to be part of a team, to improve and learn new skills, and to experience the excitement and challenge of competition. For boys, the reasons were basically the same, except that the order of importance was changed—boys rated the excitement and challenge of competition higher than girls did.

Exercising or being involved in sports can enable a child to maximize his or her potential for a healthy life. However, this does not guarantee that a child will become a star athlete or that he or she will develop a perfectly proportioned body (18). Children should be encouraged to participate, and the positive outcome of their involvement should reinforce their ongoing participation.

WHY CHILDREN STOP PARTICIPATING

The age when the most children participate in sports is between 10 and 13 years of age; subsequently, the level of participation slowly drops until age 18, where only a small percentage continue to remain involved in organized sports (17). Dropout rates for organized sports programs for youths average 35% for any given year. In an in-depth study of 50 children who stopped swimming, the major reasons were that they had other things to do and that their interests had changed. Other reasons included that the child was "not as good as I wanted to be," that it was "not enough fun," that the child "wanted to play another sport," that he or she "didn't like the pressure," "boredom," that he or she "didn't like the coach," that "training was too hard," and that the sport was "not exciting enough" (19). Seventy percent cited involvement in another sport as the reason for discontinuing swimming. However, almost 30% cited negative factors from parents and coaches that influenced their decision to stop participating in the sport.

The concept of perceived competence has gained the interest of researchers who are studying why youths do not participate in sports or why they drop out of them. Children who do not believe that they can learn a new sport or that they can perform it well do not continue involvement, whereas those who do have a higher self-perceived ability continue in the sport (20,21).

Coaching styles that enhance skill development and foster excitement and personal success should be implemented.

PSYCHOLOGIC STRATEGIES FOR ENHANCING PERFORMANCE IN THE YOUNG ATHLETE

Clearly, the physical impact of performance enhancement can be reflected in the improved outcome of athletes in their designated fields. Also important is an understanding of psychologic factors impacting sports performance. Athletic demands in the areas of training can vary, depending on the sport and coach. Through coach effectiveness training (CET), coaches are encouraged to reduce criticism and "crack the whip" behavior by instituting team rules early and by bolstering compliance. The promotion of cardiovascular endurance, muscular strength, and flexibility should occur only when the young athlete is developmentally ready to handle the training. Proper diet, as it relates to body composition, should be reviewed with a sports nutritionist for and with any athlete who is preparing for elite competition (22).

IS COMPETITION A GOOD THING FOR CHILDREN?

Basketball is a sport in which success, as symbolized by the championship, requires that the community goal prevail over selfish impulses...The less conflict there is off-court, the more inevitable friction of competition can be minimized...teams develop when talents and personalities mesh.
                                        —Bill Bradley

Competition is more than a single event; it encompasses a number of stages or events. Martens (23) defined the competitive process as consisting of the following four stages: objective competitive situation, subjective competitive situation, response, and consequence of the response (Fig. 9.2). In the objective competitive situation, individual performance is compared with some quantifiable standard of excellence of which the evaluator is aware. For true competition to exist, a second person must be involved. The subjective competitive situation is defined by how a person perceives his or her ability to compete. The person may enjoy competition and may try to "make a race" out of every situation, while another individual may not. In the third stage, the response, the person evaluates the situation and then decides either to tackle it or to avoid it. Internal factors that affect this response are motivation, confidence, and perceived ability. External factors are time, weather, and the talent level of the opponents. In the final stage of the competitive process as proposed by Martens, the participant must face the consequences. These may be ei-

ther positive or negative (e.g., success or failure). However, the young athlete's perception of these outcomes has true consequence for him or her. For instance, a loss might not be that serious to a young basketball player if he or she is praised for his or her efforts in play (e.g., for playing against taller opponents). Perceptions of success and failures can be altered if the sport's rules are modified, especially for young players. Examples of these modifications include the following:

- Lower the basket in basketball.
- Do not keep official score.
- Rotate positions on the team.
- Allow a player to stay at bat until he or she hits the ball into fair territory.
- Use smaller balls for volleyball, football, and basketball.

Competition is a process. Too much competition may cause poor outcomes, but too little competition may also have negative consequences. For example, the swimmer who competes 3 days per week may experience psychologic stress and fatigue leading to losses and poor performance. The swimmer who competes once a month, on the other hand, may not have the drive to perform well.

A blend of competition and cooperation is optimal. Orlick (24) studied this relationship and found that five relationships between competition and cooperation exist. These include (a) competitive means—competitive ends, or individual winning; (b) cooperative means—competitive ends, or team sports; (c) individual means—individual ends, or cross-country

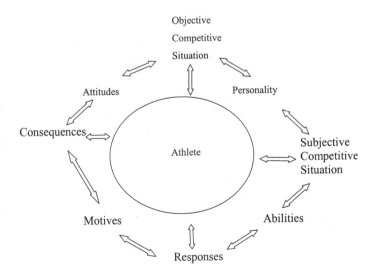

FIG. 9.2. The competitive process shows the relationship between objective and subjective response and the consequences of the response.

skiing; (d) cooperative means—individual ends, in which athletes watch each other and provide feedback; and (e) cooperative means—cooperative ends, in which everyone works towards a common goal. The final relationship is difficult to institute in the current competitive setting. The typical competition, in which talented athletes are chosen for teams and those who are not as talented are "cut," does not promote cooperation. In fact, the fun of the sport is taken away. Some children have become conditioned to win at all costs, and they have learned that enjoyment of the sport is not a high priority.

Coaches and others involved in youth sports need to focus on cooperation, competition, and the enjoyment sports can provide for their young participants. Some recommendations to implement a cooperative approach for the young participant include the following:

- Blend competition and cooperation when coaching players on physical skills.
- Remember that competition is a process.
- Individualize instruction so that each person's needs are met.
- Promote cooperation by building trust and open communication between teammates.
- Structure games for children in such a way that they include both competitive and cooperative elements.
- Give positive feedback and encouragement to young athletes, regardless of the outcomes.
- Curtail aggressive competition as it will ultimately cause others to compete.
- Step back and establish broad goals to get groups to cooperate when competition leads to extreme rivalry.
- Offer opportunities for both skill acquisition and skill practice in competition.

EFFECTS OF SPORTS-INDUCED STRESS AND BURNOUT IN CHILDREN

The fast-paced growth of organized sports for children and adolescents can be interpreted as both a security and a liability for youth. Bonuses include the increased safeguards for preventing injuries within each particular sport and the greater number of attempts that are made to match the child with a particular sport in which he or she can excel. The liability is that children may be exposed to inappropriate and excessive training by inexperienced or unqualified adult supervisors. The injury risk can increase from acute trauma incurred in a situation where the young athlete is unprepared or unprotected. Injuries also may increase from repetitive overuse. Because of the potential for injuries and the expectation of high performance, the enjoyment of children in the sport of their choice can be impaired (25,26). Competitive stress lessens the enjoyment of sports, causes impaired performance, and contributes to young athletes dropping out of sports. It also can cause sleep deprivation, which can put youngsters at greater risk for sustaining athletic injuries (27).

An extremely important relationship in sports psychology is that of arousal and anxiety and performance. Most people recognize that, when they are extremely nervous, they do not perform as well on a particular task. Some degree of nervousness or anxiety, however, is necessary for the athlete to perform well. What is the optimal amount of nervous tension for performance and when is it deleterious? Figure 9.3 portrays the inverted U theory. It illustrates that, when an athlete is in a low arousal state, performance may suffer because he or she is not "psyched up" or ready. Then, as arousal increases, so does performance, but only to a certain point. If further increases in anxiety occur, the athlete's performance declines (28).

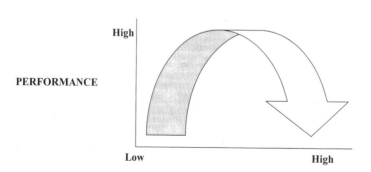

FIG. 9.3. The inverted U arousal–performance relationship.

How does arousal, stress, or anxiety—all these term are interchangeable in this context—influence performance? When children experience stress, their heart rate increases, and they complain of aches and pains and muscle soreness. They feel that they are "too tensed up" and "not quite right." Suddenly, they feel that they cannot play or practice anymore, and they often want to stay home. When an individual feels muscle soreness and tension, his or her coordination does suffer. With the ensuing decrease in coordination, performance is impaired.

What else is affected during arousal? The more anxious a child athlete is, the less ability he or she may have to pay attention. For instance, a child may be so nervous about finally being able to play in right field in softball because she wants to please everyone. This child's focus is too broad. Therefore, when the fly comes towards the child, she then sees it too late and drops the ball. In this example, the child appeared not to be paying attention at all, but instead she was hypervigilant. The more anxious the athlete is, the greater the likelihood is that a downward spiral may occur. Other manifestations of heightened arousal may cause an athlete to pay attention to inappropriate cues. He or she may be watching the goalie, while a charging halfback then steals the ball. In other situations, the athlete's attention may be too focused, almost as if he or she is looking through a small tube. As a result, he or she cannot get a broad picture of the playing field, and performance suffers.

Coaches and trainers can utilize the knowledge of arousal stress and anxiety by using the following five guidelines (29):

1. Identify the optimal combination of arousal-related emotions needed for the best performance.
2. Recognize how personal and situational factors interact to influence arousal and performance.
3. Identify signs of increased arousal and anxiety in sport and exercise participants.
4. Tailor coaching and instructional practices to individuals.
5. Develop confidence in performers to help them cope with increased stress and anxiety.

Although involvement in sports may have many beneficial psychologic effects, detrimental effects may result if the coaching staff is nonsupportive or abusive or if the child and/or family have unrealistic expectations (30). Factors associated with stress in a young athlete are overtraining, high self expectation (or another imposed expectation), a "win at all costs" attitude, parental pressure, long repetitive practices with little variety, and inconsistent coaching prac-

tices. Other factors causing stress in young athletes are overuse injuries incurred from excessive practice, inordinate time demands, and extensive travel commitments. One must recognize that, for these children, affection from others is based on their ability to win and that being loved can only happen if they are perfect (31). Physical signs and symptoms of stress in the young athlete are depicted in Table 9.6 (32).

Although high levels of stress are experienced by youths in sports, the level of stress experienced by young athletes is generally the same as that found in any of the other achievement-oriented activities in which children participate, such as chess, drama, and music (33). Learning to understand the stress experienced by youth in order to delineate the foci for intervention strategies is important. These strategies may be utilized in other areas of the lives of busy young people.

The question of the long-term effects of anxiety remains unanswered, but it is certainly relevant. Another question centers around how to determine which specific athlete is at risk for high stress or anxiety. Sports psychologists have evaluated self-esteem measures and the results of personality testing to determine if a specific personality type is more susceptible to the pressures of athletic competition. These results are summarized in Table 9.7.

One should find the young athlete who sees his or her sports involvement as a defining personal characteristic extremely worrisome. To a certain extent, these young athletes are one-dimensional, they have a difficult time making decisions, and they lack the internal motivation to succeed. These young athletes need to be evaluated and nurtured so that they do not experience burnout and its potential for devastating long-term effects.

TABLE 9.6. *Physical signs and symptoms of stress*

Increased heart rate
Increased blood pressure
Increased respiratory rate
Decreased adaptive performance
Inability to concentrate
Sleeping difficulties
Cold, clammy hands
Headache
Constant need to urinate
Negative talk about self
Increased muscle tension
Consistently performs better in noncompetitive practices
Constantly sick

TABLE 9.7. *Characteristics of children at risk for heightened competitive state anxiety*

High anxiety trait disposition
Low self esteem
Low performance expectations relative to his or her team
Low self performance expectations
Frequent worries about failure
Frequent worries about adult expectations and social evaluation by others
Less perceived fun
Less satisfaction with his or her performance, regardless of winning or losing
Perceived importance to parents of his or her participation in the sport

From Weinberg RS, Gould D. *Foundations of sport and exercise psychology.* Champaign, IL: Human Kinetics, 1995:457, with permission.

POSTINJURY STRESS

In adults, as well as young athletes, responses to injuries may lead to feelings of identity loss. Children may also feel fear and anxiety regarding the possibility or speed of recovery. Young athletes also may be concerned about whether they will be replaced in the line-up. Because athletes cannot practice and compete when injured, they have plenty of time to fret and worry. They can lose confidence in their abilities if they have not been able to play, placing them at risk for further injury. Many athletes cannot modify their personal expectations, and they think that immmediately on their return to play they should be able to perform at preinjury levels, putting them at risk for further injury. Problems with adjusting can be noted by identifying athletes who are angry, and confused, or withdrawn; who experience rapid mood swings; who feel denial or guilt about letting other teammates down; and who dwell on minor physical complaints (34). Athletes who respond well to their own internal motivation for improvement and who are compliant with the rehabilitation seem to have the quickest recovery and the least psychologic impairment from the injury.

Coping with setbacks is part of any involvement in sports. The typical responses include the five coping stages of grief—denial, anger, bargaining, depression, and acceptance. The order of experiencing these coping stages can be varied. Even the most well adjusted young athlete should be allowed to experience all of the emotions and should be supported through this process (35).

Nonpunitive guidelines for dealing with injured athletes should be set before injuries occur. Injured athletes may need temporary withdrawal from or a reduction in practice time, but they should not be dropped from the team. Unfortunately, some athletes will return to participation in the sport with pain and incomplete rehabilitation.

STRATEGIES FOR REDUCING BURNOUT IN YOUNG ATHLETES

Athletes can be taught to cope with stress through the use of a positive and constructive attitude in a supportive environment. Adult anxiety reduction techniques utilizing progressive muscle relaxation, breathing exercises, mental imagery, systematic desensitization, and biofeedback can be adapted for children (29,36).

Teams that are coached by individuals who have been trained to build self-esteem and cooperation derive more enjoyment from sports. Lower dropout rates and better peer relationships are seen with the same win/loss records (37,38). Understanding which of the successful coaching strategies have been effective in supporting athletes during practice and game situations is important. A good play should be reinforced, so that the athlete knows that his or her efforts are appreciated and supported. The efforts of youth who are trying their best should never be taken for granted. After a mistake, a child should never be punished or yelled at, nor should he or she be shown disapproval. A mistake should be gently corrected by explaining how it could have been done in a different way. Clear expectations will lead to positive results. Running laps or nagging the team may result in chaos and a lack of team spirit. Instruction should be given in a positive manner and should, if possible, be accompanied by demonstration. However, abundant praise can also become meaningless. A coach should be supportive, but not excessively so, as praise then loses its effectiveness (22).

Stress management clearly is beneficial to young athletes, as it may reduce susceptibility to injury and, at the same time, enhance performance in a given sport (34,36).

Learning stress management techniques and using behavior modification to help with changing undesirable habits represents the psychologic component of most health-related fitness programs. Stress management is incorporated because the diseases targeted for prevention are related to psychologic stress in various ways. In Table 9.8, strategies to help reduce stress are incorporated into a fitness program.

TABLE 9.8. *Keys to success of a health-related fitness program*

Motivated adult involvement is essential for children's fitness programs.

Achievable goals for the individual over both short- and long-term intervals (e.g., at the end of the first week, walking one block at least three times per week; at the end of the first month, walking for 30 min/d at least four times per week; at the end of 6 mo, walking 30 to 60 min/d at least five times per week).

Daily charting of progress in each component of the fitness program for each individual involved in the program.

Appropriate recognition and predetermined awards for achievement of various levels of goals.

Varying the type of activities that are chosen helps to keep the program fresh and interesting decreases overuse injuries.

Make the program a family priority.

*From the Utah Governor's Council on Health and Physical Fitness. Governor's Family F.U.N. Awards Program. Salt Lake City, UT: Utah Govenor's Council.

EFFECTIVE PRACTICES FOR COACHING CHILDREN

The following 11 coaching practices are recommended for the purpose of helping youth excel in self-development through sports (39):

1. Catch athletes doing things correctly; praise them and encourage them frequently. Focus on giving positive feedback with a smile and a pat on the back, rather than on reminding them of errors that they have made.

2. Give praise sincerely. When the athlete knows that he or she has done poorly, insincere praise destroys the credibility of the coach. Acknowledging a less than optimal performance with words like "Stick with it; it is hard out there" is okay.

3. Set expectations, but make them realistic. These should be appropriate to the child's age and ability. Coaches should not expect a 12-year-old to perform as athletically as a 16-year-old.

4. Praise efforts, as well as outcomes. Most teams lose once in a while; many lose a lot. Players still try hard, and that effort should be rewarded. Sportsmanship should be praised, as should poise and respect.

5. Maximize the participation of all players, all equipment, and all of the talent in each practice. Instructions and expectations should be clear, and they should be identified early. The coach should demonstrate his or her expectations. Athletes need to see that they are improving. All of the positive talk will not help until each player feels that he or she is getting "better."

6. Modify skills and activities so that players learn at an age-appropriate level. Batting tees can be utilized, balls can be decreased in size, baskets can be lowered, and the field length can be shortened; all of these efforts can enhance performance successes. The purpose of these measures is to increase safety and to minimize personal injuries.

7. Adapt rules so that everyone gets to play and have fun. This is especially important with younger children and nonelitist teams. Coaches can pitch to their own teams, scores do not need to be kept, and fouls should not be called unless they are obvious. This will keep games exciting and will decrease stress.

8. Praise the proper technique. If a basket is made with an off-balance throw and the player is rewarded, the player has learned nothing, except that making a basket is the most important thing. Instead, a proper shooting technique should be praised, even if a basket is not made.

9. Use a positive sandwich approach as follows:

Positive sincere remark
Corrective information
Positive encouraging remark

When young athletes learn a sport, they make many mistakes. In order to give them negative feedback, first say something encouraging, such as, "Nice try. You were really swinging hard." Then, provide constructive criticism, "Next time, you might want to try putting your hands closer together." The final remark should also be positive and encouraging, "This is a tough sport, but you'll get it."

10. Establish a place where learning new skills is not feared. Everyone needs to make mistakes to learn, but these mistakes should never be laughed at. How else can individuals grow?

11. Smile, laugh, be a cheerleader for the young athletes! Children love enthusiasm, and the effect can spill over into their performance and personal successes.

CONCLUSION

In spite of the potential problems associated with youth sports, the athletic environment can foster psychologic growth. Stress management can promote the achievement of cognitive coping skills. Sports psychologists, pediatricians, family practitioners, and other interested health professionals have demonstrated a growing interest in assisting youth sports programs to promote the welfare of children. The ability to handle failure, overcome adversity, and endure frustration is taught through sports. Athletes must deal with unfavorable referee calls, hostile crowds, jealousy, and people that are unlikable. To handle these parameters of the athletic environment, athletes must develop poise.

Much talk centers around what is wrong with school sports, including abusive coaches, overscheduled youth, and competitive parents. However, sports are an essential and integral part of any educational program. The obvious benefit of sports comes from the development of confidence and self esteem. Participation can build character and provide a forum where teamwork and dedication are fostered. In an athletic program that encourages youth to be "the best that they can be," true success is not measured by the team's victories, but by the commitment members make to reaching team goals.

The young athlete has many unique qualities that can be enhanced to promote lifelong involvement in sports that is both rewarding and satisfying. They are willing to become involved in activities that they do not associate with pain or injury. In many ways, the young athlete is in a better psychologic position than the older athlete for handling not being the best or even losing. They are also more capable of winning with grace.

The approaches for counteracting stress-inducing factors in youth sports may require evaluating the meaning of the sport to the child and his or her parents. Some families' lives are built around youth sports, and winning becomes the reason for living. Correspondingly, a loss may be psychologically catastrophic. Parents and coaches can be part of this problem, yet both need to be piece of the solution.

Sport programs needs to be administrated by coaches and parents with goals and objectives that are outlined before the season begins. Especially in elite athletes, exploitation by coaches and parents and the loss of self-image with injury or failure in competition are devastating (12). Many examples of burnout and "acting out" behaviors in child athletes have been related to excessive pressure. The physician is in an ideal position to identify and intervene if these situations arise.

REFERENCES

1. Martens R. Youth sports in the USA. In: Weiss MR, Gould D, eds. *Sport for children and youths*. Champaign, IL: Human Kinetics, 1986:27–33.
2. DuRant RH. The pre-participation examination of athletes. *Am J Dis Child* 1985;139:657–661.
3. Skinner A. Time out: criticism not withstanding school sports are still the best game in town. *American School Board Journal* 1988;175:22–23.
4. Suinn RM. Psychological approaches to performance enhancement. In: May JR, Asken MJ, eds. *Sport psychology*. New York: PMA Publishing Corporation, 1987: 41–57.
5. Larson GA, Zaichkowsky LD, Starkey C. Psychological aspects of athletic injuries as perceived by athletic trainers. *The Sport Psychologist* 1996;10:37–47.
6. Johnson MD. Disordered eating in active and athletic women. *Clin Sports Med* 1994;13:355–369.
7. Dummer GM, Rosen LW, Heusner WW, et al. Pathogenic weight control behaviors of young competitive swimmers. *The Physician and Sports Medicine* 1987;15: 75–86.
8. Rosen LW, Hough DO. Pathogenic weight control behavior of female college gymnasts. *The Physician and Sports Medicine* 1988;16:141–146.
9. Ryan J. *Pretty girls in little boxes*. New York: Warner Books, 1995.
10. American Psychiatric Association. *Diagnostic and statistical manual of mental disorders*, 4th ed. Washington, D.C.: American Psychiatric Association, 1994.
11. Root MPP. Persistent disordered eating as a gender-specific post traumatic stress response to sexual assault. *Psychotherapy* 1991;28:96–102.
12. Kaye WH, Weltsin TE. Neurochemistry of bulimia nervosa. *J Clin Psychol* 1991;52:21–28.
13. Drinkwater BL, Nilson K, Chesnut DH et al. Bone mineral content of amenorrheic and eumenorrheic athletes. *N Engl J Med* 1984;311:277–281.
14. Kreipe RE, Birndorf SA. Eating disorders in adolescents and young adults. *Med Clin North Am* 2000;84: 1027–1049.
15. Kreipe RE, Dukarm CP. Outcome of anorexia nervosa related to treatment using an adolescent approach. *J Youth Adolesc* 1996;25:483–497.
16. Tofler IR, Stryer BK, Micheli LJ, et al. Physical and emotional problems of elite female gymnasts. *N Engl J Med* 1996;335:281–283.
17. Ewing ME, Seefeldt V. *Participation and attrition patterns in American agency sponsored and interscholastic sports: an executive summary. Final Report*. North Palm Beach, FL: Sporting Goods Manufacturing Association, 1989.
18. Jopling RJ. Health related fitness as preventative medicine. *Pediatr Rev* 1988;10:141–148.
19. Gould D, Martens R. Attitudes of volunteer coaches toward significant youth sports issues. *Research Quarterly* 1979;50:369–380.
20. Weiss M, Chaumeton N. Motivational orientations in sports. In: TS Horn, ed. *Advances in sport psychology*. Champaign, IL: Human Kinetics, 1992:61–99.
21. Fox K, Goudus M, Biddle S, et al. Children's task and ego profiles in sports. *Br J Educ Psychol* 114;64:353–361.
22. Smoll FL, Smith RE. Psychology of the young athlete. *Ped Clin North Am* 1990;37:1021–1046.
23. Martens R. *Social psychology and physical activity*. New York: Harper & Row, 1975.
24. Orlick T. *The cooperative sports and games book*. New York: Pantheon, 1978.
25. Micheli LL. Sports injuries in children and adolescents. *Clin Sports Med* 1995;14:727–745.
26. Morgan WP. Selected psychological factors limiting

performance a mental health model. In: Clark OH, Eckert HM, eds. *Limits of human performance*. Champaign, IL: Human Kinetics, 1985.

27. Watson MD, Di Martino PP. Incidence of injuries in high school track and field athletes ad its relation to performance ability. *Am J Sports Med* 1987;15:251–254.

28. Landers DM, Boucher SH. Arousal performance relationships. In: Williams JM, ed. *Applied sport psychology: personal growth to peak performance*. Palo Alto, CA: Mayfield Publishing Co, 1986.

29. Weinberg RS, Gould D. *Foundations of sport and exercise psychology*. Champaign, IL: Human Kinetics, 1995.

30. Begel FL. An overview of sport psychiatry. *Am J Psychiatry* 1992;149:606–614.

31. Gould D, Feltz D, Horn T, et al. Reasons for attrition in competitive youth swimming. *J Sport Behav* 1982,5: 155–165.

32. Ahern DK, Lohr BA. Psycho-social factors in sports injury rehabilitation. *Clin Sports Meds* 1997;16:1–10.

33. Heil J. Mental training in injury management. *Psychology of sports injury*. Champaign, IL: Human Kinetics, 1993:151–174.

34. Williams JM, Tonymon P, Wadsworth WA. Relationship of life stress to injury in intercollegiate volleyball. *J Hum Stress* 1986;12:38–43.

35. Hergengroeder AC. Prevention of sports injuries. *Pediatrics* 1998;101:1057–1063

36. Orlick T. *Freeing children from stress: focusing and stress control activities for children*. Willits, CA: ITA Publications, 1992.

37. Salokun SO. Positive change in self-concept as a function of improved performance in sports. *Percept Mot Skills* 1994;78:752–754.

38. Martens R. *Joy and sadness in children's sports*. Champaign, IL: Human Kinetics, 1978.

39. Smoll FL, Smith RE, Barnett NP, et al. Enhancement of children's self esteem through social support training for youth sport coaches. *J Appl Psychol* 1993;78:602–610.

10

Medical–Legal Issues in Pediatric Sports Medicine

Lauren M. Simon

As the field of sports medicine has grown, so has the number of medical–legal considerations encountered by sports medicine practitioners. In the sports medicine milieu, many people are involved in various aspects of providing medical care to athletes and physically active youth. In addition to physicians, athletic trainers, nurses, therapists, psychologists, nutritionists, and others may be part of the sports medicine provider-team. The array of services provided to athletes include primary care, preventive care, treatment of injuries, and rehabilitation. The legal questions surrounding duties, responsibilities, and the provision of services by the various members of the sports medicine team are constantly evolving. This discussion focuses primarily on the role of the sports medicine physician and the legal regulations affecting the medical care in the practice of sports medicine.

THE TEAM PHYSICIAN

Many sports medicine practitioners serve as team physicians. They come from a variety of specialties, including family medicine, pediatrics, internal medicine, orthopedics, and others. Some team physicians have completed sports medicine fellowships, although such a fellowship is not required to be a team physician (see Chapter 1). Team physicians should be competent in applying medical knowledge to athletics, and he or she should stay current on the appropriate standards of care relevant to the treatment of athletes and teams (1). A team physician consensus statement (2), which outlines the duties and qualifications of a team physician, has been developed by the collaboration of six major professional sports medicine associations in the Sports Medicine Project-Based Alliance (composed of the American Academy of Family Physicians, the American Academy of Orthopaedic Surgeons, the American College of Sports Medicine, the American Medical Society for Sports Medicine, the American Orthopaedic Society for Sports Medicine and the American Osteopathic Academy of Sports Medicine).

The duties of a team physician can vary, depending on the team that the physician is covering. One strong recommendation is that an agreement delineating the duties and responsibilities of the team physician should exist (i.e., a contract or letter of engagement) between the team physician and the team and/or the entity in charge of the team (i.e., the school, school district, university, or sports league) (1). A document that sets the parameters of the physician's role *vis-à-vis* the athletic team and its players is essential because the team physician is called upon to make decisions about an athlete's condition not only while in the controlled setting of an office but also during games that can involve reactive, high pressure situations. These on-field situations do not typically afford the physician the opportunity to inquire about the limits of his or her role with respect to a patient–athlete.

The major responsibilities of the team physician include the performance of the preparticipation physical examinations (PPE) of athletes, the treatment and management of injuries, the coordination of rehabilitation, and the return to participation (2), as well as the provision of education and counseling for athletes, teams, the athletic staff, and schools on protective equipment, nutrition, conditioning guidelines, infectious precautions, and other medical problems that could affect the athlete. The team physician also provides proper event coverage and assesses environmental concerns and playing conditions (2). An imperative necessity is the team physician's familiarity with the injury patterns common in the particular sport, his or her clear understanding of the rules concerning medication use and the athlete's ability and eligibility to play, and a cognizance of the need for and use of protective equipment. Most importantly, the physician must ensure that a well-conceived plan is in place to handle emergencies during competition and practice. This plan should identify properly trained personnel that are onsite. It should list the emergency equipment that must be at the event, as well as the medical transport system servicing the event. Moreover, the plan must describe specifically who must be contacted in case of the injury of a team player.

Medical Malpractice

The definition of what constitutes a team physician, the scope of a team physician's responsibilities, and the standard of care applied to the team physician are constantly evolving. If a team physician is sued for his or her medical treatment (or lack thereof) of an athlete and the case results in a trial, the key question is, *"Did the physician abide by the standard of care?"* Pivotal evidence at trial includes expert testimony on the issue (1). Litigation focuses on whether the team physician was negligent. For a litigant to prevail against the physician on a claim of medical malpractice, the following four elements of negligence must be established: duty, breach, causation, and damages (Table 10.1).

The first element, *duty,* refers to whether the team physician has a physician–patient relationship that results in a duty to care for the athlete in question. Where such a relationship or duty exists, the physician must competently care for the athlete at the minimum skill level of other physicians who provide medical treatment for such an injury. The second element, *breach,* connotes a failure to provide the requisite standard of care to the athlete. Much of the testimony in medical malpractice cases consists of expert witnesses for the patient–plaintiff and for the physician–defendant who attempt to demonstrate that the physician's diagnosis and/or treatment did or did not conform to the standard of care owed to the patient. The third element, *causation,* is proven if the plaintiff demonstrates that the physician's breach of the duty of care (i.e., the failure to provide the minimum skill level to the patient) resulted in (i.e., had a sufficient causal connection to) the specific harm in-

flicted on the patient–athlete. This means that medical treatment (or failure to treat) that falls below the standard of care cannot result in a finding of negligence unless the acts (or failure to act) result in harm and/or injury to the patient. For example, if the team physician failed to diagnose a fractured navicular bone in the wrist of a baseball player and the athlete subsequently had a hyperextension injury to his knee rupturing his anterior cruciate ligament that caused the player to miss the remainder of the season, then causation has not been proven. No causation exists because the treatment (actually, the lack thereof) involving the wrist did not cause the injury to the knee. The fourth element of negligence of action is *damages.* The patient–athlete must have sustained some quantifiable damage, whether physical, financial, or emotional, in order to have a viable case against the physician (1). This means that, if the team physician renders medical treatment below the standard of care (e.g., permitting an athlete to play when other qualified physicians would not) that proximately causes an injury where no damages result, the team physician should not be considered negligent. A team physician may allow an injured athlete to return to play when other physicians would not. If the athlete sustains a slightly bruised extremity that enables the athlete to continue to compete after the application of ice without sustaining quantifiable damages, then the physician has not been negligent. In short, if the team physician does what a reasonably competent team physician would have done under similar circumstances, a plaintiff–athlete will be unlikely to prevail on a claim of negligence against the physician.

Medical Malpractice Insurance

A team physician's malpractice insurance must cover the scope of the physician's practice of sports medicine. Since many patients treated by team physicians, particularly in a school setting, are minors who, in certain circumstances can file lawsuits upon reaching the age of majority, the team physician must give careful consideration to the type of insurance coverage he or she selects.

Malpractice insurance can be divided into the following two main types: "occurrence" insurance and "claims-made" insurance. Occurrence insurance provides coverage for alleged malpractice events that occur during the policy period but that can be brought to court during or after the period of the policy. By design, occurrence insurance does not require tail coverage. In contrast, a claims-made policy provides coverage for alleged malpractice events that occur

TABLE 10.1. *Elements of negligence*

1. Duty
2. Breach
3. Causation
4. Damages

and that are brought to court during the time that insurance policy is in effect. If a physician has claims-made insurance, the physician should acquire tail coverage to ensure malpractice coverage if a claim is filed at a later date.

A team physician must ensure that his practice activities are covered by the policy, and, if they are not, the physician should seek additional insurance coverage prior to engaging in an uncovered practice. Additionally, if a physician travels with a team, he or she must check the territory section of the malpractice policy to see if the locale to which the physician is traveling is within the scope of the insurance coverage.

THE TRAVELING TEAM PHYSICIAN

When a team physician accompanies a team out of state where the team physician is not licensed to practice medicine, the physician might be perceived as practicing medicine without a license. In order to avoid such a circumstance, the team physician must become familiar with the laws governing the practice of medicine in the state where he is visiting (hereafter referred to as the "visiting state"). A good resource for information concerning the visiting state is that state's medical board.

Some states allow physicians who are licensed in another state to practice medicine occasionally in their state, as long as the physician does not have an office in that state nor publically declare that they are licensed in the visiting state; other states do not allow this practice (1). The physician has the obligation to know the laws of the visiting state. Moreover, in order to ensure the safety of athletes, the traveling team physician must familiarize himself or herself with the practices and protocols of sports medicine providers in the visiting state. This must occur prior to athletes taking the field so that injuries and emergencies can be planned for and local sports medicine providers can be apprised of any special medical needs for traveling athletic team members.

Other considerations about traveling with a team arise when the team is comprised of minors. The traveling team physician should make sure that each player's parent or guardian has completed written treatment authorization forms in case the need for treatment arises and the parent or guardian cannot be reached.

GOOD SAMARITAN LAWS

Many physicians volunteer their time to perform PPEs or to serve as team physicians. Others do not volunteer their time because of the fear of liability. One of the most common questions of any prospective team physician is whether he or she is protected from lawsuits under a Good Samaritan statute. Good Samaritan statutes, which are present in some form in all 50 states, essentially protect persons offering medical assistance (i.e., who come to the aid of those in need of treatment) from liability (1).

No definitive answer exists to the question of whether a team physician is protected from liability because, in the United States, lawsuits commence easily, typically with the mere payment of a court filing fee and the service of the legal document upon the opposing party. Having a case filed does not mean that it has merit or that it will proceed to trial. For cases to be dismissed or verdicts to be in favor of the physician is not uncommon in those instances in which the doctor voluntarily came to the aid of another person in an emergency situation. In such cases, the Good Samaritan law has been successfully invoked as a defense.

The team physician must know the parameters of the Good Samaritan law in each state where he or she will be rendering athletic coverage. Some states, in order to encourage volunteer medical care by physicians, have passed Good Samaritan legislation that specifically protects from liability those physicians who volunteer as athletic team physicians and/or who render care at athletic events or in other emergency situations. California is one such state. The statute in California, as reproduced in the *California Physician's legal handbook 1999,* states the following:

> No licensee (physician), who in good faith and without compensation renders voluntary *emergency* [emphasis added] medical assistance to a participant in a community college or high school athletic event or contest, at the site of the event or contest, or during transportation to a health care facility, for an injury suffered in the course of such event or contest, shall be liable for any civil damages as a result of any acts or omissions by such person in rendering such voluntary medical assistance. The immunity granted by this section shall not apply to acts or omissions constituting gross negligence (Business & Professions Code 2398) (3).

The reader should note that the parameters of Good Samaritan laws can vary from state to state. As a general rule, however, most state Good Samaritan statutes protect a particular class of persons (i.e., some states protect all persons rendering assistance, while other statutes specifically protect particular health care providers, such as physicians and nurses) acting in "good faith," in an emergency setting, where the provider's assistance has conformed to the profession's conduct standards under the circumstances and where the assistance has been provided gratuitously (i.e., without compensation) (1). In other words, the Good Samaritan provider must offer rescue or aid with honest intentions (good faith) at an emergency scene (e.g., an automobile accident, sporting event, and other locations specified by statute, normally not a hospital or office), while performing the aid with the minimum standard of care (without negligence) and while acting gratuitously (for free). Most importantly, the team physician must ensure that he or she is not receiving "compensation" for serving as team physician because, if he or she does, the physician's protection under a state's Good Samaritan statutes could be invalidated. However, receiving a team shirt, a free meal, or a bus ride to accompany the team have not been deemed monetary compensation (1).

THE PREPARTICIPATION PHYSICAL EXAMINATION

Many school systems and states require a PPE before an athlete may participate in interscholastic athletics. Its purpose is to identify health problems or injuries that may require further evaluation or rehabilitation or that could restrict an athlete from participating in the proposed activity. According to a publication endorsed by five major medical societies (the American Academy of Family Physicians, the American Academy of Pediatrics, the American Medical Society for Sports Medicine, the American Orthopaedic Society for Sports Medicine, and the American Osteopathic Academy of Sports Medicine) (4), the objectives of PPE include (a) detection of conditions that may predispose the athlete to injury or that could be life-threatening or disabling, (b) satisfying legal and insurance requirements, (c) ascertaining the student athlete's good health, (d) counseling the student on health-related issues, and (e) assessing the student's fitness level for a specific sport. Since not all students regularly see a family physician, this may be the only opportunity for health assessment and counseling on health issues for many student athletes.

The basic components of PPE are the review of the student athlete's history, the physical examination and/or tests, and any additional evaluation as needed (see Chapter 2).

Although many physicians provide PPEs to student athletes without compensation, the Good Samaritan statutes, in most states, do not shield the physician from liability in this context because medical services are performed in a nonemergency situation. Potential liability areas for any team physician who provides physicals to students include the failure to diagnose a medical problem or injury that would necessitate barring the athlete from play, particularly problems that may result in permanent injury or death, such as arrhythmias. One of the most publicized cases involving cardiac anomalies or arrhythmias linked to sudden death in athletes was the death of basketball star Hank Gathers (5). Another anomaly associated with sudden death in athletic and other activities is hypertrophic obstructive cardiomyopathy (HOCM) (4). This can be problematic for the team physician as HOCM may be asymptomatic, and thus it is often not easily identified during the medical history and/or physical examination. Other possible medical and legal problems include the failure to identify inadequately rehabilitated prior injuries that could be aggravated by participating in a particular sport.

Several different formats can be used to conduct PPEs, such as individual visits to the doctor's office; a station examination whereby multiple athletes are seen by multiple examiners, each of whom performs one section of the exam at his or her station; or locker room *en masse* examinations. Although station-based rotations or locker room examinations may be efficiently conducted, the impersonal nature of the examination (i.e., the lack of privacy or the noise factor, which could impede a physician's ability to auscultate cardiopulmonary systems reliably), could expose the physician to liability. This is particularly relevant if the problem could have been detected in a quiet setting or if the information (i.e., preexisting injury) could have been divulged by the student athlete in a more private setting or with the taking of a more thorough history.

Preparticipation Physical Examination Standards

Many professional medical organizations have issued standards regarding PPEs that address common medical problems and whether athletes with these problems would be at risk through participation in various sports (4,6–8). In 1988, the American Academy of Pediatrics published, "Recommendations for participation in competitive sports;" and, in 1994, the American Academy of Pediatrics Committee on Sports Medicine and Fitness issued, "Medical conditions affecting sports participation" (see Chapter 2) (6). Both guides classify sports into subsets by the degree of physical contact between players and the level of strenuousness (6). The contact subsets divide sports into the following three categories: (a) contact/collision, (b) limited contact, and (c) noncontact (see Chapter 2, Table 2.8, for additional information). For instance, football and soccer are deemed contact/collision sports, while baseball and cheerleading are limited contact sports. Swimming and golf are categorized as noncontact sports.

The strenuousness subsets consist of four classifications (see Chapter 2, Table 2.9). The gradations of strenuousness are divided according to intensity and the dynamic, and static aspects of the sport. The high to moderate intensity category includes (a) high to moderate dynamic and static demand sports, such as football and water polo; (b) high to moderate dynamic and low static demand sports, such as baseball and soccer; and (c) low dynamic and high to moderate static demand sports, such as gymnastics and karate. The low intensity category includes low dynamic and low static demand sports, such as golf and bowling.

The *Preparticipation physical evaluation* (4) adopts the contact strenuousness classifications described above, and these classifications, along with the monograph's preparticipation athletic clearance guidelines, have been endorsed by the American Academy of Family Physicians, the American Academy of Pediatrics, the American Medical Society for Sports Medicine, the American Orthopaedic Society for Sports Medicine and the American Osteopathic Society of Sports Medicine. Another source for athletic clearance guidance is found in the 26th Bethesda Conference guidelines (8), which are used for clearance of cardiovascular problems. The preparticipation monograph (4) includes sample forms (i.e., history, physical, and clearance) for use in the PPE.

Thus, after consideration of the athlete's condition, the team physician should document his or her conclusions and the rationale behind those determinations in view of the sports classifications detailed above. The team physician should then summarize the findings, and, to a limited extent, given the confidentiality of medical evaluations, should share those findings with the coach or athletic staff to arrange for appropriate follow-up. The reader should note that the team physician has limits to his or her ability to disclose particular medical information to third parties, including the school, coach, and athletic staff. Confidential medical information should not be divulged unless the athlete and/or the parent or guardian has agreed to its release.

Preparticipation Physical Examination and Athletic Clearance

The four types of clearance assessments for sports participation are (a) unrestricted clearance, (b) clearance after completing further evaluation or rehabilitation, (c) restricted clearance for certain sports, and (d) not cleared for any sports. The *Preparticipation physical evaluation* (4), the 26th Bethesda Conference guidelines (8), and the 1994 American Academy of Pediatrics Committee recommendations (6) (see also Chapter 2, Table 2.10) can be used to guide clinical clearance determinations. The classification guidelines can assist in determining which activities, if any, the athlete can participate in safely (4). For example, if an athlete has an abnormality or condition, such as certain pulmonary or cardiac problems, that warrants restricted clearance from football, the athlete might be cleared for a noncontact, low dynamic and static sport, such as golf. One reason clearance decisions can restrict athletes from certain sports is that dynamic sports cause a volume load on the left ventricle, whereas static sports cause a pressure load (4).

In determining which type of clearance to give an athlete, a thorough history must be taken, and a physical examination must be performed. The recommendation is that the student's parent and/or guardian complete and sign the history form. Inquiry must be made about any medical conditions affecting the athlete, including the medications he or she uses, previous head injuries, heat injuries, exercise-related medical problems, risk factors for sudden death, and any previous musculoskeletal injuries. For female athletes, a menstrual history should also be obtained.

When the general medical and musculoskeletal examination is performed, careful evaluation should be made of previous injury sites. Additionally, the physical maturity level of the athlete must be assessed, and a sport-specific musculoskeletal evaluation should be performed.

When making clearance determinations, the physician is using his or her best medical judgment. The physician should not be significantly influenced by outside considerations. Some other special clearance decisions deserve mention, particularly those athletes with unpaired organs or cardiac abnormalities. In cases of athletes with unpaired organs or cardiac abnormalities who wish to engage in any contact/collision or limited contact sports, a thorough discussion of the choice of sport and the risks attendant to participation should occur (see Chapter 2, Table 2.10). If an athlete has only one kidney and if the athlete receives clearance to participate in a contact sport after a thorough evaluation is conducted and informed consent regarding the risks has been documented, then protective equipment for the athlete's kidney must be used. Similarly, if an athlete with one eye wants to participate in a racquet sport, protective eye-wear must be used.

The decision to exclude an athlete from participation in a particular sport, like the decision to permit an athlete to play a particular sport, can be fraught with unexpected legal repercussions. Some athletes seek legal redress to reverse determinations made by a team physician or school district. In *Pace v. Dryden Central School District* (9), a 17-year-old boy with a solitary kidney was prohibited by the school district physician from participating in high school football and basketball interscholastic athletic programs. His parents filed a lawsuit to compel the school to permit him to play (9). As part of their case, the parents submitted evidence showing that the particular health risks involved with the selected sports had been discussed with the family and that the student's own physician, as well as an urology specialist, had attested that the student's participation in contact sports was, in the opinion of the physicians, "reasonably safe." The court reversed the school district's decision and permitted the student to play (9). Most significantly, the court held that, by virtue of its legal challenge to the restriction, the family waived any future liability claim against the school district in the event that the athlete's sole kidney was injured. The import of this decision is that litigation is often inevitable, whether an athlete is or is not cleared for participation in sports. The team physician should rely on the clearance guidelines in making his or her determinations, even if they are subsequently challenged in court. If the physician succumbs to pressure and permits a clearance that does not comport with the guidelines, that litigation will ensue over the physician's allegedly improper clearance determination is quite foreseeable. However, if a court intervenes and permits an athlete to play against the team physician's advice or if the athlete has been conditionally cleared after the athlete's written waiver of the risk, the team physician continues to have the responsibility to help the athlete participate in the sport as safely as possible. Thus, if an athlete with an arrhythmia is participating in a particular sport whether by court order or by the athlete's waiver of the risks of participation, the team physician must ensure that a defibrillator is within immediate reach and that people who are trained in its use are present.

Athletes have no constitutionally protected right to participate in interscholastic sports; rather such participation is a privilege that may be withdrawn by school or voluntary association whose rules the school has agreed to follow (10). However, once interscholastic sports are offered, the athlete must be afforded due process if he or she is to be excluded from competition for medical reasons (11). Procedural due process is afforded a student if the institution has and follows published standards that give the student notice and permit a hearing on the issue (11). Even so, problems of a constitutional nature can arise when a high risk student athlete is barred from play, since "no state shall deny a citizen equal protection under the law" (11). A plethora of laws prohibiting discrimination, arbitrary classifications, and disparate treatment can be applied to the athletic context (11). Examples include the Federal Rehabilitation Act of 1973, the Individuals With Disabilities Education Act of 1989, and the Americans With Disabilities Act of 1990 (12–14). Athletes have used these laws to challenge team physicians' decisions to exclude athletes from participation. For example, in *Lambert v. The West Virginia State Board of Education* (15), a school district excluded a deaf student from participating in basketball. The student then sued, and the court held that the Federal Rehabilitation Act and the Individuals with Disabilities Education Act barred such discrimination against the handicapped student. The court ruled that the student could participate in the sport by using the services of a signer (15). In contrast, a high school football player who was restricted from playing football due to a heart defect caused by hypertrophic cardiomyopathy that was discovered after he passed out at practice, sued his high school and the Archdiocese of Cincinnati in order to permit him to play (16). The court in *Larkin v. Archdiocese of Cincinnati* (16) ruled that schools have the power to enforce medical standards, even if doing so means barring some athletes from competition (1,11,16).

RISK RELEASES AND WAIVERS OF LIABILITY

Team physicians must ensure that athletes and their parents are informed of the risks of the sport. This is usually accomplished by providing the student athlete and his parents with a written, sport-specific information packet and parent approval form. For those student athletes with known medical risks or conditions that place them at a higher risk of injury than other athletes, the condition and possible consequences of participating in that sport, with that risk or condition, must be noted on the risk release and signed by both the athlete and the parents or guardians. (The clinician should note that minors are legally not considered competent to enter into such waivers.)

Many of these forms contain provisions that attempt to absolve the school and its personnel. The rationale for these waivers (which, in essence, are contracts between the student and parents and the school) is that, if the athlete and parents are aware of the dangers inherent in a particular sport and they choose to permit the student to participate in the sport, the student (and parents) have assumed the risk and the school district, team, activity sponsor, and physician are insulated from liability. However, waivers and risk releases do not, in and of themselves, inoculate the school and any related parties from suit. As with any contract, the courts often are called upon to determine whether the waiver was valid and binding. The courts consider whether the waiver was clearly written and specific and whether it was subject to different interpretations (11). Risk releases that permit a student to play a sport commonly do not eliminate liability, if the student's injury was a result of the school's or physician's negligence in the treatment (or the lack thereof) with respect to the student's injury, not to the decision to play.

As with other medical decisions, the physician must use his or her best medical judgment in determining whether a student should be permitted to play a particular sport. Each sports medicine physician must be cognizant of the law of the state (or states) in which he or she practices as some states are more receptive to the use of waivers than others.

RETURN TO PLAY DECISIONS

Once an athlete has been cleared and participation in the sport commences, injuries may occur during practice or games. One of the roles of the team physician is to determine whether an injured athlete may safely resume participation in the sport. Some general principles that guide these decisions are the diagnosis of the injury and a determination as to whether additional play will worsen the injury or will place the athlete at additional risk of harm (1). The team physician's final decision must be based on what is best for the athlete's health. Even though pressures to minimize the time an athlete is restricted from participating in the game are often found (as typically expressed by the athlete, team, parents, or coach), the team physician must never compromise the athlete's safety. The standard of care used in making return to play decisions should be what a "reasonably prudent physician [would] do under same or similar circumstances (1)." The team physician should rely upon recognized sport-specific injury profiles and injury specific guidelines in making those determinations

(1,6–8,17). One of the most common return to play determinations concerns players with head injuries. For example, when a football player sustains a grade 1 concussion, has experienced dizziness, and has a headache but has not lost consciousness, should he be allowed to resume play?

Utilizing the "reasonably prudent physician standard," the existence of the postconcussive headache would be a significant factor that causes the athlete to be barred from play, at a minimum, for the remainder of the game (1,17).

The team physician must make sure that all team members, coaches, and sponsors are apprised—preferably in writing by the school—that the team physician makes the ultimate determination of participation and that the physician's determination cannot be overruled. An explicit statement of the hierarchy of medical decision making can assuage the return to play conflicts that invariably can arise during a game.

CONFIDENTIALITY

The communications between a doctor and patient are privileged, unless the privilege is expressly waived. Thus, confidentiality of patient information, whether the patient is an athlete or not, is sacrosanct. Care must be taken, most often in response to inquiries about an athlete's condition, not to compromise the condition of the patient–athlete inadvertently through comments to the athletic staff, press, or teammates, unless such a disclosure has been authorized by the patient and/or his or her parents. Confidentiality issues can also arise when athletes possess infectious diseases, such as human immunodeficiency virus (HIV), hepatitis, herpes simplex ,and fungal infections. Not only must the sports medicine physician be familiar with the applicable guidelines regarding the participation of athletes with infectious diseases, such as those issued by the American Academy of Pediatrics Committee on Sports Medicine and the World Health Organization; but he or she must also inform the patient–athlete about the transmission risks of the infection, and he or she should educate the athlete regarding precautionary steps with respect to transmission prevention (18). Moreover, the physician should counsel the athlete on his or her selection of sports, while at the same time respecting the athlete's confidentiality.

The American Academy of Pediatrics Committee on Sports Medicine Guidelines regarding HIV recognizes that the chance of transmitting HIV during sports is extremely low, and it recommends that HIV-positive athletes be permitted to participate in all sports (18). Thus, even though a nominal risk exists for blood exposure from the HIV-infected athlete who chooses to participate in contact sports (e.g., football or tae kwon do), the right of confidentiality protects the disclosure of the athlete's HIV status to others, including the athletic staff, unless the athlete consents to the disclosure (see Chapter 2).

DRUG USE

Drug use by athletes also raises confidentiality concerns. Due to the increasing amount of illicit drug use among athletes, drug testing has been implemented in many collegiate and professional sports and in some high school athletic programs for the purpose of maintaining competitive fairness. However, a patient–athlete's own disclosure of drug use to the team physician is privileged, unless the confidentiality is expressly waived by the patient–athlete. For this reason, the team physician ideally should not be the same individual conducting drug testing for the various school and sports governing bodies, since this could potentially compromise the trust relationship of the athlete with the team physician. Should a student athlete admit to drug use (e.g., anabolic steroids), the team physician should utilize the opportunity created by the disclosure to have an honest, balanced discussion regarding the risks and benefits of the particular drug in the hope of steering the athlete away from the use of drugs.

Drug use, whether illicit, performance enhancing, by prescription, or purchased over-the-counter, can be problematic for an athlete in competition, as well as for the athlete's team physician (see Chapter 5). The physician needs to be aware of all the drug regulations and prohibitions governing the particular competition. This knowledge is essential in order to prevent an athlete from disqualification or restricted sport participation due to a positive result on a drug test from the use of a prohibited substance. For example, an unwary team physician's proper and reasonable medical treatment (e.g., instructing an athlete with an upper respiratory infection to use a cold preparation with ephedrine) could jeopardize an athlete's career and could subject the physician to litigation by the athlete or the athlete's parents, since the drug is a banned substance for athletic competition (19). Therefore, the sports medicine physician should be familiar with the lists of banned drugs and substances for competition that are published by two of the major amateur sport governing bodies in the United States, the United States Olympic Committee and the National Collegiate Athletic Association (19) (see Chapter 11, Table 11.1 for a list of these).

RISK MANAGEMENT

The practice of sports medicine is often exciting, as well as being emotionally and professionally rewarding. Unfortunately, an increase in sports medicine litigation has occurred concurrently with the development of the field of sports medicine. In order for the sports medicine physician to deter litigation or to prevail, if litigation occurs, he or she must practice the four Cs of good risk management.

The four key components of good risk management are *compassion, communication, competence,* and *charting* (1). *Compassion* is exhibited by those physicians who foster good relationships with the athletes and athletic staff; and, perhaps not coincidentally, they are less likely to be sued, even if a bad outcome occurs. *Communication* focuses on the exchange of information between the patient and the physician. Physicians who communicate effectively are those who give athletes and parents clear information about risk of sports and risks and treatment options for conditions or injuries when securing informed consent. *Competence* means that the sports medicine physician stays apprised of all aspects of the emerging field of sports medicine and that he or she is cognizant of, and delivers, the required standard of care to the patient. The fourth component, *charting,* concerns the physician's duty to maintain particularized and complete medical records.

Meticulously prepared medical records can save a physician untold grief if litigation ensues. The team physician must ensure that an organized system for record completion, retention, and retrieval is in place. The file of a patient–athlete should, at a minimum, contain the PPE record.

Although team physicians often practice medicine on the field instead of in an office, the need for detailed medical records still exists. If treatment is rendered on the sideline when time for documentation is scarce, the physician, as well as any assisting athletic trainers, should use a notepad to document the essential medical information contemporaneously. Then, as soon as is feasible, the physician should complete the notes and then make a copy and place the document in the patient's file. The record should be legibly written and should be signed by the physician; it should contain the athlete's name, sport, date of the event, the assessment of injury or illness, immediate treatment, and further recommendations for treatment and rehabilitation (1,6).

The team physician should maintain medical records for periods of time that often exceed the student's tenure at the school or on the team. Since the ability of minors to sue for medical malpractice upon reaching the age of majority varies from state to state, the team physician should consult with an attorney before destroying any medical records.

While the four Cs of good risk management are useful for all physicians, an additional C can be added. The fifth C is a well-drafted *contract* between the team physician and the entity for which the physician is providing services. The team physician should insist upon a contract or letter of agreement that delineates the services that he or she will provide the team and what insurance coverage is in effect for those services, including games and practice sessions. If the team physician is a volunteer (i.e., providing services without remuneration), this too should be made part of the contract or agreement. Such an inclusion could prove to be pivotal evidence in litigation, if the team physician seeks to meet the requirements for a Good Samaritan defense, stemming from rendering medical care in an emergency situation. Finally, the contract or agreement should include a statement that the final decision on participation or return to play considerations is to be made by the team physician. This can serve to minimize potential conflicts on the sideline when an athlete is injured.

SUMMARY

A broad expanse of administrative, state, and federal laws govern the practice of medicine, including that of sports medicine. A physician who cares for athletes must be aware of these laws so that he or she can abide by them in the course of providing exemplary care to the pediatric athlete while executing the duties of a team physician.

REFERENCES

1. Gallup EM. *Law and the team physician*. Champaign, IL: Human Kinetics, 1995.
2. Sports Medicine Project-Based Alliance. *Team physician consensus statement*. Washington, D.C.: United States Government Printing Office, 2000.
3. Moore MA, Lee HP, eds. *California physician's legal handbook 1999*. San Francisco: California Medical Association, 1999.
4. Hawthorne S, ed. *Preparticipation physical evaluation*, 2nd ed. Minneapolis: McGraw-Hill, 1997.
5. Lavelle M. A star basketball player's death rattles the college sports world and creates a nightmare of numerous legal battles. *Natl Law J* 1991;13:1.
6. American Academy of Pediatrics Committee on Sports Medicine and Fitness. Medical conditions affecting sports participation. *Pediatrics* 2001;107:1205–1209.
7. Herbert DL, *Legal aspects of sports medicine*. 2nd ed. Canton, OH: PRC Publishing, Inc., 1995.
8. 26th Bethesda Conference. Recommendations for determining eligibility for competition in athletes with cardiovascular abnormalities [published erratum appears in *Med Sci Sports Exerc* 1994;26]. *Med Sci Sports Exerc* 1994;26:S223–S283.
9. *Pace v. Dryden Central School District*, 574 N.Y.S. 2d 142, 1991.
10. *JM, JR v. Montana High School Association*, 875 P.2d 1026, 1994.
11. Greenberg M.J., Benching of an athlete with medical problems may spur legal claims. *Natl Law J* 1993;15:29.
12. United States Congress. *The Federal Rehabilitation Act*. Washington, D.C.: United States Government Printing Office, 1973.
13. United States Congress. *The Individuals with Disabilities Education Act*. Washington, D.C.: United States Government Printing Office, 1989.
14. United States Congress. *The Americans with Disabilities Act*. Washington, D.C.: United States Government Printing Office, 1990.
15. *Lambert v. The West Virginia State Board of Education*. 447 S.E. 2d 901; 1994.
16. *Larkin v. Archdiocese of Cincinnati*. 90–3893 (6th Circuit, 1990).
17. Harmon KG. Assessment and management of concussion in sports. *Am Fam Physician* 1999;60:887–892.
18. American Academy of Pediatrics Committee on Sports Medicine and Fitness. The human immunodeficiency virus and other blood-borne pathogens in the athletic setting. *Pediatrics* 1999;104:1400–1403.
19. Potts KA, ed. *NCAA sports medicine handbook, 2000–01*. Indianapolis: The National Collegiate Athletic Association, 2000.

PART II

Medical Conditions and Young Athletes

11

Infectious Illnesses

William F. Miser

Primary care physicians often provide health care to athletes, both young and old. Most published articles focus on preventive services, such as the preparticipation physical examination (PPE), or the treatment of acute musculoskeletal injuries, such as ankle sprains. However, little is published on the most common reason young athletes seek medical care—acute febrile illnesses, especially those involving the upper respiratory tract.

Moderate exercise enhances the immune system, while intensive exercise, especially overtraining, depresses it (1–5). Athletes involved in demanding training programs are more susceptible to infections and viral illnesses than are nonathletes (6–10). Strenuous exercise during the incubation phase of an infection may actually worsen the severity of the illness (9). The athlete's desire to train through an illness or to minimize layoff time often conflicts with the need to avoid strenuous exercise during an acute illness.

Primary care physicians who care for the young athlete must recognize and correctly manage these illnesses in order to avoid unnecessary complications and to speed recovery. The therapeutic goal for the athlete is to provide as much relief as possible, without affecting performance. For example, antihistamines approved for international competition may be appropriate, but side effects, such as drowsiness, may impair performance, and the anticholinergic effects may predispose the athlete to a heat injury (11). The International Olympic Committee (IOC) disallows topical and systemic decongestants for use by world-class athletes, although they may be approved for use in other athletic competitions. The primary care physician should weigh the discomfort and the effects of acute febrile illness on the athlete against the potential side effects and the disqualifying nature of medical therapy. If the athlete has relatively mild to moderate symptoms that do not impair performance, avoiding the use of any pharmacotherapy may be beneficial. However, if the symptoms do impair performance, then therapy should be individualized.

This chapter highlights those common acute febrile upper respiratory illnesses that may occur in the young athlete. Space prohibits an exhaustive discussion of each illness, and the reader is encouraged to refer to the bibliography, which contains several excellent reviews.

THE SYMPTOMATIC TREATMENT OF FEVER

Body temperature normally varies with time of day, and it is often low in the morning and high in the early evening. The upper limit of normal body temp is 37.7°C (99.9°F) in adults and 37.9°C (100.2°F) in children, with fever being defined as a temperature greater than this upper limit (12). Usually, fever is the body's normal response to various agents, most often viral or bacterial pathogens. These exogenous pyrogens induce the body to produce cytokines, which act on the anterior hypothalamus to generate prostaglandins, subsequently resetting the thermal set point (12,13). Once it has been reset, this thermoregulatory center maintains a higher body temperature through cutaneous vasoconstriction (heat conservation) and shivering (thermogenesis) (13).

A fever actually can have beneficial effects. At 40.0°C (104°F), neutrophil function and host defenses are more active, and many pathogens, such as *Streptococcus pneumoniae*, are more susceptible to these defenses (13). Only with extremely high temperatures of greater than 42°C (107.6°F) are deleterious effects noted. However, in the athlete, any fever may result in heat-related illness during exercise (14). As needed, effective and safe antipyretics include acetaminophen (10 to 15 mg/kg orally, every 4 to 6 hours; maximum of 1 g per dose and 4 g in 24 hours) and ibuprofen (5 to 10 mg/kg orally, every 6 to 8 hours; maximum of 1,200 mg in 24 hours) (15). In addition to reducing fever, these medicines may also relieve the pain from the myalgias or headache that often accompanies an acute febrile illness.

THE COMMON COLD

The common cold, a benign, self-limited viral infection of the upper respiratory tract, causes more disability among athletes than all other diseases combined (7,8,16,17). During the 1992 Winter Olympics, upper respiratory infection (URI) prevented a number of athletes from competing, and it caused others to have subpar performances (18). The athlete with a common cold typically has one or more of the following symptoms: low-grade fever, headache, myalgias, nasal congestion, watery nasal discharge, sneezing, sore or scratchy throat, or nonproductive cough. These symptoms typically last for 1 to 2 weeks, with most athletes feeling much better within the first week.

Since the common cold is a self-limited viral illness, treatment is symptomatic, and it includes rest; heated, humidified air (19); and warm fluids. Antibiotics do not change the course or outcome of a viral URI, and thus they should not be prescribed (20–23). Although nasal secretions commonly become thicker and more mucopurulent during the natural course of an URI, antibiotics are not beneficial unless other signs and symptoms of acute sinusitis are found (see "Sinusitis" below) (23).

Most of the over 800 cold medicines available on the market include mixtures of antihistamines and decongestants. The majority of these are ineffective (16,24,25), and many are prohibited by the IOC (Table 11.1). If necessary, decongestants (pseudoephedrine and oxymetazoline), chlorpheniramine, and guaifenesin may provide some relief (26). Ipratropium bromide nasal spray may provide specific relief for the profuse rhinorrhea and sneezing associated with the common cold (27). The use of large doses of vitamin C (≥1 g per day) both to alleviate and to prevent common cold symptoms is controversial. In a recent evidence-based analysis of published studies, long-term, daily supplementation with vitamin C did not appear to prevent colds, but it did seem to have a modest benefit in reducing the duration of cold symptoms (28). Echinacea, also known as the purple coneflower, is an herbal medicine that appears to be effective for reducing the duration and the severity of symptoms of the common cold (29,30). The data to support the use of zinc gluconate throat lozenges to shorten the duration of the common cold is controversial (31–33). The home remedy of chicken soup actually improves mucociliary clearance, and it may provide some relief (16).

INFLUENZA

Influenza is an acute febrile infection of the respiratory tract that typically occurs during the winter months; it is characterized by abrupt fever, myalgias, headache, and cough. The athlete who competes in winter sports and who lives in close quarters with other athletes may benefit from vaccination against influenza. This vaccine is given annually, and it is 70% to 90% effective in preventing influenza (34,35). The virus in the vaccine is inactivated, so it cannot cause influenza or produce viremia. Those who have an anaphylactic reaction to chicken eggs, chickens, chicken feathers, or chicken dander or those who have a sensitivity to any of its components should not receive the vaccine. The vaccine also should not be administered to children with an active neurologic process or an acute febrile illness. Children younger than the age of 13 years should receive the split virus vaccine, 0.5 mL intramuscularly, while those who are older may receive either the whole or split virus. A live attenuated vaccine is nearing approval in the United States, and it may provide an alternative to the current inactivated vaccine (35).

If the athlete develops symptoms suggestive of influenza, and an influenza type A outbreak is known to have occurred in the area, the duration of the fever and symptoms may be shortened by 1 to 2 days by using amantadine (Symmetrel) or rimantadine (Flumadine) in the first 48 hours of symptoms (35). The usual dosage of both drugs is 5 mg per kg, with a 150 mg maximum daily dose for children and 200 mg for adults, given

TABLE 11.1. *Partial list of medicines permitted and prohibited by the World Anti-Doping Agency and the International Olympic Committee[a]*

Medicines that are permitted:
  Analgesics, such as acetaminophen, ibuprofen, codeine
  Antihistamines, such as fexofenadine, loratadine, cetirizine
  Anticholinergics, such as ipratropium bromide
  Cough suppressants, such as dextromethorphan
  Corticosteroids used as nasal or inhalation therapy
  Expectorants, such as guaifenesin
  Throat lozenges, such as domiphen bromide
Medicines that are prohibited:
  Caffeine[b]
  Ephedrine[b]
  Oral corticosteroids
  Propylhexedrine[b]
  Pseudoephedrine[b]

[a]This list is updated each year. For a current listing of permitted and prohibited drugs, visit the Internet Web site of the International Olympic Committee (http://www.olympic.org) or write to the United States Olympic Committee, 1750 E. Boulder St., Colorado Springs, CO 80909–5760 or the National Collegiate Athletic Association, Box 1906, Mission, KS 66201.
[b]Common ingredients found in decongestant cold and sinus medications; as a general rule, avoid combination products that may contain caffeine (analgesics), mild stimulants, such as pseudoephedrine (decongestants and cold remedies), and alcohol (many liquid cough and cold preparations).

orally in a tablet or syrup form, once or divided in two, for 3 to 5 days. Common side effects may include loss of appetite, nausea, difficulty concentrating, nervousness, insomnia, and lightheadedness. Two recently released neuraminidase inhibitors, zanamivir (Relenza) and oseltamivir (Tamiflu), are effective against both influenza A and B viruses if they are started within 48 hours of the onset of symptoms (35). Zanamivir is inhaled as a powder form through the mouth, while oseltamivir is taken orally. At this time, only zanamivir has been approved for children under the age of 18 years.

Symptoms of fever, headache, and myalgias can be diminished or relieved with the use of acetaminophen or ibuprofen. The three most common cough suppressants with proven efficacy are codeine, dextromethorphan, and guaifenesin (36). Dextromethorphan is equivalent to codeine, and it is generally safe at lower dosages, such as 15 to 30 mg, which are given orally four times a day.

SINUSITIS

Sinusitis (inflammation of the mucosa of the paranasal sinuses) or rhinosinusitis (sinusitis accompanied by inflammation of the contiguous nasal mucosa) is a common problem, especially in those athletes involved in water sports, such as swimming, diving, surfing, and water polo (37). Sinusitis should be suspected if the symptoms of a common cold fail to resolve after 2 weeks, if a purulent nasal discharge is accompanied by fever, or if pain is present over the cheek or teeth, especially if it is worsened by bending forward (38–41). The diagnosis of sinusitis is based on clinical presentation; imaging or laboratory studies are not recommended for the routine diagnosis of uncomplicated sinusitis (37). Plain sinus radiographs, such as Waters (maxillary), Caldwell (frontal), lateral (sphenoid), and submentovertical (ethmoid) views, are of limited use in younger athletes. Focused sinus computerized tomography (CT) is a more sensitive and cost-competitive alternative to plain films (42).

Analgesics are often needed for pain control. Decongestants, saline nasal spray, and hot tea with lemon are useful to promote drainage of the sinuses, and guaifenesin, 1,200 mg orally, twice per day, is effective in thinning nasal secretions (43). Avoid antihistamines because they may thicken nasal secretions. Nasal corticosteroids, used for a minimum of 3 to 5 days, are effective and safe. Distinguishing sinusitis caused by viruses (majority of cases) from that caused by bacteria is difficult clinically (44). Therefore, antibiotics are usually not required, especially if the symptoms are mild or moderate (45). Instead, antibiotics should be reserved for those who have persistent purulent nasal drainage and facial tenderness or pain, for those who have not improved after 7 days, or for those with severe symptoms, regardless of duration (44). For the majority of cases, 7 to 10 days of a first-line antibiotic (Table 11.2) is effective (44,46). If incomplete resolution or early relapse of symptoms occurs, treat the athlete with another 10-day to 14-day course of a second-line antibiotic. If no significant improvement occurs after the second course of antibiotics or if the symptoms are particularly severe, consider consultation with an otolaryngologist. The athlete should avoid diving below the water surface until the sinusitis is completely resolved.

TABLE 11.2. *Oral antibiotics used for treating acute rhinosinusitis*

Antibiotic	Dosage[a]		
	Adults (mg)	Children (mg/kg/d)	Dosing frequency[b]
Suggested primary regimen			
Amoxicillin	500–875	40–80	bid–tid
Doxycycline	100	100[c]	bid
Trimethoprim/sulfamethoxazole	160/800	6–10	bid
Second-line treatment			
Amoxicillin/clavulanate	875/125	45/6.4	bid
Cefaclor	500	40	tid
Clarithromycin extended release	1,000	15	qd
Cefuroxime axetil	250	30	bid
Cefpodoxime proxetil	200	10	bid
Cefdinir	600	14	qd
Levofloxacin[d]	500	—	qd
Moxifloxacin[d]	400	—	qd
Gatifloxacin[d]	400	—	qd

[a]Unless otherwise indicated, antibiotic is given orally for 10 d.
[b]qd, once a day; bid, twice a day; tid, three times a day; qid, four times a day.
[c]Avoid in those less than the age of 9 yr.
[d]Fluroquinolones not recommended under 18 yr of age, except in cystic fibrosis.

ACUTE OTITIS MEDIA

Otitis media refers to inflammation of the middle ear, often associated with a middle-ear effusion (47). *Acute otitis media* (AOM) is an infection of the middle ear, with the rapid appearance of symptoms and signs, such as fever, pain, irritability, decreased hearing, abnormal appearance (erythematous, bulging), and decreased mobility of the tympanic membrane.

Accurate diagnosis of AOM requires a clear and well-illuminated view of the tympanic membrane. Athletes involved in water sports are particularly prone to cerumen impaction. When attempting to remove earwax with a cotton-tipped applicator, the athlete may cause the cerumen to become impacted deep in the ear canal, thus worsening the condition (48). Therefore, athletes should be counseled against such a practice. In the absence of a known tympanic membrane perforation, a wax softener, such as olive or mineral oil, triethanolamine polypeptide oleate-condensate, or carbamide peroxide, makes cerumen removal easier (49). Earwax can then be removed by gentle warm water irrigation, suction, or cerumen curette, under direct visualization. The most valuable diagnostic test is inspection of the middle ear with a pneumatic otoscope (50). The tympanic membrane in AOM appears red, dull or opaque, and immobile. Vesicles present on the tympanic membrane (bullous myringitis) suggest a *Mycoplasma* infection.

Because of the growing worldwide occurrence of multidrug resistant bacteria and the fact that up to one-third of cases of AOM are viral in origin, a brief period of observation, consisting of a 72-hour period before prescribing antibiotics, is gaining acceptance, especially in many European countries. In several randomized clinical trials, antibiotics were shown to provide only a small benefit (51,52). If antibiotics are used, amoxicillin remains the drug of choice for most young athletes (51,53). It achieves high levels in the middle ear fluid, it is effective against most bacterial pathogens known to cause AOM, it is inexpensive, and it has a low incidence of side effects (skin rash, nausea, and diarrhea). Al-

TABLE 11.3. *Antibiotics for acute otitis media*

	Dosage[a]		
	Adults (mg)	Children (mg/kg/d)	Dosing frequency[b]
Antibiotic			
Suggested primary regimen			
Amoxicillin	500	80–90	bid–tid
Second-line treatment			
Amoxicillin/clavulanate (Augmentin)	875/125	90/6.4	bid
Sulfonamides			
Trimethoprim/sulfamethoxazole (Bactrim, Septra)	160/800	8 (trimethoprim)	bid
Erythromycin-sulfisoxazole (Pediazole)	40–50	50 (erythromycin)	qid
Cephalosporins			
First generation			
Cefaclor (Ceclor)	500	40	tid
Second generation			
Cefprozil (Cefzil)	250–500	30	bid
Cefuroxime axetil (Ceftin)	250	30	bid
Loracarbef (Lorabid)	200–400	30	bid
Third generation			
Cefdinir (Omnicef)	600	14	qd–bid
Cefixime (Suprax)	400	8	qd
Cefpodoxime (Vantin)	200	10	qd–bid
Ceftibuten (Cedax)	400	9	qd
Ceftriaxone (IM) (Rocephin)	—	50	qd
Macrolides			
Clarithromycin (Biaxin)	250	15	bid
Azithromycin (Zithromax)	500 mg, day 1; 250 mg, days 2–5	10 mg, day 1; 5 mg, days 2–5	qd

Abbreviation: IM, intramuscular.

[a]Do not exceed adult doses in children weighing more than 40 kg. Initial therapy is for 5 d; duration is 10 to 14 d for treatment failures or recurrence.

[b]qd, once a day; bid, twice a day; tid, three times a day; qid, four times a day.

From Block S. Strategies for dealing with amoxicillin failure in acute otitis media. *Arch Fam Med* 1999;8:68–78; Klein J. Clinical implications of antibiotic resistance for acute otitis media. *Pediatr Infect Dis J* 1998;17:1084–1089; and Albrant D. APhA drug treatment protocols: management of pediatric acute otitis media. *J Am Pharm Assoc (Wash)* 2000;40:599–608, with permission.

though over a dozen other clinically effective antibiotics have been approved by the Food and Drug Administration for treating AOM (Table 11.3), not one of these more expensive options has been shown to be more effective for empiric therapy of uncomplicated AOM (54). Rather, these other antibiotics are good alternatives for those who are known to be allergic to amoxicillin, who have a more severe clinical course, or who have treatment failure, which is defined as no clinical improvement after 2 to 3 days or the recurrence of AOM within 2 weeks of therapy (53). In the case of bullous myringitis, a macrolide antibiotic is the drug of choice.

Oral antihistamine–decongestant preparations are no more effective than a placebo in decreasing middle ear effusion (55). Analgesia with acetaminophen, 10 to 15 mg per kg every 4 to 6 hours, or ibuprofen, 5 to 10 mg per kg every 6 to 8 hours, is effective in relieving pain (56). Occasionally, codeine is needed for severe pain. Topical analgesia with antipyrine, benzocaine, and glycerin (e.g., Auralgan Otic), every 1 to 2 hours, effectively relieves pain and congestion within 30 minutes of administration; however, this should be avoided if the tympanic membrane has ruptured (56). During the illness, the athlete should not dive below the surface of the water. If the infection fails to clear or if an effusion persists beyond 12 weeks, the athlete should be referred to an otolaryngologist.

ACUTE PHARYNGITIS

Many causes exist for a sore throat in an athlete, the chief of which are infectious. Since over 60% of cases of pharyngitis are caused by viruses, the challenge is to determine, in a cost-effective manner, which athletes require antibiotic therapy. Group A B-hemolytic *Streptococcus* (GABHS), the most important bacteria because of its potential sequelae, can be isolated by throat culture in 30% to 40% of children and 5% to 10% of adults with sore throat, with the highest prevalence found among children from 5 to 15 years of age (57). Groups C and G streptococci, *Mycoplasma pneumoniae* and *Chlamydia pneumoniae* (TWAR), occur most commonly in adolescent and young adults, and they usually have no serious sequelae (57). In 20% to 65% of patients, no infectious pathogen can be found. Noninfectious causes to consider are postnasal drip, low humidity levels in the environment, irritant exposure to cigarette smoke or smog, and malignant disease (e.g., leukemia, lymphoma, or squamous cell carcinoma). GABHS pharyngitis is most frequently seen in late winter and early spring, while other infectious agents occur year-round. All infectious disease etiologies of sore throat are spread by close contact or by droplets.

GABHS pharyngitis can often be confused with viral pharyngitis, and even the most experienced clinician may miss the diagnosis, if it is based on clinical findings alone. The classic features of GABHS pharyngitis are a sudden onset of severe sore throat, moderate fever (39°C [102.2°F] to 40.5°C [104.9°F]), headache, anorexia, nausea, vomiting, abdominal pain, malaise, tonsillopharyngeal erythema, patchy and discrete tonsillar or pharyngeal exudate, soft palate petechiae, and tender cervical adenopathy (58). The majority of patients have mild disease, with overlap of these features and those of viral pharyngitis. The most reliable predictors of GABHS pharyngitis are the Centor criteria of history of fever, absence of cough, tonsillar exudates, and tender anterior cervical lymphadenopathy or lymphadenitis (58,59).

The gold standard for diagnosing acute GABHS pharyngitis is a throat culture, but obtaining the results may take 48 hours, and up to 10% may be falsely negative. Over 25 different streptococcal rapid antigen tests are available commercially. Most are highly specific (90% to 96%), but they are not as sensitive (41% to 93%) as throat cultures (57). No consensus is found on the best cost-effective approach to treating patients with a sore throat. Current guidelines (59) to testing for and treating GABHS pharyngitis are as follows:

1. For those unlikely to have GABHS pharyngitis (none or only one of the Centor criteria), do not test or treat with antibiotics.
2. For those young athletes with two or more Centor criteria, any of the following strategies are appropriate:
   a. Test athletes with two or more criteria using a rapid antigen test, and limit antibiotics to those with a positive test result.
   b. Test athletes with two or three criteria by using a rapid antigen test, and limit antibiotics to those with a positive test result or to those with four criteria.
   c. Do not use any diagnostic tests and limit antibiotics to those with three or four criteria.
3. Do not perform throat cultures for the routine primary evaluation of athletes with pharyngitis or for confirmation of negative rapid antigen tests when the test sensitivity exceeds 80%.

If antibiotics are used for the treatment of acute pharyngitis, penicillin remains the drug of choice; a macrolide can be used for those who are penicillin-allergic (Table 11.4). In addition to antibiotics, pain can be relieved with acetaminophen, ibuprofen, naproxen, or codeine. Avoid aspirin in children and teenagers because of the risk for Reye syndrome. Warm liquids and gargles are an effective adjuvant treatment. In those with severe inflammatory symptoms, a short course of oral prednisone or a single 10-mg injection of dexamethasone may be given (60).

TABLE 11.4. *Oral antibiotics used for treating acute pharyngitis*

Antibiotic	Dosage[a]		Dosing frequency[b]
	Adults (mg)	Children (mg/kg/d)	
Suggested primary regimen			
Benzathine Penicillin G			
≤60 pounds, 27 kg	600,000 u IM	Same	Once
>60 pounds, 27 kg	1,200,000 u IM	Same	Once
Benzathine/Procaine PCN	900,000/300,000 IM	Same	Once
Penicillin VK	500 mg total	250 mg total	bid
Penicillin, allergic			
Erythromycin estolate	Not advised	20–40	bid–qid
Erythromycin ethylsuccinate	400	40	bid–qid
Second-line treatment			
Amoxicillin	500	40	tid
Amoxicillin/clavulanate	500–875	40	bid–tid
Cephalexin	500	25–50	bid
Cefadroxil	1,000	30	qd
Cefaclor	250	20–30	tid
Cefuroxime axetil	125	15	bid
Cefixime	200	8	qd
Clarithromycin	250	—	bid
Azithromycin (5 d)	500 mg, day 1; 250 mg, days 2–5	12	qd

Abbreviations: IM, intramuscularly, PCN, penicillin.
[a]Unless otherwise indicated, antibiotic is given orally for 10 d.
[b]qd, once a day; bid, twice a day; tid, three times a day; qid, four times a day.

INFECTIOUS MONONUCLEOSIS

Infectious mononucleosis (IM) is an acute, usually self-limited, lymphoproliferative disease generally caused by the Epstein-Barr virus (EBV) (61–65). The highest incidence of IM occurs in the 15-year-old to 19-year-old age group (66). On college campuses, 1% to 3% of students each school year develop symptomatic IM. Typically, the athlete with IM experiences a 3-day to 5-day prodromal period of malaise, fatigue, myalgias, mild headache, anorexia, and nausea. This period is soon followed by moderate fever, chills, severe (sometimes incapacitating) exudative pharyngitis, and tender, enlarged posterior cervical lymphadenopathy. Clinical jaundice and a transient morbilliform rash that is similar to rubella may develop in up to 10% of athletes with IM.

During the acute phase, laboratory evaluation will reveal a modest leukocytosis of 10,000 to 20,000 cells per cubic millimeter, with a striking absolute lymphocytosis (over 50% of the total white blood cell count) and over 10% to 20% atypical lymphocytes. A transient, rarely severe, neutropenia and thrombocytopenia may occur during the second week of illness. Anemia is uncommon, and, if it is present, may suggest splenic rupture. Up to 90% of those with IM will have mild elevations of hepatic enzymes consistent with mild hepatitis by the third week of illness; this usually resolves by the fifth week.

The diagnosis of IM is confirmed by serologic tests. Up to 80% of young athletes with IM have a positive heterophile test (Monospot) by the end of the third week of illness. However, 10% will repeatedly have a negative Monospot; in these individuals, EBV-specific antibody studies are needed to confirm the diagnosis of IM.

The acute phase of IM (fever, pharyngitis, malaise, and fatigue) typically lasts for 2 weeks, and complete recovery is expected within 8 weeks. However, the highly trained athlete may take up to 3 months to attain the previous level of fitness (61). Most young athletes with IM recover without problems, but complications may occur.

Almost all athletes with IM develop splenic enlargement, although this is often missed on physical examination (67,68). The most accurate methods for detecting splenomegaly are ultrasonography, computed tomography (CT), and radionuclide scan. Spontaneous rupture of the enlarged spleen is a rare, but potentially fatal, complication of IM, typically occurring between days 4 and 21 of symptomatic illness (69,70). The characteristic pattern of splenic rupture is left upper quadrant abdominal pain, which may radiate to the top of the left shoulder (Kehr's sign), and leukocytosis with absolute neutropenia. Ultrasonography or CT confirms the diagnosis in those who are hemodynamically stable; diagnostic peritoneal lavage confirms the diagnosis in more emergent cases. Current treatment options for this complication include splenectomy; partial splenectomy; splenorrhaphy; and, in selected individuals, observation (69,71).

Therapy for the athlete with IM consists of (a) providing supportive care, (b) identifying and treating potential complications, and (c) giving safe, yet rational, guidelines for the resumption of training and competition, especially in contact sports. Since the duration of the most symptomatic part of the illness lasts for only 5 to 7 days in the majority of those with IM, treatment is primarily supportive. Analgesia with acetaminophen is preferable to aspirin, which may inhibit platelet function. All patients with IM should have a throat culture conducted, and those with GABHS (up to 30%) should be treated with penicillin or a macrolide. Avoid the use of ampicillin, amoxicillin, and amoxicillin–clavulanic acid, since these can cause a florid, diffuse maculopapular eruption in athletes with IM. Those who develop severe pharyngitis with impending airway obstruction and those who are unable to swallow liquids may require hospitalization, treatment with intravenous fluids and corticosteroids, and evaluation by an otolaryngologist. The routine use of corticosteroids in uncomplicated IM is not recommended.

During the acute phase, the athlete with IM should limit activity to what can be tolerated; strict bed rest or isolation is not required. Light duties and work typically can resume within 5 to 7 days. If the athlete develops splenic discomfort and an enlarged spleen, walking should be limited and stool softeners should be given until the symptoms resolve and the spleen returns to normal size.

The most difficult decision facing the physician is when to allow the young athlete to resume training; recommendations have ranged from 3 weeks to 6 months. The most significant complication is splenic rupture, especially in individuals involved in strenuous contact sports, such as football, ice hockey, lacrosse, rugby, wrestling, basketball, judo, karate, diving, and gymnastics. The current recommended return-to-play criteria for the athlete with IM are found in Table 11.5.

RETURN-TO-PLAY CRITERIA FOR ATHLETES WITH FEVERS

Except for those described for infectious mononucleosis, no absolute rules exist on when an athlete should return to play following a minor febrile illness. No well-controlled studies have been performed to help elicit return-to-play criteria. However, several considerations should be addressed. First, although proving that an intercurrent viral illness increases the risk of death during exercise is difficult, numerous anecdotal reports exist of young athletes dying while vigorously exercising during an acute viral illness (6,18). Certain common viruses, such as coxsackie, adenovirus, and influenza virus, may cause myocarditis with subsequent cardiomyopathy. Exercising during subclinical myocarditis has caused arrhythmia-associated deaths (72). In addition, acute illnesses, especially when they are accompanied by fever, and the medicines used to treat them, such as antihistamines, predispose the athlete to a heat injury. Therefore, severe exertion during an acute viral febrile illness or in early convalescence is potentially dangerous, and it must be avoided.

Viruses can also affect performance because of decreased endurance and isometric strength (18). Exercise during an acute illness actually prolongs the condition, and it may increase its severity. On the other hand, periods of up to 10 days of inactivity have been shown not to alter the fitness levels of endurance athletes (73).

Based upon these facts, the following general guidelines for return to training are offered. The reader should realize that they are quite conservative and that they are not based on well-controlled studies.

1. The athlete who has signs or symptoms of an impending viral infection should reduce the intensity of training for 1 to 2 days.

2. The athlete who has symptoms of a common cold, with no other constitutional symptoms such as fever or myalgias, can safely resume training a few days after the symptoms have resolved.

3. The competitive athlete who does not want to miss training days when he or she is ill should perform a neck check (74). If symptoms are confined to the head (stuffy or runny nose, sneezing, or scratchy throat) with no constitutional symptoms, the athlete can proceed through the scheduled workout at half-

TABLE 11.5. *Return-to-play recommendations for athletes with infectious mononucleosis*

The athlete may resume easy jogging or swimming but not weight lifting, diving, or other strenuous activities any time after day 21 of illness, if he or she subjectively feels ready to resume easy training and if marked or symptomatic splenomegaly is not present.

For those athletes with clinically enlarged or tender spleens, most activity and all athletic training should be restricted until the splenic discomfort and splenomegaly has totally resolved.

For those athletes *not* in strenuous contact sports, full participation can be resumed 1 mo after onset of symptoms.

For those in strenuous contact sports, especially football, early easy training is allowable, as energy permits; contact is delayed for at least 1 full mo after onset of symptoms, if no splenomegaly is present; if splenomegaly is present, ultrasonography should be done at 1- to 2-wk intervals until the spleen returns to normal size.

speed; after a few minutes, the athlete can gradually increase the intensity and can finish the workout if the symptoms improve; if the symptoms worsen, however, the athlete should rest.

4. The athlete who has suspected coxsackie virus or influenza virus infection or who has a viral infection with myalgias and fever can safely resume full training 2 to 4 weeks after the symptoms have resolved; hopefully, this additional time avoids the complications of myocarditis, cardiomyopathy, and arrhythmia.

5. The athlete who has a documented bacterial infection may resume full training once the fever has resolved and the athlete feels well.

The best way for an athlete to ensure that no training is missed is to prevent illness. This is best accomplished by eating a well-balanced diet, avoiding overtraining and chronic fatigue, spacing vigorous workouts as far apart as possible, obtaining adequate sleep, avoiding individuals who are ill, and minimizing life stresses.

HEPATITIS

Five distinct forms of infectious hepatitis are a potential concern for primary care sports medicine physicians who care for young athletes. Two of these, hepatitis D and hepatitis E, are single-stranded RNA viruses that pose a limited risk to young athletes unless they are traveling and competing extensively in international sports. Hepatitis C (HCV), which is also a RNA virus, poses little or no threat to young athletes from transmission in a sports setting. HCV is transmitted by blood-borne contamination, and, although it does cause chronic infection in patients who develop this disease, it is unlikely to be a health risk for young athletes in practice or competition.

The transmission of hepatitis B (HBV) infection in sports events has been reported in the adult and young adult populations. The exact mode of transmission is unclear, but it is suspected to be the result of blood-borne contamination from an infected teammate or competitor. Universal immunization against HBV, which is the current recommendation of the American Academy of Pediatrics, will effectively eliminate this virus as a health risk in young athletes.

Hepatitis A (HAV), a picornavirus, is the most likely etiology of infectious viral hepatitis that will be encountered in a primary care sports medicine setting. Infection by this organism occurs by fecal-oral contamination, and aquatic events in pools or open water venues that have contaminated water sources pose a higher risk for athletes in these sports. Hepatitis A immunization is not universally recommended, but it may be an important consideration for athletes who are competing in venues that have a potentially higher risk

of HAV transmission (e.g. international competition and open water aquatic events). Parents, coaches and athletes can all reduce the risk of hepatitis A transmission by paying close attention to personal hygiene, hand washing, and food handling and preparation.

If a young athlete is diagnosed with acute hepatitis, modification of the practice and competition schedule may be appropriate. Adequate rest, proper nutrition, and adequate fluid intake are important components of acute case management. Strict bed rest may result in a more rapid return to preinfection competition performance levels (75). Individuals with both active, acute hepatitis A and the chronic form of this infection may participate in sports if they feel well enough. Unlike infection with the Epstein-Barr virus, HAV does not appear to increase the risk of organ damage in competitive scenarios. As in return-to-play decisions in mononucleosis, the return of liver enzyme profiles to normal baseline levels may aid primary care physicians in determining when a return to competitive activity is appropriate. Young athletes become progressively less contagious within days of the onset of symptoms of HAV, and they pose little risk for transmission to their teammates or competitors. If a young athlete exposes teammates to HAV prior to the onset of symptoms, a postexposure prophylaxis regimen with immune globulin can be considered for significantly exposed individuals.

The American Academy of Pediatrics (76) and other professional organizations have formulated official policy statements that may be of help to the primary care physician caring for a young athlete with infectious hepatitis.

HUMAN IMMUNODEFICIENCY VIRUS

Standard precautions should be taken when caring for athletes when blood or secretions are involved to minimize the risk of transmission of human immunodeficiency virus (HIV). Coaches, trainers, and others treating athletes should be instructed in proper infection control procedures and should use them at all times (78).

Children who are HIV positive may participate in most sports most of the time. Decisions to participate should follow the guidelines discussed in Chapter 2. Young athletes may participate as their personal health allows. Any limitations to play must be individualized (e.g., a child with diarrhea should be excluded from swimming). Contact sports do pose an increased risk of transmission because of the greater possibility of injuries that could cause contact with another athlete's blood. However, studies have shown this risk to be virtually inconsequential, with a possibility of 1 in 4 million per player per game. This is significantly less than the risk of transmission for HBV, which is 1 in 20,000 per player per game. Therefore, athletes infected with HIV are permitted to participate in contact sports unless specific contraindications are present (e.g., increased bleeding tendency).

Open skin lesions may cause concern, and, thus, players are required to cover lesions appropriately. Other skin infections (e.g., exudative lesions that cannot be easily covered) may preclude participation until successfully treated.

Certain conditions may preclude participation in some sports. Athletes with thrombocytopenia, for example, would not be appropriate candidates for contact or collision sports because of the increased risk of bleeding. Other noncontact sports activities could be suggested.

Confidentiality in caring for children who are infected with HIV must be maintained. However, those physicians directly involved in making preparticipation judgements and those who are responsible for rendering medical care must be made aware of the young athlete's status in order to make proper judgments. The athlete must be aware not only of the risk that he or she is taking but also of the potential for transmitting HIV to teammates and caretakers if an injury occurs. Assisting in this is the important place of education and awareness regarding HIV and acquired immune deficiency syndrome (AIDS) in the health curriculum of many middle schools and high schools.

Common sense, familiarity with the AIDS spectrum and modes of transmission, and attention to standard precautions are important in preparticipation evaluations and the management of on-field injuries. HIV postexposure prophylaxis should be considered on an individual basis based on risk analysis (see Appendix F).

REFERENCES

1. Bury T, Marechal R, Mahieu P, et al. Immunological status of competitive football players during the training season. *Int J Sports Med* 1998;19:364–368.
2. Gabriel H, Kindermann W. The acute immune response to exercise: what does it mean? *Int J Sports Med* 1997; 18:S28–S45.
3. Garagiola U, Buzzetti M, Cardella E, et al. Immunological patterns during regular intensive training in athletes: quantification and evaluation of a preventive pharmacologic approach. *J Int Med Res* 1995;23:85–95.
4. Lewicki R, Tchorzewiski H, Denys A, et al. Effect of physical exercise on some parameters of immunity in conditioned sportsmen. *Int J Sports Med* 1987;8:309–314.
5. MacKinnon L. Special feature for the Olympics: effects of exercise on the immune system: overtraining effects on immunity and performance in athletes. *Immunol Cell Biol* 2000;78:502–509.
6. Roberts J. Viral illnesses and sports performance. *Int J Sports Med* 1986;3:296–303.
7. Strauss R, Lanese R, Leizman D. Illness and absence

among wrestlers, swimmers, and gymnasts at a large university. *Am J Sports Med* 1988;16:653–655.
8. Weidner T. Reporting behaviors and activity levels of intercollegiate athletes with an URI. *Med Sci Sports Exerc* 1994;26:22–26.
9. Fitzgerald L. Overtraining increases the susceptibility to infection. *Int J Sports Med* 1991;12:5–8.
10. Nieman D. Exercise, upper respiratory tract infection, and the immune system. *Med Sci Sports Exerc* 1994; 26:128–139.
11. Milgrom H, Bender B. Adverse effects of medications for rhinitis. *Ann Allergy Asthma Immunol* 1997;78:439–446.
12. McCarthy P. Fever. *Pediatr Rev* 1998;19:401–407.
13. Styrt B, Sugarman B. Antipyresis and fever. *Arch Intern Med* 1990;150:1589–1597.
14. Barrow M, Clark K. Heat-related illnesses. *Am Fam Physician* 1998;58:749–756, 759.
15. Kauffman R, Sawyer L, Scheinbaum M. Antipyretic efficacy of ibuprofen vs. acetaminophen. *Am J Dis Child* 1992;146:622–625.
16. Spector S. The common cold: current therapy and natural history. *J Allergy Clin Immunol* 1995;95:1133–1138.
17. Lorber B. The common cold. *J Gen Intern Med* 1996; 11:229–236.
18. Sevier T. Infectious disease in athletes. *Med Clin North Am* 1994;78:389–412.
19. Singh M. Heated, humidified air for the common cold. *Cochrane Database Syst Rev* 2000;2:CD001728.
20. Mainous A, Hueston W, Clark J. Antibiotics and upper respiratory infection—do some folks think there is a cure for the common cold? *J Fam Pract* 1996;42:357–361.
21. Dowell S, Schwartz B, Phillips W. Appropriate use of antibiotics for URIs in children. II. Cough, pharyngitis and the common cold. *Am Fam Physician* 1998;58:1335–1342, 1345.
22. Arroll B, Kenealy T. Antibiotics for the common cold. *Cochrane Database Syst Rev* 2000;2:CD000247.
23. Gonzales R, Bartlett J, Besser R, et al. Principles of appropriate antibiotic use for treatment of nonspecific upper respiratory tract infections in adults: background. *Ann Intern Med* 2001;134:490–494.
24. Smith M, Fedlman W. Over-the-counter cold medications—a critical review of clinical trials between 1950 and 1991. *JAMA* 1993;269:2258–2263.
25. Luks D, Anderson M. Antihistamines and the common cold—a review and critique of the literature. *J Gen Intern Med* 1996;11:240–244.
26. Taverner D, Bickford L, Draper M. Nasal decongestants for the common cold. *Cochrane Database Syst Rev* 2000;2:CD001953.
27. Hayden F, Diamond L, Wood P, et al. Effectiveness and safety of intranasal ipratropium bromide in common colds—a randomized, double-blind, placebo-controlled trial. *Ann Intern Med* 1996;125:89–97.
28. Douglas R, Chalker E, Treacy B. Vitamin C for preventing and treating the common cold. *Cochrane Database Syst Rev* 2000;2:CD000980.
29. Percival S. Use of echinacea in medicine. *Biochem Pharmacol* 2000;60:155–158.
30. Melchart D, Linde K, Fischer P, et al. Echinacea for preventing and treating the common cold. *Cochrane Database Syst Rev* 2000;2:CD000530.
31. Zinc for the common cold. *Med Lett Drugs Ther* 1997; 39:9–10.
32. Macknin M, Piedmonte M, Calendine C, et al. Zinc gluconate lozenges for treating the common cold in chil-

dren. A randomized controlled trial. *JAMA* 1998;279:1962–1967.

33. Marshall I. Zinc for the common cold. *Cochrane Database Syst Rev* 2000;2:CD001364.

34. Zimmerman R, Ruben F, Ahwesh E. Influenza, influenza vaccine, and amantadine/rimantadine. *J Fam Pract* 1997;45:107–124.

35. Couch R. Prevention and treatment of influenza. *N Engl J Med* 2000;343:1778–1787.

36. Croughan-Minihane M, Petitti D, Rodnick J, et al. Clinical trial examining effectiveness of three cough syrups. *J Am Board Fam Pract* 1993;6:109–115.

37. Stewart M, Siff J, Cydulka R. Evaluation of the patient with sore throat, earache, and sinusitis: an evidence-based approach. *Emerg Med Clin North Am* 1999;171:153–187.

38. Williams J, Simel D. Does this patient have sinusitis? Diagnosing acute sinusitis by history and physical examination. *JAMA* 1993;270:1242–1246.

39. Willett L, Carson J, Williams J. Current diagnosis and management of sinusitis. *J Gen Intern Med* 1995;9:38–45.

40. Lanza D, Kennedy D. Adult rhinosinusitis defined. *Otolaryngol Head Neck Surg* 1997;117:S1–S7.

41. Hadley J, Schafer S. Clinical evaluation of rhinosinusitis: history and physical examination. *Otolaryngol Head Neck Surg* 1997;117:S8–S11.

42. Burke T, Guertler A, Timmons J. Comparisons of sinus x-rays with CT scans in acute sinusitis. *Acad Emerg Med* 1994;1:235–239.

43. Ferguson B. Acute and chronic sinusitis—how to ease symptoms and locate the cause. *Postgrad Med* 1995;97:45–57.

44. Hickner J, Bartlett J, Besser R, et al. Principles of appropriate antibiotic use for acute rhinosinusitis in adults: background. *Ann Intern Med* 2001;134:498–505.

45. Snow V, Mottur-Pilson C, Hickner J. Principles of appropriate antibiotic use for acute sinusitis in adults. *Ann Intern Med* 2001;134:495–497.

46. Poole M. Antimicrobial therapy for sinusitis. *Otolaryngol Clin North Am* 1997;30:331–339.

47. O'Neill P. Acute otitis media. *Br Med J* 1999;319:833–835.

48. Macknin M, Talo H, Medendrop S. Effect of cotton-tipped swab use on ear-wax occlusion. *Clin Pediatr (Phila)* 1994;33:14–18.

49. Freeman R. Impacted cerumen: how to safely remove earwax in an office visit. *Geriatrics* 1995;50:52–53.

50. Pichichero M. Acute otitis media. I. Improving diagnostic accuracy. *Am Fam Physician* 2000;61:2051–2056.

51. Glasziou P, DelMar C, Sanders S. *Antibiotics for acute otitis media in children (Cochrane Review)*. The Cochrane Library, Issue 3. Oxford, England: Update Software, 2000.

52. Little P, Gould C, Williamson I, et al. Pragmatic randomized controlled trial of two prescribing strategies for childhood acute otitis media. *Br Med J* 2001;322:336–342.

53. Block S. Strategies for dealing with amoxicillin failure in acute otitis media. *Arch Fam Med* 1999;8:68–78.

54. Klein J. Clinical implications of antibiotic resistance for management of acute otitis media. *Pediatr Infect Dis J* 1998;17:1084–1089.

55. Albrant D. APhA drug treatment protocols: management of pediatric acute otitis media. *J Am Pharmaceutical Assoc (Wash)* 2000;40:599–608.

56. Zempsky W, Schechter N. Office-based pain management. The 15-minute consultation. *Pediatr Clin North Am* 2000;47:601–615.

57. Pichichero M. Group A streptococcal tonsillopharyngitis: cost-effective diagnosis and treatment. *Ann of Emerg Med* 1995;25:390–403.

58. Ebell M, Smith M, Barry H, et al. Does this patient have strep throat? *JAMA* 2000;284:2912–2918.

59. Cooper R, Hoffman J, Bartlett J, et al. Principles of appropriate antibiotic use for acute pharyngitis in adults: background. *Ann Intern Med* 2001;134:509–517.

60. O'Brien J, Meade J, Falk J. Dexamethasone as adjuvant therapy for severe acute pharyngitis. *Ann Emerg Med* 1993;22:212–215.

61. Maki D, Reich R. Infectious mononucleosis in the athlete—diagnosis, complications, and management. *Am J Sports Med* 1982;10:162–173.

62. Chetham M, Roberts K. Infectious mononucleosis in adolescents. *Pediatr Ann* 1991;20:206–213.

63. Haines J. When to resume sports after infectious mononucleosis—how soon is safe? *Postgrad Med* 1987;81:331–333.

64. Bailey R. Diagnosis and treatment of infectious mononucleosis. *Am Fam Physician* 1994;49:879–895.

65. Godshall S, Kirchner J. Infectious mononucleosis—complexities of a common syndrome. *Postgrad Med* 2000;107:175–186.

66. Auwaerter P. Infectious mononucleosis in middle age. *JAMA* 1999;281:454–459.

67. Dommerby H, Stangerup S, Stangerup M, et al. Hepatosplenomegaly in infectious mononucleosis, assessed by ultrasonic scanning. *J Laryngol Otol* 1986;100:573–579.

68. Grover S, Barkun A, Sackett D. Does this patient have splenomegaly? *JAMA* 1993;270:2218–2221.

69. Farley D, Zietlow S, Bannon M, et al. Spontaneous rupture of the spleen due to infectious mononucleosis. *Mayo Clin Proc* 1992;67:846–853.

70. Safran D, Bloom G. Spontaneous splenic rupture following infectious mononucleosis. *Am Surg* 1990;56:601–605.

71. Schuler J, Filtzer H. Spontaneous splenic rupture: the role of nonoperative management. *Arch Surg* 1995;130:662–665.

72. Burke A, Farb V, Virmani R, et al. Sports-related and nonsports-related sudden cardiac death in young adults. *Am Heart J* 1991;121:568–575.

73. Cullinane E, Sady S, Vadeboncoeur L, et al. Cardiac size and VO$_2$ max do not decrease after short-term exercise cessation. *Med Sci Sports Exerc* 1986;18:420–424.

74. Eichner E. Neck check. *Runner's World* 1992;27:16.

75. Harrington D. Viral hepatitis and exercise. *Medicine Sci Sports Exerc* 2000;32:S422–S430.

76. Committee of Sports Medicine and Fitness, American Academy of Pediatrics. Human immunodeficiency virus and other blood-borne viral pathogens in the athletic setting. *Pediatrics* 1999;104:1400–1403.

77. Dominguez K. Management of HIV-infected children in the home and institutional settings. *Pediatr Clin North Am* 2000;47:203–239.

12

Dermatology

Arnold M. Ramirez and Daniel J. Van Durme

ACNE MECHANICA AND KELOIDALIS

Acne is a common condition in the adolescent population. However, in the young athlete, two variants, acne mechanica and acne keloidalis, can be especially problematic.

Acne mechanica is one of the more prevalent dermatoses among athletes, and it usually presents with mild to moderate inflammatory lesions consisting of papules or pustules. It can progress to nodules and cysts in severe cases (Fig. 12.1) (1). Acne mechanica is typically found in athletes wearing heavy protective equipment (mainly football and hockey players), and it can

also be a result of contact between other athletic apparel or equipment (e.g., spandex and plastic-covered weight benches) and underlying skin. It results from the direct mechanical irritation that is most commonly seen with forehead guards, chin straps, or various braces. Although the mechanism for acne mechanica is unclear, it is believed to be the result of a number of factors, including pressure, friction, occlusion, and heat. A preexisting acne condition may or may not be present.

In severe cases, particularly in black athletes, the lesions of acne mechanica may progess into acne keloidalis, in which continued mechanical friction leads to the development of multiple small keloids. This is most commonly seen on the posterior neck, from helmet irritation.

Prevention and Treatment

Minimizing mechanical stress on the skin can help alleviate the symptoms and can prevent recurrences. The simplest measure is to wear a clean cotton T-shirt under uniforms and equipment. Other fabrics that wick moisture from the skin can also be used. Athletic apparel should be removed immediately after play or practice, and the skin should be washed thoroughly. Use of a back brush can be particularly useful in hard to reach areas. Benzoyl peroxide soaps or skin cleansers (5% to 10%) can be used instead of the usual soaps. Solutions containing salicylic acid and resorcinol may also be applied. Bedtime tretinoin creams can be useful in further reducing the hypercohesive keratinization of the follicles. Systemic antibiotics appear to be less effective, and they should rarely be used, unless a coexisting bacterial folliculitis that can sometimes be seen with acne keloidalis is present. Severe cases of keloidalis can be treated in the off-season with serial intralesional steroid injections. Recurrence, however, is likely with each new season.

Restrictions for Play

No contraindications to athletic participation with acne mechanica or keloidalis exist.

FIG. 12.1. Acne mechanica.

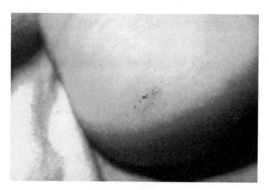

FIG. 12.2. Talon noir.

BLACK HEEL

Black heel (talon noir) results from the lateral sheering force between the epidermis and the underlying capillaries, and it is associated with sudden stops or position changes. This repetitive trauma ultimately causes rupture of the superficial capillaries, producing punctate petechiae or bluish–black macules that are typically found on the posterior aspect of the heel (Fig. 12.2). Occasionally, this lesion can also be found on the palms of weight lifters, tennis players, and golfers. Teenagers and young adults are the most likely to be affected by this condition (2). Talon noir is often confused with warts or acral lentiginous malignant melanoma. These various conditions can be distinguished by close examination of the affected area. In athletes who have talon noir, as opposed to warts or other conditions that cause pigmentary changes, close examination reveals normal skin lines; and gentle paring of the superficial epidermis (stratum corneum) will reveal that the black color is merely surface pigment. Talon noir is a self-limiting condition with spontaneous resolution in a few weeks. It causes no permanent disability, nor does it affect performance.

Prevention and Treatment

Talon noir is a self-limiting condition. Properly fitted gloves and shoes can minimize recurrence.

Restrictions for Play

No contraindications to athletic participation exists with talon noir.

BLACK TOENAIL

Another traumatic lesion that is typically found under the hallux nails is the extremely common subungual hematoma or "black toenail." Similar to talon noir, it is associated with activities that involve quick starts and stops. Repetitive jamming of the great toe into the front of the toe box of the shoe, boot, or skate causes trauma to the nail plate that may result in immediate bleeding and pain. This condition may also develop with repeated microtrauma, and, in this situation, the athlete may experience minimal discomfort. The hemorrhage results in the characteristic blue or black color under the nail. The hemorrhage may be of sufficient quantity to cause separation and loss of the nail plate (onycholysis). Although most athletes have minimal symptoms, more profuse hemorrhage into this closed space can generate enough pressure to cause significant pain. More severe cases may result in the compromise of athletic performance in the young athlete.

Prevention and Treatment

Properly fitted footwear can prevent this injury. Mild cases usually respond to rest and warm water soaks. Nails should be trimmed to minimize further trauma. In acute cases with moderate to severe pain, decompression and drainage can be accomplished by puncturing the nail with a flame-heated paperclip or an electrocautery unit.

Restrictions for Play

No contraindications to athletic participation with black toenail are found.

BLISTERS

Blisters caused by repetitive rubbing of the skin. Friction blisters form when shearing forces cause separation within the midepidermal or spinous layer, resulting in fluid formation. This fluid is usually clear; but, in more severe cases, it can also be bloody. Typically, these are seen in areas where the epidermis is thin and unconditioned (suboptimal epidermal hyperplasia in areas of maximal pressure), but they can also be found under calluses, if the frictional forces are great enough. Hyperhidrosis may contribute to the formation of blisters by allowing the skin surface to slide, thus enhancing the shearing force (3). Blisters are most commonly seen on the extremities, especially the feet of runners and athletes who are involved in a lot of quick stop-and-go movements.

Prevention and Treatment

Blisters can be treated in several different ways, depending on size and location. Small blisters usually resolve spontaneoulsy without intervention. The epidermal roof should be left intact, as it provides a natural occlusive dressing that promotes healing. Continued activity often results in rupture of an intact blister. Larger blisters are best drained at the edge with a sterile needle or scalpel, thus allowing the roof to remain. This can minimize pain and can provide a natural occlusive dressing. Drained blisters should then be covered with an occlusive pressure dressing to increase the speed of epithelialization. Hydrocolloid and hydrogel dressings, such as DuoDERM or Second Skin, are particularly useful if the roof of the blister is lost. Antibiotic ointments may also be used to prevent secondary infection.

Preventative measures are directed to interventions that attempt to decrease frictional shearing force and to condition susceptible areas. Training intensity should be gradually increased, particularly with new athletic equipment or shoes. Calluses should be pared to distribute frictional forces equally, and Vaseline or petroleum jelly can be used to keep the skin lubricated and to reduce friction. Moisture should be controlled, as much as possible, by using material that wicks perspiration from the skin and/or drying agents (e.g., chalk, powders, or even deodorants and Drysol). Soaking the feet in tea water is an inexpensive, but effective, method of treating any underlying hyperhidrosis and toughening of the skin. Three to four bags of generic black tea, in 1 quart of water, make a weak tannic acid solution that will decrease sweating and will condition the skin. This can be helpful for the athlete early in the season or with new shoes that have not yet been conditioned.

Restrictions for Play

No contraindications to athletic participation with blisters have been reported.

COLD INJURIES

Hypothermia, caused by prolonged exposure to cold ambient temperatures, can produce cutaneous injury in varying degrees. The underlying pathophysiology behind cutaneous cold injury involves the crystal formation of the intracellular fluid that punctures cells and results in cell lysis. Frostnip, the most common form of cold injury, represents superficial involvement of only the skin and the tissue immediately below it. It is most commonly seen on exposed areas of skin, such as the face, nose, cheeks, chin, and ears; and it presents clinically as numb, white patches of skin. Superficial vesiculation may result, and persistent numbness may persist for 2 to 3 days.

True frostbite involves deeper layers of injury, including subcutaneous tissue, muscle, and even bone. This type of injury can be particularly troublesome in high altitudes, where decreased oxygen tension further complicates the cutaneous anoxia caused by peripheral vasoconstriction (2). Pernio, also known as chilblains,

is another form of superficial cold injury characterized by cyanotic, subcutaneous tender nodules in exposed areas, such as the fingers and toes. It usually coincides with the first exposure to lower temperatures, and it more commonly affects younger women. Pruritus and burning are usually noted several hours later.

Prevention and Treatment

Rapid rewarming is a first-line treatment for any cold injury (see Chapter 7). However, care must be taken to insure that the possibility for refreezing has been removed prior to any rewarming procedure because subsequent refreezing greatly potentiates tissue necrosis. A circulating warm water bath, at 40.0 to 40.5°C (104 to 105°F), provides an optimum modality for rewarming. Analgesics are also helpful. Covering all exposed areas, particularly the vulnerable anterior neck, as well as limiting the amount of cold exposure, can prevent cold injuries. Layering of lightweight garments, postponing washing or showering to retain natural skin oils, and less frequent shaving of facial hair in men are additional measures to provide insulation.

Restrictions for Play

While no specific restrictions for play are seen with cold injuries, some limitations may be imposed based on the location and severity of the injury.

CONTACT DERMATITIS

Contact dermatitis is an inflammatory reaction to substances in the environment. This reaction can be classified as either irritant or allergic, but both types produce an eczematous type of inflammation that can be acute, subacute, or chronic. Contact dermatitis is characterized by erythema, wheals, and, occasionally, vesicle or scale formation. Pruritus and/or pain is common to all contact dermatoses.

Irritant contact dermatitis is the most common form. It results from absorption of an irritant through skin whose integrity has been compromised, thus causing a nonimmunologic, nonallergenic inflammatory response (4). The intensity of the response is related to the concentration of the irritant and the duration of the exposure. The amount of exposure time required to produce a response varies with an individual's ability to maintain skin integrity with repeated exposure. Thus, the length can vary from days to years of exposure, and the onset is gradual. Usually, the substances producing this type of reaction are organic solvents or detergents, as well as topical medications (e.g., tretinoin or benzoyl peroxide).

Allergic contact dermatitis, on the other hand, is a delayed hypersensitivity reaction that affects a predisposed population, usually after only a few exposures. T lymphocytes that have been sensitized will produce an inflammatory response in a well-defined or demarcated area of skin that has been in contact with the substance. Hence, the pattern of distribution can often reveal the offending substance. Reexposure can occur in the form of the same substance or with a chemically related substance (cross-sensitization). The following five main substances can produce an allergic reaction: *Rhus* (most common), dyes, nickel compounds, rubber, and chromates (leather and other metals). Nickel compounds can be a particular source of problems in athletes who may demonstrate small round eczematous patches in the area in which an equipment snap or buckle makes contact with the skin. Patch testing can be useful in determining the identity of a contact allergen if behavioral surveillance and attempts to modify exposure to offending substances prove ineffective at alleviating symptoms.

Prevention and Treatment

Avoiding the offending substance is obviously the first step. Establishing a barrier, such as a cotton T-shirt or hypoallergenic tape, between the athlete's skin and the offending agent can often accomplish this goal. If a particular snap is causing problems, a coating of clear nail polish that is reapplied periodically to the snap can resolve the problem easily. Moderate to potent topical steroids can be used if the rash is localized. Vesicular reactions should be treated with cool compresses or soaks, as well as topical steroids to promote drying. Oral antihistamines will relieve itching, and, occasionally, short courses of systemic corticosteroids can reduce the severity of symptoms if they are diffuse or generalized. Secondary bacterial infections can occur, and they should be treated with oral or topical antibiotics, depending on the area involved and the severity of the infection.

Restrictions for Play

Disqualification of an athlete is totally dependent upon the degree of skin involvement and the severity of symptoms.

CORNS AND CALLUSES

These benign lesions are hyperkeratotic reactions at specific pressure points that result in a protective thickening of the stratum corneum due to continued friction and shearing force (4). The forces can be either external, such as shoes or athletic equipment, or internal, such as bony prominences. Calluses, which are most commonly found in proximity to the metacarpal or metatarsal heads, are more broad-based. Calluses also are characterized as having a relatively even thickness

and as lacking a central core. Corns, also known as clavi, are typically sharply demarcated, and they have a central translucent core. These can be either hard or soft, and they are often found between toes (usually the fourth and fifth [soft]) or on the dorsal and/or dorsolateral surfaces of toes (hard). Both soft and hard corns may be extremely painful.

Prevention and Treatment

Primary care physicians should devote attention to ensuring the use of properly fitted equipment or footwear as this can minimize the incidence of corns and calluses. Extra padding at susceptible pressure points is also helpful. Donut pads, in particular, can alleviate pressure around bony prominences. Because calluses are a natural reinforcement for sites of cutaneous stress, intervention is not always advisable. The goals of treatment of corns and calluses are mainly to reduce discomfort and to prevent blister formation. For alleviating pain, paring and removal of the central core in corns can be easily accomplished with a scalpel. Soaking the affected area, followed by abrasive debridement with a pumice stone or the application of a keratolytic agent, can help debulk a corn or a callus. Occasionally, surgical osteotomies are necessary if an underlying bony deformity causes persistent or recurrent callus or corn formation.

Restrictions for Play

No contraindications to athletic participation exist with corns and calluses.

GREEN HAIR

Long-term exposure to swimming pool water causes the cosmetically unacceptable appearance of green hair. This condition is found in swimmers with light blond or bleached hair, and it is caused by copper ion deposition (5). Chlorine additives have little to do with this condition; the usual source of the copper is pool algaecides that contain copper sulfate as the active ingredient. This condition has no physiologic or pathologic consequence other than the bothersome cosmetic complaints.

Prevention and Treatment

The application of a 3% solution of hydrogen peroxide or a commercial chelating agent will remove the discoloration.

Restrictions for Play

No contraindications to athletic participation with green hair are found.

HERPES SIMPLEX

Herpes simplex viral (HSV) infections are extremely contagious infections of the skin and mucous membranes caused by one of two strains of the herpes virus. While type 1 is generally associated with nongenital infections and type 2 is usually found in the genital areas, either type can be found anywhere on the body if direct contact occurs. The virus is spread primarily by contact with active lesions or with secretions known to contain the virus, such as saliva or vaginal secretions. However, transmission by asymptomatic individuals is known to occur. Prodromal symptoms consist of erythema, localized pain and tenderness, and mild paresthesias or burning at the site of inoculation, and they may include fever, malaise, and lymphadenopathy (more commonly seen with the initial outbreak). Subsequently, small, tender vesicles appear in clusters on an erythematous base; these lesions then dry and heal within 7 to 10 days. Secondary or recurrent infections result from the reactivation of virus, and they can be brought about by a wide variety of stressors.

In athletes, the spread of HSV is most commonly seen in wrestlers, and thus, it is known as "herpes gladiatorum" (see Chapter 2, Table 2.10). It is spread by direct contact with an opponent's active lesion or through contact with infectious secretions on the mat (6). Other sports, such as rugby, also have been associated with the spread of type 1 HSV. Although the diagnosis of HSV infection is made clinically in most cases, it can be confirmed by a Tzanck smear of the vesicle base or by viral culture of a fresh lesion.

Prevention and Treatment

Classic treatments of HSV infections employ a variety of drying agents, such as benzoyl peroxide, alcohol, and tretinoin, to hasten healing and resolution and to minimize infectivity. These agents can be used to get an athlete back to play more rapidly. Newer antiviral therapy has proven to be more effective, and it can be used alone or in conjunction with the above methods. While three effective antiviral agents for HSV exist, only acyclovir has been approved by the Food and Drug Administration for use in children. The recommended dosage of 10 to 20 mg per kg orally, four times daily for 5 days, for varicella or herpes zoster can also be used for HSV (both types 1 and 2). Higher doses are recommended for the primary outbreak. Minimizing stress and using lip balms and sunscreens can help prevent frequent recurrences of HSV in these areas.

Restrictions for Play

Because of the highly contagious nature of this infection, athletes with acute lesions should be disqualified from participating in contact or swimming sports. Only when all of the lesions have crusted over can an athlete resume participation. Further recommendations indicate that even the crusted lesions should be covered with gas-permeable membranes and that the athlete should be on medication at the time of competition.

IMPETIGO

Impetigo is a contagious bacterial infection commonly caused by staphylococci, β-hemolytic streptococci, or both. It can present as either the bullous form or the nonbullous form. Both begin as vesicles with an extremely thin, fragile roof that either enlarges to form bullae or ruptures to expose a moist erythematous base that subsequently becomes covered by a honey-colored adherent crust. It is most commonly found on the face, but it can be found anywhere. While usually some minor trauma to the skin, such as an insect bite or scratch or friction from football helmet chin straps, has occurred, impetigo can also be found on apparently uninjured skin. The diagnosis is generally straightforward, and it is made by clinical appearance. Athletes at the greatest risk for contracting this are those who are involved in prolonged skin-to-skin contact, such as wrestlers and rugby players. Swimmers have also been found to be susceptible to transmission. Although the disease is usually self-limited, potential complications can include poststreptococcal glomerulonephritis.

Prevention and Treatment

Both topical and oral antibiotics are effective at treating impetigo. Topical mupirocin (Bactroban) cream or ointment can be effective for smaller areas that are easy to reach. Several oral regimens are also highly effective, including semisynthetic penicillins, first generation cephalosporins, and macrolides. Antibacterial soaps (e.g., Hibiclens, Betadine) and drying agents, such as alcohol or other astringents, may hasten the resolution of the condition. Topical antibiotics applied to sites of minor skin trauma can be efficacious as preventative treatment. Recurrent cases have been found to be related to the colonization of *Staphylococcus aureus*, particularly in the nares. Intranasal mupirocin can be used in this setting.

Restrictions for Play

The highly contagious nature of this infection precludes athletic competition with new or active lesions. The recommendation is that the athlete be free of any new lesions for 2 days and/or complete 3 days of antibiotics before returning to competition. All lesions must be covered during the contest.

JOGGER'S NIPPLES

This painful condition results from the repetitive friction on the areola and nipple that usually results from coarse fabrics, as well as the overlying logos on jerseys. More commonly seen in men or boys, the condition presents as denuded erosions that can bleed in severe cases (2). Long-distance runners tend to be the most predisposed to developing jogger's nipples.

Prevention and Treatment

This condition can be easily avoided by running without a shirt when possible. Other preventative measures include taping the nipples and the use of occlusive lubricating ointments, such as petrolatum. Treatment of jogger's nipple involves gentle cleansing with antibacterial soap, antibiotic creams, and a simple dressing.

Restrictions for Play

No contraindications to athletic participation result from jogger's nipples.

MILIARIA

Miliaria, or heat rash as it is more commonly known, is a disorder of the exocrine sweat glands that is characterized by obstruction that clinically presents as very tiny vesicles or erythematous papules. It is generally found in hot humid environments or after periods of exertion in predisposed individuals who perspire heavily. While it is more common in infants and children, it may occur at any age. Superficial blockage at the skin surface produces *miliaria crystalline,* in which sweat accumulates under the stratum corneum and produces vesicles with little or no erythema. The more common form is *miliaria rubra,* or "prickly heat," where occlusion occurs at the intraepithelial section. Patients usually complain of a stinging or prickling sensation with this more erythematous form of the papulovesicular rash (3).

Prevention and Treatment

The condition is self-limited, but it can be alleviated by cool water compresses and air-conditioning. Avoidance of hot ambient temperatures can prevent recurrences, and the use of a low to medium potency topical steroid is sometimes helpful.

Restrictions for Play

No contraindications exist for athletic participation with miliaria.

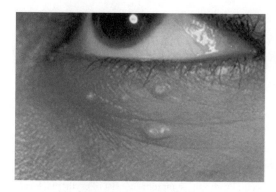

FIG. 12.3. Molluscum contagiosum.

MOLLUSCUM CONTAGIOSUM

Molluscum contagiosum is a viral infection caused by the large poxvirus, and, as the name implies, it is spread by direct contact. In older adolescents and adults, it is most often passed on by sexual contact. Within the same individual, it is spread by autoinoculation when scratched. The lesions present as discrete flesh-colored, dome-shaped papules, usually 2 to 5 mm in diameter, with classic central umbilication (Fig. 12.3). The base may or may not be erythematous, and hence the condition can often be confused with warts and herpes simplex. Commonly affected areas are the trunk, axilla, face, perineum, and thighs. The athletes most commonly affected are wrestlers, but the infection has also been found among swimmers. The diagnosis is made clinically, and it can be confirmed by biopsy.

Prevention and Treatment

Several destructive methods can be used to treat molluscum contagiosum. Curettage can be performed with or without anesthesia, but it can lead to superficial abrasions and scarring. Cryosurgery with liquid nitrogen is the treatment of choice if the lesions are few and the patient does not object to the pain. Other treatments include cantharidin and topical retinoic acid (Retin-A) (3).

Restrictions for Play

Athletes may participate if solitary or clustered lesions can be adequately covered. Athletes with diffuse lesions should be treated with curettage or cryosurgery prior to participation.

PIEZOGENIC PAPULES

Piezogenic papules are herniations of fat through connective tissue that are commonly found on the

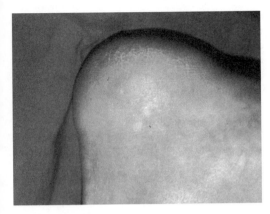

FIG. 12.4. Piezogenic papules.

mediolateral midfoot and heel. Women are more frequently affected than men, and this condition is usually seen in long-distance runners (7). These protrusions of fat appear as dome-shaped, flesh-colored papules that may only be apparent when pressure is placed on the sole of the foot, from below or upon weight bearing (Fig. 12.4). Pain may be severe, and it can preclude continuation of activity.

Prevention and Treatment

Unfortunately, no medical or surgical treatment has been demonstrated to be of definitive value. Orthotics or heel cups may have some benefit.

Restrictions for Play

No contraindications to athletic participation result from piezogenic papules.

PITTED KERATOLYSIS

Pitted keratolysis is an infectious foot disorder that is caused primarily by the *Corynebacterium* species (less commonly, it is associated with *Actinomyces*, *Dermatophilus*, and *Micrococcus*). It occurs in physically active individuals whose feet have a tendency to be excessively sweaty. The affected areas are usually asymptomatic; rarely, they may be inflamed. On evaluation, the feet generally are extremely malodorous, and they reveal marginated areas of macerated skin (a white section bordered by a deep red halo) with crater-like lesions or distinct pits that range from 1 to 7 mm in diameter and depth (7a). The lesions tend to occur on the toe pads and thicker, pressure-bearing areas of the heels and balls of the feet, and they may have a brownish color that gives the foot a dirty appearance. The differential diagnosis includes tinea pedis and plantar warts. A silver stain of a superficial biopsy of the stratum corneum is diagnostic if the clinical presentation is unclear. If left untreated, the disorder may undergo either a spontaneous remission or exacerbation, in which case, it may linger for years.

Prevention and Treatment

The warm, damp conditions that promote bacterial growth must be avoided, so the patient should be advised (a) to wear shoes made of cloth or leather; (b) to apply absorbent powder inside stockings and socks; (c) to expose the feet to air whenever possible; (d) to air out the shoes for at least 24 hours after use, preferably alternating among several pairs; (e) to avoid wearing shoes without socks; (f) to wear cotton or absorbent synthetic socks when possible (polypropylene socks worn under white cotton socks help wick moisture away from the skin); and (g) to scrub the feet with antibacterial soap, followed by rinsing, thorough drying (blow dryer if necessary), and application of an antiperspirant.

Infections resistant to the above measures can be treated with 20% aluminum chloride hexahydrate. Safe and inexpensive topical alternatives include the twice daily application of clotrimazole cream, 1%; clindamycin solution, 1%; miconazole nitrate cream, 2%; erythromycin solution, 2%; or over-the-counter benzoyl peroxide gel, 10%. Success has also been noted with the use of oral erythromycin, 250 mg, four times daily. Preventive therapy includes the use of antibacterial soap on a daily basis.

PLANTAR WARTS

Warts that occur on the plantar surface of the foot can be especially troublesome to many athletes, particularly those that run. These lesions are caused by various strains of the human papilloma virus. Plantar warts are frequently seen at points of maximum pressure, such as over the metatarsal heads and heels, during weight bearing. The macerating effect of perspiration and the exposure to the virus in locker rooms are believed to contribute to their development. Clinically, these lesions are well circumscribed, firm, and elevated, and they may have some fine, surface finger-like projections. Confluence of individual papules can result in mosaic plantar warts. These are often confused with corns and calluses, but they can be distinguished by the absence of skin lines with paring and the centrally located black dots that bleed with additional paring.

Prevention and Treatment

Conservative measures during the athletic season are key to continued participation. Hot soaks are useful to soften the superficial layers, followed by daily paring or the use of a pumice stone to decrease the callus and to reduce tenderness. Nonscarring keratolytics, such as salicylic acid, either with formalin or as a 40% plaster, can also be used nightly to diminish the volume of the wart slowly. More aggressive methods, such as cryosurgery and electrodessication, can be used for recalcitrant cases, but they should be performed in the off-season, as these more destructive methods can produce painful ulcerations that can impair mobility. Surgical excision and radiotherapy carry a significant risk of scarring that can be disabling to the athlete and that may compromise performance. Use of shower thongs in the locker room can prevent the transmission of the virus, and drying agents, such as Drysol or various foot powders, can diminish the attendant maceration.

Restrictions for Play

While no restrictions to participation are indicated, coverage of the lesions is recommended.

SOLAR URTICARIA

Solar urticaria or polymorphous light eruption is a fairly common condition that occurs in up to 10% of the population. As the name implies, the presentation can be highly variable, with the development of papules, plaques, urticaria, papulovesicular lesions, or even erythema multiforme. It may occur after 2 to 48 hours of sun exposure in any area of exposed skin, although it usually spares the face; and it usually lasts from 2 to 3 days (3). Some patients will have flu-like symptoms lasting a few hours when the problem first occurs. It may develop at any age, and it can be a source of confusion and frustration for the patient and doctor alike as the cause of this transient rash is pursued.

Prevention and Treatment

Prevention involves sun avoidance, coverage, and the frequent liberal application of a sunblock with ultraviolet protection. Treatment includes oral antihistamines and low to medium potency topical steroids. A program for hardening the skin or building up a tolerance to increasing amounts of sunlight can be pursued with the careful direction of an experienced physician.

Restrictions for Play

No contraindications to athletic participation with solar urticaria are found.

TINEA CRURIS

Jock itch is found almost exclusively in male patients, and it is often associated with untreated tinea pedis. Therefore, the evaluation should check for athlete's foot as well. Caused typically by *Trichophyton*

rubrum, the lesions appear as dull, red, dry skin with well-defined scaly borders in an anular shape. The eruptions may spread beyond the groin area to the inner gluteal areas, buttocks, and perineum, but they usually spare the scrotum. An important item in the differential diagnosis includes intertrigo of the groin, which appears as moist, nonscaling, bright red lesions involving the scrotum. The diagnosis can be confirmed with a fungal culture or a potassium hydroxide examination (7b).

Prevention and Treatment

The infection is highly responsive to topical antifungal agents applied once or twice daily for a minimum of one month. Tolnaftate cream or solution, 1%; miconazole cream, 2%; or clotrimazole cream or lotion are appropriate for dry lesions. Griseofulvin, 125 mg to 1 g per day for one month (alternatives are itraconazole, 200 mg, twice daily for seven days, and terbinafine, 250 mg, daily for two weeks), is recommended for vesicular and inflammatory infections. Daily application of miconazole powder or superabsorbent powder minimizes common recurrences, and prevention can be further facilitated by scrupulous personal hygiene, the wearing of dry, loose undergarments, regular bathing, and the drying of clothes as soon as possible following workout.

TINEA PEDIS

This common dermatophyte infection of the feet is widely seen in athletes as a result of a combination of moisture and friction. Three distinct types are seen, each of which is treated differently (8). Moccasin type includes mild erythema, mild to profuse scales, and accentuated skin lines; and it may include hyperkeratosis around the heel (Fig. 12.5). Minimal to no pruritus is observed. This often is a long-standing chronic condition in which the patient simply believes that he or she has chronic dry skin of the feet. The more symptomatic,

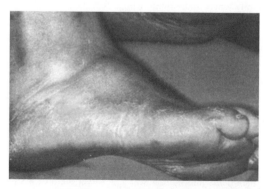

FIG. 12.5. Moccasin tinea pedis.

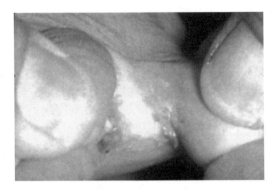

FIG. 12.6. Interdigital tinea pedis.

interdigital type consists of erosions, scaling, fissures, and maceration (Fig. 12.6). This is especially common between the fourth and fifth toes, and it causes burning, itching, and pain. It may often be more malodorous because of colonization with gram-negative bacteria. Finally, the less common vesicular or vesiculobullous tinea pedis is characterized by the sudden eruption of pruritic and painful blisters. A small single blister or larger multiloculated bullae may be found (Fig. 12.7).

Prevention and Treatment

Each type of tinea pedis requires somewhat different treatment, but the common issue in prevention is

the need to keep the feet cool and dry. Throwing out the old athletic shoes may be needed if the problem is recurrent. For the moccasin type, the athlete may use keratolytic moisturizing lotions for chronic dry skin, along with any of the over-the-counter topical antifungal creams, such as clotrimazole, miconazole, tolnaftate, or others. For the interdigital type, the individual must dry the feet first, as creams are generally not effective on macerated skin. Aluminum chloride 20% (Drysol), Burrow's solution (Domeboro), or Epsom salts soaks, two to three times daily for 15 to 20 minutes, can be effective. Then, the athlete should use talcum or antifungal powder regularly and should begin the use of over-the-counter creams when the skin is drier. Finally, the acute vesicular type should be treated like interdigital tinea pedis but with more aggressive drying of the feet (e.g., soaking three to four times daily). Carefully puncturing the painful blisters (without unroofing them) can relieve some of the pain, and a high-potency topical steroid (or even oral steroids) can help to diminish the itch and the acute inflammatory reaction. The use of topical antifungals is not as important in these cases because the acute inflammatory reaction often kills the fungi.

Restrictions for Play

While no specific restrictions are indicated, the athlete should be advised to wear shower thongs to minimize the spread to other players and to prevent recurrence.

REFERENCES

1. Basler RS. Acne mechanica in athletes. *Cutis* 1992;50: 125–128.
2. Pharis DB, Teller C, Wolf JE Jr. Cutaneous manifestations of sports participation. *J Am Acad Dermatol* 1997; 36:448–459.
3. Habif TP. *Clinical dermatology: a color guide to diagnosis and therapy*, 3rd ed. St. Louis: Mosby-Year Book, 1996.
4. Goldstein BG, Goldstein AO. *Practical dermatology*, 2nd ed. St. Louis: Mosby-Year Book, 1997.
5. Basler RS, Basler GC, Palmer AH, et al. Special skin symptoms seen in swimmers. *J Am Acad Dermatol* 2000;43:299–305.
6. Helm TN, Bergfeld WF. Sports dermatology. *Clin Dermatol* 1998;16:159–165.
7. Basler RS. Skin problems in athletes. In: Mellion MB, Walsh W, Shelton GL, eds. *The team physician's handbook*, 2nd ed. Philadelphia: Hanley & Belfus, 1997: 346–347.
7a. Ramsey ML. Pitted keratolysis: a common infection of active feet. *The Physician and Sports Medicine* 1996;24:51–52,55–56.
7b. Nowak MA, Brodell RT. Rapid diagnosis of superficial fungal infections. *Postgrad Med* 1999;105:179–180.
8. Reeves, JRT, Maibach, HI. *Clinical dermatology illustrated: a regional approach*, 3rd ed. Philadelphia: FA Davis Co, 1998.

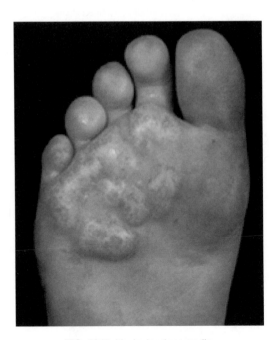

FIG. 12.7. Vesicular tinea pedis.

13

Amenorrhea in the Adolescent Athlete

Charleen L. Isé

The absence of menses can be divided into primary or secondary amenorrhea. Primary amenorrhea, or delayed menarche, is defined as the appearance of neither menses nor secondary sex characteristics by the age of 15 years or the absence of menstrual cycles by the age of 16 years, regardless of the presence of secondary sex characteristics. Secondary amenorrhea is defined as the cessation of menses for 3 to 6 months after menses has been present for 6 months (1).

Why physical training can cause menstrual disorders is not well understood. Between 2% to 5% of all reproductive age women who are not pregnant or lactating experience amenorrhea. However, in exercising women, the occurrence can be as high as 44%. Girls who begin intensive exercise prior to menarche may have their first menses delayed by 5 months for every previous year of training, when compared to sedentary controls under similar amounts of psychologic stress. The etiology is attributed to the interplay of energy expenditure and other variables, including genetics and nutrition. For example, some women continue to menstruate regularly even with low body fat levels and high exercise regimens. But exercising women also may have a shortened luteal phase (<7 days), low hormone levels, and intermittent or no ovulation. So, while some women appeared to be menstruating regularly, they may not be having normal cycles (2).

The average age of menarche is 12.8 years. Ninety percent of women cycle between 21 and 44 days, and the average is 28 days. Most menstrual disorders occur near menarche and menopause when anovulatory cycles are more common. The mean duration of menses is 5.2 days, with an average blood loss of 40 mL (3). The menstrual cycle is divided into the follicular phase, which is prior to ovulation, and the luteal phase following ovulation until the onset of menses; each lasts approximately 14 days. A complex system of hormones released by the hypothalamus, pituitary, and ovaries controls ovulation and menses (4). In response to the pulsatile release of gonadotropin-releasing hormone (GnRH) from the hypothalamus, the anterior pituitary gland releases

the following two hormones: follicle-stimulating hormone (FSH) and luteinizing hormone (LH). These two hormones act on the ovaries to produce estrogen and progesterone in a cyclical pattern, producing ovulation and the preparation of the endometrium for pregnancy. If no fertilization occurs, the endometrium sloughs and the cycle begins again. Pituitary hormones (e.g., endorphins, prolactin, and prostaglandins) also contribute to the menstrual cycle (5). In adolescent athletes, the loss of the pulsatile GnRH release is often what leads to menstrual irregularities (Table 13.1).

TABLE 13.1. *Causes of amenorrhea*

Category	Possible causes
Physiologic	Pregnancy
	Breastfeeding
	Constitutional delay
Chromosomal	Turner syndrome
	Gonadal dysgenesis
	Androgen insensitivity
Hypothalamic	Prader–Willi syndrome
	Laurence–Moon syndrome
	Female athlete triad
	Anorexia nervosa
	Psychological or physical trauma
	Depression
Structural	Imperforate hymen
	Müllerian anomalies
	Asherman syndrome
Medications	Illicit drugs
	Anabolic steroids
	Herbal products
	Hormones
	Radiation therapy
	Chemotherapy
Pituitary	Sheehan syndrome
	Pituitary tumors
Ovarian	Premature menopause
	Chronic disease
	Autoimmune disease
	Infections
Other	Thyroid disease
	Polycystic ovary syndrome
	Diabetes mellitus

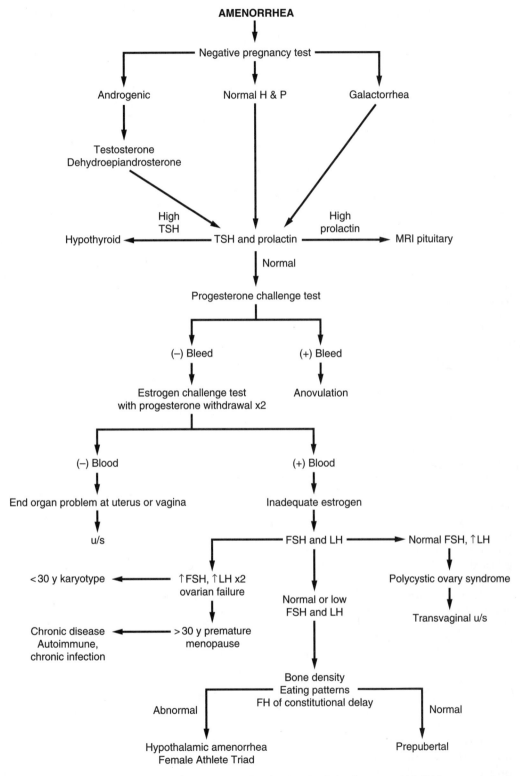

FIG.13.1. Evaluation of amenorrhea. Abbreviations: FSH, follicle stimulating hormone; H & P, history and physical; LH, luteinizing hormone; MRI, magnetic resonance imaging; TSH, thyroid-stimulating hormone; u/s, ultrasound.

EVALUATION OF AMENORRHEA

The clinician should begin the evaluation by ruling out pregnancy. Then, he or she should evaluate the patient's past, family, and social histories. The clinician must specifically look for female athlete triad (FAT) by looking for changes in weight, exercise intensity, eating habits, stress fractures, and obsessive behaviors. Endocrine symptoms (e.g., obesity, acne, striae, and hirsutism) can point to adrenal causes or polycystic ovary syndrome (PCOS). Headaches, vision changes, and galactorrhea may suggest a pituitary tumor. Constipation, fatigue, hair loss, and weight gain point to thyroid disease. A history of ambiguous or delayed gynecologic development should also be elicited. Prescribed, illegal, or over-the-counter products, including herbal supplements and anabolic steroids, can contribute to menstrual dysfunction. The examiner should question friends and teammates in an attempt to identify abnormal exercise regimens or eating patterns in an athlete. The athlete herself often fails to recognize warning signs of FAT.

The physical examination includes weight, height, body fat measurement, temperature, pulse, and blood pressure. The clinician should look for signs of secondary sex characteristics, androgen excess, endocrine abnormalities, and chromosomal anomalies. The skin of the dorsal hands and the teeth can reveal signs of induced vomiting. The visual fields should be assessed to check for pituitary tumor. A pelvic exam may reveal an imperforate hymen, absent uterus, or advanced pregnancy.

Laboratory work should begin with a test for pregnancy, the most common etiology of amenorrhea in this age group (Fig. 13.1). Next, the physician should determine thyroid-stimulating hormone (TSH) and prolactin levels. If the TSH level is abnormal, the appropriate workup for thyroid disease should be undertaken. If galactorrhea is present in an amenorrheic patient, workup for a prolactin tumor should be pursued.

Next, a progesterone challenge test should be used to determine if enough estrogen is present to proliferate the endometrium and whether the outflow tract (i.e., uterus and vagina) is competent. The patient should ingest 10 mg of medroxyprogesterone acetate orally for 5 to 10 days. If the patient bleeds within 2 to 7 days, the diagnosis is anovulation. Bleeding confirms adequate activity of the ovary (estrogen), the pituitary, the hypothalamus, and the outflow tract. If the patient does not bleed, either the outflow tract is at fault or the endometrium has not been proliferated by estrogen. The next step is the use of estrogen to cause endometrial proliferation (1.25 mg of conjugated estrogens daily for 21 days). Medroxyprogesterone acetate, 10 mg per day, is added for the last 10 days to achieve a withdrawal bleed. If no bleeding occurs, the test should be repeated. If bleeding is still not present, the problem is usually obstruction of the outflow tract. If bleeding does occur, the problem is inadequate estrogen—the hypoestrogenic state. If, after the evaluation, the clinician feels that the patient has no indication of an outflow tract problem, the trial of estrogen may be skipped.

Once low estrogen levels are detected, the clinician should check FSH and LH. High results indicate an ovarian etiology (e.g., premature ovarian failure). However, all patients under the age of 30 years with the diagnosis of ovarian failure mandate chromosomal analysis, even if they are normal in appearance, as certain chromosomal anomalies carry a significant risk of malignancy (5). If LH and FSH levels are low, the patient is either prepubertal, or she has hypothalamic dysfunction (e.g., FAT, anorexia nervosa) (5).

CAUSES OF AMENORRHEA

Many causes of amenorrhea are found in the adolescent. Structural causes, such as imperforate hymen, are easily diagnosed on physical exam by a bulging bluish mass at the hymeneal ring. Müllerian anomalies may be diagnosed by finding a complete absence of the uterus or vagina in the physical examination. However, more subtle anomalies may require gynecologic referral for ultrasound, hysteroscopy, or laparoscopic evaluation.

Asherman syndrome is due to scarring and disruption of the endometrial lining. It occurs after curettage of the endometrial lining (i.e., dilation and curettage or elective abortions). Endometritis, tuberculosis, and schistosomiasis can also cause Asherman syndrome. This syndrome is rare in the United States, but it should be considered in immigrants where abortions are the primary form of contraception (i.e., East European countries). Diagnosis is confirmed by hysterosalpingogram.

Constitutional delay is the most common cause of primary amenorrhea (5). A positive family history can be extremely helpful in differentiating this delay from FAT. Both diagnoses have low FSH, LH, and serum estradiol levels, and they do not bleed after a progesterone challenge. However, with constitutional delay, no evidence of disordered eating is found, and the bone density scan is normal. Diagnosis in the unclear case may require a several month trial of decreased activity (i.e., during off-season) to be certain.

Female Athlete Triad

FAT has the following three components: disordered eating, amenorrhea, and osteoporosis. It occurs not only in elite athletes but also in physically active girls and women. Societal and internal pressures for women to maintain unrealistically low weights for their sport encourage behaviors that lead to this disorder. Further, the belief that the cessation of menses in certain sports is a reflection of an appropriate training intensity is found among female athletes and their coaches. This is particularly true in sports where slimness (diving and swimming) or physical beauty (gymnastics, dance, and water ballet) may contribute to a better score. However, the presence of FAT is actually associated with declining performance, as well as increased injury (1). Amenorrhea is due to a decrease of the pulsatile hypothalamic GnRH release that then leads to decreased pituitary LH release and suppression of the ovarian estrogen production. One hypothesis is that an imbalance between the stress of exercise and the body's energy availability in the form of body fat and caloric intake causes the hypothalamus to malfunction (1). A recent study concluded that the hormone leptin might be the metabolic link between energy availability and the effect on the reproductive axis (6).

The prevalence of disordered eating in FAT is 15% to 62%, and it can range from restricted food intake (anorexia nervosa) to binging and purging (bulimia nervosa). The characteristics of anorexia nervosa are amenorrhea, an intense fear of weight gain, a disturbed body image, self-esteem that is influenced by weight, a denial of the seriousness of low body weight, and weight less than 85% of that expected for the individual's height and age (see Chapter 9) (7).

Anorexia nervosa exists as either the restrictive (caloric intake) or the binging and purging (similar to that seen in bulimia) form. Complications include dental, electrolyte, and cardiac problems and death. Fifteen percent of hospitalized anorexics may die of complications (8). Resumption of menses occurs at approximately 90% of the ideal body weight (4). Patients with bulimia nervosa do not have a distorted body image, but they do demonstrate at least a 3-month history of lack of control over eating with binging. Bulimics are divided into the two types of purging and nonpurging. They purge by vomiting or via the use of laxatives and/or diuretics. The nonpurging bulimic exercises excessively (7).

The amenorrheic hypoestrogenic athlete is at risk for osteoporosis and stress fractures. She has lower bone mineral density than age-matched controls due to decreased bony deposition and premature bone loss (8).

Recognizing the triad can be difficult. Table 13.2 provides an approach to the assessment of FAT. Women with one component of the triad should be screened for the other components. Athletes, their parents, and their coaches should be trained to recognize this disorder and to avoid activities that promote it. Specifically, girls should not be pressured into maintaining an unrealistic weight. They should learn basic nutrition and safe training techniques, and they should have resources for medical, nutritional, and mental health screening available (1).

Treatment requires a coordinated approach that involves the athlete, parents, coaches, the athletic trainer, a nutritionist, a psychiatrist, and the primary care or sports physician. Care can be managed as an outpatient if the athlete's life is not in danger. The hypoestrogenic athlete should be supplemented with estrogen and calcium until her menses recur. Oral contraceptives should be used if the athlete is sexually active because she still may ovulate, even though she is amenorrheic, and thus, she is at risk for pregnancy. Otherwise, 0.625 mg of conjugated estrogens daily, with 10 mg of medroxyprogesterone acetate for 10 days of each month, is used. Calcium in the form of calcium carbonate (1,500 mg per day) and vitamin D (400 to 800 IU per day) are added. Yearly bone density scans should be conducted (9).

Consultation with a nutritionist and psychiatrist is often necessary to attain a safer weight and healthier eating habits and to manage underlying psychiatric issues. Many of these patients have anxiety, depression, or obsessive compulsive disorders that improve with medications (e.g., selective serotonin reuptake inhibitors) and psychotherapy.

Controversy among experts exists as to the true cause of FAT. Do multifocal pressures from the physical activity and sporting competition cause this disorder? Or, do excessive exercise and athletic competition simply enable the expression of negative personality traits? The controversy is as yet unresolved (10).

TABLE 13.2. *Office assessment for female athlete triad*

1. Obtain a fracture and SCOFF* history.
2. Obtain and plot height and weight graphs.
3. Check for evidence of delayed puberty and hypoestrogenemia.
4. Calculate a basal metabolic index for all adolescent patients.
5. Check supine pulse following a 2-min rest; if low, measure for orthostatic changes.

*See Chapter 9, Table 9.4.

Chromosomal Anomalies

Other causes of amenorrhea include chromosomal anomalies. Turner syndrome is due to the absence of the second sex chromosome (XO or 45X), and it presents with short stature, a webbed neck, a broad chest, and an immature outflow tract. Women with Turner syndrome and other mixed gonadal dysgeneses can have either primary or secondary amenorrhea, and they may have abnormalities that predispose them to malignancies, analogous to a male with undescended testes.

Testicular feminization and/or androgen insensitivity occurs with XY karyotype and failure of virilization due to androgen receptor insensitivity. Various degrees of penetrance occur, and the presentation can range from a blind vaginal pouch and absent uterus to clitoromegaly with undescended testes. A risk of malignant transformation of these cryptorchid testes is present. A good rule of thumb is to perform a karyotype in all women who are less than 5 ft in height with primary amenorrhea and in women who are less than 30 years of age with primary amenorrhea or prolonged secondary amenorrhea (5).

Other Conditions

Ovarian failure due to chronic disease can occur with such conditions as autoimmune disease or with infections, such as mumps, gonorrhea, and tuberculosis. Ovarian failure can also result from exposure to radiation or chemotherapeutic agents.

Hypothalamic amenorrhea due to the loss of pulsatile GnRH release is important to normal menstrual function, and it can be affected by many other stresses, including uncontrolled diabetes mellitus, Cushing syndrome, and congenital adrenal hyperplasia, as well as depression, starvation, strenuous training, and severe psychologic or physical trauma or illness.

Hyperprolactinemia causes up to 20% of secondary amenorrheas. Prolactin inhibits GnRH release, causing an anovulatory state. The causes of hyperprolactinemia include pituitary adenoma, hypothyroidism, idiopathic sources, and drugs. Pituitary tumors, such as pituitary microadenomas, present with galactorrhea, headaches, and irregular menses. These can be difficult to diagnose as they may not always cause elevated prolactin levels, and these females may only exhibit galactorrhea one-third of the time. Idiopathic hyperprolactinemia acts exactly like a prolactin-secreting pituitary tumor, but pituitary magnetic resonance imaging (MRI) or computerized tomography (CT) is negative. A positive withdrawal bleed in response to progesterone, the ab-

sence of galactorrhea, and a normal prolactin level definitively rules out significant pituitary tumor (4). Bromocriptine (2.5 mg per day) will reduce the prolactin level, and it can shrink the adenoma.

Hypothyroidism causes amenorrhea because high levels of TSH cross-react in the anterior pituitary to stimulate prolactin secretion. The TSH level should be found when evaluating an elevated prolactin level. Hyperthyroidism increases testosterone–estradiol-binding globulin, thus increasing testosterone levels. Testosterone is converted to estrogen, which leads to anovulation.

Sheehan syndrome follows pituitary infarction, secondary to severe postpartum hemorrhage and prolonged hypotension. Other causes of pituitary malfunction include tumors and infections (e.g., syphilis, tuberculosis).

PCOS can be found in the patient with hyperinsulinemia, insulin resistance, abnormal hypothalamic secretion of GnRH, and high estrogen levels. This leads to anovulation, polycystic ovaries, and menstrual disorder. Clinically, evidence of androgen excess, such as hirsutism and acne, may be found. The syndrome can occur as early as menarche. Laboratory findings include an elevated LH to FSH ratio and polycystic ovaries on ultrasound (11).

Medications as Causes

Many medications can cause menstrual irregularities. Contraceptive hormones are a common cause of amenorrhea. Some athletes use contraceptive hormones to manipulate their menses relative to their competition schedule. Furthermore, athletes may take excessive doses of oral contraceptives or anabolic steroids in an effort to gain a competitive advantage. Signs of androgen excess and elevated serum androgen levels may be present (12). Phenothiazines, thioxanthenes, and other dopamine antagonists can cause a hyperprolactin state and amenorrhea. Certain herbs may interfere with the menstrual cycle due to their mild estrogenic effect. These include ginseng, black cohosh, licorice (high dose), and plant phytoestrogens (e.g., soybeans) (13).

SUMMARY

In conclusion, amenorrhea is not itself a disease, but it may be a symptom of an underlying medical condition in the adolescent athlete. While it is not an uncommon finding, it may be ignored by the patient and may be considered normal by coaches, athletic trainers, and players. In recent years, attempts have been made by groups such as the International

Olympic Committee (IOC) to recognize and address this problem. For example, all gymnasts must now be 16 years old to compete at the international level. Treating physicians must do their part to assist the athletic community in further prevention, recognition, and treatment of these conditions. Adolescent athletes and their coaches should receive specific education, proper nutrition, and training techniques regarding FAT. The primary care physician is in an ideal position to lead the care of the adolescent female athlete.

REFERENCES

1. Otis CL, Drinkwater B, Johnson M, et al. American College of Sports Medicine position stand. The female athlete triad. *Med Sci Sports Exerc* 1997;29:i–ix.
2. Bullen BA, Skrinar GS, Beitins IZ, et al. Induction of menstrual disorders by strenuous exercise in untrained women. *N Engl J Med* 1985;312:1349–1353.
3. Wiggins DL, Wiggins ME. The female athlete. II. Primary care of the injured athlete. *Clin Sports Med* 1997; 16:593–601.
4. Sulik SM, Heath CB. Menstrual disorders. *AAFP home study self-assessment*. Monograph no. 255. Leawood, KS: American Association of Family Practitioners, 2000:11–20.
5. Speroff L, Glass RH, Kase NG. Amenorrhea. In: *Clinical gynecologic endocrinology and infertility*, 6th ed. Baltimore: Lippincott Williams & Wilkins, 1999: 421–485.
6. Thong FS, McLean C, Graham TE. Plasma leptin in female athletes: relationship with body fat, reproductive, nutritional, and endocrine factors. *J Appl Physiol* 2000; 88:2037–2044.
7. American Psychiatric Association. *Diagnostic and statistical manual of mental disorders*, 4th ed. Washington, D.C.: American Psychiatric Association, 1994.
8. Smith, AD. The female athlete triad: causes, diagnosis, and treatment. *The Physician and Sports Medicine* 1996;24:67–86.
9. Joy E, Clark N, Ireland ML et al. Team management of the female athlete triad. II. Optimal treatment and prevention tactics. *The Physician and Sports Medicine* 1997;25:55–69.
10. DiPietro L, Stachenfeld NS. The female athlete triad [Letter]. *Med Sci Sports Exerc* 1997;29:1669–1671.
11. Hunter MH, Sterrett JJ. Polycystic ovarian syndrome: it's not just infertility. *Am Fam Physician* 2000;62: 1079–1088.
12. Rogol AD, Sex steroid and growth hormone supplementation to enhance performance in adolescent athletes. *Curr Opin Pediatr* 2000;12:382–387.
13. Schulz V, Hansel R, Tyler VE. Rational phytotherapy. *A physician's guide to herbal medicine*, 3rd ed. New York: Springer-Verlag, 1998.

14

Diabetes Mellitus in Young Athletes

Brian L. Mahaffey and Russell D. White

EPIDEMIOLOGY

Diabetes mellitus is a group of endocrine diseases whose incidence during the adolescent years in Western civilization is growing (1,2). Type 1 diabetes, the most prevalent type, occurs in approximately 1 in 500 adolescents. However, the incidence of type 2 diabetes is rising, secondary to increasing obesity (1). In 1994, among 10-year-olds to 19-year-olds, type 2 diabetes accounted for 33% of all new diagnoses (3,4). Athletes can be affected by diabetes mellitus, and they require modifications to care plans to maintain optimum blood glucose control. Understanding the pathophysiology, management, and certain risks that are involved with exercise help the healthcare professional assist athletes in diabetes care and management.

DIAGNOSIS

To diagnose diabetes mellitus, patients must meet one of three criteria (5). The first criterion is a fasting blood glucose level of greater than or equal to 126 mg per dL, with fasting defined as no caloric intake for 8 hours. The second criterion is a 2-hour blood glucose level of more than or equal to 200 mg per dL during an oral glucose challenge test with 75 g of glucose in liquid. The last criterion is a casual blood glucose concentration of equal to or greater than 200 mg per dL, along with symptoms of polyuria, polydipsia, and unexplained weight loss. A repeat measurement is needed with each criterion to confirm the diagnosis.

PATHOPHYSIOLOGY

Type 1 diabetes mellitus is caused by the progressive destruction of the pancreatic beta cells, either by an autoimmune or an idiopathic process (6). This leads to decreased endogenous insulin production. Thus, patients with type 1 diabetes are susceptible to hyperglycemia, weight loss, and ketoacidosis. Long term, these adolescents have the same complications

as adults, including retinopathy, nephropathy, neuropathy, and coronary and peripheral atherosclerosis (6,7). The typical onset for Type 1 diabetes mellitus occurs before 30 years of age.

A defect in both insulin secretion and its action upon the liver and peripheral muscle leads to type 2 diabetes mellitus. This is most common in patients 40 years of age or older. However, an increasing problem with obesity in adolescence is leading to a higher incidence of type 2 diabetes in youths, especially in certain ethnic groups. These adolescents are inactive and overweight, and they eat an inappropriate calorie-laden diet (3). A dominantly inherited form of type 2 diabetes in adolescence has been termed "maturity onset diabetes of the young" (MODY) (3,8). Criteria for the diagnosis of MODY includes elevated blood glucose levels, the absence of ketosis, correction of fasting hyperglycemia without insulin use for at least 2 years, and an age of onset prior to 25 years of age in at least one family member (3,8,9).

Physiologically, the regulation of blood glucose involves the coordination of the pancreas, liver, and skeletal muscle (1,3). The pancreas releases both insulin and glucagon. Insulin facilitates transfer of glucose into cells; its conversion to glycogen inhibits gluconeogenesis to spare proteins, and it also translates glucose into triglycerides in lipid tissue. Glucagon is a counterregulatory hormone that stimulates hepatic glycogenolysis and gluconeogenesis. The liver and skeletal muscle are the main stores of glycogen, and they undergo either gluconeogenesis or glycogenolysis, depending on the blood glucose level. Overall, catecholamines (e.g., epinephrine and norepinephrine), growth hormone, and cortisol help to maintain blood glucose levels by raising circulating levels. Table 14.1 summarizes this. With aerobic exercise, counterregulatory hormones balance the action of insulin to mobilize glucose for skeletal muscle use. This balance in the diabetic athlete may not be found, thus leading to problems of either lowered or elevated blood glucose levels (1,10). Most competi-

TABLE 14.1. *Regulatory hormones and actions*

Hormone	Physiologic action
Insulin	Facilitates glucose transfer into cell and promotes glycogen synthesis.
	Inhibits glucagon secretion.
	Inhibits gluconeogenesis.
	Converts glucose to triglycerides in lipid tissue.
Glucagon	Stimulates hepatic glycogenolysis and glyconeogenesis.
Catecholamines	Promotes hepatic glycogenolysis and glyconeogenesis.
Epinephrine	Suppresses insulin secretion.
Norepinephrine	Limits peripheral glucose utilization.
Growth hormone	Inhibits carbohydrate metabolism.
	Neutralizes free fatty acids.
Cortisol	Inhibits peripheral glucose utilization.
	Promotes gluconeogenesis.

tive diabetic athletes report optimal performance when they maintain blood glucose levels between 70 and 150 mg per dL (11). With type 1 diabetes, the expected decline of insulin with activity may not be seen secondary to the use of exogenous insulin. An increased absorption from injection sites may be noted with exercise, especially when insulin is injected into an exercising limb (1), Over time, patients with type 1 diabetes become desensitized to the counterregulatory hormonal system as well, causing the release of glucagon and catecholamines to be delayed. Both of these problems may lead to immediate hypoglycemia as glycogen stores become exhausted (1,12). However, if the active diabetic patient is insulin-deficient and the blood glucose level is elevated, exercise may exacerbate elevations of blood glucose, leading to ketoacidosis (12,13). In type 2 diabetes, exercise leads to improved insulin sensitivity and decreased insulin resistance at the cellular level (3,5,14,15). Resistance training with resistance to weight is key for type 2 diabetic patients to increase lean body mass and to improve insulin resistance (16).

MANAGEMENT

Management of diabetes mellitus in active young people involves coordination of preventative and treatment-oriented medical care, nutritional management, planning of exercise regimens, and the psychologic aspects of coping with a chronic disease. There-

fore, a team approach involving the patient, the patient's family, health care specialists, coaches, and the patient's peers is required. Health care specialists include the primary care physician, an endocrinologist, a dietician or diabetic educator, and an athletic trainer (5,12,14,17–19).

An athlete with diabetes should undergo the same preparticipation physical examination (PPE) as other athletes, along with a thorough assessment for retinopathy, neuropathy, and nephropathy (see Chapter 2) (1,12,20). An ophthalmoscopic examination, urinalysis, and the consideration of blood urea nitrogen and creatinine levels are appropriate, according to American Diabetes Association guidelines (5). A complete record of diabetes management, including diet and calorie intake, insulin regimen or oral medications, and the level of activity, should be obtained as well. The adolescent's level of maturity, his or her dedication to the activity, and the level of understanding of diabetes management should be assessed. Also, the social support of his or her parents, coaches, and peers is extremely important, and it plays a large role in management (1,6,12,14,17,18).

Insulin should be adjusted to achieve a preexercise blood glucose level of 120 to 180 mg per dL. Once exercise begins, patients should do self-monitoring of blood glucose (SMBG) to delineate their normal glucose response to exercise. Subcutaneous abdominal insulin injections are considered the best method for active people to achieve consistent absorption (21). Use of an intensive regimen, with short-acting insulin (regular or Humalog) and frequent SMBG, may be the best method for blood glucose control in active adolescents; but this approach can be difficult to learn. If the patient is using intermediate acting insulin (NPH) along with regular insulin, the NPH amount is often decreased by 50%, and the regular insulin amount is decreased by 25% to 75 %, depending on the time and intensity of the activity (22). The use of an insulin pump provides the best metabolic control of diabetes, and it requires a decrease of the basal infusion rate with activity (20). Performing SMBG allows the athlete to adjust the infusion rate according to the activity level. Disadvantages with the insulin pump are its cost (approximately $6,000 to $7,000), the initial difficulty of use, and the necessity to remove it for contact sports. Protective cases now exist that can withstand contact sports and water sports to a certain depth. No replacement of insulin is needed if the pump is removed for less than an hour. If the pump is removed for more than an hour, subcutaneous insulin injection with the same number of units that would have been infused during this time is required.

Adolescents with type 2 diabetes mellitus may require oral hypoglycemic agents, such as sulfonylureas and the newer biguanides and α-glucosidase inhibitors. Sulfonylureas are generally well-tolerated in adolescents, with few side effects except hypoglycemia. They work by increasing the release of insulin from pancreatic beta cells. Biguanides work by increasing sensitivity to insulin peripherally and decreasing hepatic gluconeogenesis, but they have a low incidence of associated lactic acidosis. Alpha-glucosidase inhibitors reduce the absorption of carbohydrates from the intestinal wall. All of these medicines can be used in combination to enhance the blood glucose control; however, information regarding the use of biguanides and alpha-glucosidase inhibitors in adolescents is lacking (3,5). Insulin may be used in combination with oral hypoglycemics or as monotherapy. Insulin, biguanides, and alpha-glucosidase inhibitors may require dosage adjustment to prevent hypoglycemia with exercise. The newer agents, such as metformin and pioglitazone, rarely produce hypoglycemia with exercise.

The nutritional regimen plays an important role in the treatment of both type 1 and type 2 diabetes. Patients need to have a good understanding of the basic nutritional plan, and Table 14.2 presents a summary of nutritional strategies. Carbohydrates should provide 55% to 60% of calories on average, 30% should come from fats, and proteins should not exceed 10% to 15%. Total caloric consumption should not exceed the caloric requirements calculated for an athlete's activities. One strategy used for type 1 diabetes with exercise is to increase carbohydrate ingestion by 15 g for every 30 minutes of moderate activity (12). In type 2 diabetes, weight loss should be the goal when developing a nutritional and exercise plan (3,20). Carbohydrate loading should be done cautiously in diabetic patients, and the insulin dose should be adjusted appropriately. If the diabetes is well controlled, the glycogen stores will be adequate. Fluids are an essential part of an active diabetic patient's nutritional plan (20). If carbohydrates are needed during exercise, liquid forms are easily digested, and they are converted quickly for use as fuel. As with other ath-

TABLE 14.2. *Summary of nutritional strategies**

Phase of training	Recreational athlete	Endurance athlete
Daily training	Consume <30% total daily energy from fat; 10–12% from protein; balance from CHO.	Consume <0.4 g fat/kg BW/d, 0.8–1.2 g protein; 8–10 g CHO.
CHO loading (week before event)	Not applicable.	Caution for type 1; do 90, 40, 40, 20, 20, 0 min of moderate intensity exercise per day; consume 5 g CHO/kg of BW/d during first 3 d; consume 8–10 g CHO/kg of BW during next 3 d.
Hours before event	Exercise does not need to be taken on empty stomach; work-enhancing effect of preexercise CHO meal is doubtful; consume adequate fluids.	Consume 4–5 g liquid CHO/kg 3–4 hr before event and/or consume 1–2 g liquid CHO/kg 1 hr before event. Solids may be substituted.
During event	Consume 250 ml of fluid every 20 min or at rate equal to sweat loss; fluids may be CHO or electrolyte beverages, water, or other preferred fluids.	Consume 250 ml of fluid every 20 min or at rate equal to sweat loss; preferred fluids are CHO or electrolyte (6–10% wt/vol) beverages at a rate to provide 40–65 g CHO/hr. If CHO consumption is delayed, consume 200 g of liquid CHO before completing 2 hr of exercise and then consume 40–65 g CHO/hr.
4–6 hr after event	Not applicable.	Consume 0.7–3.0 g CHO/kg *immediately* after event and every 2 hr for 4 hr; if tolerated, 0.4 g CHO/kg every 15 min after event for 4 hr.
24 hr post event	Follow daily training schedule.	Consume 8–10 g CHO/kg/d; mixed CHO foods can be consumed; high-glycemic index foods promote glycogen synthesis.

Abbreviations: BW, body weight; CHO, carbohydrate.
Individual response patterns may vary. The specific response to exercise can be monitored with self-monitoring of blood glucose (SMBG).
From American Diabetes Association. *The health professional's guide to diabetes and exercise.* Ruderman N, Devlin JT, eds. Alexandria, VA: American Diabetes Association, 1995:94, with permission.

letes, diabetics must replace fluids and carbohydrates during the hour after activity (20,23). Following the nutritional plan adequately is often a problem in the pediatric and adolescent population. Studies have shown that family and peer support of adolescents with diabetes positively influences the metabolic control of the disease process (6,14,17–19).

RISKS IN ACTIVE DIABETICS

As with all disease processes, certain hazards accompany activity in diabetes that the health care provider and the patient should understand. Patients with retinopathy should be restricted from activities that rapidly increase intraocular pressure, such as weight lifting or collision sports, (7,12,20,24). Nephropathy is rare in childhood and adolescence (7). Peripheral neuropathy also is rare in this age group, but autonomic neuropathy may cause an abnormal sweating mechanism, leading to heat intolerance. It may also slow the normal increase in cardiac output with exercise, leading to syncopal episodes.

Immediate hypoglycemia may occur if caloric intake is inadequate for the level of activity or if excessive exogenous insulin administration occurs. Conducting SMBG readings during activity can prevent this immediate hypoglycemia. Delayed, or nocturnal, hypoglycemia is a potentially serious condition in type 1 diabetes that usually occurs at night when the patient is least likely to perceive hypoglycemia. It has been reported up to 28 hours after exercise, but it usually occurs 6 to 12 hours following the activity. This results because the liver and muscle are hypersensitive to circulating insulin, and they begin extracting circulating glucose to replenish glycogen stores. The result is persistent and prolonged hypoglycemia that may take several hours to correct. Adjusting insulin dosages can be preventative, but replacing glycogen stores within 1 hour of exercise, which is known as golden replenishment period, is the best prevention (1,12,20,21,25). In type 1 diabetes, ketoacidosis may occur when an adolescent begins activity with an elevated blood glucose level secondary to dehydration and stimulation of counterregulatory hormones and is also insulinopenic. Further exercise may exacerbate ketosis; therefore, these patients require standard treatment, including fluid and electrolyte replacement, rest, and insulin (6,13).

CONCLUSION

With a team approach and good social support, adolescents who are active in sports can improve their overall health and well being. With a good understanding their treatment regimen and the potential complications of diabetes, these athletes can be as successful as their peers in any activity that they choose.

REFERENCES

1. Draznin MB, Patel DR. Diabetes mellitus and sports. *Adolesc Med* 1998;9:457–465.
2. McCarthy D, Simmet P. *Diabetes 1994 to 2010: global estimates and projections*. Melbourne: International Diabetes Institute, 1994.
3. Glaser NS. Non-insulin-dependent diabetes mellitus in childhood and adolescence. *Pediatr Clin North Am* 1997;44:307–337.
4. Fagot-Campagna A, Pettitt DJ, Engelgau MM, et al. Type 2 diabetes among North American children and adolescents: an epidemiologic review and a public health perspective. *J Pediatr* 2000;136:664–672.
5. American Diabetes Association Consensus Statement. Type 2 diabetes in children and adolescents. *Diabetes Care* 2000;23:381–389.
6. Golden MP. Special problems with children and adolescents with diabetes. *Prim Care* 1999;26:885–892.
7. Sochett E, Daneman D. Early diabetes-related complications in children and adolescents with type 1 diabetes. *Endocrinol Metab Clin North Am* 1999;28:865–882.
8. Fajans SS. Maturity-onset diabetes of the young (MODY). *Diabetes Metab Rev* 1989;5:579–606.
9. Scheuner MT, Raffel LJ, Rotter JI. Genetics of diabetes. In: Alberti KGMN, Zimmet P, Defronzo RA, eds. *International textbook of diabetes mellitus*, 2nd ed. London: Wiley & Sons, 1998:58.
10. Sutton JR. Diabetes and exercise. In: Strauss RH, ed. *Sports medicine*, 2nd ed. Philadelphia, WB Saunders, 1991:221–237.
11. Horton ES. Role and management of exercise in diabetes mellitus. *Diabetes Care* 1998;11:210–211.
12. Draznin MB. Type 1 diabetes and sports participation—strategies for training and competing safely. *The Physician and Sports Medicine* 2000;28:49–56.
13. Berger M, Berchtold P, Cuppers H-J, et al. Metabolic and hormonal effects of muscular exercise in juvenile type diabetics. *Diabetologia* 1977;13:355–1365.
14. Jones KL. Non-insulin dependent diabetes in children and adolescents: the therapeutic challenge. *Clin Pediatr* 1998;37:103–110.
15. Mayer-Davis EJ, D'Agostino R, Karter AJ, et al. Intensity and amount of physical activity in relation to insulin sensitivity. *JAMA* 1998;279:669–674.
16. Miller WJ, Sherman WM, Ivy JL. Effect of strength training on glucose tolerance and post-glucose insulin response. *Med Sci Sports Exerc* 1984;16:539–543.
17. Burroughs TE, Harris MA, Pontious SL, et al. Research on social support in adolescents with IDDM: a critical review. *The Diabetes Educator* 1997;23:438–448.
18. Anderson B, Ho J, Brackett J, et al. Parental involvement in diabetes management tasks: relationships to blood glucose monitoring adherence and metabolic control in young adolescents with insulin-dependent diabetes mellitus. *J Pediatr* 1997;130:257–265.
19. Pinhas-Hamiel O, Standiford D, Hamiel D, et al. The type 2 family—a setting for development and treatment

of adolescent type 2 diabetes mellitus. *Arch Pediatr Adolesc Med* 1999;153:1063–1067.

20. White RD, Sherman C. Exercise in diabetes management; maximizing benefits, controlling Risks. *The Physician and Sports Medicine* 1999;4:62–67.

21. Mellion MB, Berg KE. Diabetes mellitus. In: Mellion MB, ed. *Sports medicine secrets*, 2nd ed. Philadelphia: Hanley & Belfus, 1999:172–176.

22. Berger M. Adjustments of insulin therapy. In: Ruderman N, Devlin JT, eds. *The health professional's guide to diabetes and exercise*. Alexandria: American Diabetes Association, 1995:117–122.

23. Zinman B, Ruderman N, Campaigne BN, et al. Position statement: diabetes mellitus and exercise. *Diabetes Care* 2001;24:1–9.

24. Ivy JL. Muscle glycogen synthesis before and after exercise. *Sports Med* 1991;11:6–19.

25. Macdonald J. Postexercise late-onset hypoglycemia in insulin-dependent diabetic patients. *Diabetes Care* 1978;10:584.

15

Gastrointestinal Problems in Young Athletes

Russell D. White

The gastrointestinal (GI) tract is the most common site for exercise-induced medical problems, which are more prevalent among younger athletes (1–3). Symptoms increase with more strenuous activity, and they are frequently associated with running (4). Physiologically, during initial exercise, 15% of the splanchnic blood flow is shunted to exercising muscles. As core temperature increases, 20% of the splanchnic blood flow is shunted to the skin for temperature regulation and cooling; and, at maximum exercise, 80% of the splanchnic blood flow is shunted, regardless of training level (5). This vascular shunting in turn produces or exacerbates GI problems. Many of these studies of splanchnic blood flow have focused on adult athletes, but the pediatric literature is limited. Some disease states, such as functional bowel syndrome (FBS) and inflammatory bowel disease, often begin in adolescence, and they may overlap with symptoms from exercise and sports participation. Thus, GI complaints in this age group must be carefully considered and evaluated. Clinical presentations, diagnosis, and treatment of both upper and lower GI problems will be discussed.

UPPER GASTROINTESTINAL PROBLEMS

Symptoms

Upper gastrointestinal (UGI) symptoms, which are experienced by nearly one-fourth of young athletes, include heartburn, nausea, vomiting, and bleeding (2,6,7). These symptoms are more common in female athletes, similar to the pattern that is found in the general population. In two separate studies, the symptoms became more prominent in response to more strenuous exercise, thereby indicating a dose-response relationship between symptoms and exercise intensity (8,9). Although symptoms may decrease with improved conditioning, a natural attrition rate may be at work; in other words, those persons with more severe symptoms may cease exercise activity completely. While runners comprise the most studied athletes, symptoms do also occur in multisport athletes (10).

Pathophysiology

The pathophysiology of UGI symptoms has focused on (a) gastric emptying time, (b) the presence or absence of gastroesophageal (GE) reflux, (c) gastric fluid content, and (d) GI bleeding. Scientific studies of these components have been complicated by the variable osmolality and the temperature of the ingested fluid, the carbohydrate and caloric content of the ingested fluid, and the invasive methods that are required for study. For example, the introduction of a nasogastric tube to analyze emptying of the stomach may produce reflux or nausea, which can alter the acid content of the stomach.

Gastric Emptying Time

As exercise begins, mechanical abdominal contractions increase the gastric emptying rate of water until the exercise level reaches about 75% of $\dot{V}_{O_2}$ max. Above this level, the emptying rate decreases in response to increased catecholamines, reduced blood flow, and, perhaps, an increase in endogenous opioids (11,12). Emotional stress in nervous athletes also may slow gastric emptying (13). As a consequence, vomiting frequently occurs; it is influenced by the following three key factors: dehydration, high-osmolar fluids, and exercise intensity (greater than 75% of $\dot{V}_{O_2}$ max) (13,14). Finally, the rapid accumulation of lactic acid during shorter events or at the culmination of endurance events may cause vomiting.

Gastroesophageal Reflux

GE reflux and heartburn are common in the general pediatric population, they occur in 10% of recreational runners, and they are more frequent in inexperienced athletes (6). One study correlated GE reflux with the intraesophageal pH of runners monitored following a low-fat meal determined that reflux symptoms were related to air swallowing and lower esophageal sphincter relaxation during exercise (15).

Gastric Fluid Content

One study noted an increase of intragastric bile acids with exercise, with no change in gastric acidity (16).

Gastrointestinal Hemorrhage

The stomach is the most common site of exercise-induced GI bleeding, which occurs in about 20% of endurance athletes (3,13,14). Younger ages and faster running times produce more positive guaiac tests in runners (17). With running, mechanical injury to the gastric fundus occurs due to the shearing forces of the diaphragm and the gastrophrenic ligaments. This jarring action is thought to produce mucosal bleeding. This finding is less common in other sports, such as cycling or swimming. In addition, shunting of the splanchnic flow may produce relative ischemia and subsequent mucosal bleeding. While nonsteroidal antiinflammatory drug (NSAID) use is commonly associated with gastritis and peptic ulcer disease, one study found no clear relationship between NSAID use and GI hemorrhage in athletes (18).

Evaluation

A careful history should note the onset of symptoms with either rest or activity. For example, active peptic ulcer disease often occurs at rest or during sleep, and it is relieved by specific medications. The clinician should also review training intensity changes for a causal temporal relationship with symptoms. The examination should focus on localized epigastric pain, with palpation of the abdomen and evaluation of current weight versus previous measurements.

Specific studies include a complete blood count, with indices, to determine the presence or absence of anemia. Tests for liver disease should be considered. A barium swallow with an UGI series, followed by consideration of upper endoscopy with biopsy, may be indicated. Specialized studies, such as esophageal manometry and esophageal pH monitoring, are rarely necessary.

Treatment

The treatment depends on the severity and duration of symptoms. Physicians may select a specific treatment for a presumed diagnosis before initiating diagnostic studies when the symptoms are of short dura-

tion. An antireflux regimen and a temporary decrease in high-intensity exercise may be helpful. Reducing high-fat meals before exercise and ingesting low osmolar cool solutions during exercise are beneficial. One should avoid medications that may precipitate UGI symptoms (e.g., NSAIDs and salicylates).

Medications include H_2-receptor blockers or proton pump inhibitors in symptomatic athletes or in those with documented hemorrhagic gastritis (15,18). Sucralfate and antacids are helpful, but the athlete should avoid large amounts of magnesium, which may precipitate lower GI symptoms (19,20). Metoclopramide promotes gastric emptying and reduces reflux, but drowsiness or an extrapyramidal reaction may occur. A modified Nissen procedure (laparoscopic fundoplasty) may be necessary for recalcitrant cases.

LOWER GASTROINTESTINAL PROBLEMS

Symptoms

Lower GI symptoms (e.g., abdominal cramping, stool frequency, diarrhea, the urge to defecate, and bleeding) occur more commonly than UGI complaints, and they are seen more frequently in female and younger athletes (3,13,14,21). Up to 50% of runners experience these symptoms, which increase with exercise intensity. Some athletes may have underlying problems, such as FBS or lactose intolerance, which have a similar incidence (10% to 16%) to the general population (22,23). These problems often begin in adolescence, and they mimic those seen in adulthood (24).

Pathophysiology

Several theories relate the pathophysiology of lower GI symptoms to exercise. The direct effect of exercise decreases the intestinal transit time (25,26). Exercise in the upright position promotes the decreased transit time, compared to relative inactivity (27). Dietary changes alter the transit time. Due to expanding metabolic requirements with exercise, athletes increase calories and thus residue. In addition, some athletes follow a healthy lifestyle and ingest excessive amounts of fiber. The net result is a decrease in transit time (27). Finally, many performance-enhancing diets containing minerals or high-dose vitamin C promote abdominal cramping and diarrhea (28).

During strenuous exercise, an 80% decrease in splanchnic blood flow, with shunting of mesenteric blood to the exercising muscles and skin, occurs. This relative ischemia decreases GI transit time, produces cramping and diarrhea, and can cause bleeding because of mucosal and submucosal hemorrhage. Claussen (1) and Moses et al. (29) compared this ischemic state to that seen in hypovolemic shock. This ischemic change, which may progress to bowel necrosis, is exacerbated by hyperthermia (>41°C [105.8°F]) and dehydration (30). In younger athletes, this process may be enhanced by their less efficient heat exchange. This relative ischemia is related to effort level, the degree of dehydration, and the sympathetic response. In addition, endothelin-1, which is increased during dehydration and exercise, promotes further splanchnic vasoconstriction and mucosal damage (31,32).

Intestinal Fluid Shift

Intestinal fluid shift from increasing dehydration in athletes correlates highly with the frequency of symptoms. In one study, 80% of runners who experienced at least a 4% loss in body weight during competition experienced a higher incidence of GI symptoms (33). Shifts in intestinal fluid may produce intracellular electrolyte changes, thus increasing the irritability of colonic smooth muscle (8).

Autonomic Nervous System Stimulation

Autonomic nervous system stimulation with activation of the sympathetic system promotes exercise-induced vasoconstriction of the splanchnic bed. With decreased blood flow, a reduced absorption of substances (carbohydrates) from the colonic lumen, an increased osmotic load, and secondary diarrhea and cramping are noted (34).

Chemical and Neuroendocrine Agents

Chemical and neuroendocrine agents released during exercise include endogenous opioids and hormones (e.g., motilin, gastrin, glucagon, somatostatin, and vasoactive intestinal polypeptide) that increase bowel activity (35). Vasoactive intestinal polypeptide release, stimulated by mesenteric ischemia and intestinal irritation, causes colonic contraction, decreased absorption, and secretory diarrhea. Other active agents released during exercise include secretin, pancreatic polypeptide, neurokinin A, and glucagon-like peptide 1 (36). Finally, leukotrienes, which are increased with exercise, produce profound vasoconstriction and GI mucosal damage (37).

Intestinal Hemorrhage

Intestinal hemorrhage from the colon is the second most common site of exercise-induced GI bleeding,

and up to 20% of marathon runners will have blood in their stools after a race. Other sources include hemorrhoidal disease and fissures, which are found especially in those athletes experiencing diarrhea. Furthermore, blood acts as a direct irritant, stimulating bowel activity.

Mechanical Irritation

Mechanical irritation from the repetitive, high-impact activity of endurance running jars the intestines and produces mucosal injury (30,38). Rehrer and Meijer (39) measured this jarring action and found that the abdominal vibration was greater with running than with cycling. In distance runners, jarring and smooth muscle stretching of the intestinal wall increase prostaglandins (PG) that are known to produce cramping and diarrhea (40). Finally, some authors (41) have proposed that psoas muscle hypertrophy produces secondary colon compression.

Medications

Medications (e.g., aspirin and NSAIDs) taken for musculoskeletal discomfort may promote diarrhea. However, these same medications have been found to be unrelated to occult GI bleeding in some studies, and they may actually play a protective role via PG blockade (18).

Other causes

Viral, bacterial, and parasitic infections (e.g., Rotavirus, Norwalk agent, *Salmonella*, *Shigella*, toxigenic *Escherichia coli*, giardiasis, and amebiasis) may occur in the athletic population, causing lower GI symptoms. In many athletes, emotional stress increases lower GI symptoms (22). Miscellaneous medical problems, such as inflammatory bowel disease, FBS, and intestinal polyps, may occur in young athletes and may produce symptoms.

Evaluation

History

Determining what factor precipitate or exacerbate lower GI symptoms is crucial. Many systemic diseases, such as parasitic infections or inflammatory bowel disease, may have an insidious onset. Does the athlete experience baseline cramping or diarrhea that is *not* associated with exercise? Does the family have a history of lower GI problems or FBS? In children,

FBS is associated with esophageal reflux, and it is frequently precipitated by an organic cause. Reviewing the medication history may reveal the use of magnesium-containing antacids for indigestion, which secondarily produces diarrhea. Does the individual have a history of melena or hematochezia that may be producing secondary diarrhea? Does the history include weight loss or bloody mucous that might suggest inflammatory bowel disease? Finally, are fellow athletes experiencing similar symptoms, suggesting a common infection?

Examination

The physical examination includes serial weight measurements and careful evaluation for abdominal or rectal masses. Functional disease often localizes to the periumbilical area. One should search for clinical signs of hyperthyroidism, especially in female athletes.

Laboratory studies should begin with a complete blood count, a platelet count, and an erythrocyte sedimentation rate (ESR). The clinician should note that the ESR is normal in 50% of children with inflammatory bowel disease. Chemistry studies should include a chemistry panel, a liver profile, serum amylase levels, and the thyroid-stimulating hormone level. If anemia is detected on the complete blood count, a serum ferritin check is indicated. Specific stool studies include fecal occult blood, leukocytes, cultures, and examination for ova and parasites. Imaging studies include abdominal ultrasound and computerized tomography scanning. Further evaluation of the large intestine may include flexible sigmoidoscopy, air-contrast barium enema, or colonoscopy. Consultation with a specialist may be warranted.

Treatment

Nonpharmacologic treatment includes a careful review of the diet and medication history. High-residue diets and many medications actually cause lower GI problems. Caffeine-containing supplements may both increase intestinal motility and may cause diuresis. Altering the timing of food ingestion with its attendant gastrocolic reflex may eliminate bowel movements and cramping during exercise. Adherence to an elemental diet reduces symptoms in some athletes (17). Sufficient hydration with low osmolar cold fluids prior to and during exercise is crucial in preventing symptoms. Prophylactic fluid ingestion (150 to 200 mL every 15 to 20 minutes) prior to thirst stimulation is important to avoid the vicious cycle of dehydration–diarrhea–dehydration. Cool beverages that

TABLE 15.1. *Ten tips for taming the "trots"*

1. Establish a pre-run ritual.
2. Do not eat 2 to 3 hr before race.
3. Curb dietary lactose. (For some people, limit fructose.)
4. Cut fiber in diet. (Use liquid meals.)
5. Decrease intake of coffee or caffeine.
6. Avoid sorbitol or mannitol found in mints or gum.
7. Avoid large doses of vitamin C.
8. Train at different time of day. (Some athletes have only morning diarrhea.)
9. Emphasize conditioning. (Symptoms often decrease with training.)
10. Consider specific medications (loperamide).

From White RD. Reign in runner's trots. *The Physician and Sports Medicine* 1996;24:13, with permission.

contain 5% to 8% glucose and sodium (e.g., Allsport, Gatorade, and Powerade) facilitate intestinal water absorption. Often symptoms improve with a reduction of exercise intensity and then a gradual resumption.

Pharmacologic treatment must be considered with caution (42). Many medications reduce intestinal motility and decrease spasm, but they contain agents that inhibit sweating mechanisms (e.g., diphenoxylate with atropine, dicyclomine) or produce central nervous system depression (chlordiazepoxide, phenobarbital). Consequently, these agents may decrease alertness, affect athletic performance, and predispose an athlete to injury. Agents, such as loperamide and calcium-based antacids, are often well tolerated by the young athlete. Loperamide blocks calmodulin, which mediates PG and leukotriene metabolism (37). Medications containing codeine are prohibited in national and international competition. Table 15.1 summarizes specific recommendations for treating runner's diarrhea (43).

SUMMARY

The GI tract is the most common site of exercise-induced medical disorders in young athletes. The mechanism of increased PG production by the GI tract could explain the increased incidence of GE reflux, vomiting, cramps, and diarrhea seen with running activity. Motility disorders and bleeding are secondary to dehydration and the shunting of blood from the viscera. Exercise may actually be a stress test for the GI tract, since symptoms increase with training intensity. The diagnosis of exercise-induced GI problems remains one of exclusion. Nonpharmacologic measures are the primary treatment for the young athlete, followed by specific pharmacologic agents.

REFERENCES

1. Claussen JP. Effect of physical training on cardiovascular adjustments to exercise in man. *Physiol Rev* 1977; 57:779–815.
2. Worobetz IJ, Gerrad DF. Gastrointestinal symptoms during exercise and endurance athletes: prevalence and speculations of the etiology. *N Z Med J* 1985;98: 644–646.
3. Halvorsen F, Ritland S. Gastrointestinal problems related to endurance event training. *Sports Med* 1992;14: 157–163.
4. Gil SM, Yazaki E, Evans DF. Aetiology of running-related gastrointestinal dysfunction. *Sports Med* 1998;26: 365–378.
5. Costill DC. Physiology of marathon running. *JAMA* 1972;221:1024–1029.
6. Sullivan SN. The gastrointestinal symptoms of running [Letter]. *N Engl J Med* 1981;304:915.
7. Worme JD, Doubt TJ, Singh A, et al. Dietary patterns, gastrointestinal complaints, and nutrition knowledge of recreational athletes. *Am J Clin Nutr* 1990;51: 690–697.
8. Keeffe EB, Lowe DK, Goss JR, et al. Gastrointestinal symptoms of marathon runners. *West J Med* 1984;141: 481–484.
9. Riddoch C, Trinnick T. Gastrointestinal disturbances in marathon runners. *Br J Sports Med* 1988;22:71–74.
10. Putukian M, Potera C. Don't miss gastrointestinal disorders in athletes. *The Physician and Sports Medicine* 1997;25:80–94.
11. Neufer PD, Young AJ, Sawka MN. Gastric emptying during walking and running: effects of varied exercise intensity. *Eur J Appl Physiol* 1989;58:440–445.
12. Green GA. Gastrointestinal disorders in the athlete. *Clin Sports Med* 1992;11:453–470.
13. Moses FM. The effect of exercise on the gastrointestinal tract. *Sports Med* 1990;9:159–172.
14. Brouns F, Beckers E. Is the gut an athletic organ? Digestion, absorption, and exercise. *Sports Med* 1993;15: 242–257.
15. Krauss BB, Sinclair JW, Castell DO. Gastrointestinal reflux in runners. *Ann Intern Med* 1990;112:429–433.
16. Oktedalen O, Nesland A, Opstad PK, et al. The influence of prolonged physical stress on gastric juice components in healthy man. *Scand J Gastroenterol* 1988;23: 1132–1136.
17. Bounous G, McArdle AH. Marathon runners: the intestinal handicap. *Med Hypotheses* 1990;33:261–264.
18. Baska RS, Moses FM, Deutster PA. Cimetidine reduces running-associated gastrointestinal bleeding. *Dig Dis Sci* 1990;35:956–960.
19. Larson DC, Fisher R. Management of exercise-induced gastrointestinal problems. *The Physician and Sports Medicine* 1987;15:112–126.
20. Sears RJ, Sears VW, Castell DO. Effects of antacids on "runner's reflux." *Gastroenterology* 1991;100:A840.
21. Butcher J. Runner's diarrhea and other intestinal problems of athletes. *Am Fam Physician* 1993;48:623–627.
22. Priebe W, Priebe J. Runner's diarrhea—prevalence and clinical symptomatology. *Am J Gastroenterol* 1984;79: 827–828.
23. Herbst JJ. Gastroesophageal reflux. In: Behrman RE, Kliegmen RM, Jenson HB, eds. *Nelson textbook of pediatrics*, 16th ed. Philadelphia: WB Saunders, 2000: 1125–1126.
24. Latimer PR. Irritable bowel syndrome: a behavioral model. *Behav Res Ther* 1981;19:475–483.
25. Keeling WF, Martin BJ. Gastrointestinal transit during mild exercise. *J Appl Physiol* 198;63:978–981.
26. Oettle GS. Effect of moderate exercise on bowel habit. *Gut* 1991;32:941–944.
27. Bingham SA, Cummings JH. Effect of exercise and physical fitness on large intestinal function. *Gastroenterology* 1989;97:1389–1399.
28. Sharman IM. Gastrointestinal disturbances in runners. *Br J Sports Med* 1982;16:179.
29. Moses FM, Brewer TG, Peura DA. Running-associated proximal hemorrhage colitis. *Ann Intern Med* 1988; 108:385–386.
30. Fogoros FN. "Runner's trots." Gastrointestinal disturbances in runners. *JAMA* 1980;243:1743–1744.
31. Ahlborg G, Weitzberg E, Lundberg J. Metabolic and vascular effects of circulating endothelin-1 during moderately heavy prolonged exercise. *J Appl Physiol* 1995; 78:2294–2300.
32. Maeda S, Miyauchi T, Waku T, et al. Plasma endothelin-1 level in athletes after exercise in a hot environment: exercise-induced dehydration contributes to increases in plasma endothelin-1. *Life Sci* 1996;58:1259–1268.
33. Rehrer NJ, Kemenade M, Meester W, et al. Gastrointestinal complaints in relation to dietary intake in triathletes. *Int J Sports Nutr* 1992;2:48–59.
34. Mailman D. Blood flow and intestinal absorption. *Fed Proc* 1982;41:2096–2100.
35. Sullivan SN, Champion MC, Christofides ND, et al. Gastrointestinal regulatory peptide responses in long-distance runners. *The Physician and Sports Medicine* 1984;12:77–82.
36. O'Connor AM, Johnston CF, Buchanan KD, et al. Circulating gastrointestinal hormone changes in marathon running. *Int J Sports Med* 1995;16:283–287.
37. Campbell WB, Halushka PV. Lipid-derived autocoids. In: Goodman SL, Hardman JG, Limbird LE, Molinoff PB, eds. *Goodman's and Gilman's: the pharmacological basis of therapeutics*, 9th ed. New York: McGraw-Hill, 1996:601–616.
38. McCabe ME III, Peura DA, Kadakia SC, et al. Gastrointestinal blood loss associated with running a marathon. *Dig Dis Sci* 1986;31:1229–1232.
39. Rehrer NJ, Meijer GA. Biomechanical vibration of the abdominal region during running and bicycling. *J Sports Med Phys Fitness* 1991;31:231–234.
40. Hawkey CJ, Rampton DS. Prostaglandins and the gastrointestinal mucosa: are they important in its function, disease, or treatment? *Gastroenterology* 1985;89: 1162–1188.
41. Dawson DJ, Kahn AN, Schreeve DR. Psoas muscle hypertrophy: mechanical cause for jogger's trots. *Br Med J* 1985;291:787–788.
42. Sullivan S. Overcoming runner's diarrhea. *The Physician and Sports Medicine* 1992;20:63–68.
43. White RD. Reign in runner's trots. *The Physician and Sports Medicine* 1996;24:13.

16

Cardiopulmonary Problems in Children and Adolescents

George D. Harris

At least 5 million young people are actively involved in competitive athletics in the United States at the high school, collegiate, and professional level. An even larger number participate at the youth, elementary school, and junior high level.

Advances in medical and surgical management of children and adolescents with cardiopulmonary problems have allowed them to be more active and have enabled them to participate in athletics to a greater degree over the past two decades. While the prevalence of cardiovascular disease in a young athletic population remains low, some of these individuals are at increased risk of cardiopulmonary problems when their level of participation changes from the noncompetitive to the competitive arena. Despite the increased numbers of children participating in athletic activities, the risk of sudden cardiac death in athletes with underlying cardiac disease is still extremely low.

The evaluation of the athlete with a preexisting cardiovascular disorder should follow the recommendations of the 26th Bethesda Conference, which was sponsored by the American College of Cardiology and the American College of Sports Medicine in 1994. The conference provided specific recommendations on the evaluation and participation of athletes according to the type of heart disease that was present (1). The conference did not address the complex issues surrounding general preparticipation screening of athletes for cardiovascular disease, which physicians use as the basis for determining the individual's level of activity.

Not all competitive sports involve an identical type or intensity of exercise. Within the same sport, variability in the degree of physical effort required at different positions or levels of competition may exist. The demands caused by that sport can place an athlete with a cardiovascular abnormality at medical risk, due to an increased workload on the heart or the higher levels of stress on the vascular system that are caused by increases in blood flow, blood pressure, and increased body temperature. The results can be the progression of the disease, life-threatening cardiovascular alterations, or a higher risk for sudden death.

DEFINITIONS

Sports can be classified according to the type and intensity of exercise performed and also with regard to the danger of bodily injury. *Exercise* can be divided into two types—*static* and *dynamic*. These terms characterize the activity based on the mechanical action involved.

Static exercise generates a near-maximal intramuscular force or tension with relatively no change in muscle length or joint mobility. This type of exercise induces cardiovascular changes that are related to increased *pressure load* (afterload), such as mild increases in oxygen consumption, heart rate, and stroke volume, with virtually *no change in systemic vascular resistance*. The long-term effect of static exercise is left ventricular concentric hypertrophy, which may result in systolic or diastolic dysfunction in an athlete with preexisting cardiac disease.

Dynamic exercise involves changes in muscle length and joint mobility in a rhythmic fashion, with a relatively small intramuscular force; it produces a *volume load* on the heart, inducing increased oxygen consumption, heart rate, and stroke volume, with an overall *decrease in total peripheral resistance*. The long-term effects of these changes cause left ventricular hypertrophy, as well as an increase in chamber size (2).

Classification of sports is based on peak dynamic and static components during competition. The categories include low static–low dynamic, low static–moderate dynamic, low static–high dynamic, high static–low dynamic, high static–moderate dynamic, and high static–high dynamic (Table 16.1). The clas-

TABLE 16.1. *Classification of sports*

Low dynamic	Moderate dynamic	High dynamic
Low static		
Golf	Baseball	Racquetball
Bowling	Volleyball	Running (long distance)
Billards	Table tennis	Soccer
Moderate static		
Diving	Figure skating	Basketball
Archery	Football	Ice hockey
Equestrian	Running (sprint)	Running (middle distance)
High static		
Gymnastics	Body building	Boxing
Weight lifting	Wrestling	Cycling
Water skiing	Downhill skiing	Speed skating

From 26th Bethesda Conference. Recommendations for determining eligibility for competition in athletes with cardiovascular abnormalities. *J Am Coll Cardiol* 1994;24:845–899, with permission.

sification does not consider the emotional stress on the athlete, the effects of environmental factors, or the specific training regimen used by the athlete.

The child's participation needs to be evaluated on the basis of potential adverse effects of the chosen exercise or sport, the potential risks of the sport itself, and the potential risks of training. Evaluation should also be based on whether the sport is for recreational activity only or for competition (Table 16.1).

INCIDENCE AND PATHOPHYSIOLOGY

Congenital heart disease occurs in 10 per 1,000 live-born children, and it is due to interactions between genetic predisposition and environmental factors. The various congenital heart defects can be classified by anatomic and physiologic findings (Table 16.2).

Atrial septal defect, ventricular septal defect, and patent ductus arteriosus comprise the largest group of patients with congenital heart disease. In the absence of significant volume overload, pulmonary hypertension, or dysrhythmias, individuals with these heart defects may be allowed full participation in all competitive sports. Prior to any sports participation or in order to determine the restriction of any physical activity, the presence of any of these conditions warrants a complete evaluation to assess the need for surgical intervention.

TABLE 16.2. *Congenital heart lesions*

Classification	Specific manifestations
Left to right shunts	Patent ductus arteriosus
	Ventricular septal defect
	Atrial septal defect
	Coronary arteriovenous fistula
	Endocardial cushion defect
Right to left shunts	Transposition of the arteries
	Tetralogy of Fallot
	Truncus arteriosus
	Tricuspid atresia
	Total anomalous pulmonary venous return
Regurgitant lesions	Mitral valve
	Tricuspid valve
Obstructive lesions	Left side lesions—pulmonary vein, left atrium, mitral valve, hypoplastic left ventricle, left ventricular outflow, or aortic arch
	Right side lesions—systemic venous, tricuspid valve, pulmonic stenosis, or hypoplastic right ventricle
Increased pulmonary vascular resistance	
Vascular rings and slings	
Congenital coronary artery anomalies	
Ventricular malformations	
Abnormal systemic venous connections	

From Harris GD. Heart disease in children. *Prim Care Clin* 2000;27:767–784, with permission.

TABLE 16.3. *Acquired heart diseases*

Hypertension
Kawasaki disease
Acute rheumatic fever
Chronic rheumatic heart disease
Infective endocarditis
Myocarditis
Dilated cardiomyopathy
Conduction anomalies

From Harris GD. Heart disease in children. *Prim Care Clin* 2000;27:767–784, with permission.

Acquired pediatric heart disease includes a number of clinically diverse etiologies that may result in significant morbidity and mortality. Specifically, this includes hypertension, Kawasaki disease, acute and chronic rheumatic heart disease, infective endocarditis, myocarditis, and dilated cardiomyopathy (Table 16.3).

DIAGNOSIS

Everyone is encouraged to participate in routine exercise, and many children and adolescents desire to compete in organized athletics. Presently, 4 million competitive high school athletes undergo periodic medical evaluations to assess their cardiovascular, pulmonary, and musculoskeletal systems for any abnormalities that can cause harm or death if sports participation is permitted. General preparticipation evaluations for children with congenital heart disease include a complete history (Table 16.4), a physical examination, an electrocardiogram, an echocardiogram, and an exercise stress test (3). Selected patients may require cardiac catheterization (see Chapter 2).

The prevalence of *hypertension* in children and adolescents is difficult to assess. Hypertension is de-

fined as having either average systolic or diastolic values equal to or above the 95th percentile for age, sex, and height (Table 16.5). A thorough history and physical evaluation, along with limited lab testing (i.e., complete blood count, blood chemistries, urinalysis, and electrocardiogram), are necessary in an athlete with hypertension. Additional testing may include a renal ultrasound, echocardiography, and stress testing. The more common age-related causes are renal parenchymal disease, coarctation of the aorta, and renal artery stenosis in infants to children up to 6 years or age; renal artery stenosis, renal parenchymal diseases, and essential hypertension in children between the ages of 6 and 10 years; and renal parenchymal disease and essential hypertension in adolescents (3).

Relatively few congenital heart lesions have been associated with sudden death during sports participation. The most common are hypertrophic cardiomyopathy, congenital coronary artery anomalies, and Marfan syndrome. Hypertrophic cardiomyopathy is probably the most frequent cause of unexpected sudden cardiac death in young competitive athletes. (This topic is discussed in Chapters 2 and 17.)

Myocarditis is the most common acquired heart disorder. The prevalence of myocarditis in athletes is unknown. However, any individual diagnosed with myocarditis requires a thorough evaluation, including an endomyocardial biopsy. Early diagnosis and bed rest may decrease the individual's propensity for fatal dysrhythmias (4).

Supraventricular tachycardia is the most common pediatric arrhythmia; it is characterized by a fixed heart rate—usually greater than 200 beats per minute—and narrow QRS complexes on electrocardiogram. In contrast to sinus tachycardia, the heart rate does not fluctuate with agitation (5).

TABLE 16.4. *Cardiovascular conditions to inquire about in history*

Questions	Potential outcome
Is there a history of carditis?	May result in sudden death with exertion.
Is there a history of hypertension?	Those individuals with significant essential hypertension should avoid weight and power lifting, body building, and strength training. Those individuals with secondary hypertension or severe hypertension need evaluation.
Is there a history of congenital heart disease?	Those individuals with mild forms may participate fully. Those individuals with moderate or severe forms need evaluation.
Is there a history of dysrhythmia?	The individual needs further evaluation.
Is there a history of mitral valve prolapse?	The presence of chest pain, dysrhthmia, or mitral regurgitation needs further evaluation.
Is there a history of a heart murmur?	Only an innocent murmur allows for full participation. Otherwise, the murmur needs to be evaluated.

From Smith DM, Kovan JR, Rich BS, et al. *Preparticipation physical examination,* 2nd ed. Minneapolis: McGraw-Hill, 1997;32, with permission.

TABLE 16.5. *Hypertension parameters by age and sex in a pediatric patient*

Age	Female	Male
10	>122/80	>123/82
11	>124/81	>125/83
12	>127/83	>126/82
13	>128/84	>130/84
14	>130/85	>132/85
15	>131/86	>135/86
16	>132/86	>138/87
17	>132/86	>140/89

From Wilson MD. Adolescent hypertension. In: McMillan JA, DeAngelis CD, Feigin RD, Warshaw JB, eds. *Oski's pediatrics,* 3rd ed. Philadelphia: Lippincott Williams & Wilkins 1999:547–548, with permission.

TREATMENT

Sinus Tachycardia and/or Bradycardia

Treatment of sinus tachycardia and bradycardia involves evaluating and managing the underlying causes of these rhythms.

Supraventricular Tachycardia

Supraventricular tachycardia is most commonly idiopathic, or it is associated with a congenital heart defect. It occurs in one of the following three forms: (a) atrioventricular (AV) reentrant tachycardia resulting from the presence of an accessory bypass pathway (bundle of Kent), which is the most common cause of nonsinus tachycardia in children; (b) AV nodal or junctional tachycardia caused by dual AV node pathways; and (c) ectopic atrial tachycardia, secondary to rapid firing of ectopic focus in the atrium.

Most children can have supraventricular tachycardia for several hours or days without developing clinical symptoms. In those children, vagal maneuvers, such as unilateral carotid massage or the Valsalva maneuver, by taking a deep breath and forcing a cough, can be used to convert the rhythm. Crushed ice in a plastic bag or a rubber glove can be applied to the face for up to 30 seconds. If this is unsuccessful or if the patient is hemodynamically unstable, pharmacologic conversion may be indicated using adenosine (0.05 mg per kg; up to 4 mg) administered as a rapid intravenous bolus. The failure of this regimen then mandates synchronized conversion (0.5 to 1 Joule per kg) (1,1a).

Additional treatment may include digoxin, beta blockers, or esophageal overdrive pacing, along with cardiology consultation (6).

Premature Ventricular Contractions

Premature ventricular contractions (PVC) can be seen in healthy children, in those with congenital and acquired heart disease, with anxiety, and secondary to medications. PVCs can be worrisome if their occurrence increases with activity, especially if the individual becomes symptomatic. Usually, no treatment is necessary, except for addressing the underlying cardiac disease or the precipitating causes.

Management of the various conduction abnormalities is beyond the scope of this text. Thorough discussion of these can be found in a standard cardiology textbook.

Myocardial infarction in children is rare, even in children with a history of hypertension, myocarditis, and lupus. It is also rare in children who are being treated for asthma with beta agonists. However, it can occur in children with anomalous origin of the left coronary artery, Kawasaki disease, presurgical and postsurgical congenital heart disease, or dilated cardiomyopathy (6).

Treatment of congenital acyanotic and cyanotic cardiac heart disease involves consultation with a cardiologist and a cardiovascular surgeon because of the surgical interventions needed to manage the underlying defect. The exercise recommendations for some of the more common diseases are listed in Table 16.6.

TABLE 16.6. *Exercise recommendations for congenital heart disease*

Cardiac diagnosis	Sports allowed
Small ASD or VSD	All categories of static and dynamic sport classifications
Mild aortic stenosis	All categories of static and dynamic sport classifications
MVP without other risk factors	All categories of static and dynamic sport classifications
Moderate aortic stenosis	Low static/low dynamic; low static/moderate dynamic; moderate static/low dynamic
Mild LV dysfunction	Low static/low dynamic; low static/moderate dynamic; low static/high dynamic
Moderate LV dysfunction	Low static/low dynamic
Hypertrophic cardiomyopathy	None—cardiology referral
Severe aortic stenosis	None
Long QT syndrome	None

Abbreviations: ASD, atrial septal defect; LV, left ventricle; MVP, mitral valve prolapse; VSD, ventricular septal defect.

From Chiang LK, Dunn AE. Cardiology. In: Siberry G, Iannone R, eds. *The Harriet Lane handbook,* 15th ed. St. Louis: Mosby, 2000:160, with permission.

Hypertension

Hypertension is present when either the average systolic and/or diastolic blood pressure reading done on three different occasions is greater than 95% for the age, sex, and height of the individual being monitored (Table 16.4).

Nonpharmacologic treatment of hypertension includes salt restriction, aerobic exercise, weight loss when indicated, and cessation of smoking.

Pharmacologic management includes the use of calcium channel blockers, angiotensin-converting enzyme (ACE) inhibitors, diuretics, beta blockers, alpha blockers, alpha and beta blocker combinations, central acting agents, and vasodilators. Teenage female athletes who use ACE inhibitors should be aware of the contraindications for use of these medications during pregnancy. Diuretic use is dependent upon the level of athletic training and competition, since these drugs not only cause significant water loss; but they also may be contraindicated at collegiate and Olympic levels of competition due to sports regulations banning their use. Beta blockers may be contraindicated in individuals with a history of congestive heart failure, reactive airway disease, or pulmonary insufficiency or at certain levels of athletic competition because of their effects on performance capacity or on controlling tremor, such as in shooting events (i.e., to steady the trigger). Central acting agents have numerous side effects that may limit their use and compliance in this age group.

Myocarditis

Myocarditis occurs secondary to a viral (most commonly coxsackie B virus infection) or bacterial illness; an immune-mediated disease, such as Kawasaki or acute rheumatic fever; a toxin-induced condition; or a collagen vascular disease. Echocardiography reveals enlargement of the heart chambers and impaired left ventricular function. Treatment includes bedrest, diuretics, inotropes (e.g., dopamine, dobutamine), digoxin, afterload reduction, gamma globulin, and/or possibly steroids. A cardiology consultation should be ordered.

Idiopathic Dilated Cardiomyopathy

Idiopathic dilated cardiomyopathy is the most common cardiomyopathy in children, and it may represent a late sequelae of viral myocarditis, the most common form of acute myocarditis (3). The treatment is primarily supportive, and it is directed towards functional improvement of heart failure and any ar-

rhythmias. ACE inhibitors are beneficial in children with dilated cardiomyopathy.

Hypertrophic Cardiomyopathy

Hypertrophic cardiomyopathy is the single most common cardiovascular cause of sudden death in young athletes with a 4% to 6% incidence of sudden death in children and adolescents who have hypertrophic cardiomyopathy (6). Echocardiogram will reveal the extent and segment of increased contractility, the location of the hypertrophy, and the degree of obstruction. Treatment includes restriction of participation in competitive sports, except some low intensity activities; negative inotropes, such as beta blockers and calcium channel blockers; and systemic bacterial endocarditis prophylaxis. High risk individuals should be considered for implantation of a cardioverter–defibrillator (7).

RECOMMENDATIONS FOR EXERCISE

Children with surgically corrected tetralogy of Fallot or transposition of the great vessels are permitted to participate in all competitive sports if only extremely mild hemodynamic abnormalities persist. Patients who have undergone the Fontan procedure or who have any other hemodynamic abnormalities are restricted to low-intensity sports.

In the absence of myocardial dysfunction, dysrhythmias, or pulmonary hypertension, postoperative patients may participate in unrestricted sports activities 6 months following surgery. Patients with pulmonary hypertension are generally restricted from all competitive sports participation.

The most common cardiac pressure overload lesions in children include pulmonary stenosis, aortic stenosis, and coarctation of the aorta. The presence of mild stenosis, either before or after intervention, permits full participation in competitive sports 3 months after catheter balloon dilatation and 6 months after surgery. Individuals with moderate or severe stenosis are restricted to low-intensity competitive sports after a successful intervention (Table 16.6).

Children and adolescents with a history of hypertension, without any target organ damage, and with only mild to moderate blood pressure elevations should be allowed full participation in sports. With severe hypertension, the restriction of high static sports (e.g., weight lifting, rock climbing, gymnastics, and karate and/or judo) is warranted until the hypertension is adequately controlled.

All asymptomatic children without a family history of sudden death associated with mitral valve prolapse may participate in all competitive sports. Symptomatic children, those with significant mitral insufficiency, or those who have a family history are restricted to low-intensity sports (2). Restriction from all competitive sports for a minimum of 6 months, with return to activity only after an extensive evaluation, is warranted.

always have the patient's best interest at the forefront of all decision making, especially when evaluating and recommending appropriate activity levels. However, the physician should not be placed in the position of being solely responsible for whether or nor the athlete is permitted to participate. The final decision should be made jointly by the physician; player; the player's team; parents or guardians, if the player is a minor; and the sponsoring organization.

SUMMARY

All individuals are encouraged to participate in routine exercise. Many children and adolescents, including those with heart disease, desire to compete in organized athletics. Some of these selected patients may be at risk for sudden death, or they may be in danger of bodily injury from collision or the consequences of syncope.

Unfortunately, the steepest decline in physical activity for adolescent males and females occurs during the teen years. By high school, only a minority of adolescents are meeting present health-related activity guidelines (8). Inactivity in these individuals leaves them more prone to injuries during occasional evening or weekend casual sports participation.

The primary care physician should be aware of the components of the preparticipation examination and the areas of evaluation required for proper assessment of the individual with underlying cardiovascular or pulmonary disease. In addition, the physician must

REFERENCES

1. Zeppilli P, Santini C, Palmieri V, et al. Role of myocarditis in athletes with minor arrhythmias and/or echocardiographic abnormalities. *Chest* 1994;106:373–380.
1a. American Heart Association. *PALS provider manual.* Dallas, TX: American Heart Association, 2002.
2. 26th Bethesda Conference. Recommendations for determining eligibility for competition in athletes with cardiovascular abnormalities. *J Am Coll Cardiol* 1994; 24:845–899.
3. Harris GD. Heart disease in children. *Prim Care Clin* 2000;27:767–784.
4. Schamberger MS. Cardiac emergencies in children. *Pediatr Ann* 1996;25:339–344.
5. Kaminer SJ, Hixon RL, Strong WE. Evaluation and recommendations for participation in athletics for children with heart disease. *Curr Opin Pediatr* 1995;7:595–600.
6. Chiang LK, Dunn AE. Cardiology. In: Siberry G, Iannone R, eds. *The Harriet Lane handbook*, 15th ed. St. Louis: Mosby, 2000:160.
7. Maron BI. Hypertrophic cardiomyopathy. *The Physician and Sports Medicine* 2002;30:19–25.
8. Sallis JF. Overcoming inactivity in young people. *The Physician and Sports Medicine* 2000;28:31–32.

17

Sudden Death in Young Athletes

Francis G. O'Connor, Kevin DeWeber, John P. Kugler, and Ralph G. Oriscello

Sudden death in young athletes is unexpected, dramatic, and devastating. Communities are left in shock as apparently invincible athletes who represent the pinnacle of health and physical conditioning suddenly become victims of the seemingly impossible. A sudden death is equally, if not more, devastating to the primary care sports medicine community. Physicians are humbled when an asymptomatic athlete with an apparently normal clinical examination becomes the victim of sudden death.

INCIDENCE

Usually, sudden athletic death has been defined as a nontraumatic death, with symptom onset during or within 1 hour following participation in athletics and that is not the result of direct bodily injury. Fortunately, sudden death in a young athlete is a rare event. Estimates range from one death per 280,000 to one death in 735,000 persons per year, depending on the population studied (1,2). Van Camp et al. (4), from the National Center for Catastrophic Sports Injury Research, identified 160 nontraumatic athletic deaths in organized high school and college sports between July 1983 and June 1993. They calculated that male athletes had a fivefold higher risk than did female athletes, that college athletes had a twofold higher risk than high school athletes, that noncardiac causes of death accounted for 22% of cases, and that men's football and basketball accounted for 65% of the deaths.

Recent research by the Centers for Disease Control and Prevention shows that the incidence of sudden cardiac deaths in athletes between the ages of 15 and 34 years is increasing. From 1989 to 1996, the number of deaths rose 10% overall, from 2,719 to 3,000. The rate increased by 30% in young women, and it was also disproportionately higher in African-Americans than in Caucasians (3).

ETIOLOGY

Based on 20 years of research on athletic sudden death, a fairly consistent theme has evolved. Deaths in younger athletes (i.e., those under the age of 35 years) are most often associated with congenital cardiovascular structural abnormalities, while sudden deaths in older athletes are primarily associated with the consequences of acquired atherosclerotic coronary artery disease. The results compiled by Van Camp (4) in his series of 160 nontraumatic, sudden exercise-related deaths in athletes under 30 years of age list the etiologic conditions in order of decreasing frequency (Table 17.1). Of the congenital and/or structural cardiac anomalies leading to sudden death, hypertrophic cardiomyopathy (HCM) is the most common (4–7). In 1991, McCaffrey (6) reviewed seven etiologic studies of sudden cardiac death and found that HCM led the list at 24%, with coronary anomalies next at 18% and myocarditis at 12%. Arrhythmogenic right ventricular dysplasia was found to be the etiology in 6 of 22 cases of sudden death in competitive young athletes from the ages of 11 to 35 years in Northern Italy (8). This condition was much less prevalent in other studies. Next in frequency in this study was atherosclerotic coronary artery disease, which was found in 4 of 22 cases.

HCM is an autosomal dominant congenital disorder characterized by left ventricular (LV) outflow obstruction with asymmetric septal hypertrophy and marked disarray of ventricular muscle fibers. The prevalence of echocardiographically defined HCM is 2 per 1,000 young adults (9). This condition can predispose the individual to malignant ventricular arrhythmias that lead to syncope or sudden death. It is often clinically silent, but a personal history of unexplained syncope, especially effort syncope, or a family history of sudden death events is an important clinical clue. Physical examination may reveal a systolic crescendo–decrescendo murmur that is best

TABLE 17.1. *Causes of 142 nontraumatic sports deaths in college and high school athletes from 1983 to 1993*

Cardiovascular conditions	Number	Noncardiovascular conditions	Number
Hypertrophic cardiomyopathy (HCM)	51	Hyperthermia	13
Probable HCM	5	Rhabdomyolysis and sickle cell trait	7
Coronary artery anomaly	16	Status asthmaticus	4
Myocarditis	7	Electrocution due to lightning	3
Aortic stenosis	6	Arnold Chiari II formation	1
Dilated cardiomyopathy	5	Aspiration–blood–gastrointestinal bleed	1
Atherosclerosis	3	Exercise-induced anaphylaxis	1
Aortic rupture	2	Undetermined cause of death	7
Cardiomyopathy nonspecific	2		
Tunnel subaortic stenosis	2		
Coronary artery aneurysm	1		
Mitral valve prolapse	1		
Right ventricular cardiomyopathy	1		
Ruptured cerebellar arteriovenous malformation	1		
Subarachnoid hemorrhage	1		
Wolff–Parkinson–White syndrome	1		

From Van Camp SP, Bloor CM, Mueller FO, et al. Nontraumatic sports death in high school and college athletes. *Med Sci Sports Exerc* 1995;27:641–647, with permission.

heard between apex and the left sternal border. It classically increases in intensity with Valsalva or standing, and it decreases with squatting or isometric handgrip. Chest x-ray may show cardiomegaly, and electrocardiogram (ECG) may show left ventricular hypertrophy (LVH) or other changes; however, these tests may be normal, and the diagnosis is best confirmed with two-dimensional and M-mode echocardiography. Because of the high risk of sudden death in these athletes, they should be referred to a cardiologist for risk assessment and treatment. Therapeutic options can include calcium channel blockade, A-V sequential pacing, and/or septal ablation with intracardiac alcohol infusion. Most athletes with this abnormality will require exclusion from all competitive sports, except for very low-intensity activities (10).

Congenital coronary anomalies may also cause sudden death in athletes. The most common lethal abnormality is anomalous origin of the left main coronary from the right sinus of Valsalva. Screening for these conditions is difficult. Fatigue, angina, or exercise-induced syncope should prompt a more thorough evaluation. In one review of 78 cases of sudden death that were thought to be secondary to autopsy-proven coronary anomalies, 62% occurred in asymptomatic patients (11). The mechanism of death with these conditions is myocardial ischemia due to hypoperfusion of the myocardium. Coronary anomalies are detected by cardiac cathetherization; however, cardiac

magnetic resonance imaging (MRI) is an emerging noninvasive modality that may assist with diagnosis. Select cases of coronary anomalies may be amenable to revascularization procedures.

Acute myocarditis is a rare, but potentially devastating, condition that is most commonly caused by viruses. Most myocarditis patients present with sudden death secondary to a ventricular arrhythmia, and they have few, if any, prodromal signs or symptoms. Coxsackie B virus has been implicated in 50% of cases (12), but many other viruses have been implicated in fatal myocarditis cases. Chronic cocaine use has also been linked with the histologic features of myocarditis. The cardiac involvement of myocarditis is generally unpredictable, and it may include the conduction system or the myocardium, with resultant heart block or dilated cardiomyopathy with chronic cardiac dysfunction, respectively. Early symptoms, if present, may include exercise intolerance and congestive heart failure symptoms with dyspnea, cough, and orthopnea. Subtle clinical signs include tachycardia in the absence of fever, pulsus alternans, and other clinical signs of failure (e.g., S_3 gallop, soft apical murmur, distended neck veins, and peripheral edema). Athletes with diagnosed myocarditis should be withdrawn from competitive activity for 6 months, and return-to-play permission should be considered only after consultation with a cardiologist (see Chapter 2) (10). Animal research has shown that exercise during a coxsackie virus infection increases the risk of myocarditis (13). Therefore, as a precaution, the clinician should consider withholding athletes with viral infections from exercise while any systemic symptoms of infection (fever, malaise, myalgia, etc.) are present.

Congenital aortic stenosis (AS) occurs in about 2% of the population. In children, sports participation accounts for almost 20% of AS-associated deaths (14). This condition is usually due to the presence of a bicuspid aortic valve. The narrowed valve surface area causes progressive hypertrophy of the left ventricle. Over time, this can lead to myocardial ischemia from pressure overload, angina, and congestive heart failure. The murmur of AS is harsh, midsystolic, and loudest in the right second intercostal space, and it radiates into the neck. Chest x-ray may reveal a post-stenotic dilatation of the aorta and a calcified aortic valve. ECG may show signs of LV strain. Before being cleared for athletic participation, patients with this condition require cardiology consultation and a risk-stratifying workup with echocardiography or cardiac catheterization, exercise testing, and ECG.

Idiopathic concentric LVH is associated with sudden death in athletes. It can be confused with the concentric LVH seen in the athletic heart, but clinical history, in conjunction with echocardiography, can help distinguish between the two conditions. An athlete with LV wall thickness greater than 16 mm likely has HCM (15). No reliable clinical features can aid in the diagnosis.

Right ventricular dysplasia is an idiopathic cardiomyopathy that involves the right ventricle. This cardiomyopathy involves the replacement of myocardial cells with fibrous or fatty tissue, which can result in ventricular tachyarrhythmias. This condition is particularly common in Northern Italy (8). Death often occurs with exertion, and it is frequently the initial presentation of the disease. The ECG may demonstrate a right bundle branch block or ectopic beats in a left bundle branch block configuration, thus suggesting an origin in the right ventricle. The diagnosis should be clinically suspected in athletes with palpitations, syncope, or ventricular tachycardia, and it can be confirmed by echocardiography. Athletes with this condition should be precluded from competitive sports.

Acquired premature coronary artery disease can also appear in the athlete who is under the age of 30 years. A genetic predisposition, with the prevalence of other risk factors, can lead to coronary events, as in older adults. Attention to risk factors and the early symptoms of ischemia, angina, and other effort-related symptoms should be pursued just as aggressively as they are in the older athlete. Activity should be restricted until the condition is stabilized with treatment (medical and/or surgical), and precise exercise tolerance has been determined by a graded exercise test.

Heat-related illness is another common cause of sudden death in young athletes. This, in contrast to sudden death from cardiac causes, which often escape preevent detection, is entirely preventable. Heat exhaustion and heat stroke are clinical syndromes along a spectrum of severity that ranges from isolated malaise and weakness to central nervous system damage, rhabdomyolysis, and multiple organ failure. Children are at an increased risk due to greater fluid loss from their relatively larger body surface area, a decreased sweat rate, and a decreased ability for thermal homeostasis in comparison to mature athletes. Additional risk factors include obesity, sunburn, dehydration, a past history of heat stroke, cardiovascular disease, and certain medications, including antihistamines, anticholinergics, and phenothiazines. Prevention is accomplished by adequate acclimatization (1 to 2 weeks of light exercise, 60 to 90 minutes per day), attention to activity restriction guidelines based on the wet ball globe temperature readings (Table 17.2), supervision by personnel attuned to the early symptoms of heat illness, frequent water breaks,

TABLE 17.2. *Guidelines for team activities based on wet bulb globe temperature index*

°F	°C	Activity
<65	<18	Follow regular schedules; allow full access to fluids
65–72	18–22	Add quarterly fluid breaks; allow free access to fluids
73–82	23–28	Shorten games or allow unlimited substitutions; add quarterly fluid breaks; allow full access to water
82–85	28–30	Establish an alternate schedule in advance to move midday games to earlier and later hours; allow unrestricted substitution at all age levels; shorten game times; add quarterly fluid breaks; allow fluid breaks during play
>85	>30	Cancel all exertion and avoid sun exposure at rest

American College of Medicine. *Position of thermal injuries during distance running.* 1985, with permission.

and free access to fluids. Individual compliance with hydration increases when the fluid is flavored, when it has carbohydrates, and when it is cooled to about 10°C (50°F).

Under the extreme conditions of heat and altitude, some evidence suggests that individuals with sickle cell trait may be at risk for exertional rhabdomyolysis, renal failure, and death. Although death in this situation is rare, it can occur in athletes with poor physical conditioning, dehydration, or heat stress or in those who are in hypoxic states (16). Approximately 8% of African-Americans and 0.8% of other races have the sickle cell trait. These individuals are advised to acclimatize, to condition properly, and to be well hydrated to avoid the risks associated with exercising under extreme conditions.

Aortic dissection from cystic medial necrosis is the cause of sudden death in athletes with Marfan syndrome. The syndrome is estimated to occur in 1 in 10,000 Americans, and it is caused by a genetic defect that stimulates the production of a defective glycoprotein called fibrillin. Clinical clues make this a potentially screenable condition (Table 17.3). These include a family history of tall stature or sudden death before the age of 50 years, tall stature, long limbs and fingers, the ability to overlap the thumb and small finger when encircling the opposite wrist, an arm span-to-height ratio of greater than 1.05, pectus deformity, myopia, a midsystolic click, or systolic murmur on cardiac auscultation. Athletes with Marfan syndrome should not participate in collision sports, and persons with aortic regurgitation and aortic dilatation should not participate in competitive sports.

TABLE 17.3. *Features of Marfan syndrome on physical examination*

Musculoskeletal
  Tall stature
  Thin gangly body habitus
    (armspan to height ratio >1.05)
  Arachnodactyly (long thin fingers; able to wrap
    hand around opposite wrist and overlap thumb
    and small finger)
  Pectus deformity
  High arched palate
  Kyphoscoliosis
  Joint laxity
Cardiovascular
  Systolic click (mitral valve prolapse)
  Evidence of easy bruising
  Diastolic murmur (aortic regurgitation)
Ocular
  Myopia
  Retinal detachment
  Lens subluxation (need slit lamp examination)

Persons with isolated aortic root dilatation can compete in low static/low dynamic sports (e.g., golf, bowling, and billiards). Serial ultrasonography every 6 months can assist in identifying a progressive dilation of the aortic root, which may require surgical intervention (17).

Mitral valve prolapse (MVP) has a prevalence of occurrence in 4% to 7% of the population. In rare cases, it is believed to be associated with malignant ventricular arrhythmias and resultant sudden death. Athletes with MVP and the following risk factors are thought to be at risk for a sudden death event: a family history of sudden death, Marfan syndrome, complex ventricular arrhythmias, a prolonged QT interval, an individual history of syncope or disabling chest pain, or significant mitral regurgitation. These athletes should be restricted from participation in competitive athletics (10).

Wolff–Parkinson–White syndrome is characterized by an accessory conduction pathway from the atrium to the ventricle that bypasses the atrioventricular (AV) node, and it can lead to paroxysmal supraventricular tachycardia or atrial fibrillation with rapid ventricular response. These patients may have a history of palpitations or syncope, and their ECG may show a delta wave (a slurred deflection at the beginning of the QRS complex). Patients with extremely short refractory periods of the accessory pathway can develop rapid-rate atrial arrhythmias that can decompensate to a fatal arrhythmia. Younger athletes with this condition have a greater risk than do mature athletes, and affected patients require subspecialty evaluation to consider electrophysiologic testing before clearance for athletic participation is granted (18).

Prolonged QT syndrome can cause sudden exertion-related death by precipitating ventricular tachycardia. The congenital type comprises about 60% of cases, and it can be associated with neurosensory deafness. A corrected QT interval of 440 to 450 milliseconds is the upper limit of normal; QTc intervals greater than 500 milliseconds are considered to carry the greatest risk for sudden death. The diagnosis is made from a constellation of symptoms, the family history, and an abnormal ECG. To prevent sudden death, these persons should be excluded from competitive sports (10).

Exercise-induced bronchospasm (EIB) is present in about 12% to 15% of the population, but some studies have suggested that the prevalence may be much higher (19). In addition, in chronic asthmatics, the prevalence of exercise-induced symptoms is 40% to 90% (20). Sudden death due to asthma during exercise may be precipitated by cold dry air, allergens, or bronchial drying as a result of the athlete's increased ventilation during exercise. The incidence of sudden death from exercise-induced asthma is rare. Control of chronic asthma with medication and close monitoring are imperative to prevent status asthmaticus. Exercise is beneficial to patients with asthma, and activity should only be restricted until the individual has gained control over the disease. If the use of medication is unacceptable to a young athlete, changes in the sport or the position played can be entertained (21).

Commotio cordis is a cause of sudden death due to an arrhythmia, most commonly ventricular fibrillation, that is generated as a result of blunt chest trauma. The incidence is unknown, but it is most commonly seen in young adolescents in baseball. Although autopsies have failed to show any injury to the myocardium, some degree of cardiac injury is suspected to be involved. Education of coaches and players and the use of chest protectors and softer core baseballs decrease, but do not eliminate, the risk. Immediate access to an automated external defibrillator may increase the chance of a successful resuscitation (22).

Other conditions have been associated with sudden death in the young athlete with much lower frequencies. Preventable conditions, such as cocaine use and its association with coronary artery spasm (23), as well as anabolic steroid use and a potential association with HCM, should be noted (24). In addition, inflammatory coronary artery aneurysms associated with Kawasaki disease have also been reported as a cause of sudden death (25). Brugada syndrome, which is seen mostly in young adults from Southeast Asia, is a familial ECG abnormality that has been associated with syncope or sudden death from polymorphic ventricular tachycardia or ventricular fibrillation. The resting ECG is notable for right bundle branch block and the elevated ST segment in leads V1 to V3. Exercise is not a risk factor in this condition, but the condition usually does affect active, apparently healthy young men. The only treatment is an automatic, implantable cardioverter or defibrillator. Patients with a family history of early sudden death or a personal history of unexplained syncope should be evaluated for this condition.

SCREENING STRATEGIES

The impact of a sudden death in a young athlete during competition always provokes the question of what more could have been done to identify this individual who apparently had a higher risk. The use of screening tests, however, needs to be evaluated by epidemiologic criteria for determining effectiveness, not by the media and/or public consensus.

Epstein and Maron (26) have attempted to put screening strategies for the prevention of sudden death into perspective by estimating disease prevalence. They have estimated that 200,000 competitive asymptomatic athletes would need to be screened to provide a potential identification of the one athlete who would die as a result of athletic competition. If the assumption is made that a tool to screen for sudden death with a theoretic sensitivity and specificity of 99% is available, the low prevalence of disease would yield a positive predictive value of only 5%.

One of the problems with athlete screening is that "abnormalities" detected during examinations are generally variants of normal. For example, the changes that occur in the heart in response to athletic training are known as athletic heart syndrome (27). The well-trained athlete can demonstrate electrocardiographic, radiographic, and echocardiographic changes that reflect cardiac enlargement and enhanced vagal tone. In addition, the clinical examination may demonstrate bradycardia, S_3 and S_4 heart sounds, and an increased frequency of innocent flow murmurs. While clinical criteria have been developed to assist in distinguishing athletic heart syndrome from pathologic conditions, the differentiation of normal from abnormal may be extremely difficult.

As HCM is the most common cause of sudden death in the young competitive athlete, an ideal screening strategy should focus on detection of this disease. A good history and physical examination are accepted as the minimal standard for preparticipation assessment. Electrocardiography and treadmill stress testing are plagued by a high degree of false-positives primarily due to athletic heart syndrome (28), so most of the attention in the literature has been devoted to the use of echocardiography. The echocardiogram is considered to be sensitive and specific in detecting HCM. The principal concerns with echocardiogram are the prohibitive cost, and the small, but identifiable, risk of mislabeling a healthy athletic variant and of restricting an otherwise healthy athlete (29).

Several studies have applied echocardiography to screening large athletic populations. Lewis et al. (30) performed two-dimensional echocardiography on 265 college athletes of predominately African-American descent. The interventricular septum was 13 mm or more in 29 men (13%), but none had abnormal septal to posterior wall thickness ratios (normal <1.3). None of the athletes exposed to echocardiography as the initial screening test were thought to have an increased risk for sudden death.

Maron et al. (31) screened 501 college athletes with a personal and family medical history and a 12-lead ECG. Ninety athletes were subsequently triaged for echocardiography. While three athletes were identified as having interventricular septal thickening, no athlete was restricted from participation. With a fee of between $280 and $500 for the echocardiography alone, the cost to the athletic program in 1992 would have been between $25,000 and $45,000 (29).

In an attempt to evaluate the economic feasibility of a limited screening echocardiogram, Weidenbener et al. (32) performed 2,997 echocardiograms during annual athletic preparticipation examinations. The estimated total cost per athlete was $13.81, as the tests were provided free of charge. The screening echocardiogram took approximately 2 minutes and included parasternal long- and short-axis views, and the interpretation cost was estimated to be $60.00 per hour (reading 35 echos per hour). No abnormalities were uncovered that precluded athletic participation. While the authors concluded that screening echocardiograms could be incorporated into the preparticipation examination cost-effectively, they did note that additional work remained to validate the screening echocardiogram.

While the role of echocardiography in routine screening in the asymptomatic athletic population is limited by the low prevalence of disease and by cost, inroads into the molecular biology of HCM may prove to be the most concerning fact for the primary care physician. In an editorial, Fananapazir and Epstein (33) reported that recent molecular genetic studies have shed new light into the clinical spectrum of HCM. Molecular markers have demonstrated that clinical features, such as arrhythmias, myocardial ischemia, and/or diastolic dysfunction, may be present in patients in the absence of LVH, as determined by echocardiography. While the authors recognized that the medical community is far from incorporating genetic testing into routine clinical practice and screening, they do conclude that reliance solely on echocardiography provides a restricted view of the prevalence and clinical spectrum of HCM.

Maron et al. (34) published a detailed study profiling the demographics of sudden death in young competitive athletes. The most sobering aspect of the report was the review of those athletes who were victims of sudden death and who had completed the preparticipation process. Standard history and physical examination had been utilized in 115 athletes out of the 158 reviewed. Suspicion of a cardiovascular problem was found in only four (3%) of the athletes. The correct diagnosis (Marfan syndrome) was made in only one athlete, and the athlete did not withdraw completely from athletics. In 15 of the 158 athletes, symptoms led to individualized workups. These evaluations led to seven correct diagnoses and two disqualifications from competitive athletics. A retrospective review showed that 31% of the athletes with anomalous coronary arteries had symptoms (syncope or dizziness) and that only 21% of the athletes with HCM had symptoms. These medical evaluations failed to identify 47 of 48 cases of HCM.

CURRENT SCREENING RECOMMENDATIONS

A complete and careful personal and family history and a physical examination designed to identify or to raise suspicion of those conditions known to cause sudden death or disease progression in young athletes is the most practical, as well as the best currently available, approach to screening populations of competitive athletes, regardless of age. Because the majority of sudden death cases are secondary to cardiovascular conditions, the American Heart Association recommends that an examination be performed before participation in organized high school and collegiate sports. Screening should be repeated every 2 years, and an interim history should be obtained in the intervening years. Athletic screening should be performed by a healthcare worker who has the requisite training, medical skills, and background to obtain a detailed cardiovascular history reliably, to perform a physical examination, and to recognize heart disease (35).

Preparticipation physical evaluation, which is endorsed by the American Academy of Pediatrics and other bodies, contains a standardized medical questionnaire that screens for most of the causes of sudden athletic death (36). The use of this form, or one based on it, is highly recommended for preparticipation examinations. Chapter 2 also contains general recommendations for patients with specific medical problems, guidelines for the further evaluation of abnormalities, tables of sports classifications by contact categories and exertional categories, and numerous other resources.

The "focused" examination should seek those features that have been associated with common causes of sudden death in young athletes (Table 17.1). The general examination should identify the physical stigmata of Marfan syndrome (Table 17.3). The lung examination can assist in determining the current adequacy of asthma treatment. Detailed neurologic examination can be performed if the history is positive for symptoms that suggest intracranial pathology. The cardiovascular examination should include the following: precordial auscultation in both supine and standing positions to identify heart murmurs consistent with dynamic LV outflow obstruction, palpation of carotid or brachial pulse, assessment of the femoral arteries to exclude coarctation of the aorta, and brachial blood pressure measurement in the seated position.

Arterial pulse is useful in assessing cardiac rate and rhythm, as well as for providing insight into cardiac pathology. The carotid pulse provides the most accurate representation of the aortic pulse, and it is best palpated with the thumb. The brachial artery is the vessel that is the most suitable for appreciating the rate of rise of the pulse and the contour, volume, and consistency of the peripheral vessels. The normal primary wave starts with a swift upstroke to the peak of systolic pressure, followed by a more gradual decline. At the end of systole, a smaller upstroke—the dicrotic wave—occurs, caused by a rebound of blood against the closing aortic valve. Normally, the dicrotic wave is impalpable. *Pulsus bisferiens*, in which the dicrotic notch approaches the height of the primary element, can occur in AS, aortic regurgitation, and HCM. Advanced AS may manifest a *pulsus parvus et tardus*, characterized by gradual upstroke of the wave, prolonged downstroke, and a blunted peak. Suspicion of coarctation of the aorta should be raised when hypertension in the arms is coincident with weak femoral pulses or when the peak of the femoral pulse lags behind that of the radial artery. A water-hammer pulse, which is a very sharp upstroke followed by a downstroke that falls precipitously, can be seen in aortic insufficiency (37).

Cardiac palpation should be conducted routinely to evaluate cardiac dynamics. The palmar bases of the fingers are most sensitive to vibration; accordingly, the examiner should palpate the precordium with the palm of the hand. The point of maximal impulse (PMI) is caused by forward rotation of the heart during the beginning of systole. Normally, the PMI is 7 to 9 cm to the left of the midsternal line in the fifth interspace. The normal pulse is a brief tap; a forceful outward thrust may be seen in HCM. Thrills, or vibrations over the precordium, have the same significance as loud murmurs. In AS, a thrill is appreciated in the second right interspace.

Cardiac auscultation should be done carefully and systematically. Bates (38) outlined an effective and systematic cardiac evaluation as follows. Starting at the cardiac base (aortic and pulmonic areas), carefully identify S1 and S2. At the base, S2 is normally louder than S1. Identify the heart rate and rhythm. Listen in each of the valve locations. At each area, note the intensity and splitting of S1 and S2. Listen for extra sounds in both systole and diastole. Note timing, intensity, and pitch. Listen for systolic and diastolic murmurs. Note timing (early, mid, late, holosystolic), location (appropriate interspace), radiation, intensity (grade, Table 17.4), pitch (high, medium or low), and quality (blowing, rumbling, musical or harsh). Listen for other cardiovascular sounds that have both systolic and diastolic components, such as rubs and venous hums. Normal splitting of S2 is heard best along the left sternal border and is appreciated during inspiration. Splitting is thought to occur when P2 is delayed from A2, secondary to the increase in volume in the right ventricle during inspiration. A fixed S2 split can be seen in an atrial septal defect, as well as in advanced pulmonary hypertension. Paradoxical splitting—that which occurs with expiration—may be seen in left bundle branch block, AS, or HCM.

Dynamic auscultation is in important technique that alters intracardiac volume and causes changes in the characteristics of murmurs. It involves having the patient perform maneuvers, such as standing, squatting, and lying supine, during cardiac auscultation. Use of this technique should be routine when any murmur is detected. Standing decreases venous return and reduces the intensity of innocent murmurs, as well as that of the murmur of AS. Conversely, standing accentuates the murmur of obstructive HCM. In MVP, the click murmur will move closer to S1 with standing. Squatting or lying supine increases intracardiac volume and the intensity of the murmur of AS, as well as that of innocent murmurs. Squatting

TABLE 17.4. *Murmur classification*

Grade	Description
I	Faintest murmur that can be detected; often found only after close concentration and adjustment of the stethoscope
I	Faint but can be detected immediately by an experienced physician
III	Moderately loud to auscultation
IV	Loud and associated with a thrill
V	Extremely loud but still requires placement of the stethoscope on the chest wall for appreciation
VI	Can be heard without the stethoscope on the chest

or lying supine may decrease the intensity of the murmur of obstructive HCM.

Athletes who demonstrate abnormalities on either the history or the physical examination warrant a more detailed evaluation. Indications for referral would include, but are not limited to, all diastolic murmurs, holosystolic murmurs, murmurs that are grade III and above, abnormal murmur changes with dynamic auscultation, murmurs with a suspicious family history or review of systems, and murmurs about which the examiner is unclear (39). Further evaluation may include ECG, echocardiography, exercise stress testing, cardiac catheterization, pulmonary function testing, neuroimaging with computerized tomography or MRI (for neurological signs or symptoms), or other tests, as deemed appropriate. In addition, the athlete may require temporary disqualification from athletic participation pending further evaluation. As further testing has certain limitations, the authors' opinion is that athletes with unusual or suspicious findings warrant subspecialty consultation.

Cardiovascular abnormalities should be evaluated with respect to the 26th Bethesda Conference consensus panel recommendations (10) for the final determination of eligibility for future athletic competition. The Bethesda report classifies individual sports according to type and intensity of exercise and also with regard to the danger of bodily injury from collision or the consequences of syncope. This report provides useful guidance to physicians about the acceptable medical risks of athletic participation with known cardiovascular abnormalities.

CONCLUSION

Sudden cardiac death, despite the intense media attention, remains exceedingly rare. Screening strategies to identify the athlete at risk are limited by the low prevalence of disease, the inherent limitations of the tests, and the fact that most athletes are asymptomatic prior to their demise. The current consensus in the literature and the primary care sports medicine community is that screening for sudden death is best accomplished with a "focused" periodic physical examination and a targeted history that seeks to identify exercise-related symptoms and a strong family history. Despite the benign nature of most complaints in this age group, new symptoms should be carefully evaluated. Future research, including molecular genetic studies, and further efforts into refining and validating screening echocardiography offer the hope of more effective screening.

REFERENCES

1. Ragosta M, Crabtree J, Sturner WQ, et al. Death during recreational exercise in the State of Rhode Island. *Med Sci Sports Excer* 1984;16:339–342.
2. Phillips M, Robiniwitz M, Higgins JR, et al. Sudden cardiac death in Air Force recruits. *JAMA* 1986;256:2696–2699.
3. Zheng ZJ, Croft J, Giles WL. Sudden cardiac deaths are increasing in young people, especially among young women. Paper presented at the 41st Annual Conference on Cardiovascular Disease Epidemiology and Prevention, San Francisco, CA, March, 2001.
4. Van Camp SP, Bloor CM, Mueller FO, et al. Nontraumatic sports death in high school and college athletes. *Med Sci Sports Exerc* 1995;27:641–647.
5. Maron BJ, Roberts WC, McAllister HA, et al. Sudden death in young athletes. *Circulation* 1980;62:218–229.
6. McCaffrey FM, Braden DS, Strong WB. Sudden cardiac death in young athletes. *Am J Dis Child* 1991;145:177–183.
7. Burke AP, Farb A, Virmani R, et al. Sports-related and non-sports-related sudden cardiac death in young adults. *Am Heart J* 1991;121:568–575.
8. Corrado D, Thiene G, Nava A, et al. Sudden death in young competitive athletes: clinicopathologic correlations in 22 cases. *Am J Med* 1990;89:588–596.
9. Maron BJ, Gardin JM, Flack JM, et al. Prevalence of hypertrophic cardiomyopathy in a general population of young adults: echocardiographic analysis of 4111 subjects in the CARDIA study. *Circulation* 1995;92:785–789.
10. Maron BJ, Mitchell JH, Raven PB. 26th Bethesda conference: recommendations for determining eligibility for competition in athletes with cardiovascular abnormalities. *Med Sci Sports Exerc* 1994;26:S261–S267.
11. Taylor AJ, Rogan KM, Virmani R. Sudden cardiac death associated with isolated congenital coronary artery anomalies. *J Am Coll Cardiol* 1992;20:640–647.
12. Bresler MJ. Acute pericarditis and myocarditis. *Emerg Med* 1992;24:35.
13. Gatmaitan BG, Chason JL, Lerner AM. Augmentation of the virulence of murine coxsackie virus B-3 myocardiopathy by exercise. *J Exp Med* 1970;131:1121–1136.
14. Lambert EC, Menon VA, Wagner HR, et al. Sudden unexpected death from cardiovascular disease in children. A cooperative international study. *Am J Cardiol* 1974;34:89–96.
15. Pelliccia A, Maron BJ, Spataro A, et al. The upper limit of physiologic cardiac hypertrophy in highly trained elite athletes. *N Engl J Med* 1991;324:295–301.
16. Kerle KK, Nishimura KD. Exertional collapse and sudden death associated with sickle cell trait. *Am Fam Physician* 1996;54:237–240.
17. Salim MA, Alpert BS. Sports and Marfan syndrome. Awareness and early diagnosis can prevent sudden death. *The Physician and Sports Medicine* 2001;29:80–93.
18. Goldman L, Braunwald E, eds. *Primary cardiology.* Philadelphia: WB Saunders, 1998.
19. Weiler JM, Metzger WJ, Donnelly AL, et al. Prevalence of bronchial hyperresponsiveness in highly trained athletes. *Chest* 1986;90:23–28.
20. McFadden ER. Exercise-induced airway obstruction. *Clin Chest Med* 1995;16:671–682.
21. Lillegard WA, Butcher, JD, Rucker KS. *Handbook of sports medicine. A symptom-oriented approach.* Boston: Butterworth-Heineman, 1999:302.

22. Vincent GM, McPeak H. Commotio cordis. A deadly consequence of chest trauma. *The Physician and Sports Medicine* 2000;28:31–39.
23. Cantwell JD, Rose FD. Cocaine and cardiovascular events. *The Physician and Sports Medicine* 1986;14:7.
24. Mochizuki RM, Richter KJ. Cardiomyopathy and cerebrovascular accident associated with anabolic-androgenic steroid use. *The Physician and Sports Medicine* 1988;16:109.
25. Burke AP, Farb A, Virmani R. Causes of sudden death in athletes. *Cardiol Clin* 1992;10:303–317.
26. Epstein SE, Maron BJ. Sudden death and the competitive athlete: perspectives on preparticipation screening studies. *J Am Coll Cardiol* 1986;7:220–230.
27. Huston TP, Puffer JC, Rodney WM. The athletic heart syndrome. *N Engl J Med* 1985;313:24–32.
28. Spirito P, Maron BJ, Bonow RO, et al. Prevalence and significance of an abnormal S-T segment response to exercise in a young athletic population. *Am J Cardiol* 1983;51:1663–1666.
29. Farenbach MC, Thompson PD. The preparticipation sports examination: cardiovascular considerations for screening. *Cardiol Clin* 1992;10:319–328.
30. Lewis JF, Maron BJ, Diggs JA, et al. Preparticipation echocardiographic screening for cardiovascular disease in a large, predominately black population of college athletes. *Am J Cardiol* 1989;64:1029–1033.
31. Maron BJ, Bodison SA, Wesley YA, et al. Results of screening a large group of inter collegiate competitive athletes for cardiovascular disease. *J Am Coll Cardiol* 1987;10:1214–1221.
32. Weidenbener EJ, Kraus MD, Waller BF, et al. Incorporation of screening echocardiography in the preparticipation examination. *Clin J Sports Med* 1995;5:86–89.
33. Fananapazir L, Epstein ND. Prevalence of hypertrophic cardiomyopathy and limitations of screening methods. *Circulation* 1995;92:700–704.
34. Maron BJ, Shirani J, Poliac LC, et al. Sudden death in young competitive athletes: clinical, demographic, and pathologic profiles. *JAMA* 1996;276:199–204.
35. Maron BJ, Thompson PD, Puffer JC. Cardiovascular preparticipation screening of competitive athletes. *Circulation* 1996;94:850–856.
36. American Academy of Family Physicians, Preparticipation Physical Evaluation Task Force. *Preparticipation physical evaluation*, 2nd ed. New York: McGraw-Hill, 1997.
37. DeGowin EL, DeGowin RL. *Bedside diagnostic examination*, 4th ed. New York: Macmillian, 1976.
38. Bates, B. *A guide to physical examination*, 2nd ed. Philadelphia: Lippincott, 1979.
39. Phleiger KL, Strong WB. Screening for heart murmurs: what's normal and what's not. *The Physician and Sports Medicine* 1992;20:71–81.

18

Exercise-Induced Bronchospasm and Asthma

Implications for the School-Aged Athlete

Mary B. Cataletto

The psychosocial and cardiovascular benefits of exercise and sports participation in school-aged children are well known. The presence of asthma does not need to exclude these children from participation, but it does require early identification and special consideration to optimize their success (i.e., exercise without asthma symptoms). Despite advances in asthma identification and care, studies continue to show that asthmatics are less fit and less active than their nonasthmatic counterparts (1) and that teachers are more likely to consider them "out of shape." In one study, only 34% of teachers were aware of the relationship between exertion and wheezing, and, although 69% of these teachers had had asthmatic children in their classes, only 5% believed that they had adequate knowledge about asthma (2).

Asthma is an inflammatory disorder of the airways (3) that affects approximately 7% of all United States children. Exercise is a common trigger for bronchospasm in these children (up to 95%) (4,5), as well as for many children (40%) with allergic rhinitis (4,5). While the lay press heralds the Olympic gold medals and accomplishments of many talented athletes with asthma, clinicians should not be lulled into a sense of complacency. Status asthmaticus can be fatal if it is not recognized or if it is inadequately treated. Rossini et al. (6) reported demographic data on asthma-related deaths during sporting activities. Deaths from asthma followed trauma and cardiac causes in frequency, and they occurred more often in teenaged males involved in high intensity sports (basketball, football, and track). Eighty-four percent had a prior history of asthma, and 50% of these were using β-agonist therapy. Essentially, none of these used inhaled corticosteroids on a regular basis.

PATHOPHYSIOLOGY AND CLINICAL PRESENTATION

Exercise-induced bronchospasm (EIB) occurs more frequently in both allergic and asthmatic patients. In some patients, it is the only manifestation of airway hyperreactivity. With exertion, airway hyperreactivity may manifest as a cough, wheeze, shortness of breath, or chest pain. Pathophysiologic studies have shown that an underlying inflammatory process occurs in the airway of each asthmatic that combines with mucosal edema and bronchospasm to cause the symptoms described as an asthmatic response. Exercise may trigger these responses through a number of pathways. Although some controversy remains, both heat and water losses in the airway are believed to play a role in the mediator release, thereby causing symptoms (7).

Typically, the clinical scenario of EIB begins between 5 to 10 minutes after strenuous exertion. Patients may describe shortness of breath or chest tightness, or they may report increased cough or audible wheezing. Less frequently, they may complain of "being out of shape," of variable performance, or of a prolonged cough after exertion ("locker room cough") that resolves with rest (8). Concurrent with these symptoms, spirometry typically shows a decrease of at least 15% from baseline forced expiratory volume at 1 second (FEV_1) (5). FEV_1 is an airflow measurement taken 1 second into expiration, following maximum inspiratory effort. Decreased values may be seen either with increased airway resistance or decreased lung elastic recoil. Return to baseline values occurs approximately 30 to 90 minutes later in patients who have normal baseline pulmonary function. Figure 18.1 shows a diagrammatic representation of an exercise test in a patient with EIB (9).

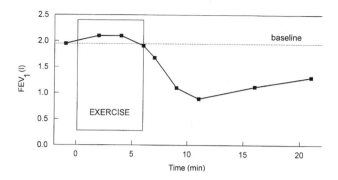

FIG. 18.1. Diagrammatic representation of exercise-induced bronchospasm. (From Bierman CW, Pearlman DS, eds. *Allergic diseases from infancy to adulthood.* Philadelphia: WB Saunders, 1988:597–606, with permission.)

Some patients (40% to 50%) may experience a refractory period following a short period of exercise. Prostaglandin release is the candidate that is most likely responsible for this persistent response, which may last up to 4 hours (10). This refractory period, however, is protective only for exercise, and thus, it does not protect the athlete from bronchospasm triggered by other factors (e.g., pollens and air pollution) (11).

The late phase response is currently under debate (4). It occurs 4 to 12 hours after the initial episode, and whether it represents a specific late phase response or indicates that baseline asthma in poor control is not clear.

DIAGNOSIS

Many children with EIB are diagnosed on the basis of history and response to therapy. Peak expiratory flow rate (PEFR) monitoring has also been used as a diagnostic tool. Although peak flow monitoring is inexpensive, easily available, and easy to use, peak flows are effort-dependent, and they are used more frequently to monitor patients with an established diagnosis. The danger of using peak flow measurements alone as a diagnostic tool is that the clinician may misdiagnose shortness of breath with exertion as EIB, thus misdiagnosing a child with poor fitness or cardiac, pulmonary, or subtle muscle disease. The elements of diagnosis include history, physical examination, pulmonary function testing, and response to therapy. Additionally, when the examiner is in doubt, an exercise challenge test may help clarify the diagnosis.

History

In the child who has already been diagnosed with asthma, the history will assist the clinician in tailoring an asthma action plan. For those athletes present-

ing for the preparticipation physical examination (PPE), an exercise-focused respiratory history will help direct the evaluation. Questions regarding shortness of breath, cough, wheezing, and chest pain (both at rest and with exertion) are essential elements of the preparticipation evaluation. If routine play activities elicit asthma symptoms, children should be evaluated to improve baseline control. The basic elements of EIB history, which are presented below, are also summarized in Table 18.1.

Environment

Exercise in cold, dry environments is more likely to precipitate asthmatic symptoms than is exercise in warm, humidified areas (e.g., ice skating versus indoor swimming). Likewise, exposure to high pollen counts in allergic athletes and to environmental air pollution can be problematic (12). For indoor activities, consider air quality (e.g., dust, smoke, etc.). The importance of avoiding both active and passive exposure to cigarette smoke should be emphasized.

Type of Activity

Participation in any sport may elicit asthmatic symptoms; however, different activities have differ-

TABLE 18.1. *Elements of history in exercise-induced bronchospasm*

1. Environment
2. Type of activity
3. Level of cardiovascular fitness
4. Obesity
5. Concomitant allergic symptoms and/or upper respiratory tract infection
6. Associated stressors/competition
7. Baseline asthma control
8. Therapeutic response

TABLE 18.2. Activities associated with exercise-induced bronchospasm

Basketball
Cross-country cycling
Ice hockey
Long-distance running
Rugby
Soccer

ing potentials for eliciting bronchospasm. For example, high intensity, moderate-to-high endurance activities (e.g., basketball, cross-country cycling, ice hockey, ice skating, long-distance running, rugby, and soccer) are more likely to be associated with bronchospasm than are activities that require short bursts of activity, such as sprinting or baseball, or than those that are low intensity, such as golf (Table 18.2). The level of intensity and endurance also impact the propensity of symptoms to occur (12,13).

Level of Cardiovascular Fitness

While improved fitness is associated with better control of asthma, fitness appears to be related to an improved workload at a specific level of intensity rather than to an improvement in baseline lung function (14).

Obesity

The overall incidence of asthma is increased, and cardiovascular fitness is decreased in obese children (4,15). A recent study by Castro-Rodriguez et al. (16) found that childhood obesity, especially in girls, was associated with a sevenfold increase in the development of asthma by early adolescence.

Concomitant Allergic Symptoms and/or Upper Respiratory Tract Infections

Poorly controlled allergy symptoms with nasal congestion and/or obstruction or upper airway inflammation secondary to infection (e.g., upper respiratory infection and sinusitis) are associated with increased airway hyperresponsiveness (9).

Psychologic Stress

Hyperventilation associated with anxiety or stress can trigger bronchospasm. Anxiety and panic disorders can also exist as comorbid conditions, and they should

be addressed. These disorders are more frequent in patients with chronic respiratory disorders (17).

Baseline Asthma Control

Athletes who have symptoms more than twice a week and peak flow or FEV_1 less than 80% of the predicted value and PEFR variability greater than 20% are classified as having persistent asthma. They require treatment with controller medications on a daily basis (18).

Therapeutic Response

The patient's response to short-acting β-agonists or cromolyn should be noted. Most patients (80% to 95%) with EIB will have a therapeutic response to short-acting bronchodilators, such as albuterol (19). Cromolyn or nedocromil may also be effective in a smaller percentage of patients (19).

For many student athletes, a focused respiratory history will raise EIB as a diagnostic consideration. However, asthma is often missed, even in elite athletes (5). A high index of suspicion should be maintained when evaluating athletes who train and compete in cold air environments and in high endurance sports.

Physical Examination

The physical examination should include a comprehensive respiratory examination with an evaluation for signs and symptoms of chronic respiratory disease and evidence of atopic disease. The PPE is discussed in greater detail in Chapter 2 of this text.

Pulmonary Function Testing

Baseline pulmonary function testing, as well as testing for bronchodilator responsiveness, is often used to identify the asthmatic patient. In these children, exercise testing is unnecessary (9). In children with normal pulmonary function at rest and symptoms of exercise-induced respiratory symptoms, an exercise challenge can be helpful (5). The exercise challenge is most commonly administered in a pulmonary function laboratory where the athlete exercises on either a cycle ergometer or a treadmill in a controlled environment. Alternatively, intermittent spirometric measurements over time may be taken with free running, although these results are not considered as reproducible as in-lab studies (5). Characteristic falls in FEV_1 of more than 15% are consistent with a diagnosis of EIB (5,9).

CLASSIFICATION OF ASTHMA SEVERITY

The National Asthma Education and Prevention Program sponsored by the National Heart, Blood, and Lung Institute (18) released a series of guidelines by which asthmatic symptoms can be classified and approached. These guidelines convey important considerations for optimizing the baseline asthma control of student athletes. The guidelines also stress the importance of the formation of a partnership among the clinician, the patient, and his or her family to improve the patient's quality of life and to increase the number of symptom-free days.

Table 18.3 summarizes the four categories by composites of subjective and objective findings. Mild intermittent asthma is characterized by normal spirometry and normal level of activity between episodes. Intermittent symptoms (fewer than two times per week) require rescue therapy with a short-acting bronchodilator. Patients with mild persistent asthma have symptoms more than two times per week but less than once a day. Activity may affect symptoms, and peak flow variability ranges between 20% and 30%. Moderate persistent asthma occurs in patients with daily symptoms; flare-ups may last longer, and nighttime symptoms occur more than once a week. Activity levels are often affected. Severe persistent asthma is the most limiting category. Exercise is limited because of persistent daily symptoms, and frequent nighttime disruptions because of cough or wheeze occur. In any given patient, many variables may influence their category of classification at a given time. These include respiratory tract infections, the seasonal changes, and exposure to environmental pollutants.

TREATMENT

Therapeutic plans are individualized for each athlete, and they should take into consideration the baseline respiratory status and the particular sport. In addition, since asthmatic episodes are unpredictable, each asthmatic child should have an asthma action plan. By the time a child has reached school age, most are able to perform the peak flow maneuver; these measurements can provide objective data to help guide treatment. The traffic light with red, yellow, and green corresponding to stop, caution, and go, respectively, provides an easy visual way for patients to remember the plan (18). Green signifies "all clear." Peak flow rates are greater than 80% of his or her personal best, and the athlete is symptom free. Yellow signifies caution. Peak flow rate falls between 50% and 80% of the individual's personal best, indicating the need for a therapeutic response. This initially may be a short-acting bronchodilator, but it may also include adding or modifying the doses of controller medication. The red light signifies danger. The peak flow rate is less than 50%, and the athlete is symptomatic. This category also requires a therapeutic response, and a measurement in this range emphasizes the importance of having an asthma action plan, so that each patient and caretaker knows how to handle an acute emergency.

Nonpharmacologic Measures

While medications constitute the mainstay of therapy for exercise-induced asthma, nonpharmacologic measures can also be employed to modify the bronchospastic response associated with exercise (Table 18.4). Environmental modifications can be very helpful when choosing an activity for a persistent asthmatic (e.g., indoor swimming versus a cold air sport). For instance, this option may help with a child recovering from an acute asthmatic exacerbation or in the case of an allergic asthmatic during the height of pollen season. Cross training is a valuable adjunct for maintaining fitness in an athlete who has recently experienced an exacerbation of his or her asthma. Particularly following a respiratory infection, training limits should be considered. Warmups are recommended, as they may allow the child to take advantage of the refractory period (5,13). Stretching and short sprints may be employed. Cool downs of approximately 10 to 30 minutes may include stretching and jogging. During cold weather, the use of facemasks that cover both the nose and mouth will help warm environmental air before it reaches the airway (4).

Medications

Asthma medications are classified into the following two major groups: controllers and relievers (18). Both may be used in the treatment of children with EIB. Asthma education is critical to the implementation of an effective asthma action plan and the therapeutic partnership.

Children who report asthma symptoms more than twice a week require controller therapy. Medications in this class include corticosteroids, leukotriene modifiers, nedocromil, cromolyn, and theophylline. Long-acting β-agonists (e.g., salmeterol) may complement and work synergistically with inhaled corticosteroids to provide an improved baseline, as well as extended exercise coverage. They are not substitutes

TABLE 18.3. *Stepwise approach for managing asthma in adults and children older than 5 years of age*

Goals of asthma treatment

- Prevent chronic and troublesome symptoms (e.g., coughing or breathlessness in the night, in the early morning, or after exertion)
- Maintain (near) "normal" pulmonary function
- Maintain normal activity levels (including exercise and other physical activity)
- Prevent recurrent exacerbations of asthma and minimize the need for emergency department visits or hospitalizations
- Provide optimal pharmacotherapy with minimal or no adverse effects
- Meet patients' and families' expectations of and satisfaction with asthma care

	Classify severity of asthma			Treatments[c]		
	Clinical features before treatment[a]			Treatment goal		
	Symptoms[b]	Nighttime symptoms	Lung function	Long-term control	Quick relief	Education
Step 4: Severe persistent	Continual symptoms Limited physical activity Frequent exacerbations	Frequent	forced expiratory volume at 1 s (FEV$_1$)/peak expiratory flow rate (PEFR) ≤60% predicted PEFR variability >30%	Daily medications: Antiinflammatory: **inhaled corticosteroid (high dose)** *and* Long-acting bronchodilator: either **long-acting inhaled** β$_2$**-agonist**, sustained-release theophylline, or long-acting β$_2$-agonist tablets *and* Corticosteroid tablets or syrup long term (make repeat attempts to reduce systemic steroids and maintain control with high-dose inhaled steroids)	Short-acting bronchodilator: **inhaled** β$_2$**-agonists** as needed for symptoms Intensity of treatment will depend on severity of exacerbation Use of short-acting inhaled-β$_2$-agonists on a daily basis, or increasing use, indicates the need for additional long-term–control therapy	Steps 2 and 3 actions plus Refer for individual education and counseling

continued on next page

TABLE 18.3. Continued

| | Classify severity of asthma | | | Treatments[c] | | |
| | Clinical features before treatment[a] | | | Treatment goal | | |
	Symptoms[b]	Nighttime symptoms	Lung function	Long-term control	Quick relief	Education
Step 3: Moderate persistent	Daily symptoms Daily use of inhaled short-acting β₂-agonist Exacerbations affect activity Exacerbations ≥2 times per wk; may last days	>1 time per wk	FEV_1 or PEFR >60% <80% predicted PEFR variability >30%	Daily medication: Either **Antiinflammatory: inhaled corticosteroid (medium dose)** or Inhaled corticosteroid (low-medium dose) and add a long-acting bronchodilator, especially for nighttime symptoms; either **long-acting inhaled β₂-agonist,** sustained-release theophylline, or long-acting β₂-agonist tablets If needed **Antiinflammatory: inhaled corticosteroids (medium-high dose)** and Long-acting bronchodilator, especially for nighttime symptoms; either long-acting inhaled β₂-agonist, sustained-release theophylline, or long-acting β₂-agonist tablets	Short-acting bronchodilator: **inhaled β₂-agonists** as needed for symptoms Intensity of treatment will depend on severity of exacerbation Use of short-acting inhaled β₂-agonists on a daily basis or increasing use indicates the need for additional long-term–control therapy	Step 1 actions plus: Teach self-monitoring Refer to group education if available Review and update self-management plan
Step 2: Mild persistent	Symptoms >2 times per wk but <1 time per d Exacerbations may affect activity	>2 times per mo	FEV_1 or PEFR ≥80% predicted PEFR variability 20%–30%	One daily medication: **Antiinflammatory: either inhaled corticosteroid** (low doses) or **cromolyn or nedocromil** (children usually begin with a trial of cromolyn or nedocromil) Sustained-release theophylline to serum concentration of 5–15 β/mL is an alternative, but not preferred, therapy Zafirlukast or zileuton may also be considered for patients ≥12 years of age, although their position in therapy is not fully established	Short-acting bronchodilator: **inhaled β₂-agonists** as needed for symptoms Intensity of treatment will depend on severity of exacerbation Use of short-acting inhaled β₂-agonists on a daily basis, or increasing use, indicates the need for additional long-term–control therapy	Step 1 actions plus: Teach self-monitoring Refer to group education if available Review and update self-management plan

Step 1: Mild intermittent	Symptoms <2 times per wk Asymptomatic and normal PEF between exacerbations Exacerbations brief (from a few hours to a few days); intensity may vary	≤2 times per mo	FEV_1 or PEFR ≥80% predicted PEFR variability <20%	No daily medication needed	Short-acting bronchodilator: **inhaled β_2-agonists** as needed for symptoms Intensity of treatment will depend on severity of exacerbation Use of short-acting inhaled β_2-agonists more than 2 times per wk may indicate the need to initiate long-term–control therapy	Teach basic facts about asthma Teach inhaler/spacer/holding chamber technique Discuss roles of medications Develop self-management plan Develop action plan for when and how to take rescue actions, especially for patients with a history of severe exacerbations Discuss appropriate environmental control measures to avoid exposure to known allergens and irritants

[a]The presence of one of the features of severity is sufficient to place a patient in that category. An individual should be assigned to the most severe grade in which any feature occurs. The characteristics noted in this figure are general, and they may overlap because asthma is highly variable. Furthermore, an individual's classification may change over time.

[b]Patients at any level of severity can have mild, moderate, or severe exacerbations. Some patients with intermittent asthma experience severe and life-threatening exacerbations separated by long periods of normal lung function and no symptoms.

[c]Preferred treatments are in bold print.

Step down
→ Review treatment every 1 to 6 mo, a gradual stepwise reduction in treatment may be possible.

Step up
← If control is not maintained, consider step up. First, review patient medication technique, adherence, and environmental control (avoidance of allergens or other factors that contribute to asthma severity).

Note:

- The stepwise approach presents general guidelines to assist clinical decisionmaking; it is not intended to be a specific prescription. Asthma is highly variable; clinicians should tailor specific medication plans to the needs and circumstances of individual patients.

- Gain control as quickly as possible; then decrease treatment to the least medication necessary to maintain control. Gaining control may be accomplished by either starting treatment at the step most appropriate to the initial severity of the condition or starting at a higher level of therapy (e.g., a course of systemic corticosteroids or higher dose of inhaled corticosteroids).

- A rescue course of systemic corticosteroids may be needed at any time and at any step.

- Some patients with intermittent asthma experience severe and life-threatening exacerbations separated by long periods of normal lung function and no symptoms. This may be especially common with exacerbations provoked by respiratory infections. A short course of systemic corticosteroids is recommended.

- At each step, patients should control their environment to avoid or control factors that make their asthma worse (e.g., allergens, irritants); this requires specific diagnosis and education.

- Referral to an asthma specialist for consultation or comanagement is *recommended* if difficulties are found in achieving or maintaining control of asthma or if the patient requires step 4 care. Referral may be *considered* if the patient requires step 3 care (see also component 1-Initial Assessment and Diagnosis).

TABLE 18.4. *Management options for the treatment of exercise-induced asthma*

Nonpharmacologic	Pharmacologic
1. Environmental modification	1. Short-acting β-agonists
2. Appropriate choice of activity	2. Long-acting β-agonists (e.g., Salmeterol, Formoterol)
3. Warm-ups/cool downs	3. Cromolyn sodium, nedocromil
4. Training and conditioning	4. Leukotriene modifiers (e.g., Singulair, Accolate)
5. Facemasks	5. Inhaled corticosteroids

for inhaled corticosteroids. However, in the child who has only exercise-induced symptoms with normal pulmonary function, salmeterol may be used as prophylaxis. It is particularly useful when exercise takes place over hours (e.g., competitions, meets, and after school practices). Montelukast, a leukotriene modifier, has been shown to have a bronchoprotective effect against a cold air challenge in preschool children, as well as some exercise protection in school-aged children (20). This agent may be used in children as young as 2 years of age.

Rescue therapy is most commonly provided by a short-acting β-agonist, such as albuterol (5). Other drugs in this class include metaproterenol sulfate, bitolterol mesylate, pirbuterol acetate, and terbutaline. For athletes with normal baseline function and EIB, prophylaxis is most often achieved via the use of a short-acting inhaled β-agonist. It is given 15 to 30 minutes before exercise, and it is effective in 90% patients with EIB. These agents have a rapid onset of action, and they provide maximum protection within the first 1 to 2 hours, although they may remain effective for up to 3 to 6 hours (19). Long-acting β-agonists, such as salmeterol, have been used in children who require more sustained protection. Salmeterol is effective up to 10 to 12 hours (5), and it is available in both a diskus and a metered-dose inhaler. Concerns about the development of tachyphylaxis have been expressed. The clinician should consult the *Physician desk reference* for doses indicated by age. Formoterol is another long-acting β-agonist, but it has a shorter onset of action (approximately 15 minutes). It has recently been approved for exercise prophylaxis in patients who are 12 years of age and older. As with all medications, the risk benefits should be considered, and the precautions should be discussed with patients. Cromolyn sodium or nedocromil may be used as second line therapy for exercise prophylaxis, although the effectiveness is not as widespread as the short-acting bronchodilators. Combination with one of the short-acting β-agonists improves efficacy, and this may be used as an option in patients who fail to achieve control with single drug therapy (19).

The recommendation is that doses should be given 15 to 30 minutes prior to exertion (5). When the individual's inhaler technique is suboptimal, commercially available spacer devices should be used to improve drug delivery. Techniques employed to improve asthma control at baseline (e.g., inhaled corticosteroids and combination therapy) may also be indicated for athletes with moderate to severe EIB who do not respond to the above measures (21). When the clinician is caring for competitive athletes, he or she should refer to governing or regulatory agencies for lists of allowed, restricted, and banned medications.

CONCLUSION

A high suspicion for hyperreactive airways disorder should be maintained when evaluating student athletes. This includes preparticipation questionnaires about cough, wheezing, shortness of breath, fatigue, or chest pain following exertion. Particular attention should be paid to those athletes involved in cold air sports (e.g., ice skaters) and high endurance sports. The physical examination should include a comprehensive respiratory exam with evaluation for signs and symptoms of chronic respiratory disease and evidence of atopic disease. In cases where asthma is suspected, pulmonary function testing is indicated. When pulmonary function at rest is normal and the diagnosis remains in question, a therapeutic drug trial and/or exercise challenge test may help clarify the cause of the athlete's symptoms. Once a diagnosis of asthma or EIB is made, the physician and athlete should work together to tailor an asthma action plan that will allow the athlete to optimize participation in the sport of his or her choice.

REFERENCES

1. Clark C, Cochrane L. Physical activity and asthma. *Curr Opin Pulm Med* 1999;5:68–75.
2. Bevis M, Taylor B. What do school teachers know about asthma? *Arch Dis Child* 1990;65:622–625.
3. Busse W, Lemanski R. Asthma. *N Eng J Med* 2001;344: 350–362.

4. Hough DO, Dec KL. Exercise induced asthma and ana-phylaxis. *Sports Med* 1994;18:162–172.

5. Randolph C. Exercise induced asthma: update on patho-physiology, clinical diagnosis and treatment. *Curr Probl Pediatr* 1997;27:53–77.

6. Rossini G, Crocetti J, Rogers J, et al. Asthma deaths as-sociated with sporting events. *Am J Respir Crit Care Med* 2000;161:A623.

7. McFadden E. Exercise induced airway narrowing. *Al-lergy Principles and Practice* 1998;2:953–962.

8. Kyle J. Exercise pulmonary syndromes. *Med Clin North Am* 1994;78:413–421.

9. McFadden E. Exercise induced airway obstruction. *Clin Chest Med* 1995;16:671–682.

10. Smith B, LaBotz M. Pharmacologic treatment of exer-cise induced asthma, sports pharmacology. *Clin Sports Med* 1998;17:343–363.

11. Cabral AL, Conceicao GM, Fonseca-Guedes CH, et al. Exercise induced bronchospasm in children. *Am J Respir Crit Care Med* 1999;159:1819–1823.

12. Johnson R. Exercise induced asthma. In: Sallis R, Mas-simino F, eds. *Essentials of sports medicine*. New York: Mosby, 1997:64–68.

13. McFadden ER, Gilbert I. Exercise induced asthma. *N Eng J Med* 1994;330:1362–1367.

14. McArdle W, Kalch F, Kalch V. Exercise physiology. In: McArdle W, Kalch F, Kalch V, eds. *Exercise physiology: energy, nutrition and human performance*, 4th ed. Philadelphia: Williams & Wilkins, 1996:228 .

15. Kaplan TA, Montana E. Exercise induced broncho-spasm in nonasthmatic obese children. *Clin Pediatr* 1993;32:220–225.

16. Castro-Rodriguez JA, Holberg CJ, Morgan WJ, et al. In-creased incidence of asthma like symptoms in girls who become overweight or obese during the school years. *Am J Respir Crit Care Med* 2001;163:1344–1349.

17. Wamboldt M, Wamnoldt F. Psychiatric aspects of respi-ratory symptoms. In: Taussig L, Landau L, eds. *Pedi-atric respiratory medicine*. New York: Mosby, 1999: 1222–1234.

18. National Asthma Education and Prevention Program. *Expert panel report 2: guidelines for the diagnosis and management of asthma*. NIH Publication no. 97-4051. Bethesda, MD: National Heart, Lung, and Blood Insti-tute, 1997.

19. Rupp N. Diagnosis and management of exercise in-duced asthma. *The Physician and Sports Medicine* 1996;21:1–10.

20. Bisgaard H, Nielsen K. Bronchoprotection with a leukotriene receptor antagonist in asthmatic preschool children. *Am J Respir Crit Care Med* 2000;162:187–190.

21. Storms W, Joyner D. Update on exercise induced asthma: a report of the Olympic exercise asthma summit confer-ence. *The Physician and Sports Medicine* 1997;25:45–55.

19

Exercise-Induced Anaphylaxis

Mary B. Cataletto

Anaphylaxis is an acute medical emergency that can be caused by a variety of triggers. Exercise-induced anaphylaxis (EIA) is a relative newcomer that was first reported as a clinical entity by Matthews and Pan in 1970 (1). Classic, variant, and overlap forms of EIA have been described. Idiopathic anaphylaxis, food-induced anaphylaxis, and EIA may occur in the same child, and they are not mutually exclusive. Recognition of this entity on the playing field is critical, as prompt treatment may be lifesaving.

EIA is a form of urticaria (2). In contrast to the other urticarias in this class, it is seen with greater frequency in patients with allergic disease (50% to 66%) (3,4), and its occurrence is often unpredictable (2,5,6). EIA with no triggers other than exercise is the most common form. However, food-dependent subtypes have been described. Table 19.1 lists some of the foods commonly linked to EIA. Postprandial EIA has also been described (6a). This occurs in patients who exercise within several hours (generally fewer than 4 hours) of eating, regardless of their food choice. Episodes may also occur when an individual exercises after ingesting certain drugs, such as aspirin, nonsteroidal antiinflammatories, and certain cold preparations.

While the exact pathogenesis of EIA remains unclear, the clinical picture is similar to that of other type I hypersensitivity reactions. EIA is believed to result from the release of chemical mediators from mast cells and basophils.

Wade et al. (7) reported an epidemiologic study of patients with EIA. The age of onset varied between 4 and 74 years of age, with a median age of onset of 24.7 years. Episodes were more likely to occur if exercise took place in a humid environment or in those at the extremes of the temperature range. Food intake within 3 to 4 hours prior to exercise and aspirin ingestion in sensitive patients were found to increase the likelihood of occurrence. Shadick et al. (8) performed a similar questionnaire to look at the natural history of EIA over a 10-year period, and they found that the frequency of episodes tended either to stabilize or to de-

crease over time, largely as a result of diagnosis and the appropriate modification of exercise patterns.

CLINICAL SYNDROME

The clinical prodrome typically begins within the first 10 minutes of exercise, with fatigue and a generalized sensation of warmth. Pruritic erythematous lesions, which coalesce, occur. Moderate to large (10 to 15 mm) urticarial lesions and angioedema then become the predominant features. Respiratory symptoms result from upper airway edema and laryngospasm, and they may include a sensation of choking, audible stridor, and respiratory distress. Wheezing is a less frequent and inconsistent finding. Nausea, gastrointestinal colic, and vomiting can occur, and severe cases may result in cardiovascular collapse. Headaches have been described for up to 72 hours after an event (4). Serum histamine and tryptase levels are transiently elevated, and these can be useful for determining whether anaphylaxis has occurred (9), if the diagnosis is in doubt. In addition to environmental factors and prior food and medication ingestion, the type of exercise has also been implicated in the occurrence of EIA. Jogging is most frequently cited

TABLE 19.1. *Most commonly reported food triggers for exercise-induced anaphylaxis*

Shellfish
Alcohol
Tomatoes
Cheese
Celery
Strawberries
Milk
Wheat products
Peaches

From Shadick NA, Liang MH, Partridge AJ, et al. The natural history of exercise-induced anaphylaxis: survey results from a 10-year follow-up study. *J Allergy Clin Immunol* 1999;104:125, with permission.

(4,7,8), followed by aerobics, brisk walking, dancing, cycling, racket sports, swimming, and skiing (7,8). Less strenuous activities have also been reported to trigger episodes, but these reports are less frequent (< 2%) (8). The variant form of this syndrome is distinguished by skin lesions that are punctate and urticarial and that measure from 2 to 4 mm (4,10). This form occurs infrequently (i.e., approximately 10% of patients with EIA have this variant of the syndrome). It is also distinguished from the classic form by its precipitating factor, which is exercise alone. As with classic EIA, cardiovascular collapse may occur (10). Prompt recognition and treatment are essential.

ronment with capabilities for resuscitative emergencies. The most important historical features include the precipitating factors, the presence of hives, compatible pulmonary symptoms, and the clinical course of the event. The differential diagnoses include cholinergic urticaria and mastocytosis (10). The presentation of EIA is distinct from exercise-induced asthma, in which the primary symptoms are cough, wheezing, and shortness of breath and which does not produce the characteristic skin lesions EIA (10). In contrast to cholinergic urticaria, the hives in EIA are not precipitated by elevations in the core body temperature (2).

DIAGNOSIS

On the playing field, the diagnosis of anaphylaxis is usually clear-cut because of its symptoms and onset, which have been described above. In the office setting, the diagnosis of EIA is generally made by the history (4,10). In cases where questions exist, methacholine skin challenges, passive warming tests, exercise challenge, and skin prick tests may be helpful in evaluating the differential diagnosis (10). Exercise challenges should only be done in a controlled envi-

TREATMENT

Treatment of EIA is best accomplished initially by early recognition and management with medication and subsequently by vigilance and anticipatory guidance. Athletes with EIA should be taught to recognize the early warning signs (4). General guidelines for athletes with EIA are summarized in Table 19.2, and they include the following: waiting for 4 to 6 hours after a meal before exercising (4), avoiding foods or drugs known to trigger the condition before exercise

---

TABLE 19.2. *Treatment of anaphylaxis*

1. Immediate measures
   a. Administer aqueous epinephrine, 1:1,000, 0.3–0.5 mL (0.01 mL/kg in children, maximum of 0.3 mL/dose) subcutaneous (SC) or intramuscular (IM). Repeat as necessary every 15–20 min (×2) to control symptoms and maintain blood pressure.
   b. Provide aqueous epinephrine, 1:1,000, 0.1–0.3 mL in 10 mL of normal saline (1:100,000) intravenous (IV) over several minutes; repeat as necessary for anaphylaxis not responding to therapy. A dilution of 1:10,000 for IV infusion may be necessary.
2. General measures
   a. Place subject in recumbent position and elevate lower extremities.
   b. Establish and maintain airway (endotracheal tube may be necessary).
   c. Administer oxygen.
   d. Place a normal saline IV for fluid replacement and venous access. If severe hypotension exists, rapid infusion of volume expanders is necessary (colloid-containing solutions or saline).
3. Specific measures
   a. Aqueous epinephrine, 1:1,000, 0.1–0.3 mL, at reaction site delays antigen absorption.
   b. Give diphenhydramine (Benadryl), 5 mg/kg/d in divided doses, with maximum daily dosage of 300 mg for children and 400 mg for adults.
   c. Use a short-acting β-agonist (albuterol, [Xopenex]) may be used for bronchospasm.
   d. Administer dopamine (400 mg in 500 mL) in 5% dextrose in water [D5W], 2–20 μg/kg/min, if hypotension persists, with the rate titrated to maintain adequate blood pressure.
   e. Providing cimetidine (Tagamet), 300 mg, or ranitidine (Zantac), 50 mg, by IV over 10–15 min may also be useful. Rapid administration of cimetidine may cause hypotension, but ranitidine may be diluted to 20 mL and injected as a bolus over 5 min. Cimetidine use in children is discouraged, due to limited data.
   f. Give glucagon, 1–5 mg (20–30 μg/kg [maximum 1 mg] in children) by IV over 5 min and follow with an infusion of 5–15 μg/min. This may be useful when a β-blocker complicates anaphylaxis.
   g. Administering glucocorticoids, such as methylprednisolone (1–2 mg/kg for 24 hr), is usually not helpful in acute anaphylaxis, but it may be useful in delayed onset or protracted anaphylaxis.

From Kemp SF. Anaphylactic and anaphylactoid reactions in children and adolescents. *Pediatr Asthma Allergy Immunol* 2000;14:39, with permission.

(4,8,11), and modifying or avoiding outdoor exercise during pollen allergy season in pollen-sensitive patients (8) and around menses in young women affected with the syndrome (11). Use of a buddy system is important, especially in the case of long-distance runners or athletes who jog at off-hours or in remote areas. The partner should be trained in the use of the EpiPen kit, which the athlete should carry during training and exercise (4). Such patients should be advised to wear a MedicAlert identification. These can be obtained through Medicalert, Inc. (For the necklace and bracelet, call 1-800-432-5378; for sports band emblems, call 1-800-633-4025.) Patients who require emergency treatment with epinephrine should be taken to the nearest medical facility for evaluation.

Premedication with sodium cromoglycate or an antihistamine has had variable results (2,4,6,8,11), and it cannot be relied upon for prevention. Patients should be advised to stop exercising when they first experience any symptoms of EIA (11). However, once symptoms have reached the urticarial stage, medical intervention is required. Patients who have systemic reactions should be medicated with epinephrine and an H-1 antagonist. If this is not effective, the administration of epinephrine can be repeated, and an H-2 blocker may be added. In patients who present with dermatologic symptoms alone, hydroxyzine hydrochloride may be given (25 mg intramuscularly [i.m.] or by mouth [PO]), depending on symptom severity; alternatively, diphenhydramine hydrochloride may be administered (age 6 to12 years, 12.5 to 25 mg; over 12 years of age, 25 to 50 mg) (10). Terfenadine and acrivastine have also been used with variable success (10).

Acute anaphylaxis is a medical emergency. The time to intervention with appropriate treatment and supportive measures can be critical. The earlier that the patient receives treatment, the better the outcome is. Each school physician and each coach must have a protocol in place for the occurrence of EIA. Table 19.3 provides a sample treatment protocol for anaphylaxis (12). Severe manifestations of anaphylaxis include airway symptoms, and it may present as acute angioedema. Cardiovascular collapse can quickly ensue. After beginning with epinephrine, cardiopulmonary resuscitation is managed using the fundamental tools of basic life support. The first priority is airway management. Airways are evaluated as open, maintainable, and unmaintainable; and they are handled accordingly. If the patient is breathing, attention to the work of breathing and the airway sounds will direct the treatment. For example, if the patient has progressively worsening stridor, airway intervention with intubation may be necessary. In the emergency department, racemic

TABLE 19.3. *Anticipatory guidance*

1. Avoid exercise for 6 hr following meals or the ingestion of known triggers.
2. Modify or avoid exercise during pollen season if the patient is pollen-sensitive with a history of exercise-induced anaphylaxis.
3. Learn to identify prodromal symptoms; stop exercise when they are identified.
4. Prepare an anaphylaxis plan with the primary care physician.
5. Use the buddy system.
6. Discuss MedicAlert identification with the primary care physician.
7. Carry Benadryl and epinephrine.
8. Establish a treatment protocol with coaches and team physicians.

epinephrine may be given. Supplemental oxygen is necessary whenever the airway is compromised or if the work of breathing is acutely increased.

Intravenous lines should be placed for access and for fluid administration as indicated by the patient's clinical condition. Chest compressions are administered according to the American Heart Association pediatric guidelines. Guidelines for fluid administration are outlined in Table 19.3. The appropriate sized EpiPen (EpiPen contains a single dose of 0.3 mg of 1:1,000 strength epinephrine; EpiPen Jr. contains a single dose of 0.15 mg of 1:1,000 strength epinephrine and is recommended for children weighing less than 30 kg or in heavier patients in whom the full dose is contraindicated) should administered. It is given i.m., and it can be administered through the clothing. A second injector should be available, in case it is needed. Antihistamines should be administered to all patients with anaphylaxis. While epinephrine autoinjectors are often preferred because of their easy availability, ease of use, and rapid onset, the potential for underdosing and overdosing exists because of the weight spectrum seen in pediatrics (13). Epinephrine inhalations have not been shown to be effective substitutes (14). The combination of an H-1 and an H-2 blocking agent is superior to a single agent. The combination therapy should be continued until symptoms resolve. Corticosteroids are effective in preventing a late phase response.

Although EIA does not occur frequently in children, untreated anaphylaxis can result in significant morbidity and mortality. The diagnosis should be considered in all children presenting with urticaria and respiratory symptoms associated with exercise and in those children who become acutely hypotensive with exercise.

REFERENCES

1. Matthews KP, Pan PM. Postexercise hyperhistaminemia, dermatographia and wheezing. *Ann Intern Med* 1970;72:241–249.
2. Sheffer A, Soter N, McFadden ER, et al. Exercise induced anaphylaxis: a distinct form of physical allergy. *J Allergy Clin Immunol* 1983;71:311–316.
3. Kaplan AP. Urticaria and angioedema. In: Middleton E, Reed C, Ellis EF, et al, eds. *Allergy principles and practice*. New York: Mosby, 1998:1111.
4. Castells M, Horan R, Sheffer A. Exercise induced anaphylaxis. *Clin Rev Allergy Immunol* 1999;17:413–424.
5. Castells M, Horan R, Ewan P, et al. Anaphylaxis. In: Holgate S, Church M, Lichenstein L, eds. *Allergy*. New York: Mosby, 2001:163–173.
6. Hough D, Dec K. Exercise induced asthma and anaphylaxis. *Sports Med* 1994;18:162–172.
6a. Novey H, Fairshter R, Salness K, et al. Postprandial exercise induced anaphylaxis. *J Allergy Clin Immunol* 1983;71:498–504.
7. Wade J, Liang M, Sheffer A. Exercise induced anaphylaxis: epidemiologic observations. In: Tauber AI, Wintroub BU, Simon AS, eds. *Biochemistry of the acute allergic reaction—Fifth International Symposium*. New York: Alan R. Liss, Inc., 1989:175–182.
8. Shadick NA, Liang MH, Partridge AJ, et al. The natural history of exercise induced anaphylaxis: survey results from a ten-year follow-up study. *J Allergy Clin Immunol* 1999;104:123–127.
9. O'Dowd L, Zweiman B. Anaphylaxis. In: *UptoDate Online* 2000. Accessed May 2002.
10. Volcheck G, Li J. Exercise induced urticaria and anaphylaxis. *Mayo Clinic Proc* 1997:72:140–147.
11. Kyle J. Exercise induced pulmonary syndromes. *Med Clin North Am* 1994;78:413–421.
12. Kemp SF. Anaphylactic and anaphylactoid reactions in children and adolescents. *Pediatr Asthma Allergy Immunol* 2000;14:33–45.
13. Simons FE, Peterson S, Black C. Epinephrine dispensing for the outpatient treatment of anaphylaxis in infants and children: a population based study. *Ann Allergy Asthma Immunol* 2001;86:622–626.
14. Simons FE, Gu X, Johnston L, et al. Can epinephrine inhalations be substituted for epinephrine injections in children at risk for systemic anaphylaxis? *Pediatrics* 2000;106:1040–1044.

20

Obesity

Kim Edward LeBlanc

The disturbing trend toward increasing body weight in the United States spares no particular group. In fact, obesity has become the most common metabolic disorder in the United States, and its incidence is increasing. Furthermore, the World Health Organization identifies a "global epidemic of obesity." Commonly, overweight and obese children and adolescents grow up to be overweight and/or obese adults, or, to state this another way, obese adults often have a history of childhood obesity. Therefore, beginning the treatment for obesity in the younger years would seem prudent. As with any other disease state, prevention is the best method for decreasing the rate of obesity and for halting the spread of this disease state.

DEFINITION

Multiple ways of defining obesity exist, and, therefore, no universally accepted definition has been formulated. Most researchers and clinicians use body mass index (BMI) to define obesity. Using this method, obesity in children is defined as BMI greater than the 85th percentile, with severe obesity defined as BMI greater than the 95th percentile. Some experts use a weight for height greater than 120% of ideal body weight (1). Strict definitions may not always prove entirely useful, however. Extremely muscular children or adolescents may have a BMI that would place them in the obese category, without any evidence of excessive body fat. Furthermore, African-American children generally have less body fat than white children (2).

EPIDEMIOLOGY

The incidence of pediatric obesity is steadily increasing at an alarming rate. Recent data indicates that, based on the definition as a BMI greater than the 95th percentile, 11% of 6-year-old to 11-year-old children and 10.8% of 12-year-old to 17-year-old children are obese. If the 85th percentile is used, the incidence increases markedly to 22.3% and 21.7%, respectively. This compares to 5.2% and 15.1% in the 1960s when the 95th and 85th percentiles are applied

to the data as standards (3). Moreover, certain populations (e.g., Native American, Hispanic, and African-American) tend to have more obesity than others (4).

PATHOPHYSIOLOGY

Simply stated, obesity is excess body fat. Obesity results whenever an imbalance of energy intake and energy expenditure occurs (i.e., if the individual eats more calories than he or she consumes, his or her body fat composition increases). Therefore, body fat content is determined by energy balance. This is the determining factor in whether body fat increases, decreases, or remains the same.

Fat cells increase in both number and size during childhood. Formerly, the thinking was that, once adulthood was realized, the number of fat cells remained the same with only an increase in cell size. However, evidence now supports the concept that this is not the case. New fat cell growth (e.g., hyperplasia) does occur in adults. This means that an obese child will be able to increase the cell number into his or her adult life, compounding the problem of obesity management even further. Moreover, the number of fat cells remains constant, while the size (but not the total number) of fat cells may diminish. Therefore, the prevention of the initial development of fat cells during the childhood years is extremely important.

Some endogenous causes of obesity, such as hypothalamic disorders or genetic syndromes, are observed. Managing some of these requires the assistance of an endocrinologist. However, in the pediatric population, organic causes of obesity are rare. The primary care physician should be able to rule out most of these disorders with a thorough history and physical examination.

CONSEQUENCES OF OBESITY IN CHILDHOOD AND ADOLESCENCE

Many well-known health consequences of obesity are observed in this younger population. These have both short-term and long-term adverse effects. A number of medical conditions have been associated with obesity in children, including sleep apnea, pseudotumor cerebri, and a slipped capital femoral epiphysis. In addition, these children are prone to suffer psychologic stresses and the potential for impaired emotional development (5). Other significant concerns include the development of such diseases as hyperlipidemia, insulin resistance, heart disease, hypertension, and cholelithiasis. For example, in a recent report, over 90% of type 2 diabetes mellitus patients were associated with a BMI greater than the 95th percentile (6).

Obese children tend to become obese adults. However, in early childhood, less correlation is seen between the child's weight and adult obesity. At this age, the parents' weight is a more reliable predictor of the child's future weight. By the time the child has reached the second decade of his or her life, the child's own weight does become important in predicting the likelihood of his or her potential for being an obese adult (7).

EVALUATION OF THE OBESE CHILD

As was noted above, several morbid states are associated with obesity in childhood. The possible presence of these entities must be assessed when evaluating an obese child. This includes assessing orthopedic problems, cardiovascular risk factors, and skin problems (e.g., intertrigo), as well as possible psychologic or emotional difficulties. In particular, screening tests should be performed to assess the possibility of diabetes mellitus, insulin resistance, or hyperlipidemia.

During the physical examination, several details can be used to characterize the obesity as idiopathic or endogenous. In the *idiopathic* type of obesity, these include normal or advanced bone age, normal mental functioning, a positive family history of obesity, stature above the 50th percentile usually, and an otherwise normal physical examination. These are contrasted with the findings noted in *endogenous* obesity, which include delayed bone age, mental impairment, negative family history in general, stature less than the 5th percentile, and associated stigmata on physical examination (1).

Assessing the child's level of physical activity is crucial. Coincident with this should be a determination of how much time the child spends watching television or using the computer.

Dietary history is important for ascertaining the knowledge base and the perceptions of both the child and parents. Often, misconceptions, as well as erroneous nutritional beliefs and trends, may be uncovered.

TREATMENT

As with many diseases, prevention is the best way to manage obesity. This should be addressed during well-child examinations and during other visits throughout the child's life. Once obesity has been diagnosed, a plan should be established to achieve success in weight loss. Although many aspects are part of losing weight, five basic elements must be included in any weight loss plan. These include the following: (a) parental and family participation (e.g., parents should buy the food and monitor television and computer use), (b) reasonable and attainable weight loss goals (loss of 1 lb per week), (c) medical nutritional therapy (the focus should be education of the child and family, with avoidance of strict dietary regimens), (d) focus on avoiding high-fat foods and the use of healthy snacks, and (e) behavior modification and increasing physical activity (begin slowly with the goal of 20 to 30 minutes of daily activity, *excluding* school activity) (8).

The success or failure of any therapeutic intervention depends on its effect on overall energy balance. Less intake, more energy expenditure, or preferably both should be part of the regimen. Regardless of what is done, this element must be included for any real hope of success.

Healthy People 2010 has been used to describe the initiative suggested by many of the nation's leading health experts to assist health professionals in this difficult endeavor. This has been supported by the Centers for Disease Control and Prevention, as reported by Anderson (9). Healthy People 2010 helps to assist patients and physicians alike with enhancement of the effort to achieve a healthier and less overweight society.

ROLE OF PROPER NUTRITION AND EXERCISE IN MANAGING CHILDHOOD OBESITY

Although dietary caloric restriction is one of the essential components of any successful weight loss program, one must temper this course of action with the knowledge that some accommodation must be made for the growing child and young athlete. All children and, in particular, young athletes must maintain adequate nutrition. This is critical for the maintenance of health and for assuring optimal performance.

Some caloric restrictions may be required in order to achieve weight loss of between ½ and 1 lb per week. In addition, exercise should be incorporated into the weekly routine of the child or adolescent. This should be done at least three times a week (preferably every school day), for a minimum of 20 to

30 minutes of aerobic activity. In order to lose 1 lb of weight, a deficit of 3,500 calories must be accumulated over time. This should be a combination of decreased caloric intake and increased energy expenditure. In this population, having more activity with less dieting is preferable as the principal mode of achieving a caloric deficit.

For the active and growing athlete, some special considerations should be remembered. Children and adolescents must maintain a positive nitrogen balance (i.e., they must take in more protein than they expend) to insure proper growth and development. This translates into an increased protein requirement for this age group. In the growing athlete, the situation becomes complicated because exercise has significant effects on protein metabolism. Following exercise, protein degradation is enhanced, while the synthesis of protein is diminished. If an adequate recovery time is allowed, this process is reversed. The primary care physician should be mindful of this process when counseling these pediatric patients. The recommended daily allowance (RDA) for protein in adults is 0.8 to 1.0 g per kg of protein per day, according to a 1989 recommendation from the National Research Council. These requirements are increased in childhood and adolescence. Children between the ages of 7 and 10 years should consume 1.1 to 1.2 g per kg per day, while the recommendation for those between the ages of 11 and 14 is 1.0 g per kg per day (10). Adult levels begin at the age of 15.

Fat is the major storage form of energy in the body. Along with carbohydrates, it is the primary fuel supply for exercise metabolism. Consequently, fat is a requirement in the diet. Some evidence indicates that children use relatively more fat and less carbohydrates than do adolescents or adults. The significance of this is not clear at this time. However, no evidence suggests that children and/or adolescents should consume more than 30% of their dietary intake as fat. If weight loss is to be achieved, limiting fat intake to lesser amounts would be a prudent starting point (11).

Regardless of age, carbohydrates remain the critical nutrient for the exercising individual. Carbohydrates represent the major fuel for muscle contraction. Children use more energy per kilogram of body weight during various athletic events than adults do. Therefore, the carbohydrate and energy requirements of children and adolescents should be increased. In general, children between the ages of 8 and 10 years should add 20% to 25% to adult values, and children between the ages of 11 and 14 years should add 10% to 15% to adult values for energy expenditure (11). Here too, if weight loss is to be achieved, using rea-sonably lesser amounts will help attain this goal. Beyond the age of 14, the amounts should be the same as those recommended for the adult.

RISKS OF THE EXERCISING OBESE CHILD

As with any age group, physical activity may make the child susceptible to injury. This is particularly true for someone who has been sedentary and who is not accustomed to exercise. These patients, along with their parents, should be advised to progress slowly in achieving higher levels of fitness. The overweight child, in particular, may have some problems with endurance, balance, and muscle use, leading to an increased risk of overuse injuries, as he or she endures the stresses of physical activity, as well as the added stress of excess weight. An overweight child may complain more of muscle strains and joint aches and pains. In addition, an overweight child may complain more of dyspnea and easy fatigability. These complaints should be expected, and anticipatory guidance should be given.

CONCLUSION

While physiologic responses to exercise in children and adolescents may be similar to adults, the differences must be taken into account when making dietary intake recommendations. Obese children should be encouraged to exercise and to follow proper dietary regimens. Any successful weight loss program must include the participation and support of parents and coaches. Goals should be easily attainable and realistic, and they should be clearly stated. Beginning these recommendations at an early age will help in the prevention of adult obesity and the attendant comorbid conditions (e.g., diabetes, hypertension, hyperlipidemia).

REFERENCES

1. Williams CL, Campanaro LA, Squillace M, et al. Management of childhood obesity in pediatric patients. *Ann N Y Acad Sci* 1997;817:225–240.
2. Dietz WH, Bellizzi MC. The use of body mass index to assess obesity in children. *Am J Clin Nutr* 1999;70:123S–125S.
3. Troiano RP, Flegal KM, Kuczmarski RJ, et al. Overweight prevalence and trends for children and adolescents. The National Health and Nutrition Examination Surveys, 1963–1991. *Arch Pediatr Adolesc Med* 1995;149:1085–1091.
4. Moran RC. Evaluation and treatment of childhood obesity. *Am Fam Physician* 1999;59:861–868.
5. Jelalian E, Saelens BE. Empirically supported treatments

in pediatric psychology: pediatric obesity. *J Pediatr Psychol* 1999;24:223–248.

6. Rosenbloom RL, Joe JR, Young RS, et al. Emerging epidemic of type 2 diabetes in youth. *Diabetes Care* 1999;22:345–354.

7. Whitaker RC, Wright JA, Pepe MS, et al. Predicting obesity in young adulthood from childhood and parental obesity. *N Engl J Med* 1997;337:869–873.

8. Barlow SE, Dietz WH. Obesity evaluation and treatment: Expert Committee recommendations. *Pediatrics* 1998;102:E29.

9. Anderson RE. Healthy people 2010. *The Physician and Sports Medicine* 2000:28:7–93.

10. Ziegler PJ, Khoo CS, Kris-Etherton PM, et al. Nutritional status of nationally ranked junior US figure skaters. *J Am Diet Assoc* 1998;98:809–811.

11. Bar-Or O. Nutrition for child and adolescent athletes. *Sports Science Exchange* 2000;13:1–4.

21

Epilepsy and the Young Athlete

William Michael Brown

Epilepsy is a common neurologic disorder that affects more than 1 million people in the United States today. It has been characterized as recurrent seizures that are unrelated to fever or an acute cerebral insult. Epilepsy has been well documented since ancient times. Studies have shown that approximately 10% of the population will have a seizure at some point in their lifetime and that about 3% will develop epilepsy by the age of 70 (1). However, most people who develop epilepsy have their first seizure when they are young. Although seizures rarely occur during or immediately following exercise, young athletes typically have been unfairly limited or restricted because of their epilepsy. In actuality, a regular exercise program is now felt to be beneficial in controlling seizures, and most people with epilepsy can participate in physical activity safely.

COMMON TYPES OF EPILEPSY IN YOUNG ATHLETES

The diagnosis of epilepsy requires at least two documented seizures. Generally speaking, seizures can be divided into three main categories: partial, generalized, and unclassified (Table 21.1). An understanding of the type of seizure disorder is necessary in order to make an accurate prognosis for the athlete. The patient with generalized tonic–clonic epilepsy has a condition that is usually readily controlled with anticonvulsants, whereas the patient with partial seizures may fare less well. One must realize that most children diagnosed with epilepsy at an early age will become free of seizures and that anticonvulsant medication will be discontinued by adulthood.

GENERAL OVERVIEW OF THE TREATMENT OF EPILEPSY

The goals in managing patients with epilepsy are straightforward as follows: (a) eliminate seizures completely; (b) avoid medication side effects; and (c) restore patients to physical, mental, and social health (2). Although both medical and surgical treatments of epilepsy have made significant advances in the past 5 to 10 years, antiepileptic drugs remain the cornerstone of therapy (Table 21.2). For most types of seizures, multiple antiepileptic drugs are available, but the potential side effects to the athlete must be considered.

EFFECTS OF ANTIEPILEPTIC DRUGS ON EXERCISE PHYSIOLOGY

The following two questions can be used to explore this topic: (a) how do antiepileptic drugs affect exercise physiology and (b) does exercise affect the action of antiepileptic drugs? Undoubtedly, all antiepileptic drugs have both common and rare side effects, and these differ depending on the mechanism of action of

TABLE 21.1. *International classification of epileptic seizures*

Partial seizures
  Simple partial (consciousness retained)
    Motor
    Sensory
    Autonomic
    Psychic
  Complex partial (consciousness impaired)
    Simple partial, followed by impaired
      consciousness
    Consciousness impaired at onset
  Partial seizures with secondary generalization
Generalized seizures
  Absences
    Typical
    Atypical
  Generalized tonic–clonic
  Tonic
  Clonic
  Myoclonic
  Atonic
  Infantile spasms
Unclassified seizures

TABLE 21.2. *Antiepileptic agents*

Agent	Decade of clinical introduction
Phenobarbital	1910s
Phenytoin	1930s
Primidone	1950s
Carbamazepine	1960s
Diazepam	1960s
Ethosuximide	1960s
Valproate	1960s
Clonazepam	1970s
Lorazepam	1970s
Felbamate	1990s
Gabapentin	1990s
Lamotrigine	1990s
Oxcarbazepine	1990s
Tiagabine	1990s
Topiramate	1990s
Vigabatrin	1990s
Zonisamide	1990s

the drug. The most commonly reported side effects to this category of drugs are sedation, cognitive dysfunction, ataxia, dizziness, diplopia, nausea and vomiting, headache, and fatigue. These side effects may be detrimental to athletic participation, but tolerance to these effects usually develops over time. Meanwhile, the liver is almost exclusively the site of metabolization of antiepileptic drugs. Since exercise is thought to induce the activity of hepatic enzymes, concern has been raised about the effects of exercise on antiepileptic pharmacokinetics. Most studies have not shown a significant fluctuation in serum levels of antiepileptic drugs with either exercise or athletic training (3).

EFFECTS OF VARIOUS STIMULI IN PROVOKING SEIZURE ACTIVITY

Although multiple factors are clearly known to provoke seizure activity, exercise is not one of them. In actuality, a regular physical exercise program may help in preventing seizure activity and may aid in improving seizure control (4). Of all the stimuli known to provoke seizure activity, fatigue is the one most likely to occur with exercise. In addition to fatigue, the clinician should always be concerned about the possibility of alcohol or drug use or abuse. Although head trauma during physical activity is considered a minor stimulus, it cannot be ignored. Hyperventilation, hyperthermia, and photic stimulation have also been reported to increase the risk of seizure activity. As with diabetic therapy, the likelihood of a young or adolescent athlete neglecting to take the prescribed medications should be anticipated, and counseling should be initiated early to prevent such events (5).

RESTRICTIONS FOR EXERCISE IN YOUNG ATHLETES WITH EPILEPSY

Over the past 30 years, recommendations concerning athletes with epilepsy have changed radically. In the late 1960s, initial recommendations for those with epilepsy were to avoid not only contact sports but noncontact sports as well. As medical knowledge and experience with athletes with convulsive disorders improved, the medical community now not only realizes the benefits of regular exercise for those with epilepsy, but it also understands the potential psychologic consequences of limiting athletic participation (6). Still, the need for some restrictions does exist in certain situations. Common sense is an integral ingredient when evaluating the need for athletic restrictions. Since the fact that regular physical activity will not precipitate seizures is now known, athletes with infrequent and well-controlled seizures probably will not require any limitations. On the other hand, athletes with frequent seizure activity or newly diagnosed epilepsy should have appropriate restrictions in place until seizure control has been established (see Chapter 2) (7). The recommendations of numerous neurologists, sports medicine physicians, and primary care physicians are compiled in Table 21.3.

Common sense must prevail in making these decisions. Epileptic athletes should only participate in aquatic sports when a trained lifeguard is present. Recreational swimming does carry a fourfold increased risk of drowning for epileptics, when compared to the general population (1). Falls, which are always possible in sports involving heights, may lead to extremely serious injuries, and thus they may re-

TABLE 21.3. *Recommendations for athletic participation for well-controlled epilepsy*

Recommended	Questionable or with limitations	Contraindicated
Baseball	Climbing	Boxing
Basketball	Diving	Motor sports
Cycling	Swimming	Automobile
Football	Water polo	Motorcycle
Gymnastics	Water skiing	Boat racing
Horseback riding		Scuba diving
Karate		Ski jumping
Long distance running		Sky diving
Skating and/or rollerblading		
Snow skiing		
Soccer		
Wrestling		

quire setting certain limitations or taking special pre-cautions. Clearly, certain sports, such as motor sports, are contraindicated—not only because of the risk posed to the athlete, but also because of the risk to the other participants and spectators.

TREATMENT APPROACH TO THE YOUNG ATHLETE WITH EPILEPSY

First and foremost, the treatment approach to the young athlete with epilepsy should consist of getting the convulsive disorder under excellent control. The athlete must be completely convinced of the impor-tance of strict adherence to, and compliance with, his or her anticonvulsant medication regimen. However, even when compliance is excellent, breakthrough seizures can occur, and they should be anticipated. Athletic trainers and coaching personnel should be familiar with an athlete's convulsive condition, and they must be trained in the use and administration of antiepileptic medication, as well as in basic medical care and cardiopulmonary resuscitation. The most common serious injuries from generalized tonic–clonic seizures include inferior dislocation of the shoulder, as well as fractures of the humeral neck, femoral trochanter, clavicle, and ankle. Thus, the care of such injuries must be understood, and appropriate medical supplies for their treatment should be present (6). As was stated above, personnel trained in aquatic lifesaving techniques must always supervise aquatic sports. Young athletes with epilepsy should be en-couraged to participate in activities that do not pose a threat to themselves or to spectators. Medically trained personnel should be present and prepared to intervene when necessary (see Chapter 27).

SUMMARY

Without a doubt, numerous pieces of evidence exist to support the belief that exercise itself does not act as a seizure precipitant. In fact, ample studies demon-strate the potential seizure protection that is offered by regular physical exercise. The most serious hazard of epilepsy is often not the seizures *per se*, nor the per-ceived risk of injury during athletic competition, but

rather, it is the associated emotional aberrations that are prone to develop in patients with this disorder (8). When the proper precautions are taken, specific limi-tations are followed, and common sense is applied, the young athlete whose convulsive disorder is under ex-cellent control should never be denied the opportunity to experience the physical, mental, and psychologic benefits of physical exercise and athletic competition.

ADDITIONAL READING

American Academy of Pediatrics Committee on Children with Handicaps. Sports and the child with epilepsy. *Pedi-atrics* 1983;72:884–885.
Bennett DR. Epilepsy and the athlete. In: Jordan BD, Tsairus P, Warren RF, eds. *Sports neurology*. Rockville, CO: Aspen Publishers, 1989:116–126.
Gates JR. Epilepsy and sports participation. *The Physician and Sports Medicine* 1991;19:98–104.
Kemp AM, Silbert JR. Epilepsy in children and the risk of drowning. *Arch Dis Child* 1993;68:684–685.
Meythaler JM, Yablon SA. Antiepileptic drugs. *Phys Med Rehabil Clin N Am* 1999;10:275–300.
Nakken KO. Physical exercise in outpatients with epilepsy. *Epilepsia* 1999;40:643–651.
Starreveld E, Starreveld AA. Antiepileptic drugs. Status epilepticus current concepts and management. *Can Fam Physician* 2000;46:1817–1823.

REFERENCES

1. Gates JR, Spriegel RH. Epilepsy, sports, and exercise. *Sports Med* 1993;15:1–5.
2. Bazil CW, Pedley TA. Advances in the medical treat-ment of epilepsy. *Ann Rev Med* 1998;49:135–162.
3. Nakken KO, Bjorholt PG, Johannessen SI, et al. Effect of physical training on aerobic capacity, seizure occur-rence, and serum level of antiepileptic drugs in adults with epilepsy. *Epilepsia* 1990;31:88–94.
4. Bennett DR. The athlete with epilepsy. In: Mellion MB, ed. *Sports medicine secrets*. Philadelphia: Hanley & Belfus, 1994;184–186.
5. Howe WB. The athlete with chronic illness. In: Birrer RB, ed. *Sports medicine for the primary care physician*, 2nd ed. Boca Raton, FL: CRC Press, 1994:197–205.
6. Cantu RC. Epilepsy and athletics. *Clin Sports Med* 1998;17:61–69.
7. Commission of Pediatrics of the International League Against Epilepsy. Restrictions for children with epilepsy. *Epilepsia* 1997;38:1054–1056.
8. Livingston S. Epilepsy and sports [Editorial]. *Am Fam Physician* 1978;17:67–69.

22

Renal Problems

Edward R. Gillett and Rachel A. Dunnagan

Even with wide fluctuations in a person's activity level and fluid intake, the kidneys precisely regulate body fluid volume and osmolality, maintain the body's electrolytes and pH, and process metabolic end products. They also produce and secrete important hormones, such as renin, erythropoietin, and the metabolically active form of vitamin D (1). Strenuous exercise may markedly affect renal function. The physician must determine whether this effect is physiologic or pathologic.

IMPACT OF EXERCISE ON RENAL FUNCTION

The kidneys typically receive 20% of the cardiac output, and they consume approximately 10% of the oxygen needed for resting metabolism (2). Oxygen consumption increases with exercise, but renal perfusion decreases as adrenaline and noradrenalin activate the sympathetic nervous system and cause vasoconstriction (3). The extent of change is relative to the intensity of the exercise. Strenuous exercise can reduce renal flow by up to 75% (3). Subsequently, the glomerular filtration rate (GFR) decreases, and the filtration fraction (FF) increases. Circulating levels of antidiuretic hormone increase, causing both urine flow and water excretion to decrease. Renin release increases with adrenergic stimulation, and, consequently, angiotensin and aldosterone increase. Increased aldosterone contributes to sodium retention by decreasing filtered sodium excretion and increasing tubular absorption. This minimizes excretion of sodium and other urinary electrolytes, such as chloride, calcium, phosphorus, and potassium (3,4). In addition, strenuous exercise can produce renal abnormalities secondary to trauma.

SPECIFIC RENAL PROBLEMS

Proteinuria

Proteinuria is one of the most common nonpathologic renal abnormalities found in athletes of all ages.

Alyea et al. (5) found proteinuria in 70% to 80% of the athletes studied. Other sources have reported it in up to 100% of runners (6). Evidence of exercise-induced proteinuria has been recognized for almost a century, but Gardner (4) did not coin the phrase "athletic pseudonephritis" to distinguish between similar urinary findings in healthy athletes versus patients with renal disease until 1955. These findings can include proteinuria, myoglobinuria, hematuria, and casts. When the above abnormalities are mild, asymptomatic, and transient, athletic pseudonephritis is the most likely etiology. This phenomenon has been well documented in children. Houser et al. (7) studied urinary protein excretion in children at rest, with normal daily activities, and after strenuous exercise. A statistically significant increase in postexercise protein excretion in both sexes was noted.

Even in the absence of exercise, proteinuria can be a normal finding in children and adolescents (8). Protein leaks from the tubules in an amount that decreases relative to a child's body surface area as that child ages and the kidneys mature. By the age of 16 years, physiologic proteinuria can average 83 mg per day and can range from 22 to 181 mg per meter squared per 24 hours (8). Approximately 10% of healthy adolescents have been estimated to have mild proteinuria.

One must always investigate proteinuria, as it may herald a serious underlying condition. Evaluation usually begins with urine dipstick analysis. This result can be falsely negative in dilute urine that has a specific gravity of less than 1.010. It can be falsely positive if the urine is contaminated with blood, mucus, pus, semen, or vaginal secretions or if the pH is greater than 7.0 (8). The dipstick can detect as little as 30 mg per dL of protein. The results correlate with the following protein amount (in mg per dL): 1+ = 30; 2+ = 100; 3+ = 300; 4+ = 1,000.

A positive urine dipstick should be repeated after rest on two occasions. The estimation is that 30% to 50% of resting dipstick urinalyses will be negative (8). Transient asymptomatic proteinuria is benign, largely due to increased glomerular permeability and decreased tubular resorption; it is commonly seen with normal daily activity and exercise (7). Patients with transient asymptomatic proteinuria can be reassured and followed routinely. No special precautions or activity restrictions are required.

If, on the other hand, two or more of three urine samples are positive for protein, a more detailed evaluation is indicated. The physician should obtain a thorough history, with attention to any injuries, signs of physical abuse, chronic problems, or recent throat or skin infections. The family history should be

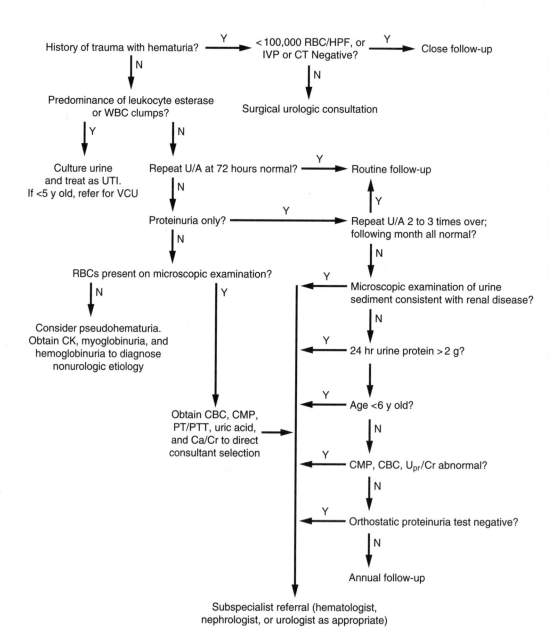

FIG. 22.1. Athlete presenting with initial episode of proteinuria or hematuria. Abbreviations: Ca/Cr, calcium to creatine ratio; CBC, complete blood count; CK, creatine kinase; CMP, chemistry metabolic profile; CT, computed tomography; HPF, high powered field; IVP, intravenous pyelogram; PT/PTT, prothrombin time/partial thromboplastin time; RBC, red blood cell; U/A, urine analysis; U$_{pr}$/Cr, urinary protein to creatine ratio; UTI, urinary tract infection; VCU, voiding cystourethrogram; WBC, white blood cells.

searched for clues that suggest polycystic kidney disease, lupus, or other renal problems. The use of medications, over-the-counter drugs, supplements, and illegal substances should be noted. The physical examination should include investigations for hypertension, pallor, skin lesions, edema, abdominal masses, and genitourinary (GU) tract abnormalities. Laboratory studies commonly begin with a microscopic urinalysis and the determination of the urinary protein to creatinine ratio (UPr/Cr). This ratio is indicative of renal function and can be used to estimate 24-hour urine protein as follows (9,10):

$$\text{total urine protein (gm/m}^2 \cdot \text{day)} = 0.63 \times (\text{UPr/Cr}).$$

The UPr/Cr and subsequent calculation is often easier to obtain and more accurate than a 24-hour collection of urine from a pediatric patient, although both methods are acceptable. Other helpful studies include serum electrolytes, blood urea nitrogen (BUN), creatinine (Cr), protein, albumin, complement (C3), and complete blood count (CBC).

If all of the above tests are normal in a child older than 6 years of age who displays persistent proteinuria, the most likely diagnosis is orthostatic or postural proteinuria. This is verified by collecting urine immediately upon awakening that is protein-free, followed by collecting urine with a UPr/Cr of less than 1.0 (or a 24-hour urine protein of less than 1 g) over the next 12 hours. The prognosis for orthostatic proteinuria is excellent, and these children may be followed yearly.

If the orthostatic test is negative or if the child is younger than 6 years of age, a renal ultrasound may detect anatomic abnormalities, such as polycystic kidney disease, renal dysplasia, or hydronephrosis. If any of the other blood tests are abnormal, the likelihood of glomerular disease is higher. Electrolyte abnormalities indicate more serious renal disease. An elevated Cr can be seen with several forms of nephropathy and nephritis. Low serum protein and a UPr/Cr greater than 3.0 suggest nephrotic syndrome. A low C3 level may be seen with lupus or acute glomerulonephritis. All of these findings warrant consultation with a pediatric nephrologist for further evaluation and possible renal biopsy (Fig. 22.1).

Hematuria

Blood in the urine is another common finding in pediatric athletes. This may be microscopic or grossly visible. The occurrence may be asymptomatic, or it may accompany flank pain, pelvic pain, or dysuria. In athletes with no underlying GU abnormalities, hematuria commonly follows strenuous exercise, and it re-solves within 48 to 72 hours. Hematuria has been specifically linked to running, swimming, rowing, boxing, soccer, football, lacrosse, hockey, and track. It has been reported in ranges of 11% to 100% of athletes. The extent of hematuria increases with the intensity and duration of activity (9).

Exercise-induced hematuria affects both males and females through traumatic and nontraumatic effects on the GU system. The renal vasculature, renal parenchyma, bladder, and urethra sometimes undergo direct trauma, which can cause insignificant changes or life-threatening conditions. (Chapter 31 provides additional information.) Even in the absence of obvious injury, the GU system can suffer repetitive microtrauma from high impact or high stress activities. For example, a completely empty bladder is commonly contused internally as the posterior wall repeatedly hits the fixed trigone, and bleeding ensues. Alternatively, nontraumatic etiologies exist. As exercise intensity increases, renal perfusion decreases, thereby creating an environment of relative hypoxia. Red blood cells (RBCs) then leak through a more permeable glomerulus. This increased permeability may be further exacerbated as the sympathetic nervous system induces renal vasoconstriction and increases filtration pressure (9).

Although exercise-induced hematuria is of concern to the athlete and family, it usually is a benign self-limiting condition. The first episode of hematuria, therefore, does not require a work-up. Repeat episodes require more thorough investigation, since this benign condition could herald an underlying abnormality. For example, cases of covert bladder cancer have been discovered in young men with recurrent exercise-induced hematuria (10). Although bladder cancer is rare in young people, the possibility should be considered. A large differential diagnosis for pediatric hematuria exists. Neiberger (11) published an excellent mnemonic that utilizes the alphabet to order it in the following categories: *A*natomy; *B*oulders; *C*ancer; *D*rug-related; *E*xercise; *F*oreign body, *F*amilial, and *F*actitious; *G*lomerulonephritis; *H*ematology; and *I*nfection.

Evaluation begins with a thorough history and physical examination similar to that previously discussed, with attention to the above differential. Pertinent positive findings should guide the workup. Otherwise, analysis can begin with the urine dipstick study, and it is followed by microscopic confirmation. The absence of actual RBCs indicates pseudohematuria. Pseudohematuria can be caused by drugs (rifampin and phenazopyridine hydrochloride), foods (beets and berries), artificial food coloring, myoglobinuria, and hemoglobinuria. False positive results are also possible with a high specific gravity, a pH less than 5.1, menstrual blood, or hematospermia (9,12).

True hematuria requires three or more RBCs per high-powered field on microscopic examination of a spun urine sediment (12). Urinalysis that confirms hematuria without finding any other abnormalities in an asymptomatic child should prompt two repeat urinalyses on samples obtained 1 to 3 months apart. If the repeat studies are negative, the patient and family can be reassured, and the patient should be followed routinely. If the hematuria occurred in the setting of strenuous exercise and no other confounding variables are present, the hematuria will likely clear within 72 hours with rest. If recent athletic activity involved flank trauma in an asymptomatic child, close, careful follow-up is appropriate. If the child has pain, ecchymosis, tachycardia, hypotension, or any other signs that are a cause for concern, he or she requires immediate imaging and surgical evaluation. Similarly, if any suspicion of nonaccidental trauma exists, intervention should be immediate.

Persistent hematuria without trauma may indicate a urinary tract infection (UTI). Other dipstick findings may include leukocyte esterase, nitrites, white blood cells, or bacteria, but a culture should be ordered, even without these findings. Remember that the definitive diagnosis of UTI in a child requires urine by catheterization or suprapubic aspiration in children who are unable to obtain a clean catch midstream specimen (13). If cystitis is confirmed in a child younger than 5 years of age or if pyelonephritis is found in any child, an ultrasound and a voiding cystourethrogram should be performed to check for obstruction, anatomical abnormalities, and vesicoureteral reflux (14). In the adolescent athlete, the clinician should consider chlamydia and other sexually transmitted diseases.

Additional studies may be helpful. Ultrasound, intravenous pyelogram, and other imaging studies can detect anatomic abnormalities, arteriovenous malformations, nephrolithiasis, and neoplasms. A spot urine calcium to Cr ratio (UCa/Cr) greater than 0.2 may indicate hypercalcinuria (9). Medications can lead to elevated BUN and Cr levels. Nonsteroidal antiinflammatory drugs and dietary supplements (e.g., creatine) are possible culprits in the athlete with otherwise unexplained interstitial nephritis and papillary necrosis (12,15). Foreign bodies in the urethra, familial causes (e.g., Alport syndrome), and factitious hematuria should be considered. An elevated BUN or Cr level and late physical examination findings (e.g., hypertension, pallor, fever, or rashes) suggest glomerulonephritis. In poststreptococcal glomerulonephritis, antistreptolysin-O or anti-DNAase B titers should be

positive. With lupus, the antinuclear antibody titer (ANA) may be positive, and the complement levels may be low.

Serum studies such as the CBC, hemoglobin electrophoresis, prothrombin time (PT), and partial thromboplastin time (PTT) are useful in diagnosing hematologic causes of hematuria. Hemoglobin SS, AS, or SC may cause hematuria from sickling in the renal medulla. Sickling may be precipitated by dehydration or altitude training (16). Platelet abnormalities, such as thrombocytopenia and disseminated intravascular coagulation, may cause hematuria. Coagulopathies indicated by abnormal PT or PTT can contribute to hematuria in athletes taking hepatotoxic substances. Renal vein thrombosis also should be considered when an athlete with a hypercoagulable state develops hematuria, thrombocytopenia, or flank mass (16).

Most causes of hematuria in the pediatric athlete that are not explained by exercise will require follow-up with a subspecialist. Consultation also may be necessary if the etiology remains unclear despite an appropriate workup.

Acute Renal Failure

Significant renal damage can occur with exercise. Acute renal failure is the most consequential problem and, fortunately, the least common. Other serious disorders include rhabdomyolysis and acute tubular necrosis (ATN). These conditions should be suspected in the athlete with no history of trauma who complains of bilateral flank tenderness or who is found to have myoglobinuria, significant proteinuria (4+), sustained oliguria, azotemia, electrolyte abnormalities, or an elevated creatinine phosphokinase level following strenuous activity (3). Risk factors include extreme exertion by underhydrated and unconditioned athletes who are further stressed by heat or who have a history of prior heat-related illness. Under these conditions, renal ischemia, metabolic acidosis, and myolysis occur, with toxic effects on renal tubular epithelial cells. Patients who develop rhabdomyolysis or ATN require hospitalization and aggressive intervention. They may not develop complications, but even those with renal failure usually recover fully (4,17). Patients with permanent disease require lifelong dialysis or renal transplantation.

PREPARTICIPATION PHYSICAL EXAMINATION

Overall, extremely few renal system conditions prevent a child athlete from participating in sports. A child with only one functioning kidney should be discouraged from contact sports. Such a patient and his or her family must be counseled in detail about the risks of participation. A child with mild renal disease can play sports, but he or she requires close follow-up and periodic evaluation of renal function. All children and their parents should be taught the importance of safety, conditioning, and hydration.

SUMMARY

When signs or symptoms of renal problems develop in the pediatric athlete, a logical evaluation based on a broad differential diagnosis should follow. Benign exercise-induced conditions are common, but unrelated disorders may also be uncovered. Serious permanent exercise-related problems rarely occur. Most athletes ultimately return to their normal activities without restrictions. While the renal system is highly complex, it is also quite forgiving to the stresses imposed by exercise.

REFERENCES

1. Koeppen BM, Stanton BA, eds. *Renal physiology,* 2nd ed. St. Louis: Mosby-Year Book, 1997:95–116.
2. Lynch JM. Renal and genitourinary problems. In: Mellion M, ed. *The team physician's handbook*, 2nd ed. St. Louis: Hanley & Belfus, 1997:280–284.
3. Cianflocco AJ. Renal complications of exercise. *Clin Sports Med* 1992;11:437–451.
4. Gardner KD. Exercise and the kidney. In: Appenzeller O, ed. *Sports medicine*, 3rd ed. Baltimore: Urban & Schwarzenberg, 1988:189–195.
5. Alyea EP, Parish HH, Durham NC. Renal response to exercise- urinary findings. *JAMA* 1958:167:807–813.
6. Helzer-Julin M. Proteinuria, hematuria, and athletic pseudonephritis. In: Mellion MB, ed. *Sports medicine secrets*. Philadelphia: Hanley & Belfus, 1999:200–202.
7. Houser MT, John MF, Kobayashi A, et al. Assessment of urinary protein excretion in the adolescent: effect of body position and exercise. *J Pediatr* 1986:109:556–61.
8. Loghman-Adham M. Evaluating proteinuria in children. *Am Fam Physician* 1998;58:1145–1152.
9. Gambrell RC, Blount BW. Exercise-induced hematuria. *Am Fam Physician* 1996;53:905–911.
10. Eichner ER, Scott WA. Exercise as disease detector. *The Physician and Sports Medicine* 1998;26:41–52.
11. Neiberger RE. The ABC's of evaluating children with hematuria. *Am Fam Physician* 1994;49:623–628.
12. Thaller TR, Wang LP. Evaluation of asymptomatic microscopic hematuria in adults. *Am Fam Physician* 1999; 60:1143–1154.
13. American Academy of Pediatrics, Committee on Quality Improvement, Subcommittee on Urinary Tract Infection. Practice parameter: the diagnosis, treatment, and evaluation of the initial urinary tract infection in febrile infants and young children. *Pediatrics* 1999;103: 843–852.
14. Hellerstein S. Urinary tract infections in children: why they occur and how to prevent them. *Am Fam Physician* 1998;57:2440–2446.
15. Graham AS, Hatton RC. Creatine: a review of efficacy and safety. *J Am Pharm Assoc (Wash)* 1999;39:803–810.
16. Bergstein JM. Nephrology. In: Behrman RE, Kliegman RM, Jenson HB, eds. *Nelson's textbook of pediatrics*, 16th ed. Philadelphia: WB Saunders, 2000:1573–1596.
17. Sinert R, Kohl L, Rainone T, et al. Exercise-induced rhabdomyolysis. *Ann Emerg Med* 1994;23:1301–1306.

23

Hematology in Young Athletes

Brian L. Mahaffey

In an active population, people, regardless to age, depend on their ability to improve their conditioning by improving their oxygen delivery system. This ability to deliver oxygen to vital tissues depends on red cell mass and function (1). Time and time again, a slight drop in hemoglobin has been shown to affect performance adversely. Many different reasons exist for a drop in hemoglobin. It can be related to a decrease in red blood cell (RBC) production or to an increase in RBC destruction or loss. A decrease in hemoglobin may also be congenital or acquired. Anemia is defined as a decrease in the circulating RBC mass to below age-specific and gender-specific limits (2,3). This can lead to clinical symptoms at rest, as well as to a noticeable decrease in performance.

Most adolescent athletes will develop anemia secondary to nutritional deficiencies, silent blood losses, or as a response to activity (Fig. 23.1). A much less common finding is an adolescent with congenital anemia who wants to participate in sports. The prevalence of anemia in sports is difficult to obtain secondary to the lack of adequate control groups. Studies on the frequency of anemia in sports with nonathlete control groups show that mean hemoglobin levels in athletes tend to be slightly lower than those in a control population (1,4). This, however, may be a false anemia that occurs secondary to physiologic responses to exercise.

SYMPTOMS

Commonly, active patients have no symptoms associated with anemia. However, they may complain of fatigue with activity or of a decrease in their performance level (3,5,6). Dyspnea with exertion may exist. Clinical signs are usually not found unless the anemia is severe. The most sensitive (74%) and specific (96%) signs are pale conjunctivae and nail beds (6). Orthostasis may also be noted. Most anemias are found with laboratory tests that drawn either for screening purposes or for other suspected diseases (2,3,5). Some authors suggest that routine screening

of athletes, especially females, should be conducted for hemoglobin levels (7).

PSEUDOANEMIA

Vigorous exercise can lead to athletic pseudoanemia secondary to an increase in plasma volume as a normal physiologic response. Because the RBC mass does not change, athletes tend to have a slightly lower hematocrit and hemoglobin than the normal population, due to dilutional reasons (1,4,8). To compensate for plasma volume loss, the body releases renin, aldosterone, and vasopressin to conserve water and salt. This allows the plasma volume to increase, leading to higher stroke volume and a lower chance of thrombus formation (1,8). Normal drops in hemoglobin range from 0.5 g per dL for moderate exercise to 1.0 g per dL in elite endurance athletes (4).

"FOOT-STRIKE" HEMOLYSIS

"Foot-strike" hemolysis is one anemia associated with athletes. Although it was initially seen as an intravascular hemolysis secondary to ground impact of the foot in running, it has now been found in swimmers, rowers, dancers, and weight lifters. Rarely, foot-strike hemolysis causes a clinically relevant anemia (4). Possible explanations for the cause of this include the theory that the RBCs become fragile with exercise, that hemolysis results from the temperature effects of exercise, or that exercises causes the destruction of older RBCs (1). Treatment usually consists of cushioned shoe inserts with activity.

IRON DEFICIENCY DISEASE

Iron deficiency anemia is the most common anemia in an active population, similar to its incidence in the general population. Iron deficiency is the most common nutritional deficit in the United States, whether with or without anemia (1). Iron deficiency anemia is particularly common in menstruating fe-

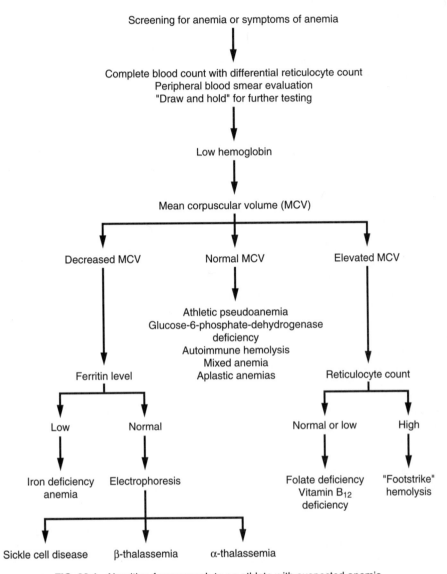

FIG. 23.1. Algorithm for approach to an athlete with suspected anemia.

males (20% of general population) and in adolescents (1,6,9,10). The rate of hemoglobin iron needs per unit of body weight is quite high during adolescence. (Only toddlers have a higher rate.) White females have a higher incidence of iron deficiency secondary to menstruation. Males require more iron at adolescence, secondary to gains in muscle mass and myoglobin (6). Multiple studies have shown that iron deficiency is common in athletes; however, iron deficiency anemia is extremely uncommon, with levels of incidence of approximately 0% to 3% (1,7). As athletes enter adulthood, men rarely display iron defi-

ciency unless gastrointestinal (GI) bleeding is present, whereas women continue to be highly susceptible to this deficiency secondary to menstruation (4). The avoidance of red meat may also induce an iron deficient state in athletes (1,4,6,8).

Diagnosis of an iron deficient state or of iron deficiency anemia is based on serum blood tests that consider RBC indices and hemoglobin levels. Classically, the mean corpuscular volume (MCV) is low, with hypochromic microcytic red cells seen on a peripheral blood smear. The serum ferritin concentration is low (1,4,6,8). If, in addition to these findings, a patient's hemoglobin is below reference levels for his or her age, the diagnosis of iron-deficiency anemia is made. The best serum test for iron levels is that of ferritin, as it has a linear relation with bone marrow hemosiderin granules. Hemosiderin granules are considered the gold standard (1).

Iron deficiency is treated with oral iron supplementation. The standard protocol consists of ferrous sulfate (325 mg, one to three times daily) with meals. Side effects can include GI distress and constipation, and these can lead to noncompliance (1,9). Drinking citric acid juices with iron tablets can help improve the absorption from the GI tract (1,6). Nutritional changes, such as increasing the young athlete's intake of red meat and of the dark meat of poultry, using cast-iron cookware when preparing acidic foods (e.g., tomato sauces), and eating legumes with chicken or seafood (iron absorption from legumes is increased with animal protein), are helpful (1,4,8).

For many years, iron supplementation was felt to be inappropriate for iron deficiency without anemia. Prophylactic iron treatment is not recommended because of the possibility of iron overload. In adult males, iron deficiency is less common than is hereditary hemochromatosis (1). However, some authors have begun to recommend iron replacement in situations of low or borderline ferritin levels with borderline hemoglobin levels (4,5,7,8). These recommendations are based on evidence that endurance improves with increases in the ferritin level (9,11). If serum ferritin is under 20 µg per L, treatment with a daily ferrous sulfate tablet is appropriate, and the level is rechecked within 1 to 2 months. If a hemoglobin increase of 1 g per dL occurs, this result indicates that the patient had a "relative" anemia and that treatment should continue. Any athlete with hemoglobin levels below 13.5 g per dL is considered to have anemia, and he or she should be treated long term. During a preseason physical, a screening test for hemoglobin and ferritin levels can be done. However, screening is recommended by some authors only in female athletes, unless a male has evidence of GI blood loss (7).

SICKLE CELL DISEASE

Sickle cell disease and anemia are the most common hereditary hematologic diseases. Sickle cell anemia (Hb SS) affects approximately one in 375 persons of African descent (12,13), and 8% of the African-American population carries the gene for sickle cell disease. Individuals with this gene are considered to have sickle cell trait. As at least 50% of these individuals' hemoglobin is normal, which leads

to rare clinical problems (13). Over 50,000 persons in the United States are affected by the most common form of the disease, Hb SS (14). Multiple combinations of abnormal hemoglobin types, which were caused of the migration of multiple gene pools to the United States (15), are classified under Hb SS. Therefore, sickle cell diseases are best classified by genotype (14).

The diagnosis may be made at any age, and it is usually established by hemoglobin electrophoresis, liquid chromatography, or DNA analysis. Anemia may not be present in all cases at diagnosis, even though the hemolysis is occurring (13). Neonatal screening has been widely implemented in the United States as a result of a study showing an 84% decrease in the incidence of pneumococcal sepsis in young infants with screening (16,17). The use of universal screening versus targeted screening is still debated because of the costs of the former (14).

Sickle cell disease is characterized by acute episodes of capillary and arteriole occlusion with sickled RBCs (13,14). Hb SS forms rigid polymers that deform the corpuscles, causing adherence to the vascular endothelium, occlusion, and the release of cytokines from white blood cells (13,14,18). Adherence and occlusion leads to hypoxia and pain, with tissue ischemia and infarction. This is called a sickle cell event. Physical exertion, which leads to acidosis, hypoxia, and dehydration, is a known precipitating event, as are cold temperatures and underlying infections. Altitudes greater than 10,000 ft have also been shown to cause sickling (8,18). Long-term effects on organs may result from vasoocclusion, and the organs most commonly affected are the spleen, kidney, lung, bone, retina, and brain (13,18). Long-term anemia may lead to high-output cardiac failure. Encapsulated bacterial infections may be overwhelming, which can lead to splenic infarction (19). The cause of sudden death on exertion in sickle cell disease is a controversial issue. No evidence, however, indicates that acute death is associated with any of the typical complications seen in sickle cell events (18). However, cases of fulminant rhabdomyolysis and death with sickle cell trait carriers have been reported (8,18).

Acute chest syndrome is the leading cause of death in patients with sickle cell disease, and repeated events may lead to chronic lung disease (14,19,20). This syndrome occurs in 50% of patients with sickle cell disease (20). Death rates with acute chest syndrome are four times higher in adults than they are in children (14). The syndrome is characterized by chest pain, cough, progressive anemia, hypoxia, and new pulmonary infiltrates on chest radiographs. Patients may or may not have fever (20). Only 3.5% of acute chest syndrome episodes are associated with bacteremia (14).

Treatment of sickle cell disease includes both primary and secondary prevention. Management of sickle cell disease has progressed from merely managing an acute event to actually anticipating and preventing these events and their complications.

Primary prevention begins with newborn screening. Education of both the patient and his or her parents is important, and taking the time to do so results in a higher rate of follow-up for appointments (14). Fluid intake of 1.5 to 2 times the normal child's maintenance fluid intake should be calculated and followed (13,14), as adequate hydration has been shown to prevent vascular occlusion (21). Immunizations are important in sickle cell patients. Patients should also receive pneumococcal vaccine, beginning in early infancy and continuing every 4 to 5 years throughout life. Infections may lead to severe complications in sickle cell disease, so prevention is key. Prophylactic penicillin should begin at 2 months of age and should continue until the child is 5 years old. If a patient has had a splenectomy, the continuation of penicillin is appropriate (13,14). Folate supplementation is recommended to prevent megaloblastic changes (14).

Secondary prevention deals with the early detection and prompt treatment of an acute sickle cell event. The ability to recognize the clinical signs of an event and to respond quickly is crucial. Acute splenic sequestration and acute chest syndrome can rapidly be fatal (14,19,20). Pain is felt to be related to vasoocclusion and subsequent ischemia, and thus it should be treated according to its severity. Meperidine hydrochloride is not recommended because sickle cell patients are at risk for seizures as a result of its metabolite, normeperidine (14,19). The use of patient-controlled analgesia (PCA) has been shown to be extremely effective for pain control, and it automatically limits the amount of drug that is used (19). The use of intravenous fluids for rehydration is necessary to maintain a normovolemic state (14,19,20). Supplemental oxygen may need to be administered to maintain arterial oxygen pressure (PaO$_2$) between 70 to 100 mm Hg. Pulse oximetry in sickle cell patients should not be relied upon because use of this technique may underestimate peripheral oxygenation (19). Empiric antibiotic coverage should be initiated to cover any community-acquired pathogens (19,20). Medicines that have demonstrated their effectiveness in sickle cell events include β-agonists and corticosteroids. Hydroxyurea has been shown to reduce the frequency of acute events and acute chest syndrome by 50%, but it may lead to bone marrow depression (14,19). Nitric oxide may be beneficial in acute chest syndrome, but further study is needed to establish the efficacy of this particular intervention (22). Transfusions, both simple and exchange, may be required to maintain a hemoglobin level of 10 g per dL. Transfusions should be followed with caution because of the increase in blood viscosity that can result, thus worsening oxygen delivery. Transfusions may also lead to iron overload (14,20). Bone marrow transplantation may be curative in children with sickle cell disease who are less than 16 years of age (14).

Health care providers, parents, coaches, and the patient should be cautious with regard to sickle cell disease and exercise. Moreover, patients with sickle cell trait should also maintain appropriate precautions in order to avoid acute rhabdomyolysis. However, limited studies have shown no effect on exercise performance with sickle cell trait (18). Prompt recognition of fatigue and dehydration is important, as is decreasing activity levels with viral and bacterial infections. Temperature increases and altitude changes should be avoided (8,18), and changes in exercise intensity should be gradual.

OTHER ANEMIAS

Other types of anemia can affect an active young person. These include acute or chronic blood loss from multiple etiologies, other hemolytic anemias (thalassemias and glucose-6-phosphokinase dehydrogenase [G6PD] deficiency), and decreased RBC production (megaloblastic and aplastic anemias). As these are rare in a sports medicine setting, they are not discussed. Diseases of the platelets may also be seen in the active patient. No relation between exercise and the development of thrombocytopenias is apparent (23–25).

RHABDOMYOLYSIS

Rhabdomyolysis, which has already been discussed, is related to hematology as well. This relatively common entity involves damage to the skeletal muscle sarcolemma and leakage of its contents into the intravascular space. The chemicals that are released in the process include electrolytes, muscle enzymes, and myoglobin, a molecule that is closely related to hemoglobin in both structure and function. Rhabdomyolysis is commonly seen with orthopedic trauma, heat illness, drug and alcohol intoxication, compartment syndromes, prolonged seizure activity, both viral and bacterial infections, and congenital myocyte metabolic diseases (26–29). The hereditary deficiency of carnitine palmitoyl transferase II leads to recurrent rhabdomyolysis in childhood (29). The development of rhabdomyolysis from exertion is rare in childhood, but it becomes more prevalent through adolescence and adulthood (levels of 40% have been recorded in new military recruits with initial training) (26).

Rhabdomyolysis is recognized by muscle weakness, myalgias, and dark urine. A urinalysis that reveals high levels of hemoglobin with little or no RBCs is consistent with myoglobinuria. Serum creatinine phosphokinase (CPK) is the most sensitive test for muscle injury, and levels at least five times the normal are required to diagnose rhabdomyolysis (26,27). CPK levels peak at 24 to 36 hours postinjury, and they decrease by 40% over every subsequent 24-hour period (26). The disappearance of myoglobin in the urine signals the end of muscle injury (29). Electrolyte abnormalities are common in rhabdomyolysis. Hyperkalemia, hyperphosphatemia, hypercalcemia, and hyperuricemia result directly from the muscle damage and leakage into the intravascular space (26,27,29). Acute renal failure (ARF), which is caused by acute tubular necrosis (29), may occur. The incidence of ARF is higher in patients with CPK levels greater than 15,000 units per L (26,27). The severity of ARF correlates better with electrolyte elevations than with the level of CPK. The mortality rate of rhabdomyolysis is much higher if ARF occurs (27).

Treatment of rhabdomyolysis begins with adequate support of the patient's respiratory and circulatory systems. Thorough assessment for signs of continuing muscle injury should be conducted, and appropriate treatment should be initiated. Intravenous normal saline is administered at a rate that maintains the urine output above 200 mL per hour. A urinary catheter is necessary for assessing input and output levels. Mannitol or furosemide can be given for diuresis to convert a patient from an oliguric to a nonoliguric ARF. Accomplishing this lowers the mortality rate. Alkalization of the urine with sodium bicarbonate protects the kidneys from myoglobin. Treatment of the other electrolyte abnormalities should be according to standard protocols and should include the use of electrocardiac monitoring for hyperkalemia. Dialysis may be required in severe cases. A gradual return to activities can be accomplished. The patient needs to be educated regarding symptoms to prevent recurrence. If the patient does have a recurrent episode of rhabdomyolysis, a full evaluation for a congenital muscle enzyme deficiency should be completed (26).

CONCLUSION

Overall, hematology problems in young active people can range from minimal problems that may cause a decreased performance to life-threatening diseases that can be acute or chronic. An excellent understanding of these entities and their pathophysiologies can lead to improved health and athletic performance in these patients.

REFERENCES

1. Balaban EP. Sports anemia. *Clin Sports Med* 1992;11: 313–323.
2. Brill JR, Baumgardner DJ. Normocytic anemia. *Am Fam Physician* 2000;62:2255–2264.
3. Cotran RS, Kumar V, Robbins SL. Diseases of red cells and bleeding disorders. In: Robbins SL, Cotran RS, Kumar V, eds. *Pathologic basis of disease*, 4th ed. Philadelphia: WB Saunders, 1989:657–702.
4. Eichner ER. Anemia and blood doping. In: Sallis RE, Massimino F, eds. *Essentials of sports medicine*. Saint Louis: Mosby, 1997:35–38.
5. Eichner ER. Coping with anemia. *Sports Medicine Digest* 2000;22:57–58.
6. Wharton BA. Iron deficiency in children: detection and prevention. *Br J Haematol* 1999;106:270–280.
7. Eichner ER. Anemia in female athletes. *Sports Medicine Digest* 2000;22:42–43.
8. Eichner ER. Anemia, athletic pseudoanemia, and sickle cell disease. In: Mellion MB, ed. *Sports medicine secrets*, 2nd ed. Philadelphia: Hanley and Belfus, 1999: 197–200.
9. Beard JL, Tobin B. Iron status and exercise. *Am J Clin Nutr* 2000;72:594S–597S.
10. Beard JL. Iron requirements in adolescent females. *J Nutr* 2000;130:440S–442S.
11. Hinton PS, Giordano C, Brownlie T, et al. Iron supplementation improves endurance after training in iron-depleted, non-anemic women. *J Appl Physiol* 2000;88: 1103–1111.
12. Berg AO. Sickle cell disease: screening, diagnosis, management, and counseling in newborns and infants. *American Board of Family Practice* 1994;7:134–140.
13. Wethers DL. Sickle cell disease in childhood. I. Laboratory diagnosis, pathophysiology, and health maintenance. *Am Fam Physician* 2000;62:1013–1020.
14. Simon K, Lobo ML, Jackson S. Current knowledge in the management of children and adolescents with sickle cell disease. I. Physiological issues. *J Pediatr Nurs* 1999;14:281–295.
15. Nagel RL. Origins and dispersions of the sickle cell gene. In: Embury SH, Hebbel RP, Mohandas N, et al. *Sickle cell disease: basic principles and clinical practice*. New York: Raven Press, 1994:353–380.
16. Gaston MH, Verter JI, Woods G, et al. Prophylaxis with oral penicillin in children with sickle cell anemia: a randomized trial. *N Engl J Med* 1986;314:1593–1599.
17. Consensus Conference. Newborn screening for sickle cell disease and other hemoglobinopathies. *JAMA* 1987; 258:1205–1209.
18. Kark JA, Ward FT. Exercise and hemoglobin S. *Semin Hematol* 1994;31:181–225.

19. Wethers DL. Sickle cell disease in childhood. II. Diagnosis and treatment of major complications and recent advances in treatment. *Am Fam Physician* 2000;62: 1309–1314.

20. Yale SH, Nagib N, Guthrie T. Acute chest syndrome in sickle cell disease: curtail considerations in adolescents and adults. *Postgrad Med* 2000;107:215–222.

21. Warth JA, Rucknagel DL. Painful crisis and dense echinocytes: effects of hydration and vasodilators. *Prog Clin Biol Res* 1987;240:429–449.

22. Sullivan KJ, Goodwin SR, Evangelist J, et al. Nitric oxide successfully used to treat acute chest syndrome of sickle cell disease in a young adolescent. *Crit Care Med* 1999;27:2563–2568.

23. Ware RE. Autoimmune hemolytic and thrombocytopenic disease in the adolescent patient. *Adolesc Med* 1999;10:377–384.

24. George JN, Raskob GE. Clinical decisions in idiopathic thrombocytopenic purpura. *Hosp Pract* 1997;32:159–176.

25. Dror Y. Essential thrombocythaemia in children. *Br J Haematol* 1999;107:691–698.

26. Moghtader J, Brady WJ, Bonadio W. Exertional rhabdomyolysis in an adolescent athlete. *Pediatr Emerg Care* 1997;13:382–385.

27. Veenstra J, Smit WM, Krediet RT, et al. Relationship between elevated creatine phosphokinase and the clinical spectrum of rhabdomyolysis. *Nephrol Dial Transplantation* 1994;9:637–641.

28. Singh U, Scheid WM. Infectious etiologies of rhabdomyolysis: three case reports and review. *Clin Infect Dis* 1996;22:642–649.

29. Watemberg N, Leshner RL, Armstrong BA, et al. Acute pediatric rhabdomyolysis. *J Child Neurol* 2000;15: 222–227.

24

Scoliosis

Kim Edward LeBlanc

Apparent scoliosis may present quite frequently in an athletic setting. However, most of these cases will involve acute asymmetry of the back. In the athletic arena, the usual etiology is pain due to muscular causes. These types of scoliosis are quite obvious, and they resolve spontaneously.

Although idiopathic scoliosis is only seen in 2% to 3% of the normal adolescent population (1), it will be seen in children and adolescents who participate in sports. It occurs in neurologically normal and healthy individuals.

Although back pain is a common complaint that is often noted in athletics, scoliosis is not one of the causes of this discomfort. Therefore, the clinician should remember that idiopathic scoliosis is not a painful condition. When a child or adolescent presents with complaints of back pain, a thorough evaluation should be initiated, as this pain should not be attributed to scoliosis.

DEFINITION

Scoliosis has been defined as lateral curvature of the spinal column that is persistent and that is greater than 10 degrees in the coronal plane. An important consideration in this entity is etiologies that can be both nonstructural and structural. Nonstructural causes will correct with either side bending or traction, such as during radiographic examination. Structural causes result in a lateral curvature that is fixed and persistent, even with rotation. Idiopathic scoliosis is the most common cause of this latter type of deformity; this condition has no known cause, and it occurs more frequently in girls.

Classically, idiopathic scoliosis has been described according to the time of first discovery. Hence, infantile idiopathic scoliosis is defined as an age of onset of less than 3 years old. The idiopathic juvenile form is noted between the ages of 3 years to 10 years, while the idiopathic adolescent type is detected between the age of 10 years and skeletal maturity (2). These distinctions are used because they are felt to coincide with periods of rapid growth of the spine. However, to a certain extent, this is only partially true as the juvenile type actually occurs during a period of relatively little spinal growth.

Dickson et al. (3) proposed another method of classification in 1984. The premise of the authors was that the juvenile type is so uncommon that it does not warrant a separate category. Consequently, they suggested distinguishing only two categories as follows: early onset (< 5 years of age) and late onset (> 5 years of age). Moreover, the use of this classification does have applicability from a cardiovascular standpoint. Many life-threatening cardiopulmonary abnormalities have been observed to have an association with scoliosis in children who develop large curves before 5 years of age (2,4). The early onset group is also at risk for developing pulmonary artery hypertension, restrictive pulmonary disease, and cor pulmonale (2,4). In the adolescent form of idiopathic scoliosis, or late onset form, pulmonary function remains normal even if the curve magnitude exceeds 100 degrees (2).

PHYSICAL FINDINGS IN THE YOUNG ATHLETE WITH SCOLIOSIS

As with all diseases, a thorough history and physical examination is required in any patient with suspected scoliosis. For cases that are noted acutely, other disease processes must be considered. Conditions other than idiopathic scoliosis can cause an apparent spinal asymmetry. Some of these diseases may be relatively benign, such as leg-length discrepancy or abnormal posture. However, any painful condition that produces spinal asymmetry must be scrutinized because idiopathic scoliosis does not cause pain unless muscle complaints (e.g., spasm) are present. A rapid and/or painful onset of scoliosis should prompt the examining physician to consider such entities as tumors, fractures, nerve root irritation, or infections (e.g., Pott disease or discitis).

On physical examination, evidence of spinal curvature is seen. The findings include asymmetry of the posterior thorax on forward bending (this is usually the most consistent abnormality), asymmetry in the levels of the shoulders, asymmetry of the crease at the waist, and the prominence of one iliac crest. In ideopathic scoliosis, the neuromuscular examination should be normal, as no coexistent neuromuscular condition should be found.

Certain findings on physical examination may suggest a nonidiopathic cause of the deformity, including possibilities such as café au lait spots, midline hairy patches, dimpling of the sacrum, foot deformity, or asymmetry of shoe size.

RADIOGRAPHIC EVALUATION

Radiographs of the entire vertebral column are necessary in the complete evaluation of a patient with suspected scoliosis. The most important views to obtain are the standing posteroanterior (PA) and lateral radiographs of the entire spine. The amount of curvature is determined by the Cobb method, as Figure 24.1 depicts. Using this method, the degree of curvature is determined by measuring the angular relationships between the most tilted vertebra at either end of the apparent curve. A line is drawn across the proximal endplate of the superior end vertebra and the distal endplate of the inferior end vertebra, and lines perpendicular to these are drawn. The angle at the intersection of the perpendicular lines determines the degree of curvature. In most cases, no further studies are necessary. Therefore, imaging studies should be reserved for patients with suspected nonidiopathic causes of curvature.

TREATMENT

Widespread school screening in the United States allows the most successful treatment—early detection and intervention. Early intervention will minimize the potential complications of this disorder. The most

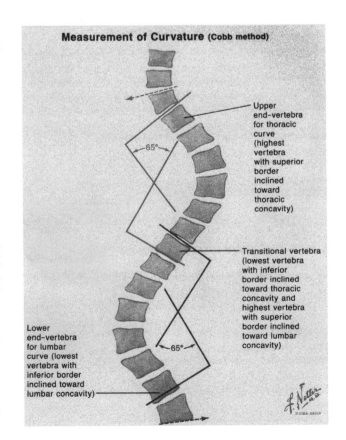

FIG. 24.1. Measurement of curvature (Cobb method). (From ICON Learning Systems, LLC, with permission.)

common approach for idiopathic scoliosis in this population of patients is nonsurgical treatment.

Curvature of less than 30 degrees rarely progresses upon reaching skeletal maturity. However, curves greater than 45 degrees at the time of skeletal maturity tend to progress later in life. With progression, the patient will be more likely to develop complications of scoliosis (e.g., cor pulmonale or restrictive lung disease).

Curvatures that are less than 10 degrees when measured radiographically and that are not progressive require no treatment or referral to an orthopedist. If the progression or stability of the curvature is in doubt, repeat radiographs should be obtained every 4 to 6 months, depending on the age of the child. This is particularly important in the child or adolescent who is entering a period of rapid skeletal growth. Curvatures greater than 10 degrees, particularly those that may be progressive, should be referred to an orthopedist for initial evaluation and possible treatment. The primary care physician may also opt to follow this patient, if no signs of progression are seen in the early stages—even in a skeletally immature individual. However, this patient should be followed by periodic physical and radiographic examinations until the time of skeletal maturity.

During the period of observation, if the curve should progress more than 5 degrees or if, on initial examination, the curvature is greater than 25 degrees, orthopedic referral is essential. Bracing therapy may be initiated for such findings.

Consistent with the philosophy of nonoperative intervention, brace therapy is the most desirable form of treatment. The brace, also known as a spinal orthosis, consists of a polypropylene shell that is shaped in such a manner to provide a corrective force to the spine. The patient should wear the brace 23 hours a day until reaching skeletal maturity (1). Surgical intervention is reserved for insistences in which the curve progresses to between 45 to 50 degrees, as the patient is at high risk for further progression.

SCOLIOSIS AND ATHLETICS

As a general rule of thumb, an athlete with idiopathic scoliosis should not be excluded from participation in sports. Most sports are not contraindicated (5). A specific exercise and/or training program should be integrated into the sports training. In addition, participation in the chosen sport should be modified based on the severity of the disease and/or its progression. Generally, even if an athlete requires the use of a brace, he or she may participate in any sport that is not impeded by the bracing device (5). However, athletes that have required surgical intervention, whether instrumentation or fusion, should be excluded from participation in contact sports. In addition, some have been suggested that, following fusion, gymnastics and diving should be disallowed as well (6).

RISKS AND BENEFITS OF EXERCISE WITH SCOLIOSIS

In spite of being afflicted with scoliosis, patients should attempt to maintain an active lifestyle. This is beneficial both physiologically and psychologically. These patients will be able to enjoy life, as well as the benefits of exercise. Unfortunately, no data suggests that maintaining an active lifestyle and having increased fitness levels alters the course of the disease.

Patients with scoliosis may be more prone to muscle strains or ligamentous sprains, depending on the severity of the deformity, and they should be cautioned accordingly.

Athletes with scoliosis should maintain proper muscle balance and strength.

CONCLUSIONS

Idiopathic scoliosis may be seen in the athletic population. Anyone presenting with painful spinal asymmetry should be thoroughly evaluated for a nonidiopathic cause of the scoliosis. Physical examination and radiographs are necessary to categorize individual treatment plans that are based on the degree of curvature. Once this has been determined, an appropriate treatment plan may be initiated.

In general, participation in sports should be allowed, as long as the physical encumbrance of a brace is not an impediment (see Chapter 2). Once surgery has been performed, the young athlete is restricted from participating in contact sports.

The key to treatment is early detection. Therefore, each and every primary care physician should actively evaluate patients for this deformity.

REFERENCES

1. Boachie-Adjei O, Lonner B. Spinal deformity. *Pediatr Clin N Am* 1996;43:883–897.
2. Dobbs MB, Weinstein SL. Infantile and juvenile scoliosis. *Ortho Clin North Am* 1999;30:331–341.
3. Dickson RA, Lawton JO, Archer IA, et al. The pathogenesis of idiopathic scoliosis: biplanar spinal asymmetry. *J Bone Joint Surg* 1984;66:8–15.

4. Pehrsson K, Larsson S, Oden A, et al. Long-term follow-up of patients with untreated scoliosis: a study of mortality, causes of death, and symptoms. *Spine* 1992; 17:1091–1096.

5. Smith DM, Kovan JR, Rich BS, et al. *Preparticipation physical evaluation*, 2nd ed. Leawood, KS: American Academy of Family Physicians, American Academy of Pediatrics, American Medical Society for Sports Medicine, American Orthopedic Society for Sports Medicine, American Osteopathic Academy of Sports Medicine, 1997.

6. Omey ML, Micheli LJ, Gerbino PG. Idiopathic scoliosis and spondylolysis in the female athlete. *Clin Orthop* 2000;372:74–84.

25

Special Considerations for Athletes with Disabilities

Jack M. Levine

A major responsibility for healthcare providers is assisting children with disabilities so that they are able to participate in athletics. Investigating the whole spectrum of athletic possibilities, as well as evaluating the wide range of abilities and disabilities, presents a unique challenge and makes decision-making particularly complex. Often, the clinician finds that he or she must encourage children with disabilities to participate in sports. This sometimes must be done in the face of overprotective attitudes in both parents or guardians and other healthcare providers. Therefore, a creative approach is essential. Frequently, cooperation and collaboration with therapists and other healthcare providers, as well as with schools and community programs, is necessary.

Currently, between 15 million to 20 million children in the United States have a chronic health condition. Severe health conditions that are likely to require extensive daily caretaking affect between 1 million and 2 million children (1). Approximately 5% to 10% of children in the United States are thought to have some functional limitation due to chronic medical issues or disabilities (2). A wide range of disabilities with varying prevalence are found (Table 25.1) (3–7). A growing number of children is totally or partially dependent on technologic intervention, such as ventilators, and these individuals present special complex challenges (8). This dictates the need for a wide variety of sports programs.

The "medical home," a concept of the American Academy of Pediatrics (AAP), is directly applicable to children with disabilities (9,10). General medical care for all children needs to be accessible, family-centered, continuous, comprehensive, coordinated, compassionate, and culturally competent. Within this framework, the healthcare provider can help children with disabilities and their families to be-

come meaningfully involved in athletic activities. Comprehensive primary care should include the discussion of athletic participation and regular exercise (11). Families of children with disabilities consistently report the importance of community-based recreation programs (12,13). However, decisions about athletic participation must also be respectful of the family's desires and consistent with its values. Activities that are discussed need to be functional within the child's life and meaningful within the family context (14).

The primary care provider must often communicate with other professionals, both medical and nonmedical, to ensure successful sports participation. Coordination and consultation with therapists, psychologists, physiatrists, neurologists, neurosurgeons, and orthopedists are often necessary.

A wide range of appropriate sports activities exists for children with disabilities, and all opportunities should be explored (15). The desired athletic program may be part of a school physical education program, community recreation initiatives, or a social program. When discussing sports programming, the issue of inclusion versus participation in a special program often arises (16).

TABLE 25.1. *Occurrence of childhood disabilities*

Disability	Occurrence (per 1,000)
Attention deficit/ hyperactivity disorder	75–100
Learning disability	75–100
Mental retardation	10–30
Cerebral palsy	2.3
Spina bifida	0.6
Duchenne muscular dystrophy	0.3 (males)

CHILDREN WITH DISABILITIES

Children with disabilities have many complex medical problems (Table 25.2) (17,18). These issues can cause difficulty in decision-making with regard to athletic participation, as well as for designing well-run programs. Appropriate and accessible facilities and personnel to assist in toileting are essential for adequate programming. Difficult-to-control seizure disorders, while uncommon, are quite problematic for children in special athletic programs. Orthopedic issues, such as scoliosis, hip subluxation, dislocation, or "brittle bones" (e.g., osteogenesis imperfecta and osteoporosis), need special consideration. Feeding difficulties may be important if snacks are served at activities. Attention deficit/hyperactivity disorder (ADHD) and depression are frequently seen in children with disabilities.

Complicated psychosocial and family issues are common in the lives of children with disabilities (19,20). Some children suffer from anxiety, depression, or sadness. Self-esteem issues are common, and they often impact decision-making. Different ways of dealing with the issues of independence and separation may interfere with athletic participation. Many children with disabilities live in relative social isolation yet have almost no privacy in their personal lives because of their need for constant supervision. Peer relationships may be difficult to maintain. School, family, and social lives may be disrupted because of frequent hospitalizations. Behavioral and psychologic problems are common, and they affect athletic participation.

Families may be under pressure because of financial demands and difficulty in obtaining needed services (e.g., medical services and transportation). Parents and guardians often suffer from lack of privacy and social isolation. Families may be suffering from anxiety, sadness, and depression. Many parents need, but may not receive, guidance in dealing with issues of separation and independence, social problems, and transition issues. Marital stress and sibling issues are frequent.

SPORTS PROGRAMS AND ACTIVITIES

Benefits

Sports activities and exercises are particularly important to children with disabilities (21). The psychosocial benefits are well known (22). Parents report marked increases in self-esteem. Increased socialization and opportunities for conflict resolution are highly positive experiences. Sports allow children to feel good and to take pride in their accomplishments and to exhibit courage to themselves and others. Overall enjoyment and exposure to positive adult role models are additional benefits. As with all children, sports also become an outlet for physical energy and aggression. A frequently mentioned study (23) found that social competence correlates with the amount of time that a child with a disability spends in the Special Olympics (SO), regardless of age and intelligence quotient (IQ). Furthermore, SO athletes had more positive self-perceptions.

Regular physical exercise is particularly beneficial to the development of children with physical disabilities (21). The known benefits of cardiopulmonary fitness, decreased body fat, increased flexibility, and increased muscle strength and endurance are critical to many children with disabilities (24). Some children require extra energy because of their use of wheelchairs and orthotics. Awkward gait patterns are extremely tiring. Daily activities can be exhausting. Moreover, preventing obesity is important for children who use crutches to ambulate or who bear weight on weakened extremities. Preventing osteoporosis and strengthening bone structure and function is another critical aspect of exercise for children. Children with scoliosis and thoracic deformities may have comprised cardiopulmonary functioning, and thus they may greatly benefit from fitness programs. Increased mental alertness and psychologic well being are further benefits. Children who participate regularly in sports demonstrate less anxiety and depressive symptoms (24).

Challenges

In spite of the increase in athletic programs for children with disabilities, many obstacles and diffi-

TABLE 25.2. *Associated problems of children with disabilities*

Cognitive delays
Communication deficits
Learning problems
Seizure disorders
Toileting difficulties
Visual impairment
Hearing impairment
Feeding difficulty
Emotional and behavioral problems
Orthopedic problems
Other medical issues (cardiac, pulmonary, and renal)

culies exist. Often, disability-specific opportunities for children are lacking (22). Many times, widely differing groups of children are combined into programs without regard to their physical and/or mental characteristics. For example, in a wheelchair basketball program, a child with spastic quadraparetic cerebral palsy with upper and lower extremity involvement is unable to compete fairly with a child with only lower extremity paralysis secondary to spinal cord injury. Often programs emphasize winning and outcome, rather than participation and social experience. This limits participation to the "best" and most competitive athletes. Other characteristics of poorly run programs include unrealistic parental expectations or a lack of family support, inadequately trained coaches, inadequate transportation and toileting facilities, and a lack of medical support. Adolescents are often unwilling to participate in such athletic programs. Some become self-conscious, and they may lose their motivation.

Other medical considerations may also interfere with the success of special sports programs (21). Cardiac problems are more common in certain disabilities, such as Duchenne muscular dystrophy (DMD), and these can lead to serious complications. On occasion, medical conditions contraindicate too much exercise. This could be the case in certain children with severe pulmonary compromise secondary to scoliosis or severe anemia. Children with DMD may have decreased strength, and they therefore can easily overexercise. They may need to participate in repetitive, low intensity, aerobic activities (24). Environmental factors also need to be considered, especially in children who may have thermoregulatory difficulties (e.g., familial dysautonomia), severe dermatologic disorders, and limb deficiencies. Disability-specific injuries include fractures in children with osteogenesis imperfecta, as well as overuse injuries, such as tendonitis, in children with tonal abnormalities. Extra care must be taken to avoid damage to ventriculoperitoneal (VP) shunts, central lines, and gastrostomies.

Program Availability

In recent years, both a legal and social impetus to create special programs for children with disabilities has occurred (25). Section 504 of the Rehabilitation Act of 1973, PL 94-142, the Individuals With Disabilities Education Act, and the Americans With Disability Act have all helped in the dramatic increase in programs. Nevertheless, funding issues and liability factors can still interfere with program implementation.

A wide range of school and community programs is available for children with disabilities (15). Both the family and the child must be involved in choosing an activity that best meets their needs. This activity can often be part of a comprehensive plan that includes health, educational, and rehabilitative components. Adapted physical education programs are often part of special education programming, and they should be included in the individualized education plan (26). These are specialized programs for children who cannot participate in regular physical education. Advocacy by the primary care physician, however, may be necessary to ensure that the appropriate services are being delivered in a professional manner. Children may, in addition, be included in scholastic intramural programs, interscholastic sports, or community recreation leagues. The goals of integrated programs vary from intense competition to individual participation. Acting as a team manager may be extremely fulfilling for some adolescents (27). Many communities and organizations have special recreation leagues and programs for competitive participation. Input from physical and occupational therapists is often invaluable for planning appropriately.

Modifications that consider the cognitive, physical, behavioral, and sensory domains are usually necessary for sports programs to be effective for children with disabilities (28). Children with learning issues may have problems understanding rules, socializing, and participating fully. Regular sports activities with extra support from coaches, teachers, and counselors may suffice to meet the needs of some athletes. Children with ADHD are often able to participate fully in regular programs as long as they have some modifications.

Special Olympics

Children with significant developmental delay (i.e., below average scores on intelligence tests) often need specially adapted programming. The SO is the most widely known and most successful of these programs (29,30). The first SO games were held in 1968 under the auspices of Eunice Kennedy Shriver and the John P. Kennedy foundation. The goals of SO are for children with developmental disabilities to have the opportunity to strengthen character, to develop physical skills, to display their talents, and to fulfill human potential Participants must be 8 years old or older. No fee is charged for involvement. SO provides instruction, training, and competition to developmentally disabled athletes. Participation in activities is based on ability, and the activities can include aquatics, track and field, gymnastics, bowling, skiing, volleyball, soccer, basketball, floor hockey, figure and speed skating, golf, cycling, tennis, and roller-skating. The program now consists of 1 million participants, with 500,000 volunteers and 100,000 coaches, in every state of the United States and in many other countries. The principles of SO include activities that are appropriate for the participant's age and ability; the use of local volunteers; a family-oriented approach; and equality, respect, and acceptance for all. The rules are adapted, and the goal is to experience the joy of participation, rather than that of winning. Some children, like those with severe pervasive developmental disorder, may not be able to participate in SO.

The SO motor activities training program (MATP) focuses on basic sensorimotor activities for those children whose level of functioning does not allow them to participate fully in SO (14). The purpose of this program is to improve coordination and body control, to increase exposure to sports and recreation, to provide integration into community programs, to improve sensory awareness and self concept, and to prepare children for SO.

Modifications

Modifications for physical disabilities include special skis and bicycles, adaptive bowling equipment, and wheelchair sports of all types. Adaptive winter sports, such as skiing, snowboarding, skating and sledding, are particularly popular (31). Wheelchair and adaptive sports include biking, bowling, floor hockey, fishing, hiking, races and events, golf, baseball, and basketball (32,33,34). Wheelchair basketball can also be played with adapted baskets of varying heights and sizes. Special sleds and sticks are used in ice hockey (35). Aquatic sports, such as swimming, waterskiing and boating, with special flotation devices and other adaptive equipment are especially well received because no undue pressure is placed on joints and bones (36).

An integral part of all successful programs is psychosocial support and positive emotional experiences. Children must have the opportunity for success. Providing a sports experience that is age appropriate and that is geared towards the child's functional level can help to assure a positive experience. (22).

Modifications for sensory impairment are, of course, essential. Programs of this type often stress multisensory experiences. Special adaptations include the use of a "beeper ball," brightly colored equipment, sign language, easily read signs, and other visual prompts. Goalball, which uses a ball with four bells inside, is a unique sport for the visually impaired that has developed into an internationally popular event that is now enjoyed by all individuals (37).

Model Programs

Additional popular sports opportunities for children with disabilities include Challenger Little League baseball (38), soccer (39), horseback riding (40), dance (41), tennis, table tennis, and karate. The Empire State Games for the Physically Challenged is an innovative model program in New York State that has been extremely successful (42). Participants include children from 5 to 21 years of age. Both competitive and noncompetitive sporting events are offered. The classifications for participants are amputee, blind and visually impaired, cerebral palsy, deaf and hearing impaired, Les Autres (i.e., osteogenesis imperfecta, muscular dystrophy, arthrogryposis, dwarfism, and cardiac and pulmonary disorders), and spinal cord injury. Extensive care is taken to make the competition fair. Nine categories are found in the amputee classification, including all combinations of upper and lower limb deficiencies. Three categories of blind and visually impaired are established. The eight categories for cerebral palsy range from severe spasticity (necessitating a power wheelchair) to nonambulatory to ambulating with assistive devices to hemiplegia. Les Autres and spinal cord injury classifications are also divided into multiple categories.

PREPARTICIPATION PHYSICAL EXAMINATION

The primary care provider is called upon to evaluate a child with a disability for sports participation. An in-depth evaluation of the child and the activity is necessary, and this task can be quite complex. The AAP has formulated general guidelines for counseling children and adolescents about sports participation (11). The first consideration is the appropriateness of the suggested activity and its availability. The activity needs to be proper for the child's age and developmental level, and it must be functionally useful. Furthermore, it must have some meaning to the child and family. In addition, the child should be involved in the decision-making process. The practical aspects of participation, such as transportation and finances, must be considered. If possible, the activity should stress fundamental skills and, in addition, should improve the child's self-sufficiency (14). Cognitive ability, social and behavioral skills, and physical and sensory limitations must all be considered. Discussion and coordination with appropriate personnel, including therapists (occupational, physical, and speech), vision specialists, physical education teachers, psychologists, neurologists, orthopedists, physiatrists, and other professionals, are often necessary. Practical aspects of participation may include a need for adaptive equipment and modifications. Risks should be discussed openly and candidly, and recommendations for appropriate equipment (e.g., glasses and helmets) should be made.

The preparticipation examination is well described, and it is fairly standard (see Chapter 2) (11). The history includes cardiac symptoms, injuries, previous surgery, seizures, and past participation experiences. Any medications should be reported, and their effects must be evaluated. A complete physical examination is necessary, and it should include a blood pressure check and a careful cardiac evaluation. Particular attention should be paid to the neurologic and orthopedic exam and any limitations found on these. Vision and hearing should be evaluated. Special problems, such as a single testicle or kidney, VP shunt, or gastrostomy, must be addressed.

CHILDREN WITH SPECIFIC DISABILITIES

Cerebral Palsy

A large number of children with cerebral palsy participate in sports activities, and they need special considerations (43). Decreased exercise tolerance and a possible lack of flexibility secondary to the tonal problems of spasticity, athetosis, and ataxia have to be addressed. A successful, well-planned program avoids overuse, and it should include flexibility and strength training (44). Contractures can limit range of motion and strength. Persistent primitive reflexes (especially startle and asymmetric tonic neck) can interfere with performance. Consultation with a physical therapist or a physiatrist may be necessary. Modifications are often made because of cognitive, communication, and perceptual deficits. Seizures, while they can be common in cerebral palsy, are not usually a problem in athletic participation. Some medications used to treat spasticity may cause weakness and fatigue (24). Anticholinergics (for saliva control) may lead to temperature dysregulation, including overheating and excessive sweating.

Down Syndrome

Children with Down syndrome need complete preparticipation evaluations. Particular attention needs to be paid to ligamentous laxity and hypotonia. In particular, pes planus and other foot problems are common. Foot orthotics may be necessary. Congenital heart disease and obesity are other common problems that could require special attention (45). The most controversial aspect of sports participation for children with Down syndrome is atlantoaxial instability (AAI) (46). Its occurrence is especially common (15% of children with Down syndrome are affected).

AAI is defined as increased mobility at the articulation of the first and second cervical vertebrae. Fortunately, symptomatic AAI is uncommon. Cervical radiographs are of limited predictive value, but the neurologic examination is diagnostic. Neurologic findings of significance include easy fatigability, abnormal gait, difficulty walking, neck pain, limited neck mobility, torticollis, incoordination, clumsiness, increased reflexes, clonus, positive Babinski sign, sensory changes, and weakness. Clearly, a careful neurologic evaluation or referral to neurologist and/or neurosurgeon may be necessary for complete evaluation. The American Academy of Orthopedic Surgeons suggests that an initial screening x-ray be conducted for diagnostic purposes and follow-up, if needed (47). The SO still requires cervical x-rays before participation. The most recent recommendations suggest avoiding activities such as tumbling, diving, gymnastics, football, and soccer in the presence of AAI.

Spina Bifida

Children with spina bifida warrant special consideration when they participate in sports activities (48). Excessive concerns over spinal cord involvement, which is central to the disability, are usually unnecessary, and children with spina bifida generally tolerate sports well. Any considerations of spinal cord involvement, such as tethering, should be conducted in coordination with a neurologist or neurosurgeon. While damage to a VP shunt is possible, it is uncommon. Regular athletic helmet recommendations should be followed (see Chapter 8). The existence of the Arnold-Chiari malformation is of concern, similar to AAI in Down syndrome. Cervical spine precautions should be followed, and the same sports as in AAI should be avoided if the Arnold-Chiari malformation is present. Cognitive and learning problems, which are common in athletes with spina bifida, may require adaptations to the rules. The musculoskeletal characteristics of spina bifida, including varying degrees of paralysis of the lower extremities, may be a problem. Osteoporosis and the lack of sensation make the legs especially vulnerable to injury. Modifications for wheelchair and orthotics should be considered. While bowel and bladder dysfunction may be a nuisance during athletics, they are usually not major problems. They do, however, dictate the need for accessible and appropriate toileting facilities. The use of anticholinergic medications for bladder control can lead to overheating. Modifications for sensory and visual perceptual impairments may be necessary.

Duchenne Muscular Dystrophy

Athletic participation should be encouraged throughout the life of children with DMD. Common factors affecting athletics are underlying muscle weakness, obesity, respiratory compromise, and the possibility of overwork weakness (49). The goals of athletic participation with DMD have to be modified. Maintenance of strength becomes a primary goal. Building up strength in children with progressive neuromuscular disorders is difficult and often impractical. Low impact aerobic exercise, such as walking, swimming, and stationary bicycling, seems to be effective, and they will improve cardiovascular performance, increase muscle efficiency, and, ultimately, will help to fight fatigue. It is also beneficial in fighting depression, maintaining ideal body weight, and improving pain tolerance (24). Consultation with therapists is often necessary in the presence of progressive muscle weakness.

Children with DMD should not exercise to exhaustion, due to the risk of muscle damage. The warning signs of overwork include feeling weaker, rather than stronger, within 30 minutes following exercise or excessive muscle soreness 24 to 48 hours following exercise. Other warning signs include severe muscle cramping, heaviness in the extremities, and prolonged shortness of breath.

Because of the X-linked recessive inheritance pattern of DMD, overwhelming family issues often impact the child's participation. These include the presence of another affected male family member, feelings of guilt and/or depression, and other psychosocial issues. Significant contractures and profound proximal weakness often require extensive athletic modifications. Scoliosis and restrictive pulmonary disease may impact endurance as well. Cardiopulmonary consultation is often needed for sports participation because of the possibility of cardiomyopathy from primary cardiac disease and chronic pulmonary disease.

CONCLUSION

Children with disabilities have the right to participate in sports programs. Athletic participation is ex-tremely beneficial to children with disabilities. Special modifications and adaptations are often necessary. A wide array of athletic opportunities is available for children with disabilities. Healthcare providers should be actively involved in encouraging participation that is meaningful to the child and his or her family. In so doing, careful evaluation is essential. Coordination and cooperation with various other professionals in the life of the child is often necessary as well. Successful sports participation for children with disabilities is well worth the extra effort.

REFERENCES

1. Palfrey J, Haynie M. Managed care and children with special health care needs: creating a medical home. Elk Grove Village, IL: American Academy of Pediatrics, 1998.
2. Hack CH. Paradigms of care for children with special healthcare needs. *Pediatr Ann* 1997;26:674–678.
3. Bax M, Whitmore K. Prevention and management of specific learning disorders. In: Whitmore K, Hart H, Willems G, eds. *A neurodevelopmental approach to specific learning disorders*. London: MacKeith Press, 1999:280–292.
4. Lipkin PH. Epidemiology of the developmental disabilities. In: Capute AJ, Accardo PJ, eds. *Developmental disabilities in infancy and childhood*. Baltimore: Paul H. Brooks, 1991:43–68.
5. Boyle CA, Yeargin-Allsopp M, Doernberg NS et al. Prevalence of selected developmental disabilities in children 3–10 years of age: the metropolitan Atlanta developmental disabilities surveillance program 1991. *Mor Mortal Wkly Rep* 1996;45:1–14.
6. Liptak GS. Neural tube defects. In: Batshaw ML, ed. *Children with disabilities*, 4th ed. Baltimore: Paul H. Brooks, 1997:529–552.
7. Aicardi J. *Diseases of the nervous system in children. Clinics in developmental medicine*. No. 115 of 118. London: MacKeith Press, 1992.
8. Levine JM. Including children dependent on ventilators in school. *Teach Exceptional Child* 1996;28:25–29.
9. Sia C, Peter M. *The pediatrician and the new morbidity*. Honolulu, HI: Hawaii Medical Association, 1989.
10. American Academy of Pediatrics Committee on Children with Disabilities. General principles in the care of children and adolescents with genetic disorders and other chronic health conditions. *Pediatrics* 1997;99:643–644.
11. American Academy of Pediatrics Committee on Sports Medicine and Fitness. *Sports medicine: health care for young athletes*, 2nd ed. Elk Grove Village, IL: American Academy of Pediatrics, 1991.
12. Liptak GS, Revell GM. Community physician's role in case management of children with chronic illnesses. *Pediatrics* 1989;84:465–471.
13. Garwick AW, Kohrman C, Wolman C et al. Families' recommendations for improving services for children with chronic conditions. *Arch Pediatr Adolesc Med* 1998;152:439–448.
14. Exceptional Parent Fitness Column. Motor activities

and sports skills: age appropriate, functional and fun. *Exceptional Parent* 1990;20:50–52.

15. Burton SS. Sports: more than winning. *Exceptional Parent* 1987;17:35–36.

16. Burkor CK. We want to play too! including all children in youth sports and complying with the ADA. *Exceptional Parent* 1998;28:72–75.

17. Shapiro BK, Palmer FB, Wachtel RC, et al. Associated dysfunctions. In: Thompson GH, Rubin IL, Bilenker RM, eds. *Comprehensive management of cerebral palsy.* New York: Grune & Stratton, 1983:87–96.

18. Taft LT, Matthews WS. Cerebral palsy. In: Levine MD, Carey WB, Crocker AC, eds. *Developmental-behavioral pediatrics,* 2nd ed. Philadelphia: WB Saunders, 1992: 527–534.

19. Pimentel AE. The family system in developmental disabilities. In: Capute AJ, Accardo PJ, eds. *Developmental disabilities in infancy and childhood.* Baltimore: Paul H. Brookes, 1991:189–196.

20. Perrin JM. Chronic illness. In: Levine MD, Carey WB, Crocker AC, ed. *Developmental-behavioral pediatrics,* 2nd ed. Philadelphia: WB Saunders, 1992:304–308.

21. Nelson MA, Harris SS. The benefits and risks of sports and exercise for children with chronic health conditions. In: Goldberg B, ed. *Sports and exercise for children with chronic health conditions.* Champaign, IL: Human Kinetics, 1995:13–30.

22. Colon KM. Sports and recreation: many rewards, but barriers exist. *Exceptional Parent* 1998;28:56–60.

23. Dykens EM, Cohen DJ. Effects of Special Olympics International on social competence in persons with mental retardation. *J Am Acad Child Adolesc Psychiatry* 1996;35:223–229.

24. Carter GT. Rehabilitation management in neuromuscular disease. *J Neurol Rehabil* 1997;11:69–80.

25. Rieser L, Cohn SD. Legal issues regarding children with chronic health conditions. In: Goldberg B, ed. *Sports and exercise for children with chronic health conditions.* Champaign, IL: Human Kinetics, 1995: 65–76.

26. Lytle RK. Learning movement through play. *Exceptional Parent* 2000;30:32–37.

27. Andrews V. A varsity letter. *Exceptional Parent* 1992; 22:22–24.

28. Lamphear NE, Liptak GS, Weitzman M. Impact of chronic health conditions in childhood. In: Goldberg B, ed. *Sports and exercise for children with chronic health conditions.* Champaign, IL: Human Kinetics, 1995:3–12.

29. Exceptional Parent. Special Olympics. *Exceptional Parent* 1990;20:24–26.

30. Privett C. The Special Olympics: a tradition of excellence. *Exceptional Parent* 1999;29:28–36.

31. ABLEDATA. *Database of Assistive Technology. Winter sports and recreation equipment.* Fact sheet no. 16. Washington, D.C.: National Institute on Disability and Rehabilitation Research, 1993.

32. Chamalian D. Tee time for all. *Exceptional Parent* 2000; 30:74–77.

33. Mayo R. Easy riders. *Exceptional Parent* 2000;30: 55–57.

34. Broadrick T. Play ball! *Exceptional Parent* 1997;27: 40–43.

35. Broadrick T. Hockey time is here! *Exceptional Parent* 1998;28:54–55.

36. ABLEDATA. *Database of Assistive Technology. Aquatic sports and recreation equipment.* Fact sheet no. 15. Washington, D.C.: National Institute on Disability and Rehabilitation Research, 1992.

37. Chamalian D. Gooaaaaal! Ball. *Exceptional Parent* 2000;30:32–33.

38. Stolting J. The challenge to be great. *Exceptional Parent* 1998;28:42–45.

39. Chamalian D. "Top" of their game. *Exceptional Parent* 2000;30:90–92.

40. Pianoforte K. Horsin' around. *Exceptional Parent* 2000; 30:80–83.

41. Shea A. A moving experience. *Exceptional Parent* 1998; 28:53–55.

42. Empire State Games for the Physically Challenged. *Long Island regional competition.* NY State Office of Parks, Recreation, and Historic Preservation, 1998.

43. Mushett CA, Wyeth DO, Richter KJ. Cerebral palsy. In: Goldberg B, ed. *Sports and exercise for children with chronic health conditions.* Champaign, IL: Human Kinetics, 1995:123–134.

44. Little J, Gaebler-Spira D. Cerebral palsy and sports. *Exceptional Parent* 1996;26:53–55.

45. Pueschel SM. The child with Down syndrome. In: Levine MD, Carey WB, Crocker AC, eds. *Developmental-behavioral pediatrics,* 2nd ed. Philadelphia: WB Saunders, 1992:221–228.

46. American Academy of Pediatrics Committee on Sports Medicine and Fitness. Atlantoaxial instability in Down syndrome: subject review. *Pediatrics* 1995;96:151–154.

47. Goldberg MJ. Participating in Special Olympics. *Am Acad Orthop Surg Bull* 1995;43:3.

48. Duncan CC, Ogle EM. Spina bifida. In: Goldberg B, ed. *Sports and exercise for children with chronic health conditions.* Champaign, IL: Human Kinetics, 1995: 79–88.

49. Kilmer DD, McDonald CM. Childhood progressive neuromuscular disease. In: Goldberg B, ed. *Sports and exercise for children with chronic health conditions.* Champaign, IL: Human Kinetics, 1995:109–121.

PART III

Musculoskeletal Conditions and Young Athletes

26

Principles of Healing and Rehabilitation

Kenneth L. Taylor-Butler and Gregory L. Landry

PRINCIPLES OF INJURY

Physical activity and exercise are important to the physical health of young individuals. For many young people, physical activity is achieved by participating in sports. Some of the corporal benefits of exercise have been known since ancient times; these include weight reduction, increased physical work capacity, and increased muscular endurance. Modern knowledge of favorable changes in blood lipid and lipoprotein content reinforces the benefit of exercise. These separate components combine to offer improved physical health for the participant. Exercise is also beneficial to the individual's mental health. For instance, exercise is an important adjunct to the treatment of depression and anxiety, and it promotes healthy sleep patterns. Young people function better in school when they exercise regularly.

When an injury occurs, the benefits of exercise are interrupted. Physicians with an interest in sports medicine need to understand the ramifications of injuries and rehabilitation. Several principles have been utilized to facilitate the individual's return to participation. One of the most important principles is keeping the patient active while the injury is healing. For centuries, healers of many traditions have used exercise as a form of rehabilitation. Ancient Greek athletes had trainers and physicians who were fluent in the use of massage, diet, weightlifting, and other modalities to help restore athletic performance to its highest level.

Primary care physicians in the modern era should be comfortable responding to the variety of medical and surgical needs with which their active patients present. Exercising children and adolescents will often have injuries that are unique to their age group. The physician who has a solid understanding of the anatomy and biomechanics of children and of how they differ from adults aids the performer's timely and appropriate return to activity. Most athletic injuries do not require surgery; instead, they require the knowledge of anatomy and physiology, medications that are used judiciously, and therapeutic exercise.

One major distinction between the pediatric musculoskeletal system and that of adults that must be acknowledged is the presence of physes (growth plates). Growth plates transform the bones of children into dynamic structures, with longitudinal growth taking place at both the proximal and distal ends of long bones. The growth plate distinguishes the bones of children and adolescents from those adults, confirming the dictum that "children are not small adults." The growth plate is often the weakest link in the musculoskeletal system when it is subjected to stress. The ligaments and periosteum are often more stable than the growth plate.

Bone is softer in adolescents and children than in adults, so the fracture patterns are different from those of adults. The pediatric skeleton has a better blood supply that reduces the time of healing for fractures, as compared to adults. In most cases, fractures heal better and faster, and fewer radiographic signs after healing are found in children and young adults. Bones that are growing are resilient, and they can be bent quite vigorously before breaking.

In describing musculoskeletal injuries and the principles of rehabilitation in children, one must begin with a discussion of terminology for growing bones (Fig. 26.1). The *diaphysis* is the center of the long bone shaft. The *metaphysis* is the part of the long bone that extends from the diaphysis toward the articular surface. It is located just proximal to the growth plate, the *physis*. The physis is also called the epiphyseal growth plate, and it is under compressive forces in the long bones. The *epiphysis* is the end segment of the long bone that supports the articular cartilage. Occasionally, practitioners use the term epiphysis incorrectly when they are describing the epiphyseal growth plate. An *apophysis* is a bony prominence that is associated with the attachment of a muscle–tendon group. It is a traction physis that responds to the traction forces of a large muscle and tendon. In the immature skeleton, the apophysis is connected to the bone through a physeal plate. Eventually, the physeal plate between the ossification center and the shaft of

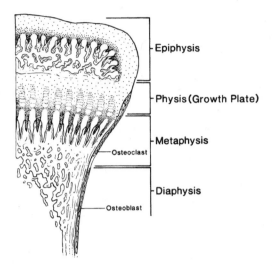

FIG. 26.1. Anatomy of normal prepubertal tubular bone. Note that the bone is divided into four segments, each of which may be involved in skeletal dysplasias either separately or in combination. (From Oski FA, DeAngelis CD, Feigin RD, et al., eds. *Principles and practice of pediatrics*, 2nd ed. Philadelphia: JB Lippincott Co, 1994, with permission.)

the bone will disappear as bony fusion is completed. *Endochondral ossification* is the progressive replacement of a preexistent and continuously dynamic cartilage with osseous tissue.

Connective tissue must be able to withstand various types of stress or *loads (Fig. 26.2).* One type of stress is *traction.* If a wire is pulled hard enough, it

will break. A thicker wire of the same material will withstand greater pulling forces. The greater strength of the thicker wire is based on its greater cross-sectional area. However, the tension in either wire, when it breaks, is the same. This is the limit of the *tensile stress.* Muscles, tendons, and ligaments all have tensile stress. Exceeding this limit will cause tissue damage (1).

Another type of force is *compression.* Thin ice cracks under the weight of a person wearing a stiletto heel, while the same person wearing wider heels will not crack the ice. The total force acting on the ice is the same in both cases, but, in the latter case, the compressive force per unit area is smaller. In a joint in which a meniscus is injured or surgically removed or if the joint is unstable from ligamentous injury, parts of the articular cartilage can be subjected to more compression than is normal because the compression forces are no longer distributed equally throughout the joint (1).

Compression and tensile stress combine when the tissue is bent. A stick that is bent has compressive force on the inside and tensile stress on the outside. An old dry brittle stick will break directly across, whereas a pliant moist stick may fold as a result of the compressive stress on the inside. This illustration may explain why children with bones that are pliable experience a *greenstick fracture* (defined under "Fracture Patterns" below).

Another type of stress is twisting or *torsion force.* Torsion is the force that is exerted on a screw by a screwdriver. If the tensile stress of the screw is low (e.g., because the metal quality is poor), a spiral frac-

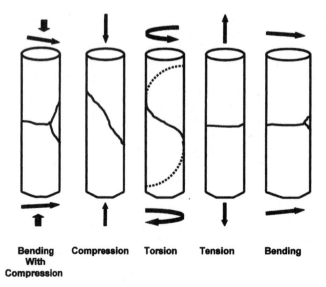

Bending
With
Compression   Compression   Torsion   Tension   Bending

FIG. 26.2. Various fracture patterns are seen in long bones, arising from different load patterns acting on the bone. (From Carter D. The biomechanics of bone. In: Nahun AM, Melvin J, eds. *The biomechanics of trauma.* Stamford, CT: Appleton & Lange, 1984:1590, with permission.)

ture will develop. The spiral fracture is seen in the skier whose foot is fixed in a boot while his or her body spins in a tumbling fall. The spiral fracture also may be seen in a child whose extremity is twisted violently. The clinician should note that the presence of a spiral fracture is often associated with child abuse, and the investigation should take this into account.

Shear stress is another important type of force when it relates to menisci or articular cartilage. When the blades of a pair of scissors cut paper, the blades exert shear stress on the paper. In the same way, the femur and the tibia can exert shear stress on a meniscus if the femur rotates counterclockwise (medially), while the tibia is stationary or rotates clockwise (laterally). This type of injury can also develop in the lumbar spine as spondylolysis (1).

Understanding these stress loads is important, because their application, either in one load or in repeated episodes, is the preceding event for tissue injury. A single load that is beyond the strength limit of the tissue (i.e., tensile stress) is the most common cause of tissue failure (i.e., macrotrauma). Repetitive smaller loads may strengthen the tissue, making it more resilient to heavier loads, if enough time is allowed for healing. Repetitive small loads that exceed the body's ability to heal the damage may eventually result in fatigue and wear on the tissue, causing pain and injury. Repetitive microtrauma is the cause of the overuse injuries that are being seen with increasing frequency in young athletes.

When done properly, training of the body tissues delays the onset of fatigue. Through adaptation to repeated loading, the body responds to physiologic stress with stronger tissue and delayed fatigue. Increasing the strength and endurance of the musculature can reduce the risk of fatigue injuries to the skeleton if a suitable training level is selected and the training loads are increased gradually over many weeks. The stressed muscular tissue responds and adapts to tolerate the increased workload. However, if training levels exceed the tissue's reparative abilities, pain and injury will develop. If pain is ignored and training persists at excessive levels, further injury results.

Understanding the development of overuse injuries through overtraining is important for all physicians who provide care to athletes of all ages. Sport injuries due to fatigue and repeated overloading of tissues are common, and they may become chronic. Young athletes may confuse the discomfort of training with the pain associated with injury. Many of these injuries heal with "relative rest," in which the injured area is not stressed beyond its limits. Relative rest provides reduced stress to the painful body part, while main-

taining fitness for the rest of the body. For example, an athlete with an ankle sprain can often safely ride a stationary bicycle to maintain some degree of cardiopulmonary fitness.

PATHOPHYSIOLOGY OF INJURY: INFLAMMATORY PROCESS

The inflammatory process is a significant part of healing for most injuries. The initial phases of inflammation allow tissue repair, and they are critical to definitive healing. When the process is interrupted or it goes on unproductively, acute injuries may not heal optimally, thus resulting in prolonged disability.

The first 7 days after an injury are an important period of inflammatory activity. Tissue damage produces hemorrhage that allows the infiltration of cellular elements to occur rapidly. The cellular elements are the chemical mediators of the inflammatory response, and they are necessary to heal the injury. Unfortunately, they also contribute to the pain and edema that occur after injury, thus interfering with the functional rehabilitation of the injury. These cellular elements can be categorized as vasoactive substances, chemotactic factors, and degradative enzymes (2).

The vasoactive substances—histamine, prostaglandins, kinins, and anaphylatoxins—cause vasodilation and increased vascular permeability. They trigger edema by relaxing the contractile elements in the endothelial and periendothelial cells, which leads to dilation of the vessels and the leakage of fluid. Prostaglandins, which are derived from arachidonic acid, cause vasodilation and increase the sensitivity of the tissue to painful stimuli. Chemotactic factors allow reparative cells to move toward the center of inflammation. Degradative enzymes are released in inflammatory exudates, and they lead to the chemical destruction of damaged tissues (2).

The goal of treatment during the first phase of inflammation, especially the first 72 hours, is to reduce additional bleeding and to limit pain and the amount of edema to allow early mobility. This goal is usually achieved by remembering the elements of the pneumonic RICE—relative *r*est, *i*ce, *c*ompression, and *el*evation.

The second phase of the inflammatory process involves the proliferation of collagen produced by the fibroblasts and cellular fibrin matrix. Collagen is laid down in a random pattern. Stretching the collagen tissue forces the collagen fibrils to become aligned in an organized pattern. This organization promotes better range of motion (ROM) and reduced scar formation. Stretching the ligamentous tissue causes the proliferation of elastin fibrils, increasing the strength of the collagen. Elastin fibers are the principal component of ligaments, and they provide tensile strength to the tissues. Excessive immobilization of ligamentous tissue causes the absence of elastin fibrils and resultant poor tensile strength. Treatment during this phase of inflammation is designed to optimize the proliferation of collagen and to strengthen it (2).

Loss of motion, joint effusion, and prolonged inflammation all contribute to pain with the concomitant loss of muscular strength and muscular atrophy. The longer that muscles are not used, the more likely the loss of strength is, which, in turn, is accompanied by a delay in the return of the athlete to maximum performance.

The inflammatory process needs to proceed in order to allow the tissues to heal. If that process is shortened, the restorative purpose of inflammation will be lost. On the other hand, excessive edema or prolonged inflammation lengthens the process, producing pain, weakness, loss of motion, and scar formation. Early mobilization is desirable whenever possible because it allows the strengthening of ligaments and tendons; this aids in ensuring that collagen and elastin fibers are deposited and aligned appropriately. Early mobilization improves chances for success of functional rehabilitation.

TYPES OF ACUTE INJURIES

Lacerations

Physicians must adhere to several principles of wound management when treating lacerations. The primary goal of wound care is to return the tissue to approximately the preinjury state, so that it will function normally with a cosmetically pleasing and minimal scar. Wounds should be closed primarily whenever possible, and wound closure should be performed under little or no tension to the tissue to prevent tissue necrosis and to provide a flat scar.

When examining any laceration, the clinician should document that all deeper structures have full function. Any compromise in neurovascular integrity requires an immediate surgical consultation. If no neurovascular compromise or injury to a tendon has occurred, the skin surrounding the laceration should be cleansed with an appropriate antiseptic solution (e.g., Hibiclens). In most cases, the region should be anesthetized using lidocaine infiltration into the subcutaneous tissue. Lidocaine with epinephrine or a topical preparation that contains tetracaine, adrenaline, and cocaine (T.A.C.), for example, can be used

in a highly vascular area. Once anesthesia is achieved, the wound should be irrigated with saline. Any necrotic tissue or foreign bodies should be removed to maximize healing.

A discussion of techniques for laceration repair is beyond the scope of this chapter. The use of tissue glue (e.g., 2-octylcyanoacrylate [Dermabond]) and staples, however, warrants some discussion. Tissue glues can be considered if the lesion is nonmucosal—in other words, if it is on the face, torso, or extremity. Glues can be considered if the wound is shallow or after deep sutures are placed if minimal skin tension is present. Minimal skin tension implies that the wound gap is less than 0.5 cm. In addition, the length of the wound should ideally be less than 8 cm.

Tissue glues are contraindicated in the presence of a mucosal laceration or if the patient is not cooperative (i.e., he or she is capable of pulling at the laceration repair). A heavily contaminated wound is not eligible for tissue glue. Therefore, glue should not be considered for human and animal bite wounds. Hand and joint lacerations also do not lend themselves to adhesive closure because repeated movement and frequent hand washing disrupts the integrity of the glue.

The major advantages to utilizing tissue glue are its speed and pain control. Tissue glues can be applied much more quickly than performing suturing procedures. Less pain is involved, so anesthetics are unnecessary. In addition, the risk to healthcare workers of needle stick injuries is reduced because no needles are required. If proper wound selection occurs, tissue glue is as effective as sutures in effecting proper wound closure without significant scarring. No reports of toxic effects or the carcinogenic potential with glue exist. Because of the speed of proper application, the rate of wound infection may actually be decreased. The cost of wound management is also reduced, since follow-up visits for suture removal are not needed; in addition, the adhesive itself is low cost.

A disadvantage of tissue glue is that wound strength on the first day is significantly less than with sutures. For this reason, wound dehiscence is the most common complaint from patients. The clincian must also recognize that accidental spills can result in adherence of uninvolved tissues (3).

Stapling wounds is another option for wound closure in the outpatient setting. This is faster than placing sutures, but its use is limted because accurate alignment of wound edges is not always ideal. Thus, selecting the location for staple use is important for achieving successful results. The scalp, arms, trunk, and legs are the best sites for surgical staples.

Abrasions

Abrasions are defined as superficial removal of the granular and keratinized cells of the skin. They result from contact between skin and the environment. Several colloquial names are known, including road rash, strawberries, rug burn, mat burn, and so forth. Since the surface epithelium is removed, thereby exposing nerve endings, these lesions are exquisitely sensitive. On examination, the lesion will show punctate bleeding and exudate.

Treatment of abrasions usually involves cleaning the wound to prevent tattooing from retained foreign materials, as well as infection. Cleaning is best accomplished with soap and water or, if circumstances allow, hydrogen peroxide, Surclens, or normal saline. The application of topical antimicrobial agents is controversial. However, the prudent course is to avoid such measures because of the potential detriment to fibroblast function and chemotactic factors. Once dry, a nonadherent dressing (e.g., Tegaderm) should be applied to the wound. The purpose of the dressing is to provide a barrier against bacteria and the environment. In some cases, Duoderm, a hydrocolloid dressing, can be applied to absorb the exudate. It can be left in place for up to 7 days.

Contusions

Contusions are most often the result of a direct blow to a body part that damages the underlying tissue. Pain and edema are common, and, if enough bleeding occurs, a hematoma develops. The initial treatment of a contusion consists of elevation of the affected area, ice, and application of pressure (compression). These modalities are used to prevent further bleeding and to promote absorption of blood.

Certain patterns of bruising should alert the practitioner. When bruises occur in unusual areas or if the pattern of bruising is not consistent with the history that is provided, then the possibility of nonaccidental injury (i.e., abuse) should be considered and appropriate steps should be taken.

When a hematoma develops, complications may follow. They include infection, necrosis of the overlying skin, acute compartment syndrome, blood loss (if the hematoma is large enough), and myositis ossificans. *Myositis ossificans* results from chronic inflammation and calcification of a hematoma. Myositis ossificans occurs when the usual inflammation following a hematoma does not allow the development of orderly scar formation. Instead, osteogenesis develops within the muscle. The condition occurs most often following contusion of the quadriceps muscles. Steps for prevention include passive stretching of the involved muscles and the avoidance of early irritation (4).

Abrasions and contusions are relatively common occurrences among active children. They are usually self-limiting; however, the clinician should care for abrasions carefully to prevent infection. For contusions, ice, rest, and compression should be used for at least 72 hours following the injury to prevent further bleeding.

Sprains and Strains

Ligaments restrict abnormal movement and excessive ROM at the joints and bony articulations. They consist of collagen fibers in semiregular bundles and elastin fibers for flexibility. An excessive load on a ligament or joint capsule can cause it to tear, resulting in an injury known as a sprain. (A strain is an injury to a muscle or tendon.)

Sprains are common, and they are usually graded 1, 2, or 3. Grade 1 injuries involve stretching the ligament without significant instability. When the ligament is tested, no laxity is detectable when compared to the same ligament in the contralateral extremity. Grade 1 sprains result in mild levels of soft tissue swelling and pain. Grade 2 injuries have more torn tissue with slight instability. When the ligament is tested, more laxity than normal is apparent, but the endpoint is definite, implying that some fibers remain intact. Greater soft tissue swelling occurs, and a joint effusion may develop. Grade 2 injuries often require some assistance (external support) for stabilizing the joint. Grade 3 injuries involve complete tearing of the ligament with joint instability. When the ligament is tested, the endpoint is "mushy," implying that other tissues (rather than the ligament) are providing stability. This injury may require constant external support for days or weeks following the injury.

As the clinician plans the rehabilitation of a sprain, the grade of injury and its location will determine the speed of the rehabilitation program. If the joint is relatively stable (e.g., grade 1 or mild grade 2), a more rapid progression in rehabilitation is possible.

Tendon Injuries

Tendons form a critical component of the locomotive network connecting muscles to bones. Tendons are composed of regular bundles of collagen fibers, the connective tissue around the tendon (tendon sheath), and the areolar tissue that provides spaces for the vasculature and nerve supply. The vascular supply of most tendons is marginal, which results in slow healing of injuries to them. Macrotrauma to a tendon, such as a tendon rupture, is rare in young athletes with healthy tendons. It is more common in adults with chronically painful tendons.

The tendon *sheath* (the synovium) can develop inflammation, swelling, and sometimes adhesions; this is called *tenosynovitis*. If tenosynovitis is left untreated, the result can be shortening of the tendon, limiting joint motion (4).

In young athletes, tendon injuries (strains) are often the result of overuse. Repeated tensile stress and tractional forces ultimately compromise the tendon integrity. Poorly conditioned and inflexible muscles lead to early muscle fatigue, with resultant increased tensile strength in the tendon. Tendonopathy is a distinct pathologic condition, and this term is more appropriately applied to tendon pain in most cases because the injury is due to the microscopic breakdown of tissue. Even though tendon pain is often called tendonitis, most overuse injuries actually involve very little inflammatory response in the tendon. When left untreated over years, normal tendon tissue becomes replaced with scar tissue, resulting in chronic pain and weakness.

Tendons can be injured through disruptions in the kinetic chain. For example, a knee injury that results in an alteration in gait can lead to an injury of the Achilles tendon. In order to properly rehabilitate any tendon injury, the treating physician needs to be cognizant of injuries elsewhere in the kinetic chain. The goal of treatment is to reduce the pain and stress to the tendon, which includes addressing other injuries that may put more stress on a particular tendon.

The treatment for most tendon injuries involves relative rest, ice, compression, and elevation (RICE). After the initial treatment addresses the first phase of inflammation and pain is under control, a flexibility program must be instituted. When ROM is restored and the tendon is no longer tender, a strengthening program is also instituted. Before returning to running sports, eccentric exercises are introduced. These exercises load the tendon while it is being stretched. (Concentric exercises load a muscle and tendon while it is being shortened.) Eccentric loading is thought to be more stressful to tendons, and thus it may play an important role in producing the injury and in providing optimal rehabilitation before resuming high performance activities. Strengthening exercises of the juxtaarticular musculature should also be part of the regimen to reduce the load to the injured tendon. For example, strengthening the quadriceps and gluteal muscles will help the jumper with Achilles tendinopathy (5).

Fracture Patterns

Simple Fractures

Simple fractures usually occur in adults with mature long bones, producing a through-and-through crack across the cortex and marrow.

Comminuted Fractures

With high-energy trauma, bone is crushed or the break consists of numerous cracks with fragments of bone. This type of fracture is known as a comminuted fracture. It can occur in growing bones, but it is more likely to occur in more mature bones.

Greenstick Fractures

Since younger patients' bones are more pliable, long bone fractures may be greenstick fractures, in which the periosteum allows the bone to bend while maintaining its overall shape. The bone is incompletely fractured, with a portion of the cortex and periosteum remaining intact on the compression side. Since the cortical bone is plastically deformed, an angular deformity is common (6).

The initial examination is often straightforward, with a bony abnormality that is fairly obvious. The patient often is in muscular spasm, and he or she is apprehensive. The primary concern for treatment is maintaining comfort levels. Early in the course of rehabilitation, pain control involves the application of a splint, the use of analgesic medication, and ice. Because anatomic reduction is not needed for healing or future function, closed treatment is generally the treatment of choice for most greenstick fractures.

In young children, simple greenstick fractures may heal in 3 to 6 weeks, whereas most simple fractures in adults take at least 6 weeks to heal. Before returning to sports, the youngster should have full ROM and full strength of the injured extremity, in comparison to the uninjured contralateral extremity.

Torus Fracture

The torus fracture is a compressive plastic deformation of a single cortex in the immature metaphyseal bone. It is also referred to as a "buckle fracture," where a compression load does not result in a complete fracture but results, instead, in a buckle, thereby producing a small protuberance of bone beyond the edge of the periosteum. The phenomenon creates a relatively stable injury. The buckle fracture can be subtle, and it is usually best visualized on the lateral radiograph. It may not be seen on initial radiographs, but the clinician should maintain a high index of suspicion for any alteration in the normally smooth contour of the cortex. This fracture is treated primarily by protecting the injured area from additional trauma by means of casting, splinting, or simply a wrap with activity modification. The typical duration for this protection is usually 3 to 4 weeks or until the bone is no longer tender. As the child matures, the metaphyseal bone becomes more rigid, and torus fractures become less common.

Epiphyseal Growth Plate Fractures

A fracture through the physis of a long bone can lead to the growth arrest for that bone. This decreased longitudinal growth can result in malformation of the adjacent articular surface or angular deformities. Any physeal fracture with displacement has a higher risk for growth disturbance. Patients with fractures involving the physis and, in particular, those with a displaced fracture that involves the physis should be referred to an orthopedist for definitive treatment.

Physeal fractures can be categorized utilizing the Salter-Harris classification system as follows (Fig. 26.3):

I: fracture only through the physis, without metaphyseal or epiphyseal involvement.

II: fracture through the physis and exiting out through the metaphysis with a fragment.

III: fracture through the physis and exiting out through the epiphysis into the joint with a fragment.

IV: vertical fracture through the epiphysis and physis, and out through the metaphysis.

V: axial compression crush injury to the physis, not evident on initial plain x-rays.

In general, the higher the class of fracture is, the greater the likelihood is of disruption of bony growth (7).

Generally speaking, in the Salter-Harris classification system, progressive amounts of energy are expended in order to cause the progressive categories of injury. Hence, type I or type II fractures involve low levels of trauma, and they have an equally low incidence of growth arrest. These are best treated with immobilization. Type III or type IV fractures have a greater chance for growth arrest. If the fracture is displaced, it will require reduction and close follow-up to watch for possible physeal arrest. Type V fractures will likely require operative reduction, and they carry the highest risk of growth arrest.

Apophyseal Fractures

Apophyses are areas of great stress, and they can be acutely injured by forceful contraction of a muscle tendon unit. Since the growth plate is weaker than the muscle and tendon, the bone is avulsed from the metaphysis. For example, a teenage sprinter with an acute pop and pain over the anterior hip has likely avulsed the iliac apophysis from the anterior superior iliac spine with a contraction of the sartorius muscle. An acute injury can occur with almost any apophysis, and some of these injuries require immediate orthopedic consultation (8).

Overuse Injuries

Overuse injuries are the result of repetitive microtrauma to a body tissue that has been insufficiently repaired. These injuries are seen with increasing frequency as children and adolescent performers push their bodies to extend their abilities. The most common contributor to their incidence is an error in training—increasing the intensity and frequency of training too rapidly. Quantifying the training load and the changes over time can be helpful. For example, in the runner, this is usually expressed as miles run per week. In gymnastics, it is discussed in terms of hours in the gymnasium per week. The primary care physician providing care for these athletes should consider several additional factors in the pathogenesis of the injury. Some authors have called the following factors the six S's that most often result in overuse injuries: shoes, surface, speed, structure, strength, and stretching. Improperly fitted or old shoes without adequate support are common causes of overuse injuries in the lower extremities. Shoes often lose their shock-absorbing qualities before much evidence of wear can be seen. For running shoes, this occurs after they have been used for about 500 miles, but some individuals need new shoes even more frequently. Training on rigid surfaces (e.g., concrete) is more stressful to the body than is training on surfaces that offer some shock absorption. (e.g., grass). Sudden increases in speed during training are another important risk factor. For example, a tennis player who spends more time practicing his or her serve has a higher risk for injury. Adolescents are subject to growth spurts, whereby bones grow much more quickly than the associated muscle–tendon units. Young athletes are probably more vulnerable to injury both during and immediately following these growth spurts. This constitutes an important time to pay attention to stretching and flexibility, as well as to the proper strength-

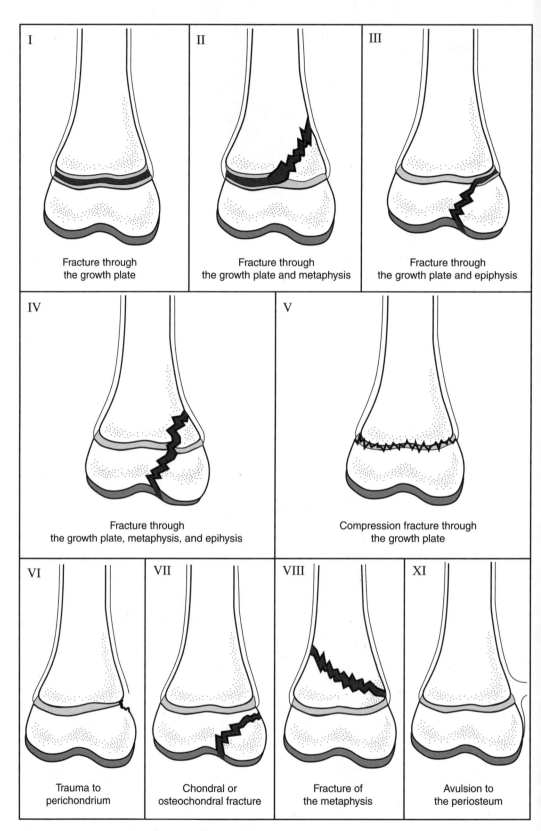

FIG. 26.3. Salter-Harris classification of epiphyseal growth plate fractures.

ening of various muscle groups, to prevent overuse injuries.

Stress Fractures

Stress fractures are fatigue fractures due to repetitive stress that cumulatively leads to mechanical failure. They represent a process rather than an event. Bone, like any viable tissue, responds to stress as part of its development. It follows Wolff's law, which states that a tissue remodels itself to withstand the mechanical demands placed upon it. If the physical demands exceed the reparative abilities of the bone, then a fatigue fracture of the trabecular or cortical bone develops.

Stress fractures are thought to result from direct loading during athletic activity or from loading by an adjacent muscle. Muscles produce a force that is exerted on bone. If repetitive forceful muscle contractions are greater than the bone strength, a stress fracture may result. If a muscle fatigues so that it is no longer able to absorb a portion of the force of weight bearing, more stress is transmitted to the bone. This increased stress increases the likelihood of a stress fracture (1).

As with any other overuse injury, the biggest risk factor for developing stress fractures is abrupt changes in the training regimen. Stress fractures develop in the skeletally maturing adolescent when he or she begins intensive training for an activity. Other factors that alter the distribution of forces in the body include anatomic problems, such as leg length discrepancy, excessive pronation, and muscle imbalances. Mechanical problems, such as improper shoes and hard training surfaces, also enhance the possibility of stress fractures. Other relative risk factors include the female gender, Caucasian race, low bone mineral density, low calcium intake, and any alterations in gait caused by physiologic or anatomic factors. Adolescent female athletes who are amenorrheic, whether with or without a poor calcium intake, are at risk for stress fractures.

Symptoms of lower extremity stress fractures include pain with weight bearing and reduced pain at rest. Tenderness is usually well localized, and it is more severe with other injuries. Swelling is often minimal. Stress fractures that are considered high risk for nonunion include those in the anterior medial third of the tibia, the tarsal navicular, and the diaphyseal–metaphyseal junction of the fifth metatarsal (*Jones fracture*). These fractures are at high risk for nonunion because they are in hypovascular areas (6).

Radiographs of the stress fracture may show periosteal elevation and new callus formation after 2 weeks of symptoms. During the first 2 weeks of pain, plain radiographs often will be normal. If the diagnosis is suspected and a definitive test is required, radionuclide bone scanning has become the gold standard, since it is capable of showing subtle changes in bone metabolism. Technetium-99m phosphate analogues are most commonly used because they are taken up at sites of turnover of bone. The stress fracture will show up in all three phases as a focally intense fusiform area of cortical uptake. The sensitivity of the bone scan is compromised by the lack of specificity. However, uptake is also seen in other conditions, such as infections, bone infarction, periostitis, and tumors. In some settings, magnetic resonance imaging (MRI) is utilized to make the diagnosis. However, MRI is also compromised by a lack of specificity as the marrow edema that is associated with a stress fracture is also seen with infections or tumors.

Treatment requires relative rest if the athlete can walk without a limp. The young athlete with a stress fracture should be advised to cross-train for 3 to 6 weeks. As long as the activities are not painful, he or she can swim, bike, or run in water. The time to full recovery from a stress fracture is usually 6 to 8 weeks. Some stress fractures require more aggressive treatment. For example, stress fractures of the calcaneus may require 2 weeks of casting or a walking orthosis. Those athletes who are at risk for nonunion require immobilization or surgical intervention. The Jones fracture may require early surgical invention because even 8 weeks in a non–weight-bearing cast may not lead to a permanent bony union.

If the young athlete develops pain again over the stress fracture site, activity should be decreased to a level where it can be conducted without pain and that level should be maintained for at least 1 week before advancement is attempted.

Apophysitis

Injuries to the apophyseal growth plate are usually secondary to repetitive use of the muscle–tendon unit attached to the apophysis and/or a major blow directly to it. The ossified nucleus may be disrupted and may be displaced partially or completely. Tenderness of the apophysis and pain is called apophysitis. Although the term apophysitis implies an inflammatory condition, the pathophysiology is more analogous to a stress fracture and it usually involves minimal inflammation (5). Muscle attachments to the apophyses are made through interosseous extensions of its tendinous segment, which are called Sharpey fibers. This attachment is stronger than the collagenous fibers that span the physeal plate. Therefore, when powerful forces are applied, logically the forces divide through the apophyseal growth plate instead of disrupting the tendon from the apophyseal insertion.

Epiphysitis

Epiphysitis is an injury to the compression physis in the long bone due to overuse. The term is a misnomer, as this condition is not inflammation of the end of a long bone but rather a stress reaction to the epiphyseal growth plate. Persistent injury to the growth plate can affect the growth of a long bone. Despite great concern about injuries to growth plates in the legs of young runners, few cases of such injuries are found in the literature. The most frequent chronic injury to a physis occurs in gymnasts' wrists, as injury to the distal radial physis. The growth disturbance in these athletes results in ulnar deviation of the wrist that may put these gymnasts at risk for early arthritis.

Enthesopathy

Enthesopathy is an inflammatory condition of the cartilaginous attachment of the ligaments and tendons to bone. It is commonly associated with juvenile-onset seronegative spondyloarthropathy, but it has also been associated with athletic activities. Enthesopathy can occur with other conditions as well, such as ankylosing spondylitis and Reiter syndrome, and other entities with the positive genetic marker HLA-B27. The presentation will depend on which site is affected. The Achilles tendon and the plantar fascia are the most common sites for enthesopathy, and they will present with heel pain. The treatment is usually nonoperative. Relative rest, antiinflammatory medications, orthotics, and a stretching program are the primary lines of treatment (4).

PRINCIPLES OF REHABILITATION

Before determining any rehabilitation plan for a patient, the primary care practitioner must properly evaluate the injured young athlete. A complete history of the injury and a proper diagnosis will provide guidance for the rehabilitation program.

Knowing the athlete's age and gender is important, in order to be able to anticipate the presence or absence of open growth plates (physes). Knowing the particular sports or activities involved may provide a better understanding of the potential mechanism of injury. Any recent changes in the athlete's training are important, especially any increase in the type, intensity, or duration of any particular activity. Knowing precisely when and how the athlete experienced the injury and whether it was an acute trauma or an overuse injury is helpful.

The physical examination begins with *observation* of the injured individual. Posture and gait are important factors in many injuries. *Palpation* of the painful region, as well as of its surrounding joints, is important. The clinician must also examine the uninjured extremity to determine what asymmetries exist that might have predisposed the athlete to injury or that may be a result of the injury. After a complete history and physical examination, a diagnosis should be established. If the diagnosis is unclear, further diagnostic testing may be necessary to make the diagnosis certain. The rehabilitation program will only be as good as the accuracy of the diagnosis, so making the correct diagnosis is important.

At the time of initial diagnosis, having precise measurements of *active and passive ROM* is helpful. If restrictions to full ROM are present, these should be documented (e.g., swelling, pain, or mechanical locking). The presence of some restrictions may alter the treatment plan. Precise measurement at the time of diagnosis will make follow-up measurements more useful for documenting the individual's improvement over the course of the rehabilitation process. Even after taking these initial measurements, taking repeated measurements using consistent, well-defined test positions is also helpful. Using goniometers for joint ROM and tape measures for length and circumference (girth) is advisable because both instruments are practical and the measurements are then reproducible.

Isokinetic testing of an affected muscle group is a useful means for quantifying muscle performance, and it is more reproducible than the standard manual muscle strength testing. This type of testing is often done in a physical therapy or athletic training setting, and it measures torque values that can be accurately measured and graphed. The usual parameters are muscle strength (slow torque), power (maximum torque), and power endurance (the number of repetitions at a specific arc of motion). These measurements can be reproduced and computerized, and they constitute a highly accurate method of tracking improvement during rehabilitation. Unfortunately, normative data is dependent on the various companies that provide isokinetic testing equipment, so clinic measurements are primarily used to compare the injured extremity to the uninjured one and to track improvement in an objective way. Determining the presence or absence of joint stability is a vital part of assessing virtually any joint injury. Any instability may adversely affect the athlete's ability to use that joint maximally during rehabilitation. *Neurovascular assessment* is accomplished through testing of deep tendon reflexes—sensation within the affected dermatome, pulse, and capillary refill, depending on the region injured. This type of assessment offers assurance that the injury is limited to the musculoskeletal system. All of this information is documented, and it becomes important in determining the goals of rehabilitation (2,5,9).

GOALS OF REHABILITATION

At the time of injury, the physician, therapist, athletic trainer, the athlete, and his or her parents ideally will come together to generate a rehabilitation plan. They each may have their own agenda; however, certain aspects of the rehabilitation plan are universal. First, the plan should decrease *pain*. This goal can be accomplished through a variety of interventions, including medications and modalities (e.g., heat, cold, therapeutic electricity, and immobilization). (Modalities are discussed more extensively in the section that follows.) Next, the plan must promote a *normal ROM* through passive, active-assisted, or active exercises. Return of *normal muscular flexibility* and joint motion is usually necessary before the athlete begins to work on muscle *strength*. Once ROM has returned, strength is improved through the use of isometric exercise, manual resistance, and isotonic exercise programs. Regaining *sports ability* is the ultimate goal, and this is manifested by several parameters, including balance, power, coordination, endurance, accuracy, and timing. Some of these tasks can be addressed simultaneously with strength training. However, the individual must understand that these parameters often require training in a variety of sports-specific activities before returning to that sport.

MODALITIES

Modalities are physical agents that create an environment for optimal healing while reducing pain. Modalities include forms of heat, cold, light, water, electricity, and massage. The goal for the use of any of these modalities is to return the performer safely to maximum capacity in a timely manner. Modalities should not be used as a substitution for rehabilitative exercises, but rather as a means to enhance the athlete's ability to perform these exercises.

Cold

Cryotherapy is useful in both acute and chronic injuries. Depending on the manner of application, therapeutic cold can have a variety of physiologic effects. Cellular metabolism proceeds at a slower pace when the temperature is lowered. The process of histamine release that ultimately causes edema can be slowed by the application of ice. Pain perception is potentially reduced by the decrease in nerve conduction velocity after the application of cryotherapy. Muscle spasm is reduced with cold application, probably by interrupting the pain cycle and/or by reducing motor nerve activity that generates a spasm.

When cold is applied, tissues can respond in several ways. Cold stimulates vasoconstriction that reduces bleeding in the acute setting and that reduces capillary leakage in both acute and chronic injury. Some evidence indicates that cold improves proprioception, although this is controversial. With the recognition of the diversity of reactions of tissues to cryotherapy, the healthcare provider should have an understanding of its uses to get the maximum effect without developing overcooling or tissue destruction.

Cryotherapy is most useful after acute trauma, since it reduces edema and controls pain. It is also used after a workout with a more chronic injury to minimize the edema that often accompanies the microtrauma associated with exercise. Cryotherapy is contraindicated in any patient with peripheral vascular disease or Raynaud phenomenon, in which excessive peripheral vasoconstriction may result. It is also contraindicated in any patient who may develop cryoglobulinemia (e.g., multiple myeloma, leukemia, and systemic lupus erythematosis).

The different types of applications for cryotherapy include ice packs, ice baths, and ice massage. Each application has advantages and disadvantages. Some are better applied to a given body part than others; some are focal, while others are generalized. Ice packs are probably the most used in sports medicine. Crushed ice in a plastic bag works well in most cases. Chemical packs are acceptable, but they are expensive and warm up rapidly. Commercial gel packs that are kept in the freezer are convenient, but these can get super cooled, and they are more likely to cause frostbite. Having a layer of clothing or thin towel under an ice pack, especially when using gel packs, is advisable. The maximal effect of cryotherapy is acheieved in 20 minutes. After that period of time, reflex vasodilatation occurs. The advantage of ice bags is their ease of application to almost any body part. Ice baths are desirable when an entire joint, such as an ankle or elbow, needs to be treated. Although these are extremely effective, they are not tolerated by some athletes because of the discomfort at the beginning of emersion. Ice massage is most desirable for superficial injuries. Ice massage, which is commonly done with ice that has been frozen in a paper cup, may not penetrate the tissue as deeply as do ice packs. This superficial penetration is fine for tendonopathies and distal extremity injuries (5,9).

Superficial Heat Therapy

Therapeutic heat is best tolerated in the subacute and chronic phases of injury and rehabilitation. Heat produces several of the following physiologic alterations in metabolism: collagen extensibility is increased, vasodilatation and peripheral blood flow go up, and joint stiffness and muscle spasm decrease. These factors make therapeutic heat an ideal application just *prior* to exercise. Heat is almost never used immediately after exercise for any therapeutic reason. As a result of increased blood flow and vasodilatation, the permeability of vessel walls increases with a concomitant increase in edema. Therefore, heat should not be used in the presence of active bleeding, inflammation, or edema.

The healthcare provider must be able to recognize the indications listed above for heat, as well as the contraindications for its use. Anesthetic skin cannot defend itself with pain indications, and therefore this condition is a contraindication for superficial or deep heat because of the risk of a burn. Medical conditions that proscribe the use of heat include rheumatoid arthritis during the active phase, any active bleeding, impaired skin sensation or fragile skin, and circulatory disorders.

Several means are available for applying superficial heat. Hot packs, whirlpools, and paraffin baths can be applied to different body parts for various uses. Hydrocollator packs, pouches of petroleum distillate or silica gel heated in a tank of water to about 76.7°C (170°F), are often utilized. A variety of shapes and sizes that can wrap around a variety of body parts exist. Before application, they must be covered with toweling material of about 1-in. thickness to prevent burns. This type of treatment, commonly called moist heat, is used for about 20 minutes.

Whirlpools can be used to clean wounds and to relieve stiffness prior to exercise. (They can also be utilized for cold water baths.) Whirlpools are utilized less frequently in most modern athletic training areas now that other, more convenient modalities are available.

Paraffin wax baths are messy but effective for treating hand and wrist injuries. The wax is kept at about 52.2°C (126°F), and the affected part can be heated with repeated dipping and is then covered with a towel to retain the heat.

Contrast baths, in which the extremity is alternately placed in warm water and then in cold water, is often utilized for the control of edema, as well as for the treatment of joint capsule sprains. The hyperemic response that the contrast bath generates makes it potentially useful in the treatment of peripheral vascular disease.

Penetrating Heat Therapy

Deep heating modalities are known to produce higher tissue temperatures, and they should be utilized with more caution. Therapeutic ultrasound is the most commonly utilized method to provide deep heat to muscle tissues. Ultrasound potentially decreases inflammation, accelerates hematoma resorption, reduces pain and spasm, promotes healing, and increases the extensibility of scars; and it can be used for phonophoresis (ultrasound with a topical medication). As the sound waves penetrate the tissue, they are thought to produce oscillations of the tissue molecules that convert sound energy to heat. An increase in the extensibility of the tissues and in the blood flow to the tissues is observed for up to 1 hour after the application of the ultrasound. By altering the frequency of the ultrasound, the depth of penetration can be affected. Ultrasound is a common method to increase the mobility of tissues that have limited ROM.

Phonophoresis is the utilization of ultrasound to drive the molecules of different medications (e.g., hydrocortisone, salicylates, lidocaine) deeper within the body. Patients in some studies report a diminution of pain and increased ROM; however, there is limited scientific evidence supporting penetration of the medication.

Since ultrasound is a means of heating tissues, it should not be applied to edematous tissue. It is also contraindicated over skin that is anesthetic or over fluid-filled cavities (e.g., brain, eyes, or heart). It should never be utilized over a bony prominence, especially not over the epiphyseal growth plates. It is contraindicated in pregnancy, cancer, acute infections, and inflammation of any tissue.

Therapeutic Electrical Stimulation

Electricity is used therapeutically to stimulate muscles and neuronal tissue and, in various forms, to relieve pain, to aid tissue healing, and to reduce muscle spasms. Electrical muscle stimulation is used to enhance muscle contraction when reflex inhibition is present and to stimulate muscle when a limb is immobilized in order to minimize muscle atrophy. It can be used to reenforce voluntary contraction during rehabilitation. It is also used to break down adhesions within muscle (2).

Transcutaneous electrical nerve stimulation (TENS) is used for the control of pain. It is thought to work initially via the "gate control" theory of pain reduction by stimulating the large sensory nerve fiber input that suppresses the small pain nerve fibers. It provides pain relief beyond the time of stimulation, so it must relieve pain by other mechanisms as well.

High voltage, pulsed (galvanic) stimulation transmits a voltage of 100 to 500 volts. Little cutaneous stimulation occurs, so the treatment is not necessarily uncomfortable. It is used for pain relief, tissue healing, the reduction of muscle spasm, and muscle reeducation (5).

Galvanic (direct) current can directly stimulate denervated muscle, but it is more commonly used to drive ions into tissues, a process called iontophoresis. The theory is that, when a direct current is applied, the molecules of the medication move away from the electrode and into the skin. Corticosteroids are the most common medications that are used in this procedure, and anecdotal evidence of relief does exist, especially for superficial injuries (e.g., tendonopathies). Scientific evidence of the efficacy of this method is not conclusive. The modality has been reported to be clinically useful in treating bursitis, tendinitis, adhesive capsulitis, calcium deposits, and hyperhidrosis. With the use of direct current electricity, the possibility of burns is always present. Iontophoresis is contraindicated in patients whose skin is anesthetic and in those who are known to be allergic to the applied medication.

Mechanical Therapy

Mechanical therapies included in the care of athletes are massage, manual therapy, manipulative therapy, traction, and intermittent compression.

Massage

Massage involves a systematic manipulation of the soft tissues of the body. This modality involves different rates and rhythm, pressure, direction, and duration, depending on the intended effect. Basic techniques include effleurage (superficial or deep stroking), petrissage (kneading), apotement (percussion or tapping), vibration (trembling with forward and backward movement), and friction (pressure across muscles or tendons). One of the more powerful techniques of massage in sports medicine is friction (or cross-fiber) massage. In this method of massage, pressure is applied transverse to the muscle fiber, tendon, or ligament. The intention of this is to break up adhesions in the subacute and chronic phases of injury. Despite a paucity of clinical data regarding its effectiveness, this type of massage continues to gain support in clinical practice.

Contraindications to massage therapy include areas of acute injuries, hemorrhaging, infection, thromboses, nerve damage, skin disease, and soft tissue calcifications.

Manual Therapy

Manual therapy is also known as joint mobilization. This therapy uses a combination of graded oscillations and traction to joint surfaces to restore normal joint function.

Manipulative Therapy

Manipulative therapy is the use of high-velocity forceful movements at the end of a normal range of joint motion. Its use is indicated for freeing a joint from a fixed pathologic position, such as with a locked vertebral facet.

Traction

Traction is usually used for the cervical or lumbar spine in a continuous fashion or for intermittent therapy. It rarely corrects any spinal dysfunction, but it can help control pain and nerve root irritation, especially in the presence of disc pathology.

Intermittent Compression

To accomplish intermittent compression, an air-filled boot or sleeve is applied to an extremity, usually in combination with elevation. This is designed to assist venous return and to reduce edema. It is often used in combination with cryotherapy.

Water Therapy

Water therapy simply means performing exercises in the presence of water. This intervention is popular because a variety of tasks that would be much riskier on dry land can be performed safely with the buoyancy of water. For example, working on balance with a sprained ankle can begin much earlier in water after an injury than if the exercise were only done on dry land. Not all athletes are comfortable working in water (especially those who cannot swim), and water rehabilitation cannot be performed with an open wound. Water therapy requires access to a pool, and the athlete must be supervised while working out in the pool.

SUMMARY OF THE GOALS OF REHABILITATION

The goal of any rehabilitation plan is to return a young athlete to his or her maximal abilities safely. This goal is best accomplished in an orderly stepwise approach. Each step will have its own area of emphasis and ideal method of application. The first step is to *control pain and inflammation*. Rest, ice, compression, and elevation (RICE) are the primary methods for effecting this control in the early stages of bleeding, swelling, and inflammation. This first step in rehabilitation primarily addresses the first 48 to 72 hours after injury. Resting the affected area may include immobilization. Use of steroidal or nonsteroidal antiinflammatory analgesics is controversial in the early days following an injury. Many individuals need analgesia, but whether antiinflammatory medications are harmful or helpful to acute injuries is not clear.

Expanding flexibility and joint ROM is the second step in effective rehabilitation of the injury. Control of pain and edema are still important in this step. The use of additional modalities may be appropriate at this point. Ice is a modality that is useful in relieving muscular spasm and pain, which cause decreased joint ROM. A TENS unit can break the pain cycle and can prevent or minimize the development of soft tissue contracture. Electrical stimulation can be helpful as a means of limiting edema and of promoting healing. Contrast baths or the use of ultrasound will often help improve motion. To regain full joint motion and muscle–tendon flexibility, therapeutic exercises, such as stretching and ROM exercises for joints, are instituted. The restoration of *proprioception,* or the awareness of the body and its position in space, also is important during this second step of rehabilitation.

Once ROM has been regained, the next step is *improving muscular strength and endurance*. Different types of strengthening exercises are used. Static (*isometric*) exercise occurs when *the joint angles* remain constant. Dynamic exercises produce joint angle changes, and they can be categorized as passive (i.e., someone else provides the movement) or active (i.e., the patient moves) exercises. Active exercises can be *isotonic*, in which the *resistance* is constant, or *isokinetic*, in which the *speed of movement* is constant. Isokinetic testing is often used (when it is available) to assess an individual's strength before allowing his or her return to sports participation. After a specific injury, the affected limb must be at least 85% to 90% as strong as the unaffected limb before returning to a sports activity.

Exercises are divided into concentric and eccentric movements. Concentric movement is that in which the effort is exerted in shortening the length of the muscle. Eccentric movement is such that effort is exerted in resisting the lengthening of the muscle.

Exercises can also be distinguished as either open kinetic chain or closed kinetic chain. The kinetic chain concept helps to explain the relationship of one joint to the next. Open kinetic chain exercises are those that have the distal segment of the extremity swinging free in space (e.g., leg extensions on a weight machine). In closed kinetic chain exercises, the distal segment of the extremity is fixed in place (e.g., squats). Closed kinetic chain exercises have several advantages in rehabilitation in terms of stimulating proprioception and enhancing joint stability, and they have greater similarity to activity or sport-specific movement (5).

Controversy exists about what types of exercise are best for a particular injury. Different means to the same end clearly exist. However, discussing rehabilitation protocols for specific injuries is beyond the scope of this chapter.

The next step of rehabilitation involves developing *functional exercises* that promote specific activities or sport-specific biomechanical skills. One type of functional exercise is *plyometrics*, in which explosive movements are produced to improve power (e.g., repetitive jumps). This set of skills is important in any type of activity that involves quick movement. Developing joint proprioception is important for injury-free movement and reflex stabilization. This will allow the young athlete to defend himself or herself better when he or she returns to activity.

As rehabilitation continues, improving the cardiovascular endurance of the young athlete will speed the return to activity. The cardiovascular needs of a ballroom dancer, however, are different from those of a power lifter, but both performers need to prepare to endure the rigors of their respective activity. Injuries are often a result of improper form during an exercise. Fatigue promotes this improper form. Developing and improving cardiovascular conditioning is an important issue for maintaining proper form during training. A good maintenance program will help to prevent injuries by involving cardiovascular conditioning, flexibility, strengthening, and sport-specific activities.

Concluding the rehabilitation program is the decision to return to play. The underlying principle is that athletes should be able to protect themselves from recurrent injury, while they are engaged in activity at a level consistent with ability. They must be able to perform all the athletic tasks comfortably *off* the field of play before attempting them on the field of play.

In general, the objective criteria that should be demonstrated before return to play are as follows:

Full range of motion;
Normal strength, with side to side differentials of less than 10% to 15%;
Normal neurologic examination;
Absence of persistent swelling;
Absence of joint instability;
Ability to run without pain, limping, or favoring the injured extremity (without pain medication);
An understanding of the need for a proper warmup and of the use of taping and/or bracing to prevent reinjury when indicated;
Comprehension of the risk of future injury and disability.

CONCLUSION

Children are often said to be more than small adults. This adage is especially true with regard to injury and their rehabilitation. The primary care physician caring for young athletes should be knowledgeable about epiphyseal growth plate injuries and injuries to apophyses. When a young athlete is sidetracked by an injury, proper diagnosis and timely rehabilitation will return him or her safely to his or her former level of competition. The goal of rehabilitation is to decrease pain and inflammation, to establish strength and endurance, and to create a maintenance program that will prevent future recurrences. A number of modalities are useful in expediting the functional rehabilitation of the athlete. The primary care physician will be well served if he or she learns about the purpose of these modalities and makes appropriate recommendations to a certified athletic trainer or physical therapist.

ADDITIONAL READINGS

American Academy of Orthopaedic Surgeons. *Athletic training and sports medicine*. Park Ridge, IL: American Academy of Orthopaedic Surgeons, 1991.

Beaty JH, Kasser JR, eds. *Rockwood and Wilkins' fractures in children*. Vol. 3. 5th ed. Philadelphia: Lippincott Williams & Wilkins, 2001.

Zachazewski JE, Magee DJ, Quillen WS, eds. *Athletic injuries and rehabilitation*. Philadelphia: WB Saunders, 1996.

REFERENCES

1. Peterson L, Renstrom P. *Sports injuries: their prevention and treatment*, 3rd ed. London: Martin Dunitz Ltd, 2001.
2. DeLisa JA, Gans BM, eds. *Rehabilitation medicine*, 3rd ed. Philadelphia: Lippincott Williams & Wilkins, 1998.
3. Mellion M, Walsh WM, Shelton GL, eds. *The team physician's handbook*, 3rd ed. Philadelphia: Hanley & Belfus, 2001.
4. Ombregt L, Bisschop P, ter Veer HJ, et al., eds. *A system of orthopaedic medicine*. Philadelphia: WB Saunders, 1995.
5. Andrews JR, Harrelson GL, Wilk KE. *Physical rehabilitation of the injured athlete*, 2nd ed. Philadelphia: WB Saunders, 1997.
6. Greenspan A, ed. *Orthopedic radiology: A practical approach*, 2nd ed. New York: Raven Press, 1992.
7. Sullivan JA, Anderson SJ, eds. *Care of the young athlete*. Park Ridge, IL: American Academy of Orthopaedic Surgeons, American Academy of Pediatrics, 2000.
8. Reid DC. *Sports injury assessment and rehabilitation*. New York: Churchill Livingstone, 1992.
9. Anderson MK, Hall SJ, Martin M, eds. *Sports injury management*. Philadelphia: Lippincott Williams & Wilkins, 2000.

27

The Management of On-Field and Catastrophic Injuries

Keith A. Stuessi and Joseph L. Moore

Fortunately, serious or life-threatening emergencies are relatively rare in sports. For the team physician standing on the sideline, however, steps must be taken to prepare for potentially fatal injuries. Once an athlete has sustained an injury, a step-by-step assessment should be initiated, starting with the initial ABCs of pediatric basic life support—airway, breathing, and circulation—and paying special attention to the stabilization of the cervical spine. Finally, the team physician must have knowledge of treatment of specific life and limb emergencies. In this chapter, key principles for the successful management of on-field injuries are reviewed.

PREPARATION

In a recent consensus statement developed by a collaboration of six major professional societies, the importance of sideline preparedness was emphasized. The statement defined sideline preparedness as "the identification of and planning for medical services to promote the safety of the athlete, to limit injury, and to provide medical care at the site of practice or competition" (1).

Preparation begins long before the actual event, as the team physician must ensure that the proper equipment is readily available. On the day of the game, the team physician must ensure that on-site medical supplies are readily available, whether they come from the school, the emergency medical services (EMS), the team physician, or a variety of sources. Having a well-stocked medical bag is paramount in treating any injury on the field. Prior to the start of the season, the team physician and the trainer should discuss who is responsible for certain equipment on the field. Although the trainer may agree to bring certain equipment, the team physician ultimately has the responsibility for ensuring that essential equipment is on the sideline prior to competition. Tables 27.1 to 27.4 provide guidance for assembling a medical bag, as well

as for the necessary equipment one should have available on the sideline. The actual contents of a physician's medical bag depend on the event covered (1).

The team physician is the designated team leader in medical matters when he or she is present. This person must assign responsibilities, prearrange referral to emergency medical care, and ultimately direct care on the field or court. Certain states and municipalities require that the responding EMS or trauma control team take control of the victim once they are on-scene. Good communication with the EMS system will clarify this arrangement, avoiding confusion. Included in this discussion are agreements to ensure that appropriate healthcare personnel are available in the event of an emergency. Typically, this entails EMS personnel standing by, along with the appropriate equipment for performing cardiopulmonary resuscitation (CPR) and pediatric advanced life support (PALS). For high risk sports, such as football, the team physician should consider whether these personnel and ambulance transportation should be at the site of the game. For other sporting events, these personnel should be on-call for assistance. In the case of an on-field emergency, the team leader must have adequate communication with the nearest emergency room or trauma center, so that he or she is able to relay information regarding the athlete's status. Cellular phones are easily accessible, and they are quite helpful when covering any sporting event.

INITIAL ASSESSMENT

In the event of an injury, as with any emergent medical situation, the clinician starts with the simple ABCDE mnemonic—airway, breathing, circulation, disability, and exposure—for the initial patient step-by-step assessment. This constitutes the primary survey, and its intent is both to identify life-threatening conditions and to institute management (2). While the amounts of fluids, the doses of medications, and the

TABLE 27.1. *Items deemed highly desirable for the medical bag*

General	Cardiopulmonary	Head, neck, and neurologic
Alcohol swabs and providine iodine swabs	Airway	Dental kit (i.e., cyanocrylate, hank's solution)
Bandage scissors	Pediatric and adult size blood pressure cuffs	Eye kit (blue light, fluorescin stain strips, eye patch pads, cotton tip applicators, ocular anesthetics and antibiotics, contact remover, and mirror)
Bandages, sterile and nonsterile	Cricothyrotomy kit	
Band-Aids	Epinephrine, 1:1,000, in a prepackaged unit	
$D_{50}W$	Mouth-to-mouth mask	
Disinfectant	Short-acting β-agonist inhaler	Flashlight
Gloves, sterile and nonsterile	Stethoscope	Pin or other sharp object for sensory testing
Large bore angiocatheter for tension pneumothorax (14–16 gauge for older adolescents; 18–20 gauge for younger children)		Reflex hammer
Local anesthetic, syringes, and needles		
Paper		
Pen		
Sharps box and red bag		
Suture set and Steri-Strips		
Wound irrigation material (sterile normal saline, 10–50 mL syringe)		

Abbreviation: $D_{50}W$, 50% dextrose in water.
From the American Medical Society of Sports Medicine. *Sideline preparedness for the team physician: a consensus statement,* with permission.

TABLE 27.2. *Items deemed desirable for the medical bag*

General	Cardiopulmonary
Benzoin	Pediatric advanced life support (PALS) medication
Blister care materials	Lidocaine
Contact lens case and solution	Adenosine
30% ferric subsulfate solution (Monsel's solution for cauterizing abrasions and cuts)	Epinephrine
	Atropine
Injury and illness care instruction sheets for the patient	PALS equipment
	14–16 gauge catheters for adolescents
List of emergency phone numbers	Laryngoscopes
Nail clippers	Miller 2 and/or Macintosh 2 for 8–10-yr olds
Nasal packing material	Macintosh 3 for 12-yr olds
Otoophthalmoscope	Miller 3 and/or Macintosh 3 for adolescent
Paper bags for treatment of hyperventilation	Endotracheal tubes
Prescription pad	6.0–6.5 cuffed or uncuffed for 8–10-yr olds
Razor and shaving cream	7.0 cuffed for 12-yr olds
Rectal thermometer	7.0 or 8.0 for adolescents
Scalpel	Various sized oropharyngeal and nasopharyngeal airways
Skin lubricant	
Skin staple applicator	Intravenous fluid and administration set
Small mirror	Tourniquet
Tongue depressors	Bulb suction syringe
Topical antibiotics	

From the American Medical Society of Sports Medicine. *Sideline preparedness for the team physician: a consensus statement;* and the American Heart Association and American Academy of Pediatrics. *Pediatric advanced life support,* 2002, with permission.

TABLE 27.3. *Items deemed highly desirable for sideline medical supplies*

General	Head, neck, and neurologic
Access to a telephone	Face mask removal tool
Extremity splints	(for sports with helmets)
Ice	Semirigid cervical collar
Oral fluid replacement	Spine board and
Plastic bags	attachments
Sling	

From the American Medical Society of Sports Medicine. *Sideline preparedness for the team physician: a consensus statement,* with permission.

injury patterns may differ, the priorities are identical. However, with a life-threatening condition, the dictum for use of EMS personnel is "call first" rather than "call fast," as in other serious injuries.

A Represents Airway and Cervical Spine

Establishing an airway is the highest priority in any injured pediatric athlete; maintenance of a patent airway and support of adequate ventilation, with spinal stabilization, are the most important components of basic life support (BLS). The initial assessment must determine if the airway is (a) patent; (b) maintainable with head positioning, suctioning, and/or other adjuncts; or (c) unmaintainable, thus requiring further interventions (e.g., intubation or cricothyrotomy) (3). In the football player, the staff should *not* remove the helmet; instead, the clinician should simply remove the facemask. Use of bolt cutters, "trainer's angels," pruning shears, and/or snap-offs can typically accomplish this. Cadaveric studies have shown that flexion and extension forces on the neck are minimized if both the helmet and shoulder pads remain on, and the risk of further damage to the cervical spine is reduced (4). In establishing an airway, the head tilt–chin lift maneuver is usually performed; however, in any child with suspected neck injury, the jaw thrust maneuver should be performed with an individual always maintaining in-line immobilization of the

cervical spine (3). The latter technique is useful because, if done properly, the neck is not hyperextended. Airway obstruction is always a concern, and, if the tongue has caused obstruction, the above maneuvers should open the airway. Remove any visible foreign body, such as a mouthpiece, using the finger sweep method.

The pediatric airway is different from the adult airway in several key anatomic ways. First, the airway of the infant or child is much smaller than that of the adult. In children who are less than 10 years of age, the narrowest portion of the airway is below the vocal cords, compared to the teenager and adult, whose narrowest portion is at the glottic inlet (3). Additionally, the tongue of an infant (relative to the oropharynx) is larger than that of an adult. The developmental anatomic differences contribute to relatively small amounts of edema and posterior displacement of the tongue, causing *severe* airway obstruction. In addition, the pediatric patient has a higher oxygen demand per kilogram of body weight due to his or her higher metabolic rate. Therefore, hypoxemia develops much more rapidly in a child than in an adult, thus making airway support and supplemental oxygen of the utmost importance (3). Adjuncts for maintaining airway patency include placement of an oropharyngeal airway or a nasopharyngeal airway and the use of suction devices. The use of an oropharyngeal airway should be reserved for the unconscious patient, as it may induce vomiting and/or aspiration in the conscious or semiconscious patient. As Table 27.2 demonstrates, various sizes of airway adjuncts should be part of the sideline medical bag. A useful guide is that the size of the endotracheal tube should be roughly the size of the child's little finger. Finally, if supplemental oxygen is available, it should be given to all seriously injured children.

In athletics, a major concern is the athlete who is lying face down. Especially in the unconscious child, the medical staff must always assume the presence of cervical spine injury, and, therefore, care must be taken in moving the athlete. In order to be brought face-up, the log roll, which preserves the body's alignment with the head and spine during the procedure, should be uti-

TABLE 27.4. *Items deemed desirable for sideline medical supplies*

General	Cardiopulmonary	Head, neck, and neurologic
Blanket	Automated external	A sideline concussion
Crutches	defibrillator	assessment protocol
Mouthguards		
Sling psychrometer and temperature/		
humidity activity risk chart		
Tape cutter		

From the American Medical Society of Sports Medicine. *Sideline preparedness for the team physician: a consensus statement,* with permission.

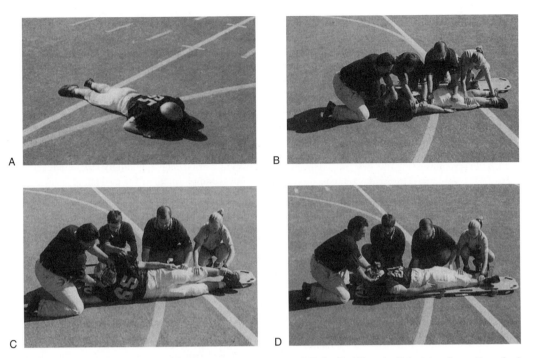

FIG. 27.1. Log roll technique. (From Garrett WE Jr, Kirkendall DT, Squire DL, eds. *Principles & practice of primary care sports medicine.* Philadelphia: Lippincott Williams & Wilkins, 2001, with permission.)

lized. To perform a log roll, the team leader stabilizes the head while his or her assistants stabilize the shoulders, hips, and knees. In one fluid motion, the child is moved to a face-up position (Fig. 27.1).

With any injury above the clavicle or in the unconscious patient, one must assume the presence of an associated cervical spine injury. Therefore, care must be taken to maintain in-line traction during the entire evaluation and treatment phase. In football players, the helmet may be taped down to the spinal board for cervical stabilization. For other athletes, a rigid cervical collar should be used; the size of the collar used should be chosen based on the athlete's age and neck size. A spine board that meets PALS guidelines (pediatric or modified) should be used on all young athletes with suspected neck and/or spinal cord injuries. As Table 27.3 conveys, these should be standard sideline equipment, especially if one is covering any of the contact sports.

B Represents Breathing and Ventilation

Airway patency does not assure adequate ventilation, and adequate gas exchange is needed to maximize oxygenation and to eliminate carbon dioxide. Once the airway is opened, the determination of whether the child is breathing is made. This is accomplished by looking for the rise and fall of the chest, listening for exhaled air, and feeling for exhaled airflow at the mouth. If no spontaneous breaths are detected, the physician or trainer gives two rescue breaths (3). If a mask with a one-way valve is readily available, this should be used.

Ventilation is then performed with either mouth-to-mouth, mouth-to-mask, or bag–valve–mask resuscitation. Of these, mouth-to-mask ventilation offers the greatest tidal volume to the patient and meets requirements for universal precautions, which are the standard of care. If the equipment is available, a more definitive airway may be established through either endotracheal or nasotracheal intubation. Table 27.2 lists the appropriate guidelines for both the laryngoscope and endotracheal tubes. One may estimate the size of the endotracheal tube that is needed by choosing a tube that approximates the diameter of the child's little finger or by using the formula (3):

$$\text{Endotracheal tube (internal diameter in mm)} = (\text{age [years]} \div 4) + 4$$
(for children older than 2 years of age).

Intubation may be difficult in the field, and it must be performed by an experienced provider.

If any signs of laryngeal edema (e.g., stridor or hoarseness) or of massive facial trauma are observed, both of which makes the use of artificial ventilation or of endotracheal or nasotracheal intubation difficult, the clinician must consider establishing a surgical airway. On the field, a needle cricothyroidotomy can be used to establish a definitive airway. This is performed initially by placing a small-bore (20- or 22-gauge) needle through the cricothyroid membrane. If air is aspirated, a large bore (12- or 14-guage) needle replaces the small bore needle, and air is again aspirated (3). The catheter is advanced, and the needle is removed. Finally, oxygen is delivered at 10 to 15 L per minute. This method may be used only for a short period of time, as carbon dioxide accumulates due to the lack of adequate exhalation.

C Represents Circulation

Assessment of circulation begins with checking the athlete's pulse, via palpation of the carotid artery. If the pulse is not present, chest compressions should begin. In a child older than 1 year of age (up to 8 years), PALS guidelines recommend using the heel of the hand over the lower half of the sternum with a compression rate of 100 times per minute (3). Compressions should be coordinated with ventilations at a ratio of 5 to 1. For pediatric patients older than 8 years of age, the compression-to-ventilation ratio is 15 to 2 for one-person resuscitation and 5 to 1 for two-person resuscitation with a compression rate of 80 to 100 times per minute (2). While ventricular fibrillation is an uncommon terminal rhythm in the pediatric age group (it accounts for only 10% of recorded terminal rhythms in children), if it is detected on electrocardiogram (ECG) monitoring, defibrillation is indicated (2). Early defibrillation has now become much easier with the use of automatic external defibrillators (AEDs) that allow nonprofessionals to defibrillate, and thus overall survival rates are improving. If the pulse is present without spontaneous breathing, rescue breathing should continue, and EMS should be activated.

In assessing circulation and overall volume status in the pediatric patient, clinical signs and symptoms, other than capillary refill, may not be helpful. In general, the pediatric patient is able to keep up with his or her vital signs until significant volume loss occurs. If signs of hypovolemia, such as altered level of consciousness, increased capillary refill, or a rapid thready pulse, are present in the athlete, begin intravenous (IV) fluid replacement immediately. Peripheral venous access should be attempted initially, and, in children older than 6 years of age, if peripheral access is unsuccessful, attempts should be made at the percutaneous central venous access or via saphenous vein cutdown. The initial fluid of choice is an isotonic crystalloid solution, such as lactated Ringer solution or normal saline. These fluids are inexpensive, and they are readily available on the field or with EMS units. They will transiently expand intravascular volume (3).

D Represents Disability

A rapid neurologic evaluation needs to be performed. Close attention should be paid to the athlete's level of consciousness, pupillary size, and reaction to light. A simple method for evaluating level of consciousness is the method denoted by AVPU, which represents the following (3):

A: alert
V: response to vocal stimuli
P: response only to painful stimuli
U: unresponsive to any stimulus

For a more detailed neurologic evaluation, the team physician may use the Glasgow coma scale, which looks at eye opening, verbal responses, and motor responses. A grading scale is used with the scores ranging from 3 (worst possible score) to 15 (best possible score); a score of less than 11 indicates severe head injury. In addition, the Pediatric Trauma score available from PALS may also be used.

E Represents Exposure

The patient must be exposed to evaluate for other injuries such as possible fractures, bleeding, and contusions. These conditions are covered elsewhere.

SPECIFIC INJURIES

After initial evaluation using the ABCDE approach, the team physician must determine further management. Ultimately, options include (a) immediate referral to the hospital for further evaluation, (b) removing the player for the remainder of the game with close follow-up, (c) observation on the sidelines with potential return-to-play, and (d) returning the athlete to play. If the athlete is going to be allowed to return to play, the team physician must ensure that the athlete can play safely, effectively, and painlessly.

Head Injury

Epidemiology

In 1996, the term traumatic brain injury (TBI) was introduced into federal law by the Traumatic Brain Injury Act. This condition has been called a silent epidemic; more than 1 million new cases of TBI occur in the United States each year and that more than 50,000 deaths are reported (5). An estimated 300,000 cases of TBI occur each year in the sports and recreation setting, with football accounting for the highest proportion of mild TBI, or concussion; the terms TBI and concussion are used interchangeably in the United States (6).

According to the National Center for Catastrophic Sports Injury Research, school sports with the highest risk of head and spine injury are football, gymnastics, ice hockey, and wrestling (7). An estimated 15% to 20% risk of minor head injury exists with each season of high school football, with more than 200,000 injuries occurring annually (8). In addition, 30% of all head injuries occurring in children are related to athletics (7). These numbers may actually be falsely low because players are unaware of the significance of symptoms and they fear to report an injury because of possible disqualification from play.

Mechanism of Injury

Three basic forces that are placed on the brain and skull are used in describing TBI. First, a forceful blow placed on the nonmoving head will usually produce injury directly under the point of impact (a coup injury). Second, if a moving head strikes a nonmoving object, maximum injury occurs on the opposite side of the impact (a countercoup injury). Finally, with skull fractures, bone may be displaced during impact and may cause direct trauma to the brain (7).

Many pathophysiologic responses to TBI are observed. Initially, cerebral edema and reduced cerebral perfusion pressure exist. Ultimately, hyperglycolysis occurs as a response to the neurochemical cascades following TBI. In all TBIs, the common finding is diffuse axonal injury and damage to the neuronal cytoskeleton, which leads to abnormal neuronal function (5). Due to damage of blood vessels in the brain, severe TBI can occur, ranging from cerebral contusion to intracerebral, subdural, and epidural hematomas, which represent neurosurgical emergencies (5).

Concussion

In 1997, the American Academy of Neurology (AAN) developed practice parameters on concussion and defined this entity as a "trauma-induced alteration in mental status that may or may not involve loss of consciousness" (9). The majority of concussions in sports occur without loss of consciousness.

Unfortunately, the effect of cumulative concussions can be catastrophic. One of the most severe complications is second impact syndrome, which results when a second concussion occurs in an athlete after the symptoms of the first concussion have not fully resolved. Since 1992, 17 cases of second impact syndrome have been reported from football alone, which translates into one to two cases per year in this sport (10). Oftentimes, the second injury appears mild, and deterioration is rapid, occurring over 2 to 5 minutes (11).

Clinically, wide variation is seen in the presentation of concussions, but more than 90% are considered mild (10). The hallmarks of concussion are confusion and amnesia, the former of which is often termed by athletes as a "bell-ring." Symptoms often include headache, nausea, dizziness, fuzzy vision, feeling "foggy" or "not sharp," difficulty with concentration and memory, and emotional lability. Signs observed by the trainer or physician include the player having a blank stare; confusion about assignments and plays; disorientation to the game, opposing team, and score; displays of incoordination; any deviation from typical behavior; and any loss of consciousness (9).

Over the past 27 years, at least 14 return-to-play scales have been published, but three of them are the most common ones used in the evaluation of concussion (12). Unfortunately, these guidelines are not evidence-based, which makes return-to-play decisions difficult. In 1986, Cantu (13) published guidelines based on his clinical experiences and on a review of the existing literature on head injury. In 1991, the Colorado Medical Society (14) published guidelines that were more rigorous than the Cantu guidelines. In 1997, the AAN published its own guidelines (9), which were amendments to the Colorado Guidelines. All of the grading systems promote the use of uniform terminology and place more emphasis on the loss of consciousness than on other markers of concussion.

Table 27.5 reviews the three grading systems and their diagnostic criteria.

On-Field Management

The ABCDE assessment should be used in any evaluation of serious head injury. On the field, the team physician or trainer can do a quick assessment by checking pupillary size and reaction, having the athlete move his or her extremities for motor function and asking the player his or her name to test speech and orientation. If any abnormalities are noted at this

TABLE 27.5. *Grading system for concussions*

Guideline	Severity		
	1	2	3
Cantu	No loss of consciousness Posttraumatic amnesia lasts less than 30 min	Loss of consciousness lasts less than 5 min **or** Posttraumatic amnesia lasts longer than 30 min	Loss of consciousness lasts longer than 5 min **or** Posttraumatic amnesia lasts longer than 24 hr
Colorado	Confusion without amnesia No loss of consciousness	Confusion with amnesia No loss of consciousness	Loss of consciousness of any duration
Practice parameter of the American Academy of Neurology	Transient confusion No loss of consciousness Concussion symptoms or mental status changes resolve in less than 15 min	Transient confusion No loss of consciousness Concussion symptoms or mental status changes last longer than 15 min	Loss of consciousness, whether brief or prolonged

From Collins MW, Lovell MR, Mckeag DB. Current issues in managing sports-related concussion. *JAMA* 1999; 282:2283–2285, with permission.

point, then serious head or neck injury should be suspected, and the athlete needs to be stabilized and transported on a backboard. For any unconscious patient, airway evaluation comes first, and adequate ventilation needs to be maintained.

After the basic evaluation, the athlete should be evaluated for his or her level of consciousness, orientation, confusional state, posttraumatic amnesia and retrograde amnesia. If no loss of consciousness has occurred and the patient has a normal neck exam, he or she may be taken to the sidelines. On the sidelines, the neurologic evaluation is performed in more detail, paying special attention to orientation, immediate memory, concentration, and delayed recall. In 1997, the AAN developed the Standardized Assessment of Concussion in football players (15). This is a simple and effective way to evaluate an athlete, and it is graded on a total of 30 points. This can be repeated to ensure that the athlete has returned to baseline neurologic status before sending him or her back into the game. In addition to the above evaluation, the physician must continue to look for any worsening signs or symptoms of concussion; if symptoms are worsening, the patient should be transported for further evaluation.

Return to Play

Table 27.6 summarizes return-to-play recommendations from the three widely used guidelines. In general, for a mild concussion (grade 1), if the athlete is asymptomatic for 15 to 20 minutes, he or she can be tested exertionally to assure no recurrence of symptoms. If the examination is normal, the athlete may return to play in that game. For a grade 2 concussion,

the athlete should be removed from the activity. These athletes should be frequently evaluated for the evolution of symptoms. The clinician should consider sending the athlete for further evaluation, if symptoms worsen or persist for more than 1 week. The athlete may return to play when he or she is asymptomatic for 1 full week. In the event of a grade 2 concussion on the same day as a grade 1 concussion, the athlete should be removed from activity until he or she is asymptomatic for 2 full weeks.

Under the Colorado and AAN guidelines, an athlete with a grade 3 concussion should be transported to the hospital for further evaluation. How soon the athlete may return to activity (i.e., 1 to 2 to 4 weeks) depends on the guideline that the clinician is following. The clock for return to play starts as soon as the athlete is asymptomatic. Close follow-up is needed in any concussion, typically within 24 hours after the injury occurred.

Neck Injury

Neck injuries account for high morbidity in children. Contact sports, such as football, rugby, wrestling, gymnastics, and ice hockey, put the athlete at risk for cervical trauma. The highest risk of spinal cord injuries comes from football, which accounts for over 50% of all spinal cord injuries in high school and college athletics. While spinal cord injury is relatively rare among children less than 11 years of age, the rate of injury increases between 15 and 18 years of age (16). This is most likely due to the fact that, at young ages, the weight, speed, and, ultimately, the force of impact is low in comparison to older, skeletally mature athletes (7).

TABLE 27.6. *Return to play guidelines*

Guideline	Severity		
	1	2	3
Cantu	Athlete may return to play that day in select situations, if normal clinical examination at rest and with exertion. If symptomatic, athlete may return to play in 7 d	Athlete may return to play in 2 wk if asymptomatic at rest and with exertion for 7 d	Athlete may return to play in 1 mo if asymptomatic at rest and exertion for 7 d
Colorado	Remove athlete from contest and evaluate immediately and every 5 min. Permit athlete to return if amnesia or symptoms do not appear for 20 min after	Remove athlete from contest and disallow athlete to return. Examine athlete the next day. Permit athlete to return to practice after 1 wk if asymptomatic	Transport athlete to hospital. Perform neurologic examination and observe overnight. Permit athlete to return to play after 2 wk if asymptomatic
American Academy of Neurology	Examine athlete immediately for mental status changes. Return to contest if no symptoms or mental status changes appear by 15 min	Remove athlete from game and disallow to return. Examine athlete on site for symptoms and mental status changes. Athlete can return in 1 wk if asymptomatic	Remove athlete from game and transport to hospital. Perform neurologic examination and observe overnight. Permit athlete to return to play if asymptomatic after 1 wk (loss of consciousness was brief) or 2 wk (loss of consciousness was prolonged)

From Collins MW, Lovell MR, Mckeag DB. Current issues in managing sports-related concussion. *JAMA* 1999; 282:2283–2285, with permission.

Certain differences in the location and types of fractures are seen in children versus adults. Children under the age of 8 years tend to experience higher level (C-2 or C-3) cervical spine fractures because the fulcrum is higher (16). In addition, due to greater ligamentous laxity and the developing ossification centers in the spine, children are more susceptible to spinal cord injury without radiographic abnormality, whereas adults will sustain fractures. Additionally, more odontoid fractures are seen in children, due to bony weakness and developing ossification centers.

On-Field Immobilization and Examination

As outlined above, the initial management of neck injuries begins in the primary survey. Any physician covering sporting events must be familiar with cervical spine stabilization and the log roll technique (Fig. 27.1). A conscious athlete who complains of neck pain, numbness, or weakness should be treated as if he or she harbors an underlying unstable spinal injury. Any unconscious participant should be considered to have a potential spinal cord injury until examination has proven otherwise, and appropriate BLS procedures should be performed.

In moving such an athlete, maintaining the airway with cervical spine control is crucial. If possible, a hard collar should be placed before initial transport. One person should be in charge of immobilizing head and neck, while at least four others take care of trunk and other body parts. All elements obstructing the face, such as face guards, should be removed, but the helmet should be left on during transport. As was indicated above, a device, such as bolt cutters or a trainer's angel, should be available to cut away all obstructive facial gear.

The actual procedure for immobilization and transport should be practiced with the medical team members prior to the start of the season. The team leader is placed at the head of the injured athlete, and he or she is in charge of calling out commands. The person in charge should control head and shoulders by cradling the head between his or her forearms; clasping the trapezius, clavicle, and scapula; and gripping the trapezius inside the shoulder pads. Other members of the team are positioned with one on each side of the shoulders and one on each side of the waist. If another individual is available, a member should support the legs and feet. At the direction of the team leader, the members of the team should reach under the athlete, clasp hands, and lift the injured athlete in unison onto a backboard. If the athlete is initially injured in the prone position, he or she should be log rolled and placed in the supine position, followed by placement of a cervical collar (Fig. 27.1). Rolling onto a long spine board should be done when possible so that immobilization of the entire spine may be accomplished. Most EMS teams have spinal boards equipped with cervical head immobilizing units. If none is available, sand bags, towels, or other weights may be placed on either side of the head.

If the young athlete is conscious, he or she should be questioned to determine the following:

1. The mechanism of injury;
2. The presence of any cervical pain;
3. The presence of neurologic symptoms, including paresthesias, weakness, or dysesthesia;
4. Any past history of neck injuries.

Depending on the above data, the physician can proceed with further physical examination (17).

The initial examination of the neck begins with palpation. Attention should be given to any localized midline vertebral tenderness; any palpable deformity, including posterior "step-off"; prominence of a spinous process; and any localized edema. If any of these conditions are present, the clinician should assume cervical spine injury and should immobilize the athlete as described above. If these conditions are not present, a complete neurovascular exam of the upper and lower extremities should be performed, paying particular attention to any loss of sensation and/or weakness. Next, the athlete should proceed to gentle active range of motion of the neck in all directions (passive range of motion should not be performed in a suspected cervical spine injury). If these tests show no defects, the athlete may then sit up, and a repeat examination may be performed (18). In the absence of abnormal findings, the athlete may be safely transported to the sideline for further testing. At this time, the clinician has the athlete actively extend the neck and laterally rotate and laterally bend the head toward the side. The examiner then conducts a Spurling maneuver where downward pressure is applied to the top of the head. Pain or numbness down the ipsilateral arm indicates neural foramina nerve impingement, while pain and numbness down the contralateral arm indicates brachial plexus injury due to stretching of the plexus.

While a universal algorithm for immobilizing an athlete with suspected neck injury does not appear to exist, multiple papers in the literature provide recommendations for immobilization in conscious athletes

(18). The American Academy of Pediatrics (AAP) recommends immobilization of the cervical spine and transportation for further evaluation if paresthesias, paralysis, neck pain at rest, or severe neck pain with gentle motion against examiner's hand are present (19). The degree of cervical pain as an indication for immobilization has been debated; however, most authors agree that a significantly decreased cervical range of motion or the presence of cervical spasm is worrisome, and these should lead to immobilization and further workup (18). Ultimately, if the athlete is sent for further evaluation, radiographs are needed, and computerized tomography is useful in identifying occult fractures (17).

Return-to-play guidelines after neck injury are based on clinical examinations, imaging studies, and the athlete's performance. Cantu (7) recommends that an athlete should not return to competition after a neck injury until "he or she is free of neck or arm pain, has full range of neck motion without discomfort or spasm, and has neck strength in flexion, extension, and on each side has returned to preinjury levels" (7). In addition, he recommends that lateral neck radiographs, if they are originally abnormal, demonstrate the return of normal lordotic curvature and that magnetic resonance imaging (MRI) shows no significant disk disease or functional spinal stenosis (7).

Specific Neck Injuries

Acute Cervical Sprains and Strains

Injury or tearing of the muscle and ligamentous components of the neck are commonly seen in contact sports. The mechanism of injury may be due to flexion, extension, compression, rotation, or any combination of these. Athletes will typically complain of pain localized to the affected muscles with the absence of neurologic dysfunction, such as numbness or weakness. On physical examination, decreased range of motion in all planes, paraspinous muscle tenderness, and spasm will be found. On-field management includes a thorough sideline evaluation, and any athlete exhibiting less than full pain-free range of motion should be excluded from further play. Treatment includes rest, ice, nonsteroidal anti-inflammatory medications, and muscle relaxants. A course of physical therapy including range of motion, stretching, and strengthening exercises may be needed. The athlete should be withheld from contact sports until the examination is normal and he or she is pain free (20).

Cervical Fractures

Fractures of the cervical spine require immediate attention. These fractures can be stable, with integrity of the spine preserved, or unstable, with excess movement between adjacent osseous elements. Clinically, the athlete will have local tenderness, and, less often, a palpable deformity will be found. Pain will be localized to the injured vertebrae, and a step-off deformity may be noted. Swelling and ecchymosis may be noted on the physical examination, and pain will accompany attempted motion. If any of these conditions are present, the steps for immobilizing the neck that were outlined above should be taken (use the log roll if necessary), and transportation on a spine board to the nearest neurosurgical facility should be arranged.

Brachial Plexus Injuries: Burners and Stingers

Burners and stingers are terms used by athletes, trainers, and physicians to describe a set of symptoms that involve pain or burning and/or paresthesias running down an arm that are occasionally associated with weakness. In adolescents, these most commonly occur from a traction injury to the brachial plexus, whereas, in adults, the etiology is usually compression at the neural foramen (16). Typically, the symptoms last from seconds to minutes, and they rarely persist for longer periods of time (e.g., days). The symptoms are most often purely sensory, and they most commonly involve the C-5 and C-6 dermatomes (i.e., the lateral forearm extending into the thumb) (7). In addition, weakness may be present but may not be severe. The most common muscle groups include the deltoid, biceps, supraspinatus, and infraspinatus.

In general, the athlete should be held from contact and collision sports until all symptoms, including weakness, resolve. When stingers are not associated with neck pain or the limitation of neck movement and if all sensory and motor symptoms clear within minutes, the athlete may return to competition (7). If the symptoms persist for a prolonged period of time, the clinician should withhold the athlete from competition until symptoms have been resolved for at least 24 hours; further imaging studies (MRI) should be contemplated to rule out the presence of a herniated disc or a foramenal stenosis (see Chapter 28). If the symptoms continue for more than 2 weeks, electromyography (EMG) can be used to assess the degree and extent of injury. Unfortunately, EMG is not accurate until at least 14 days postinjury (21).

Prevention of brachial plexus injuries in football involves the use of properly fitting equipment and modifications of the shoulder pads (see Chapter 8). These can include the use of lifters, supplemental pads at the base of the neck, modified A-frame shoulder pads with thicker padding at the base of the neck, and a collar roll attached to the posterior aspect of the shoulder pads to limit lateral neck flexion and extension. In addition, coaches can examine and adjust the athlete's blocking and tackling techniques to help prevent recurrences.

CATASTROPHIC SPORTS MEDICINE EMERGENCIES

Sudden Death

Fortunately, sudden death in the young athlete is rare. Sudden death can be classified as either traumatic or nontraumatic. Traumatic deaths in children most commonly occur following blunt trauma to the chest while playing either baseball or hockey (22). Cardiac concussion, or *commotio cordis*, occurs in individuals who are free of structural cardiac disease. Unfortunately, children seem to be the most vulnerable to *commotio cordis*, as one study indicated that 70% of the deaths from this condition occurred in children less than age 16 years (22). The exact mechanism of death is unknown, but it is thought to result from dysrythmias, particularly ventricular fibrillation, induced by a nonpenetrating precordial blow during the "vulnerable phase" of heart repolarization (23). Most of the time, the athlete will suffer instantaneous cardiac arrest, but, sometimes, the child will continue with brief periods of activity (e.g., rising, standing, or walking a few steps) before he or she collapses and experiences an ensuing cardiac arrest (22).

Nontraumatic causes of death in persons under the age of 35 years are most commonly due to hypertrophic cardiomyopathy (HCM) or coronary artery anomalies (24). Van Camp et al. (24) define nontraumatic sudden death as an event where symptom onset occurs during or within 1 hour of participation in athletics but not as the result of direct bodily injury. In high school athletes, the incidence of nontraumatic sports deaths in males has been estimated as 6.60 per million athletes per year and, in females, as 1.16 per million athletes per year (24). While these events are rare, the death of a young athlete can have a devastating impact on both the community and the clinician.

HCM is autosomal dominant, and it is characterized by asymmetric septal hypertrophy, left ventricular outflow obstruction, and pathologic specimens that show a marked disarray of ventricular muscle fibers (25). Unfortunately, screening for HCM is extremely difficult (see Chapters 2 and 17). The American Heart Association currently recommends preparticipation cardiovascular screening with a complete personal and family history and cardiovascular examination (see Chapter 16). Pertinent features in the history include a family history of HCM, premature sudden death, recurrent syncope or lethal arrhythmias, or a personal history of syncope or exertional chest pain (16). Cardiac examination may range from normal to a grade 3 or greater systolic murmur that increases with Valsalva and/or standing. If any of these findings is present, the athlete should be withheld from participation in sports, and a further workup should be instituted, including the use of the gold standard for the diagnosis of HCM—echocardiography.

For life-threatening events (i.e., sudden death from any etiology), the initial treatment includes CPR and, if possible, early evaluation of cardiac rhythm (i.e., with an AED), followed by appropriate medication and early defibrillation. Unfortunately, the success rate for resuscitation of these patients is quite low.

Seizures

Seizures that occur during exercise appear to be uncommon. Seizure during exercise may be secondary to head trauma in contact or collision sports, and, in an athlete with known history of epilepsy, seizures may be precipitated by hyperventilation or subtherapeutic levels of medication. In an adolescent athlete who participates in endurance events, such as marathons or triathlons, potential causes of seizures include electrolyte abnormalities (e.g., hyponatremia, hypomagnesemia, or hypoglycemia) (26).

Regardless of the cause of the seizure, treatment of status epilepticus remains the same (see Chapter 21). As was emphasized earlier, maintaining airway and breathing is of the utmost importance, as is providing supplemental oxygen to the patient. Depending on the equipment available on the sideline, these may be the only possible interventions. If the physician is able to obtain IV access and medications are available, then the administration of medication may be appropriate. Correction of hypoglycemia is warranted if it is detected or suspected (27). Initial pharmacologic therapy includes benzodiazepines—either lorazepam (Ativan), 0.05 to 0.1 mg per kg IV (up to 4 to 6 mg total), or diazepam (Valium), 0.3 mg per kg IV (0.5 mg per kg rectally; up to 6 to10 mg total). Repeat doses may be given every 5 to 10 minutes after the initial dose. If the seizure persists for more than 15 minutes, the clinician should load the patient with ei-

ther phenytoin, 15 to 20 mg per kg IV, at a rate not to exceed 1 mg per kg per minute or phenobarbital, 15 to 20 mg per kg IV, at a rate not to exceed 1 mg per kg per minute (27). Once the patient is stabilized, he or she should be transported to the nearest facility for further observation and workup.

Syncope

Syncope in the child or adolescent is generally a benign event; however, exercise-induced syncope may be an indicator of significant conditions that may place the young athlete at risk for sudden death. Syncope is defined as "a sudden and temporary loss of consciousness, in the absence of head trauma, that is associated with loss of postural tone with spontaneous recovery" (25,28). Exercise-associated collapse describes athletes who are unable to walk or to stand unaided as a result of light-headedness, dizziness, faintness, or syncope (25). Exercise-related syncope either occurs during athletic participation or immediately after a period of exercise. The timing of the event is important in determining its potential causes.

The differential diagnoses for syncope is lengthy, with etiologies stemming primarily from cardiac, heat regulation, or electrical abnormalities. Particular attention should be paid to athletes who have a family history of sudden death, as this occurrence may be an indicator of conditions such as HCM, prolonged QT syndrome, or coronary artery anomalies. The most common cause of exercise-related syncope in young adults, however, is neurocardiogenic syncope (25). In neurocardiogenic syncope, loss of consciousness occurs due to sudden reflex vasodilation, bradycardia, or both. In the young athlete, heart rate and stroke volume increase during exercise, and increased cardiac output is maintained during exercise by muscle contraction. After exercise, decreased muscle activity leads to decreased venous return, so when the heart attempts to contract forcefully, mechanoreceptors are stimulated and vagal reflexes trigger vasodilation and bradycardia, leading to hypotension and ultimately to syncope (25). The diagnosis may be difficult, and other more serious causes must be ruled out. Management of neurocardiogenic syncope focuses on altering training techniques and on behavior modification; pharmacologic therapy may be necessary (25).

Upon obtaining the history of syncope, determining whether the event occurred during or immediately after exercise is important. In general, syncope that occurs during exercise is a much more ominous sign, as this suggests a potential arrhythmic or cardiac etiology (25). Seizures can mimic a syncopal episode, and determining whether tonic-clonic activity or a postictal state occurred can be helpful in making this diagnosis. Once the history is obtained, the evaluation of exercise-related syncope needs to focus on the physical examination, paying special attention the vital signs and the orthostatic, cardiac, and neurologic examinations. Initial acute management of a syncopal episode includes the ABCs of PALS. Ultimately, these athletes may need further evaluation and testing (e.g., ECG, echocardiogram, or exercise stress testing) based on the history and physical examination. If any potential life-threatening abnormalities are suspected, referral to the appropriate specialist is warranted and the athlete must be restricted from any further competition until the cause has been determined (25).

Heat Illness

Heat-related illness is an important entity with which primary care physicians need to be familiar (see Chapter 7). Several differences between children and adults make children more susceptible to heat injury. First, children produce more metabolic heat per mass unit than adults do when exercising. Also, children have a slower rate of acclimatization, their core temperature rises faster during dehydration, and, due to their smaller respiratory and circulatory systems, children are less efficient and less able to adapt to exercise (16). Finally, children typically do not voluntarily drink enough liquids, which leads to dehydration and ultimately predisposes them to heat illness.

Heat illness is a spectrum, ranging from heat cramps in the most mild form to heat exhaustion, which presents as weakness, dizziness, headache, and profuse sweating, to the most severe form of heat illness, heat stroke. Heat exhaustion is the most common disorder seen in children, and, in this condition, core temperatures typically range from 38°C (100.4°F) to 40.5°C (104.9°F) (16). Heat stroke implies the possibility of end organ damage, and, if not treated promptly and aggressively, it may lead to rhabdomyalisis, renal impairment, hypokalemia, and liver damage. Typically, the athlete will display mental status changes that range from confusion to coma (16).

On-field management includes monitoring the initial vital signs and obtaining the rectal temperature. Initially, the patient should be moved to a cool area, and clothes and protective equipment should be removed to increase evaporative cooling. If cold packs are available, they may be placed at the axillae, groin, and neck. Spraying with a fine mist of water may assist in cooling. If the patient is able to tolerate liquids by mouth, he or she should attempt to drink. If the young athlete is unable to tolerate oral liquids, an IV should be started, and IV fluids, typically 5% dextrose normal saline (D5NS), should be administered (16). The goal is to lower the temperature to 38.9°C (102°F). When the core temperature is at 38.9°C (102°F), cooling measures should cease to prevent the development of hypothermia. In any child with heat illness, the clinician should consider transport for further observation, and, in the case of heat stroke, the athlete most likely requires observation in the hospital to monitor renal, hepatic, and electrolyte status.

As with other injuries mentioned in this chapter, the best treatment is prevention. Acclimatization is essential, and athletes should train in similar environments for at least 2 weeks prior to competition (16). Practices should be held during periods of cooler temperatures and low humidity. Humidity is a major factor in calculating the wet bulb globe temperature, which can be used to help determine potential risk for heat illnesses (see Chapter 7). Finally, maintaining adequate hydration is essential for preventing heat illness. Children should take water breaks every 20 to 30 minutes, and, for every 1 lb of weight lost during practice or games, approximately 16 oz of fluid should be ingested (16).

Anaphylaxis

Anaphylaxis is the systemic reaction that results from exposure to air-borne allergens, bee stings, food allergies, and drugs. Signs of anaphylaxis include apprehension, generalized urticaria, wheezing, cyanosis, and, eventually, loss of consciousness. Anaphylaxis results from decreased peripheral resistance with bronchospasm and possibly laryngeal edema. Unfortunately, no prior history of similar reaction may be found in some cases.

Management of this condition begins with the ABCs and with the use of supplemental oxygen and fluid replacement. If an allergen was injected (e.g., insect sting), the stinger should be removed and ice should be applied to the area. A tourniquet may be applied above the bite, which may slow the systemic distribution of the allergen. The tourniquet may be loosened after improvement or briefly at 3-minute intervals. Epinephrine (1:1,000, in a dose of 0.01 mL per kg; maximum of 0.3 mL) should be given intramuscularly for any case of suspected anaphylaxis. Administration may be repeated every 15 to 20 minutes, as needed for a maximum of three doses. Vital signs should be monitored closely, with special attention to blood pressure. These athletes must be transported to the nearest emergency department as soon as possible.

FACIAL AND LIMB EMERGENCIES

Eye Injuries

Approximately 1.5% of all sports injuries involve the eye, with basketball and baseball being most frequently associated with these injuries (29). Other high-risk sports include racquet sports, hockey, soccer, wrestling, and boxing. Wrestling and boxing are dangerous because no known protective eyewear exists. Children are at particular risk for eye injuries because of their aggressive play and their unfamiliarity with potential for harm that it may cause. The most common mechanisms of sports eye injuries include lacerations from flying objects, blunt injuries due to force being transmitted from a small object to the globe, and head trauma with huge forces that causes ocular injury (29).

As with most other athletic injuries, prevention is the best medicine. Data published by the AAP and the American Academy of Ophthalmology on "protective eyewear in young athletes" contain sport-specific recommendations for eye protection (see Chapter 8) (30). These eye protectors must shift the force of impact from the eyes and face to the skull while not increasing risk of injury to the brain. In addition, the recommendation is that polycarbonate or CR-39 lenses be used, as these provide the best impact resistance (30).

In preparticipation screening examinations, children and adolescents with visual acuity of less than 20/40 should be referred for further evaluation, but they should not be excluded from participation (see Chapter 2). The one-eyed athlete (defined as visual acuity < 20/200 in one eye) is able to participate in most sports, but eye protection is mandated for many of them (30). Evaluation by an ophthalmologist is recommended for these athletes prior to participation in sports.

The usual mechanism of injury is direct trauma, either with another player's fingers and/or hand or from equipment, such as a ball or racquet. The size of the object relative to the orbit will determine the type of injury incurred. Signs and symptoms of serious injury include pain, decreased visual acuity, diplopia, flashing lights, and a foreign body sensation in the eye (29). The physical examination should focus on the symmetry of the two eyes, with special attention devoted to any evidence of ptosis or proptosis of the globe. Extraocular movements and pupillary size should be evaluated. The globe and sclera should be examined for corneal defects, lacerations, and hyphema. Finally, the examiner should palpate the orbital rims for any evidence of step-off deformities or tenderness.

In general, unless the injury is minor and the examination is normal, the athlete should be sent to a treatment facility for further detailed evaluation. Indications for immediate removal from play include trauma that results in visual impairment, pain, evidence of laceration, or obvious deformity. Injuries requiring emergency referral include chemical injury, ocular perforation or globe rupture, blow-out fracture, laceration of the globe or the lacrimal drainage system, and the presence of an intraocular foreign body (16). Prior to transport, a sterile eye patch may be placed on the eye. To ensure that the patch does not put pressure on the eyeball, the clinician should cover it with a hard shield. In the case of a chemical injury, immediate sideline treatment with irrigation of the affected eye with lactated Ringer's or normal saline solution is recommended.

Injuries to the Nose

Nasal Contusion or Fractures

The nose is the most commonly injured structure on the face. Depending on the mechanism of injury, a simple fracture with deviation may be present after a lateral blow, or a more complex comminuted fracture of bone and cartilage may be observed after a direct blow to the nose. Symptoms and signs include severe pain, a feeling of a "crack" at the time of injury, and epistaxis. On examination, the clinician should look for obvious deformity. Oftentimes, a great degree of swelling occurs, making the determination of the extent of deformity difficult. The examiner should pay special attention to the presence of a septal hematoma and or a cerebrospinal fluid leak, as these require transportation for further evaluation. If a septal hematoma is seen on examination, referral for drainage and anterior packing is necessary to prevent subsequent infection and cartilage necrosis (31). In general, if the deformity is obvious, a displaced fracture may be quickly reduced on the field. However, if the amount of swelling is large and the deformity is not obvious, a referral to a head and neck surgeon within 2 to 5 days is indicated; closed reduction can be performed at 5 to 10 days postinjury, as the swelling improves (31). The athlete should be removed from the game, and return to play should be delayed for 1 week. External protective devices are required for 2 to 4 weeks after a nasal fracture.

Epistaxis

Epistaxis is commonly seen in contact sports, although an athlete may develop spontaneous epistaxis secondary to dry nasal mucosa. Anterior epistaxis in Keisselbach's plexus accounts for 90% of all nosebleeds, with the posterior epistaxis accounting for the remaining 10% (31). When conducting the examination, the clinician should look for the source of bleeding. Anterior nosebleeds typically drip from the nares, while posterior nosebleeds drain into the posterior oropharynx.

Treatment of anterior nosebleeds initially involves the athlete sitting forward with the neck extended and gently blowing out of each nostril to remove clots. The anterior nares are pinched between thumb and index finger for 5 to 10 minutes, and, if topical decongestants are available, these may be applied (31). If nasal packing is necessary, use petroleum jelly gauze, a pledget, or a tampon. These can be soaked with neo-synephrine to cause vasoconstriction. If, after these maneuvers, the bleeding still is not controlled, the athlete should be transported to the emergency department for further treatment. The athlete may return to play when hemostasis is achieved.

In the event of a posterior nosebleed, the child should be referred to the emergency department promptly for further treatment, as conservative measures are unlikely to stop the bleeding.

Extremity Injuries

This chapter initially discussed the initial ABCDEs for evaluation of an athlete who was injured. During the secondary survey, special attention should be placed on the evaluation of the extremities. In particular, muscular, tendinous, ligamentous, osseous, neurologic, and vascular systems should be evaluated. In extremity injuries, the history is especially important in determining the mechanism of injury, as this may differentiate fractures from dislocations from simple sprains and strains.

On the initial physical examination, the examiner should assess the extremities for color or perfusion, lacerations and hemorrhage, and deformities (e.g., angulation or shortening, swelling and any discoloration, or ecchymoses) (32). A rapid visual inspection is necessary in the primary survey to identify sites of major external bleeding. By contrast, a pale or ashen distal extremity is indicative of a disruption of arterial flow. Inspection of the entire body for any lacerations is necessary, as this may be important for determining the presence of an open versus a closed fracture. Finally, an examination of spontaneous extremity movement provide evidence for determination of neurologic and/or muscular impairment.

Initial treatment consists of covering any wound with a moist dressing, and, if indicated, pressure may be directly applied to reduce any bleeding. Burns should be covered with a clean, dry linen cloth. If evidence of fracture is present, the extremity should be immobilized with a splint, with a neurovascular status check conducted both before and after placement of the splint. In general, for any dislocation, reduction should be attempted as soon as possible, paying particular attention to neurovascular status. For any significant injury, especially one involving neurovascular structures, early transportation is necessary. For simple sprains and strains, rest, ice, compression, and elevation can be accomplished on the sidelines, with further evaluation later to rule out potential fractures. Indications for immediate removal from play include obvious deformity, crepitus, a loss of range of motion, loss of sensation, effusion, pain on use, instability of the joint, open wounds, or significant tenderness or swelling.

Open Fractures

Open fractures are defined as fractures in which the fractured bone is exposed to the external environment. Significant soft tissue injury is often associated with these fractures. This fact, along with the risk of bacterial contamination, makes open fractures prone to complications from infection and at higher risk for delays in healing and return to full function. Wounds should be covered with a sterile dressing that has been soaked in either saline or betadine (32). The fracture should be immobilized with a splint, while taking special care not to pull exposed bone back into the soft tissue. The wound should not be probed, as this increases the risk of infection. The athlete should be transported immediately to the hospital for definitive treatment, including antibiotics, tetanus, and surgical repair.

Traumatic Amputation

Obviously, amputation is both physically and emotionally traumatic for a child. The proximal stump should be initially irrigated with lactated Ringer's solution, and a sterile pressure dressing should be applied to provide hemostasis. The amputated limb should be thoroughly irrigated with lactated Ringer's solution, wrapped in sterile gauze, placed in a bag, and transported on crushed ice with the patient.

Dislocation

Table 27.7 shows common deformities associated with dislocations. As was mentioned above, reduction

TABLE 27.7. *Common joint dislocation deformities*

Joint	Direction	Physical exam findings
Shoulder	Anterior	Squared off, slight abduction, arm held at player's side
	Posterior	Locked in internal rotation, adduction
Elbow	Posterior	Olecranon prominent posteriorly
Hip	Anterior	Flexed, abducted, externally rotated
	Posterior	Flexed, adducted, internally rotated
Knee	Anterior and/or posterior	Loss of normal contour, extended
Ankle	—	Externally rotated, prominent medial malleolus
Subtalar joint	Lateral most common	Laterally displaced os calcis

should be attempted as soon after the injury as possible to prevent the severe muscle spasm that often accompanies these injuries. In general, most dislocations can be reduced by exaggerating the injury and gently bringing the affected part back to anatomic alignment. If the physician or trainer is not comfortable with the reduction, the athlete should be splinted and transported to the nearest facility for definitive care. Perhaps the most important point to remember is that neurovascular status must be rechecked after reduction, and the information obtained should be relayed to the accepting physician.

CONCLUSION

Advance preparation by the team physician is critical for treating a life-threatening or limb-threatening injury. Preparation begins with having adequate supplies available to treat such injuries and ends with developing and rehearsing preinjury plans for dealing with potential life-threatening emergencies. A systematic step-by-step assessment is conducted on every injured athlete, beginning with the ABCDEs, and, in the case of a life-threatening injury, ending with transportation to an emergency medical facility. Determination of return to play ultimately rests on the team physician, and, if he or she has any doubt, holding the athlete out for further observation continues is the best course of action. Ultimately, the team physician has to ensure that the athlete can play safely, effectively, and painlessly.

REFERENCES

1. American Medical Society of Sports Medicine. *Sideline preparedness for the team physician: a consensus statement.*
2. American Heart Association and American Academy of Pediatrics. *Pediatric advanced life support,* 1997.
3. American College of Surgeons Committee on Trauma. *Advanced trauma life support for doctors,* 6th ed. Chicago: American College of Surgeons, 1997.
4. Gastel JA, Palumbo MA, Hulstyn MJ, et al. Emergency removal of football equipment: a cadaveric cervical spine injury model. *Ann Emerg Med* 1998;32:411–417.
5. Kelly JP. Traumatic brain injury and concussion in sports. *JAMA* 1999;282:989–991.
6. Sports-related recurrent brain injuries—United States. *Mor Mortal Wkly Rep* 1997;48:224–227.
7. Cantu RC. Head and spine injuries in youth sports. *Clin Sports Med* 1995;14:517–532.
8. Warren WL, Bailes JE. On the field evaluation of athletic head injuries. *Clin Sports Med* 1998;17:13–16.
9. American Academy of Neurology Quality Standards Subcommittee. Practice parameter: the management of concussion in sports [Summary statement]. *Neurology* 1997;48:581–585.
10. Harmon KG. Assessment and management of concussion in sports. *Am Fam Physician* 1996;60:887–894.
11. *Guidelines for the management of severe head injury.* Brain Trauma Foundation, 1995.
12. Collins MW, Lovell MR, Mckeag DB. Current issues in managing sports-related concussion. *JAMA* 1999;282:2283–2285.
13. Cantu RC. After a cerebral concussion. *The Physician and Sports Medicine* 1986;14:75–83.
14. Colorado Medical Society. *Report of the sports medicine committee: guidelines for the management of concussion in sports.* Denver: Colorado Medical Society, 1991.
15. McCrea M, Kelly JP, Kluge J, et al. Standardized assessment of concussion in football players. *Neurology* 1997;48:586–588.
16. Luke A, Mitchell L. Sports injuries: emergency assessment and field-side care. *Pediatr Rev* 1999;20:291–301.
17. Nichols AW. Cervical spine injuries: on-field management. In: Sallis RE, Massimino F, eds. *ACSM's essentials of sports medicine.* St. Louis: Mosby, 1997.
18. Haight RR, Shiple BJ. Sideline evaluation of neck pain. *The Physician and Sports Medicine* 2001;29:45–62.
19. American Academy of Pediatrics Committee on Sports Medicine and Fitness. Head and neck injuries. In: Dyment PG, ed. *Sports medicine: health care for young athletes,* 2nd ed. Elk Grove Village, IL: The Academy, 1991:236–249.
20. Moore J, Rice EL. Neck injuries. In: Mellion MB, Walsh MW, Shelton GL, eds. *The team physician's handbook,* 2nd ed. Philadelphia: Hanley & Belfus, 1997.
21. Cantu RC. Stingers, transient quadriplegia, and cervical spinal stenosis: return to play criteria. *Med Sci Sports Exerc* 1997;29:233–235.

22. Maron BJ, Poliac LC, Kaplan JA, et al. Blunt impact to the chest leading to sudden death from cardiac arrest during sports activities. *N Engl J Med* 1995;333: 337–342.

23. Futterman LG, Myerburg R. Sudden death in athletes, an update. *Sports Med* 1998;26:335–350.

24. Van Camp SP, Bloor CM, Mueller FO, et al. Nontraumatic sports death in high school and college athletes. *Med Sci Sports Exerc* 1995;27:641–647.

25. O'Connor FG, Oriscello RG, Levine BD. Exercise-related syncope in the young athlete: reassurance, restriction or referral? *Am Fam Physician* 1999;60:2001–2008.

26. Ogunyemi A, Gomex MR, Klass DW. Seizure induced by exercise. *Neurology* 1988;38:633–634.

27. Siberry GK, Iannone R, eds. *The Harriet Lane handbook*, 15th ed. St. Louis: Mosby, 2000.

28. Driscoll DJ, Jacobsen SJ, Porter CJ, et al. Syncope in children and adolescents. *J Am Coll Cardiol* 1997;29: 1039–1045.

29. Christensen GR. Eye injuries in sports: evaluation, management, and prevention. In: Mellion MB, Walsh MW, Shelton GL, eds. *The team physician's handbook*, 2nd ed. Philadelphia: Hanley & Belfus, 1997.

30. American Academy of Pediatrics and American Academy of Ophthalmology. Protective eyewear for younger athletes [Policy statement]. *Pediatrics* 1996;98: 311–313.

31. Stackhouse T, Howe WB. On-site management of nasal injuries. *The Physician and Sports Medicine* 1998;26: 69–74.

32. Halpern BC, Cardone DA. Injuries and emergencies on the field. In: Mellion MB, Walsh MW, Shelton GL, eds. *The team physician's handbook*, 2nd ed. Philadelphia: Hanley & Belfus, 1997.

28

Head Injuries

Margot Putukian and Kimberly G. Harmon

Head injuries are common in sports, and they can have significant short- and long-term consequences if they are not appropriately managed. Detecting these injuries early, evaluating them properly, and making appropriate return-to-play decisions remain paramount priorities for the physician who is taking care of young athletes. This chapter discusses the spectrum of head injuries that commonly occur and presents guidelines for appropriate evaluation and treatment of these injuries in the athletic realm. In addition, it discusses the ongoing evolution of the clinical decisions that are involved in returning the athlete to competitive activity. Although treatment of these injuries must be individualized, basic treatment guidelines can help avoid the complications and sequelae of head injury.

Head injuries that occur on the athletic field generally are mild. While catastrophic head injuries are less common, the primary care physician who provides care for practice and competitive events must be aware of the potential risk of, and be prepared to manage, a severe head injury. Physicians also need to be aware of the risk of injuries that can occur concomitantly with head trauma. For example, intracranial vascular injuries can occur in sport-related head trauma, either with or without a skull fracture. Cervical spine injuries are a catastrophic injury that can occur concomitantly with head trauma, and they must be vigilantly looked for and ruled out as part of the initial assessment of the head-injured athlete. Other complications of head injuries include the "second impact syndrome" (SIS) (1,2), repetitive and/or cumulative injury, and postconcussive syndrome. The morbidity associated with these injuries can have a significant impact on the lives of young athletes.

Repetitive injuries may be associated with cumulative injury to the brain, or posttraumatic encephalopathy—this has been described in boxers as the "punch drunk syndrome" (3). The suggestion has been made that cumulative repetitive head trauma may increase the risk for development of Alzheimer's disease (3,4,5). The degree of risk for immediate or delayed cognitive loss secondary to repetitive head trauma is an issue that is currently the subject of ongoing debate and research in the sports medicine community. Furthermore, the degree to which a younger athlete has a greater or lesser risk of neurologic, psychologic, or cognitive deficits than an adult athlete with a similar head injury history is even more controversial. The discussion of repetitive head trauma is especially relevant to young soccer players because the repetitive heading of the ball in soccer is a sport-specific skill. Repetitive head injuries in young athletes are discussed in further detail at the end of the chapter.

Many head injuries in sports are not reported to the medical or coaching staff. This may be especially true in younger athletes because of the lack of availability of medical staff for practice and competitive events at this level of competition. In certain sports, such as football and rugby, head injuries are often dismissed as insignificant or as an expected component of the sport. In a study of rugby athletes in Great Britain, 56% of 544 athletes were found to have sustained at least one head injury associated with amnesia after an event. However, only 38 of 58 athletes who had experienced posttraumatic amnesia lasting more than an hour were admitted to a hospital for treatment (6). Detecting head injuries, maintaining a high index of suspicion for other associated injuries, and maintaining appropriate management skills are all essential for the physician who is caring for young athletes (7).

OVERVIEW

Epidemiology

According to the National Head Injury Foundation, sports cause 18% of head injuries, compared to motor vehicle accidents (46%), falls (23%), and assaults (10%). Traumatic brain injuries in the United States accounted for approximately 500,000 hospital admissions or deaths in 1984, and from 3% to 10% of these occurred during a sport or recreational activity (8). In football, head injury has been shown to cause 19% of all nonfatal injuries (9) and 4.5% of all high school sports injuries (10,11). At the elementary, junior, and high school level, football accounts for the highest incidence of head injury of any sport (12).

The mechanism for head injury in most sports that are tracked by the Injury Surveillance System (ISS) of the National Collegiate Athletic Association (NCAA) is player-to-player contact. The exceptions to this statistic are field hockey, in which the mechanism is contact with the stick, and women's lacrosse, women's softball, and men's baseball, in which the mechanism of injury is contact with the ball. These data help determine not only which sports are at risk for head injury, but they also assist sports medicine physicians in guiding changes in rules and equipment in an attempt to affect injury rates in the future.

Comparing the 1995 to 1996 data to that of previous years demonstrates that, for many sports, the incidence of head injuries and concussions is increasing. This increase may be due to multiple factors. A true increase in these types of sports-related injuries might be occurring. However, the increase may also be due to a heightened awareness of these injuries by coaching and medical personnel, an improvement in the medical supervision and athletic training coverage of sports, and better reporting and tracking mechanisms, especially at the collegiate level. Mild head injuries that were previously undetected or ignored are now more likely to be detected and documented by an attentive staff who understands the importance and significance of these injuries.

The clinician must also be aware of the inherent bias in the data system that is now utilized to monitor head injuries in sports. The incidence of injury, as well as the definition of injury used, may be different at the university level than at other levels of competition or in other age groups. Medical services available to collegiate athletes may differ from those that are available to professional athletes or school-aged athletes, and the basis for the decisions to return these athletes to play may also vary.

The epidemiology of head injuries can be useful in making recommendations to improve the safety for a particular sport. Recommendations, however, must be thoroughly supported by reliable data. For example, many authors have expressed the opinion that the sports of women's lacrosse and field hockey should incorporate helmets into their requirements for protective equipment. The desired outcome is to decrease the risk of head injuries and thus make the sport safer.

In actuality, the injury data for these particular sports indicate that the risk of head injury is relatively low. If these athletes were required to use helmets with face shields, the risk for facial lacerations, nasal fractures, and other facial and dental injuries might decrease, but the concussion rate would probably not change significantly.

One should also remember that decreasing the risk of one injury by making changes in rules of play or equipment regulations might inadvertently increase the risk of other potentially catastrophic injuries. For instance, in the example given above, adding helmets might create an increase in aggressiveness and in feelings of invulnerability that might change the sport and that potentially may increase the incidence of head and neck injuries. Thus, that rule and equipment changes be made using injury data appropriately and effectively is essential. Participants in the sport also want changes in regulations that increase the safety of the sport without changing the nature of the sport unduly.

For ice hockey and football, the use of helmets has decreased the frequency of head injury (13,14). In football, the decrease in head injuries has been 50% since 1976 (15), which has been attributed to both improvements in helmet design and fit, as well as to rule changes that forbid spearing. The benefit of helmets in ice hockey in preventing head injury has been controversial. Helmets with face masks have reduced the incidence of orofacial trauma. However, the incidence of cervical spine injuries that result from axial loading injuries when helmeted players collided with the barriers surrounding the field of play in ice hockey has increased significantly. A study by Pforringer and Smasal (16) found that, of 246 head injuries in ice hockey, 75% were due to violence outside of game play (e.g., high sticking, deliberate pushing, or fist fights). This study suggests that enforcement of existing rules may play an important in protecting athletes from head injury.

The use of helmets in baseball and softball is an example of how injuries can be decreased by using protective equipment. Helmets in these sports are used by athletes when they are batting and running bases, and this use does not affect the sport in a significant manner. The use of helmets in these sports has been well proven to be an effective tool for decreasing head injury, and, given that most of the injuries in these sports are due to contact with the ball (17), these interventions are appropriate.

Bicycling is another sport that is both recreational and competitive and in which the use of helmets makes a significant difference in safety. This decrease in the risk of injury is especially seen in the pediatric population. The large number of injuries that can be prevented by cycling helmets is due, in part, to the popularity of bicycling. It is also due to the "field of play" that is involved in cycling—the surface (hard pavement), speed, and environment (motor vehicles). When a fall from a bicycle occurs, the chance of head injury is 50%; and, if a bicyclist is traveling at 20 miles per hour, the trauma has a higher risk of resulting in a fatality (18). In the United States, 1,300 deaths of cyclists occur annually. The majority of these fatalities is secondary to head injuries. In addition, the risk of brain injury is decreased by 88% when an approved helmet is used (19). These data alone support the mandate for the use of helmets by all bicyclists.

Definitions

Head injuries are often defined as either focal brain injuries or diffuse brain injuries. Focal injuries include subdural hematoma, epidural hematoma, cerebral contusion, and intracranial hemorrhages, including subarachnoid hemorrhage and intracerebral hemorrhage. Focal injuries are usually due to blunt trauma, and they are often associated with loss of consciousness (LOC) and focal neurologic deficits. Focal injuries can occur in a variety of settings, and they can be missed if LOC is brief or if no LOC occurs. Early detection and treatment of these injuries is paramount to successful recovery if significant bleeding occurs.

One of the most common focal brain injuries that occurs in sports is subdural hematoma, in which venous blood is disrupted and blood accumulates in a low pressure setting. These injuries are often associated with LOC, and they may or may not demonstrate an associated slow deterioration in mental status and focal deficits. Subdural hematomas are three times more likely to occur than epidural hematomas. Simple subdural hematomas are not associated with underlying cerebral contusion or edema, and they have a mortality rate of approximately 20%. Complex subdural hematomas do involve these complications, and their mortality rate is greater than 50% (Figs. 28.1 and 28.2).

In the young athlete, subdural hematomas are often more symptomatic than a similar injury in an older athlete; he or she may become more symptomatic more quickly; and he or she may deteriorate faster if they are not recognized early. The anatomic basis for this difference is the fact that the subdural space is larger in the older athlete because of age-related cerebral atrophy. This allows more blood accumulation to

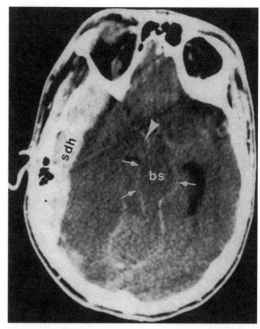

FIG. 28.1. Axial computerized tomography image demonstrating an acute subdural hematoma (*sdh*) on the right side, with herniation of the medial temporal lobe into the tentorial notch (*arrowhead*). The midbrain is outlined by subarachnoid hemorrhage in the perimesencephalic cistern (*arrows*). Abbreviation: bs, brainstem. (From Garrett WE, Kirkendall DT, Squire DL, eds. *Principles and practice of primary care sports medicine.* New York: Lippincott Williams & Wilkins, 2001, with permission.)

occur before the neurologic compromise is noticeable. Symptoms from a subdural hematoma in the young athlete generally occur as a result of compression of normal brain substance, instead of as a consequence of the mass effect, which is more common in the older individual (20).

Epidural hematomas are less common than subdural hematomas in sport-related head injuries. They are due to the disruption of the middle or other meningeal arteries, and they constitute a high-pressure vascular bleed. They classically present with initial LOC, followed by a lucid interval and subsequent apparent recovery. Within minutes to hours (rarely days), this apparent recovery period is followed by the onset of headache, deterioration of mental status, eventual LOC with pupillary abnormalities (e.g., unilaterally dilated pupil, usually ipsilateral to the bleed), and decerebrate posturing with weakness contralateral to the bleed (21). Specialists who care for this type of injury often remind physi-

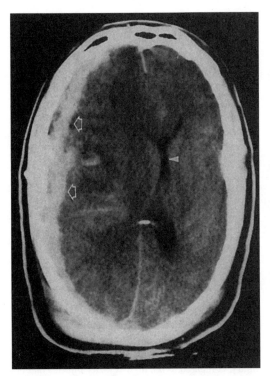

FIG. 28.2. Typical appearance of an acute subdural hematoma (*open arrows*) on axial computerized tomography imaging. The degree of shift of the midline structures (*arrowhead*) is greater than the thickness of the subdural hematoma, suggesting significant parenchymal injury to the hemisphere, in addition to the hematoma. (From Garrett WE, Kirkendall DT, Squire DL, eds. *Principles and practice of primary care sports medicine.* New York: Lippincott Williams & Wilkins, 2001, with permission.)

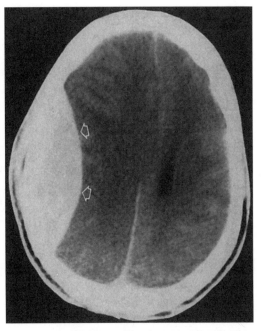

FIG. 28.3. Typical appearance of an epidural hematoma (*open arrows*) in an axial computerized tomography image. (From Garrett WE, Kirkendall DT, Squire DL, eds. *Principles and practice of primary care sports medicine.* New York: Lippincott Williams & Wilkins, 2001, with permission.)

cians that only one-third of patients present with this classic scenario (Fig. 28.3). This statistic underscores the need for a high degree of suspicion on the part of the primary care sports physician, who realizes that these vascular events may occur in the setting of mild traumatic brain injury (MTBI).

Focal injuries also include cerebral contusions, intracerebral hemorrhages, and subarachnoid hemorrhages. These injuries often present without LOC. More commonly, athletes with these injuries present with complaints that include headache, posttraumatic amnesia, and periods of confusion. Subarachnoid hemorrhages occur on the surface of the brain, and intracerebral hemorrhages are located within the substance of the brain. Both cerebral contusions and hemorrhages can be associated with hydrocephalus and changes related to a mass effect (Figs. 28.4 and 28.5).

Focal injuries can be detected by computerized tomography (CT) scanning, magnetic resonance imaging (MRI), and, to a lesser degree, electroencephalography (EEG) (22-27). In patients with persistent LOC who are admitted to an intensive care unit, the depth and severity of injury were found to correlate to MRI findings. In patients with severe clinical compromise, lesions were present 88% of the time (28).

The choice of initial diagnostic study is controversial. Many sports medicine physicians favor CT because it is more useful in detecting bleeding, as well as injury to bone. MRI is often favored for detecting subtle injuries, especially when imaging studies are being performed more than 48 hours after the incident (29–31). CT is as useful as MRI for detecting vascular injuries that require surgical management (32). When focal lesions are detected, emergent neurosurgical consultation is warranted. The time between injury and the treatment of space-occupying vascular injuries is critical for reducing morbidity.

Nonfocal injuries are classified as those head injuries that are not associated with identifiable, localized intracranial injuries. These diffuse brain injuries

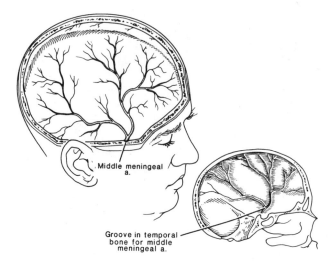

FIG. 28.4. The middle meningeal artery is tethered in a groove in the temporal bone and is easily lacerated by fractures through this bone. Hemorrhage from the middle meningeal artery causes an epidural hematoma. (From Garrett WE, Kirkendall DT, Squire DL, eds. *Principles and practice of primary care sports medicine.* New York: Lippincott Williams & Wilkins, 2001, with permission.)

represent a spectrum of injury in which the degree of brain dysfunction is related to the amount of structural or anatomic disruption. At one end of the spectrum, the anatomic integrity of the cerebral tissue is maintained. These injuries are often referred to as "nonstructural." Injuries associated with significant anatomic disruption fall at the other end of the spectrum. Diffuse axonal injury typically is associated with LOC greater than 6 hours and residual neurologic, psychologic, and personality deficits. Cerebral

concussion is also generally considered a "nonfocal" injury, although, as is discussed below, it can be associated with structural abnormalities (Table 28.1).

Concussion, or MTBI, is the most common head injury seen in athletic practice or competition. This injury, compared to the high velocity injuries that occur with motor vehicle or motorcycle accidents, is generally mild, with minimal anatomical disruption. MTBI can occur in association with the focal injuries described above. Even if MTBI is not associated with

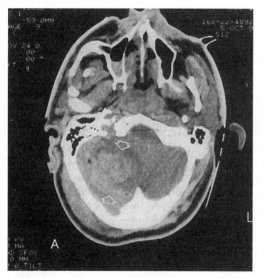
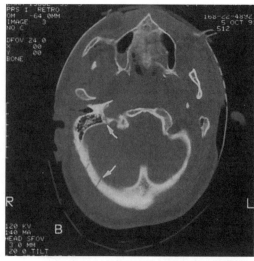

FIG. 28.5. Axial computerized tomography images demonstrate a hemorrhagic contusion of the right cerebellar hemisphere (*open arrows*) (**A**), associated with a fracture through the floor of the posterior fossa on the right side (*solid arrows*) (**B**). (From Garrett WE, Kirkendall DT, Squire DL, eds. *Principles and practice of primary care sports medicine.* New York: Lippincott Williams & Wilkins, 2001, with permission.)

TABLE 28.1. *Signs and symptoms of cerebral concussion*

Loss of consciousness
Confusion
Posttraumatic amnesia
Retrograde amnesia
Disorientation
Delayed verbal and motor responses
Inability to focus
Headache
Nausea and/or vomiting
Visual disturbances
    (photophobia, blurry vision, or double vision)
Disequilibrium
Feeling "in a fog" or "zoned out"
Vacant stare
Emotional lability
Dizziness
Slurred and/or incoherent speech
Excessive drowsiness
Symptoms consistent with postconcussive syndrome
    Loss of intellectual capacity
    Poor recent memory
    Personality changes
    Headaches
    Dizziness
    Lack of concentration
    Poor attention
    Fatigue
    Irritability
    Phonophobia and/or photophobia
    Sleep disturbances
    Depressed mood
    Anxiety

From Putukian M. Head injuries. In: Garrett WE Jr, Kirkendall DT, Squire DL, eds. *Principles & practice of primary care sports medicine.* Philadelphia: Lippincott Williams & Wilkins, 2001, with permission.

focal injuries, it can be associated with significant morbidity and mortality, especially if undetected or not treated appropriately. The remainder of this chapter focuses on such injuries.

Mechanisms and Pathophysiology

The relationship between specific traumatic forces and the type and severity of head injuries has been reviewed extensively in recent years (33). The mechanisms that account for head injury in sports can be classified as (a) impact or compressive, (b) acceleration or tensile, and (c) shearing or rotational. Impact or compressive force occurs when a stationary head is struck with a forceful blow. An example is a football player who is struck in the head; these are often called "coup" injuries, in which the maximal area injured is the portion of the brain beneath where the skull was struck. Acceleration injuries are those in which a moving head strikes a nonmoving object, such as when a basketball player dives to the ground and strikes his or her head. These injuries are often considered "contra-coup" injuries because the area of maximal injury is the brain on the opposite side of the skull from where the impact occurs. Shearing injuries occur when a rotational force is applied to the head, such as a when a boxer is struck by a left hook. These mechanisms of injury can occur in combination, and a combination of rotational and acceleration forces may be associated with significant consequences (34).

The skull can be viewed as a protective container in which the brain floats, suspended in cerebrospinal fluid (CSF). When an acceleration or rotational force is applied, the brain tissue can be injured because its acceleration lags behind that of the head so that it strikes the opposite side of the skull. The bony ridges inside the skull and the dura mater attachments form structural limitations that become points of impact (35).

The muscles of the neck function as important stabilizers of the head, and they may affect the severity of head injury. Newton's second law (mass times acceleration equals force or acceleration = force/mass) predicts that the forces acting on the head depend on whether the neck muscles are contracted when the injury occurs. If the neck muscles are rigid upon impact, the mass of the head takes on an approximation of the mass of the body. If the mass is higher, more force is required to create the same acceleration. If the neck muscles are not rigid, forces that strike the head act on the mass of the head alone, thus imparting a greater acceleration force. This principle suggests that learning and using the proper technique for sport-specific skills (e.g., tackling in football) and strengthening the neck musculature may be useful in preventing injury.

Discoveries from research involving the neurochemical and neurometabolic changes that occur with MTBI has been very exciting. When brain injury occurs in an animal model, ionic fluxes that are partially due to the release of excitatory amino acids, such as glutamate, can disrupt the cell's oxygen utilization (36,37). The cells may be mechanically normal, but they are exposed to these ionic fluxes during a concussive injury, in the setting in which increased glycolysis is needed. Since these cells are mechanically normal, the damage that has been sustained is irreversible once the insult has been removed. In animals, the increase in glucose metabolism following brain injury has been demonstrated using [^{14}C]2-deoxy-D-glucose autoradiography (38–40). This phenomenon occurs in the setting of reduced cerebral blood flow (41), and the result is an imbalance between glucose demand and cerebral blood supply. The end result is cell dysfunction, which may also place the cell at an increased risk for a second insult (42).

The data that has been obtained in human research studies appear to be consistent with the animal data. In brain-injured patients, ionic shifts that increase cerebral glucose metabolism occur (43). Alterations in glutamate, potassium, and calcium, as well as reductions in both cerebral blood flow and oxidative metabolism, occur. In severely brain-injured patients, these changes have been demonstrated by [^{18}F]fluorodeoxyglucose-positron emission tomography (FDG-PET) scanning studies (43,44).

Evaluation of the Athlete with a Head Injury

The initial evaluation and management of the head injured athlete is critical, so a well-designed protocol involving qualified medical personnel is essential (45a). The initial evaluation in the field setting should ensure that a cervical spine injury has not occurred. Subsequent to establishing the stability of the neck, the medical staff should then proceed to determine whether transporting the athlete to the sideline or to another area where detailed evaluation can be completed is safe. If any question exists as to the stability of the cervical spine, the athlete's neck should be stabilized, and the athlete should be transported to the nearest trauma center.

The sideline medical staff can determine the severity of the injury and can expedite the initial evaluation if the mechanism of injury was directly observed. If the athlete is conscious, the evaluation will be able to proceed relatively quickly on the basis of the information provided by the athlete in response to questions posed by the examiner. If the athlete is unconscious, the clinician should assume that the athlete has sustained a catastrophic cervical spine injury, and appropriate emergency procedures should be initiated immediately.

A complete neurologic examination, including a mental status evaluation, is particularly important in an athlete who has sustained head trauma. Vigilant follow-up also is essential for management and return-to-play issues. Another important aspect is individualizing treatment plans and return-to-play decisions for each athlete when possible. These management plans should consider the athlete's preexisting function, the sport in which he or she participates, the risk of recurrent injury, and the age and level of play of the participant. Precompetition information about an athlete's cognitive function, such as baseline neuropsychologic (NP) testing (see Chapter 2), may become an increasingly important tool in the assessment of head injury in sports, especially when return-to-play decisions are being made on the extent to which an athlete's neuropsychiatric parameters have returned to preinjury baseline measurements.

The first step in evaluating the head-injured athlete is the assessment of compromise in airway, breathing, and circulation. Immediately following the initial assessment, the evaluation focuses on the presence or absence of associated cervical spine and skull injuries. If the athlete is alert and responding to verbal questioning and a cervical spine injury or skull fracture has been ruled out, then a more thorough history can be obtained. If the airway, breathing, or circulation is impaired, emergency advanced cardiac life support measures should be initiated. The Glasgow coma scale (GCS) is useful in assessing and predicting long-term prognosis in the patient with a head injury (Table 28.2). For patients with a GCS that is less than 5, 80% will die or remain in a vegetative state, whereas, if their GCS is greater than grade 11, more than 90% have a complete recovery (45). Improvements in prognosis correlate with improved GCS scores, and therefore, the GCS scores should be followed serially.

Initial evaluation of the conscious athlete should include an assessment for associated injuries, such as cervical spine injuries and skull fracture. If the athlete is unconscious or if he or she has neck pain or spine tenderness, the cervical spine must be stabilized. Rigid cervical collars must be placed, and the athlete is transported on a spine board. The procedures utilized in managing a suspected catastrophic neck injury should be rehearsed in advance by the entire medical staff, and they should be performed at the physician's direction by trained medical personnel (see Chapter 27). If the mechanism of the injury puts the cervical spine at risk and the athlete is unconscious or if he or she has altered mental status, erring on the side of safety and stabilizing the cervical spine is the wisest course of action. If the athlete has a helmet in place, it should be left on, unless an airway needs to be obtained and the facemask cannot be cut away (46).

After the medical staff has determined that the cervical spine is stable, the presence or absence of an associated skull fracture should also be assessed. If any evidence for skull fracture exists or if any focal neurologic deficits are present, then the athlete should be transported to a medical facility where a CT scan should be obtained immediately (Figs. 28.6 and 28.7), and a neurosurgical consultation should be conducted, if it is indicated.

TABLE 28.2. *Glasgow coma scale*

	Score
Eye opening	
Eyes open spontaneously	4
Eyes open to verbal command	3
Eyes open only with painful stimuli	2
No eye opening	1
Verbal response	
Oriented and converses	5
Disoriented and converses	4
Inappropriate words	3
Incomprehensible sounds	2
No verbal response	1
Motor response	
Obeys verbal commands	6
Response to painful stimuli (upper extremities)	
Localizes pain	5
Withdraws from pain	4
Flexor posturing	3
Extensor posturing	2
No motor response	1
Total score = eye opening + verbal response + motor response	

From Putukian M. Head injuries. In: Garrett WE Jr, Kirkendall DT, Squire DL, eds. *Principles & practice of primary care sports medicine,* Philadelphia: Lippincott Williams & Wilkins, 2001, with permission.

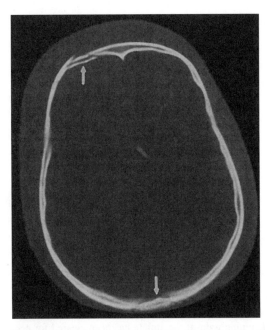

FIG. 28.7. Axial computerized tomography image of right frontal and occipital comminuted skull fractures (*arrows*). The occipital fracture is particularly ominous because it lies over the superior sagittal sinus, and it may have lacerated it, causing an intracranial hematoma. (From Garrett WE, Kirkendall DT, Squire DL, eds. *Principles and practice of primary care sports medicine.* New York: Lippincott Williams & Wilkins, 2001, with permission.)

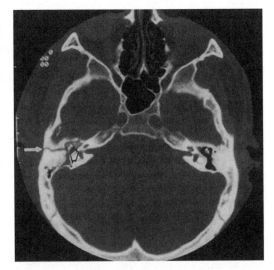

FIG. 28.6. A basilar skull fracture involving the petrous bone is seen on this axial computerized tomography image (*solid arrow*). The fracture extends into the middle ear (*open arrow*), and it can cause a conducive hearing loss by disrupting the tympanic membrane or the ossicles of the middle ear. The fracture also can cause hemorrhage into the middle ear cavity, which will result in hearing loss. (From Garrett WE, Kirkendall DT, Squire DL, eds. *Principles and practice of primary care sports medicine.* New York: Lippincott Williams & Wilkins, 2001, with permission.)

The on-field evaluation of the athlete who has sustained a head injury typically begins with questions to determine his or her orientation, memory status, and overall cognitive function. When the athlete is further evaluated on the sideline, additional questions, including the score of the game, the color of his or her teammates' jerseys, the site of the game, and previous game results, as well as questions about the events that occurred prior to the injury, are helpful. Asking teammates or coaches to help determine if the athlete can remember specific plays or defensive or offensive strategies is appropriate. Having the athlete recite the months of the year in reverse order or presenting five objects for recall several minutes later can be useful for determining his or her ability to concentrate and remember new information. For the athlete who is seen in the training room or office setting, having the trainer, teammate, coach, or family members present can be useful, especially if significant memory problems or altered levels of consciousness have occurred.

These questions help determine whether disruption in cognitive function has occurred, as well as whether memory has been affected for events prior to the injury (retrograde amnesia) or after the injury (antero-grade amnesia). Demonstrating that the athlete has difficulties answering questions or remembering a series of objects will also help parents or coaches, when they are present, understand why the athlete is being held out of competition.

The symptoms of head injury include alterations in levels of consciousness and retrograde and/or anterograde amnesia, as well as several other symptoms that are less specific to concussion. These include headache, nausea, dizziness, tinnitus, imbalance, and "feeling in a fog." Athletes may experience difficulties in gait, vision, or speech or other symptoms in association with a focal deficit. These symptoms should be assessed immediately following the injury, as well as in follow-up examinations. Deterioration in these symptoms may occur later in the course of head injury and may signify serious complications or sequelae.

A complete neurologic examination should be performed after the initial assessment has been conducted. This can be done on the sideline or in the training room if the athlete has been cleared for cervical spine injury and/or skull fracture. Pupillary response, an assessment of cranial nerve function, upper and lower motor and sensory functions, reflexes, an assessment focused on cerebellar function, and an evaluation of complex tasks, such as gait, should be checked. Any deficits should be noted, and close observation and documentation of changes in the neurologic examination should be tracked closely.

After acute symptoms have resolved, many important components affect return-to-play decisions. Determining if a previous head or neck injury has occurred is important, as is documenting when the previous injury occurred, the extent of neurologic involvement, and the clinical course for each prior injury. Previous test results, both neuropsychiatric and neuroimaging, are important components of the postinjury evaluation. Details of previous medical or surgical interventions are also important, and they preferably should be confirmed by medical record documentation, rather than by verbal report, whether from medical staff, the patient's family, or the patient's recollection.

Further diagnostic imaging is indicated when sustained loss of consciousness has occurred, when concern regarding skull fracture exists, or if any evidence for focal deficits is found. Imaging also may be indicated if an athlete has an initial lucid interval followed by a progressive decline in level of consciousness or the development of worsening symptoms. Close observation of every athlete who has sustained a head injury is important, and the athlete who has more severe symptoms warrants in-patient observa-tion. A CT scan is often considered the best initial study because of its ability to demonstrate both intracranial bleeding and fractures. These initial scans are helpful in managing traumatic brain injury in the first hours after the injury has occurred, and they may also prevent a catastrophic outcome by prompting early neurosurgical intervention if an intracranial bleed has occurred.

The athlete with head injury must be followed closely for several hours following injury, depending on the severity of symptoms. Attention to any new or resolving symptoms should be documented, including the time and date. No athlete should return to activity if any symptoms, including mild headache, are still present at rest or with exercise. If the athlete who has sustained a head injury has only mild symptoms with no deficits in memory and no decrease in the level of consciousness, the athlete should be reexamined within 15 minutes of the injury. If all of the symptoms remain clear at rest and with exercise after 15 to 20 minutes, the athlete may return to play. The athlete with persistent symptoms beyond 15 minutes postinjury or the one who has additional deficits in memory or level of consciousness should not return to competitive play for at least 24 hours. The current consensus of many sports medicine physicians is that athletes who have symptoms that persist longer than 15 minutes should be reevaluated by a physician approximately 24 hours after the injury. Additional considerations for determining clearance for competitive activity for athletes who have sustained a head injury are discussed later in the chapter.

COMPLICATIONS AND SEQUELAE OF HEAD INJURY

MTBI can be associated with sequelae and complications that can have a negative impact on long-term health. These complications include the cervical spine injuries and skull fractures that were discussed earlier. Complications and sequelae of head injury also include posttraumatic seizures, SIS, and postconcussive syndrome. Of crucial importance is the fact that the young athlete, along with his or her parents, coaches, and athletic trainers, understand these complications in order to facilitate preventive measures, prompt detection, and expedited treatment.

Skull fractures are often associated with injury to the underlying brain surface, and they may present with focal neurologic deficits or seizure activity. Seizures generally occur within 1 week of trauma, and they are seen approximately 5% of the time. Adults are more likely to develop seizures after a depressed skull fracture than children less than 16 years of age are. Risk factors for developing epilepsy after head injury include (a) seizures within 1 week of trauma, (b) posttraumatic amnesia of longer than 12 hours, (c) intracranial hemorrhage, or (d) any neurologic deficit present after injury. A normal EEG does not accurately predict whether posttraumatic epilepsy will occur (46). Cantu (47) recently reviewed the issues of participation of athletes with epilepsy in sports with a risk of head injury (see Chapter 2).

Skull fracture is associated with a 20-fold increase in the risk for intracranial hemorrhage, as compared to head injury without skull fracture (48). Skull fracture also increases the risk for intracranial infection.

Cervical spine injuries are present in 5% to 10% of patients with severe head injury (49). Cervical spine tenderness or reported neck pain in an athlete who sustains head injury mandates stabilization with a rigid collar and spine board until radiographs or imaging can rule out the presence of a fracture, instability, or another abnormality. Initially, lateral, anteroposterior, and open-mouth odontoid views should be obtained, with the lateral including the upper margin of the first thoracic vertebral body and the occiput. If these are normal, then flexion and extension lateral films must be obtained to rule out instability. CT scan or MRI can be considered if the patient has normal radiographs but neurologic symptoms related to the cervical spine persist. MRI is particularly useful in assessing cord contusion, disc herniation, or vascular lesion.

Head injury can be associated with postconcussive syndrome, a syndrome characterized by persistent headache; an inability to concentrate; irritability; fatigue; vertigo; disturbances in gait, sleep, and vision; and emotional lability. The onset of the symptoms associated with postconcussive syndrome may change widely from one case to the next. Likewise, the persistence of symptomatology and the clinical course is quite variable. To what degree the predictive significance of the duration of decreased level of consciousness or of posttraumatic amnesia is reliable in the clinical setting is unclear (50). Differentiating postconcussive syndrome from persistent symptoms associated with a particular injury and trauma-induced migraine may also be difficult.

The proposed criteria for postconcussive disorder are presented in Table 28.3. These were presented in the *Diagnostic and statistical manual of mental disorders*, 4th edition (DSM-IV), of the American Psychiatry Association, based on recommendations from Brown et al. (51). This definition uses inclusive criteria, including posttraumatic amnesia lasting more than 12 hours, head injury with loss of consciousness, and seizure activity within the first 6 months following head injury. Two of the three criteria must be present in order to make the diagnosis. Many physicians who care for athletes who have sustained a head injury feel that these criteria are too strict. Many sport medicine physicians apply the diagnosis of postconcussive disorder to any individual who has typical symptoms (Table 28.1) following head injury.

TABLE 28.3. *Proposed criteria for postconcussive syndrome*

History of head injury that includes at least two of the following:
  1. Loss of consciousness for 5 min or more
  2. Posttraumatic amnesia of 12 hr or more
  3. Onset of seizures (posttraumatic epilepsy) within 6 mo of head injury
Current symptoms (either new symptoms or substantially worsening preexisting symptoms), including:
  1. At least the following two cognitive difficulties:
    a. Learning or memory (recall)
    b. Concentration
  2. At least three of the following affective or vegetative symptoms:
    a. Easy fatiguability
    b. Insomnia or sleep/wake cycle disturbances
    c. Headache (substantially worse than before injury)
    d. Vertigo and/or dizziness
    e. Irritability and/or aggression on little or no provocation
    f. Anxiety, depression, or lability of affect
    g. Personality change (e.g., social or sexual inappropriateness, childlike behavior)
    h. Aspontaneity and/or apathy
Symptoms associated with a significant difficulty in maintaining premorbid occupational or academic
  performance or with a decline in social, occupational, or academic performance

From Brown SJ, Fann JR, Grant I. Postconcussional disorder: time to acknowledge a common source of neurobehavioral morbidity. *J Neuropsychiatry Clin Neurosci* 1994;6:15–22, with permission.

The treatment for postconcussive syndrome can be extremely difficult, and the plan often requires a multidisciplinary approach, including psychotherapy, behavioral modifications, medications, biofeedback, and physical therapy. Biochemical changes that occur in acute head injury are also possibly believed to be present in posttraumatic headache and, possibly, in postconcussive syndrome. Changes in electrolytes, excitatory amino acids, serotonin, catecholamines, endogenous opioids, and neuropeptides, in addition to impaired glucose utilization, may play a role in all of these entities (52). The use of β-adrenergic blockers and tricyclic antidepressants has had some success, and management options for postconcussive syndrome and postconcussive headaches have been extensively reviewed (53–55).

SIS, which was initially described by Saunders and Harbaugh (1), is one of the most significant concerns for primary care sports medicine physicians. This condition is caused when an individual sustains a second impact prior to full recovery from an initial insult. This second impact can result in brain swelling, persistent deficits, and even death. The symptoms from the first insult can be significant, including dizziness, vertigo, and visual motor or sensory changes; or they can consist only of a mild, persistent headache. The second impact itself may also be mild, such as a blow to the chest that imparts a force to the head (2). With SIS, the athlete often sustains the second impact and subsequently deteriorates quickly (within seconds to minutes). He or she often becomes semicomatose with rapidly dilating and fixed pupils and respiratory failure, followed by death. Although some researchers have questioned whether SIS is a true entity (56), it has been described in both adults and children, and, given its grave consequences, it should be considered when making return-to-play decisions.

The pathophysiology of SIS is thought to be due to changes in the cerebral blood flood that occur with recurrent trauma. The first impact leads to increased sensitivity in the cerebral vasculature. The second impact then results in dysfunction of autoregulation in the cerebral blood supply. This, in turn, leads to increased vascular congestion and resultant increased intracranial pressure, followed by the possible herniation of the brain, brainstem compromise, and finally coma and respiratory failure (2). The potential for SIS clearly underscores the need for close follow-up after head injury and for precluding a return-to-activity until all symptoms have been completely resolved.

A second concern after head injury is recurrent head injury and chronic traumatic encephalopathy (CTE). In the realm of athletics, CTE is believed to occur from cumulative repetitive blows to the head that result in a premature loss of normal central nervous system function. CTE can occur without a loss of consciousness, and its risk of occurrence remains difficult to predict (57). The possible occurrence of cognitive dysfunction in certain sports, such as soccer or boxing, is discussed in "Specific Sports: Implications and Debate" later in this chapter.

Classification Systems

Several classification systems describe MTBI and also provide return-to-play guidelines (35,57–61). The majority of head injuries that occur in sports are mild, especially if focal injuries or those that are associated with the complications of cervical spine injuries and/or skull fractures are excluded. Even with this restriction on the statistical data, differentiating minor from severe MTBI is one of the most difficult and important decisions facing the medical provider who is caring for an athlete at risk for head trauma. Although classification systems provide general guidelines for the primary care physician, return-to-play decisions must be individualized to ensure an expedited, yet safe, return to practice or competition.

One of the many problems with classification systems is that much of what they propose is based on assumptions that may not be correct. For example, the presence of LOC is assumed to represent a more severe injury in most classification systems. However, NP testing has demonstrated that LOC is not necessarily associated with more severe injury (62). This recent research has questioned the assumptions upon which most classification systems have been developed. This, then, underscores the need for individualization in treatment of these injuries, instead of using a "cookbook" approach.

With the plethora of classification systems that exists, healthcare professionals must understand which grading system is being utilized. Many classification systems will denote a different grade for the same injury. For example, in an athlete without loss of consciousness but significant retrograde and posttraumatic amnesia (34), the classifications include Torg grade IV, Nelson III, Cantu II, or Colorado Medical Society III. Current classification systems are not based on long-term analyses of head-injured athletes but on clinical experience instead. Therfore, using terms, such as "loss of consciousness," "retrograde amnesia," or "posttraumatic amnesia," instead of a grading system might

TABLE 28.4. *Classification systems and return to play guidelines*

Torg grades of cerebral concussion, 1982
I.   Short term confusion, no loss of consciousness (LOC), no amnesia
II. Confusion + amnesia. No LOC + posttraumatic amnesia (PTA)
III. Confusion + amnesia. No LOC + PTA + retrograde amnesia (RGA)
IV. + LOC (immediate transient) + amnesia (PTA, RGA)
V.   + LOC (paralytic coma) → coma vigil, respiratory arrest
VI. + LOC (paralytic coma) → death

Nelson classification of concussion, 1984
0.   No complaints initially, + subsequent complaints of headache (HA), difficulty with sensorium
I.   + Stunned or dazed, no LOC or amnesia, clears quick (<1 min)
II. HA, cloudy sensorium (>1 min), no LOC, + amnesia
III. + LOC (<1 min), or not comatose, grade II symptoms during recovery
IV. + LOC (>1 min), not comatose, grade II symptoms during recovery

Cantu grading system for concussion, 1986
I.   Mild: No LOC, PTA <30 min
II. Moderate: + LOC <5 min, or PTA >30 min but <24 hr
III. Severe: + LOC >5 min, or PTA >24 hr

Colorado Medical Society; guidelines for the management of concussion in sport, 1991
I.   Confusion without amnesia, no LOC
     Remove from contest
     Examine immediately and every 5 min for the development of amnesia or postconcussive symptoms at
       rest and with exertion
     Permit return to contest if amnesia does not appear and no symptoms appear for ≥20 min
II. Confusion with amnesia, no LOC
     Remove from contest and disallow return
     Examine frequently for signs of evolving intracranial pathology
     Reexamine the next day
     Permit return to practice after 1 full wk without symptoms
III. With LOC
     Transport from field to nearest hospital by ambulance (with cervical-spine immobilization if indicated)
     Perform thorough neurologic evaluation emergently
     Admit to hospital if signs of pathology are detected
     If findings are normal, instruct family for overnight observe
     Permit return to practice only after 2 full wk without symptoms

American Academy of Neurology, 1997
I.   Transient confusion, no LOC, concussion symptoms or mental status abnormalities on examination
       resolve in <15 min
     Remove from contest
     Examine immediately and at 5-min intervals for development of mental status abnormalities or
       postconcussive symptoms at rest and with exertion
     May return if abnormalities/symptoms clear within 15 min
     Second grade I concussion in same contest eliminates player from contest, returning only if asymptomatic
       for 1 wk at rest and with exertion
II. Transient confusion, no LOC, concussion symptoms or mental status abnormalities last >15 min
     Remove from contest, no return that day
     Examine on site frequently for signs of evolving intracranial pathology
     Reexamine athlete the following day
     Neurologic examination by physician 1 wk after asymptomatic before return
     Computerized tomography (CT) or magnetic resonance imaging (MRI) where HA or other symptoms
       worsen or persist >2 wk
     Following second grade 2, return to play deferred until >2 wk symptom free at rest and with exertion
     Terminating season mandated by any abnormality on CT or MRI consistent with brain swelling, contusion,
       or other intracranial pathology
III. Any LOC, either brief (seconds) or prolonged (minutes)
     Transport from field to emergency room by ambulance if unconscious or worrisome signs; consider
       cervical-spine immobilization
     Thorough neurologic examination emergently, including appropriate neuroimaging procedures
     Admit if any signs of pathology or mental status abnormalities
     If normal evaluation, may send athlete home
     Neurologic status should be assessed daily thereafter, until all symptoms have stabilized or resolved

Continued on next page

TABLE 28.4. *Continued*

Prolonged LOC, persistent mental status alterations, worsening symptoms or abnormalities on neurologic examination requires urgent neurosurgical evaluation or transfer to trauma center

After brief (sec) grade III concussion, the athlete should be held out until asymptomatic for 1 wk at rest or with exertion

After prolonged (min) grade III, athlete should be withheld from play for 2 wk at rest and with exertion

Following second grade III concussion, athlete should be withheld from play for a minimum of 1 mo without symptoms; physician may elect to extend that period beyond 1 mo, depending on clinical evaluation and other circumstances

CT or MRI recommended for athletes whose HA or other associated symptoms worsen or persist >1 wk

Any abnormality on CT or MRI consistent with brain swelling, contusion, or other intracranial pathology should result in termination of the season for that athlete; return to play in the future should be seriously discouraged in discussions with the athlete

Return to play decisions
    Cantu guidelines for return to play after concussion
      I.
        First concussion: may return to play if asymptomatic (no HA; dizziness; or impaired orientation, concentration, or memory during rest or with exertion) for 1 wk
        Second concussion: return to play in 2 wk if asymptomatic at that time for 1 wk
        Third concussion: terminate season; may return to play next season if asymptomatic
      II.
        First concussion: may return to play after asymptomatic for 1 wk
        Second concussion: minimum of 1 mo; may then return to play if asymptomatic for 1 wk; consider terminating season
        Third concussion: terminate season; may return to play next season if asymptomatic
      III.
        First concussion: minimum of 1 mo; may then return to play if asymptomatic for 1 wk
        Second concussion: terminate season; may return to play next season if asymptomatic

Colorado Medical Society Return to Play Guidelines
      I.
        First concussion: remove from contest; examine immediately and every 5 min for the development of amnesia or postconcussive symptoms at rest and with exertion; may return to contest, if amnesia does not appear and no symptoms appear for at least 20 min
        Second concussion: if in same contest, eliminate from competition that day; otherwise treat as grade I
        Third concussion: terminate season; no contact sports for at least 3 mo, and then allow only if asymptomatic at rest and exertion
      II.
        First concussion: remove from contest and disallow return; examine frequently for signs of evolving intracranial pathology and reexamine the next day; may return to practice after 1 full wk without symptoms
        Second concussion: defer return to play for 1 mo; termination of season should be considered
        Third concussion: termination of season mandated (also terminate season if any abnormality on CT or MRI)
      III.
        First concussion: transport from field by ambulance (with cervical-spine immobilization, if indicated) to nearest hospital; thorough neurologic evaluation emergently; hospital confinement if signs of pathology are detected; if findings are normal, instructions to family for overnight observation may return to practice only after 2 full wk without symptoms (no contact sports); return to full contact activity at 1 mo only if athlete has been asymptomatic at rest and exertion for at least 2 wk
        Second concussion: season terminated (also terminate if any abnormality on CT or MRI); return to contact sports should be seriously discouraged

From Putukian M. Head injuries. In: Garrett WE Jr, Kirkendall DT, Squire DL, eds. *Principles & practice of primary care sports medicine.* Philadelphia: Lippincott Williams & Wilkins, 2001, with permission.

be of more use. Most classification systems use these terms, with the presence of additional symptoms or physical findings, to differentiate the severity of injury. Examples of several well-known classification systems are presented in Table 28.4.

With more long-term prospective research on MTBIs seen in sports medicine, the hope is that a better understanding of the natural history of these injuries, as well as a standard classification system, will evolve.

Return-to-Play Considerations

The first step in treatment of the athlete with a head injury is rapid recognition that a head injury has occurred. Once the presence of an injury in the athlete is identified, the next step is ruling out associated injuries, such as cervical spine injuries, skull fractures, or intracranial hemorrhage. As was discussed earlier, close assessment for cognitive function should be made, with particular attention to difficulties with memory, as well as for the presence and persistence of symptoms. Any persistence of symptoms precludes a return to activity, as was mentioned previously. Once the athlete has become asymptomatic at rest and with exercise, a return to activity can be considered. The exact timing and progression of return-to-activity protocols continue to be controversial. Sports with a high risk for head injury, such as football, ice hockey, wrestling, soccer, gymnastics, boxing, and rugby, require different return-to-play considerations than sports such as running, tennis, or golf. Other activities with a high risk of head injury include equestrian sports and motorcycle, automobile, and boat racing, as well as skydiving.

Factors to consider when returning an athlete to sports include the specifics of the current injury, the past history of head trauma, complications of the current injury, complications of previous head injuries, the progression of the clinical course of the current injury, and the inherent risk of repeat head injury in the sport in which the athlete participates. Careful assessment of the athlete's neurologic status prior to resumption of activity should be coupled with close follow-up during the progression of the athlete's return to full competitive status. Many sports medicine physicians feel that the conservative approach to return-to-play decisions may be overly cautious, but these feelings are outweighed by the risk that is involved if an athlete returns to the sport too quickly and sustains a severe complication.

Once an athlete is asymptomatic, the progression of the return-to-play protocol may warrant a recommendation from the medical staff that an athlete remain restricted from participation for a limited period of time, based on the severity of the injury, its clinical course, and/or the previous history of head injuries. However, during this period of limited activity, the athlete may utilize the time to return to cardiovascular fitness without a significant risk for head injury.

Once the athlete is asymptomatic at rest, the athlete may progress to an exercise regimen that includes a cardiovascular challenge. If the athlete is able to exercise for 15 to 20 minutes at a pace that increases cardiac output and sweat rate without producing any abnormal neurologic signs or symptoms, the athlete may progress to sport-specific exercises and activities. The activity regimen should be individualized for each athlete, and it should still preclude a risk for head injury. For many athletes, this progression in training allows them to return to practice and to feel more confident that they are still a part of the team, while retaining relative safety in their sports activity.

If initial return-to-play activities progress successfully, the next step is allowing the athlete to participate in more aggressive practice activities with additional protection from head injury. For many sports, this can include scrimmaging with a "red cross" practice jersey or some other method to remind teammates that they should not tackle or have body contact with that player during agility drills or while participating in running–passing drills. For the basketball player, these activities may include shooting baskets or practicing ball handling. Having the athlete perform the exertional challenge and sport-specific drills on the sideline while the team is practicing helps the athlete, teammates, and coach realize that the athlete is progressing and that he or she remains "part of the team," while still providing protection from a second head injury. For sports, such as tennis or golf, that have a lower risk of head injury, the progression to full competitive activity may be more rapid.

If the athlete is able to progress to this level of activity without any abnormalities in neurologic symptoms or cognitive function, then he or she should be given clearance to return to full participation without restrictions. This progression in return-to-play protocol can occur over a short period of time, or it can be prolonged, based on the individual nature of the injury, the athlete, and the particular sport.

For focal head injuries, return-to-play guidelines that are based on clinical judgment and experience rather than long term prospective studies have been developed by Cantu (35). Lesions included in the discussion of focal head injuries include intracranial hemorrhage (i.e., epidural hematoma, subdural hematoma, intracerebral hematoma, and subarachnoid hemorrhage), as well as SIS and diffuse axonal injury. If an athlete sustains any of these injuries, he or she cannot return to play if any of the following conditions are present: (a) persistent postconcussive symptoms, (b) permanent central neurologic sequelae (e.g., organic dementia, hemiplegia, or homonymous hemianopsia), (c) hydrocephalus, (d) spontaneous subarachnoid hemorrhage from any cause, or (e) symptomatic neurologic or pain-producing abnormalities about the foramen magnum (35). If any of these focal lesions are treated surgically, continued participation in contact and collision sports should be seriously discouraged. Epidural hematoma that is not associated with any underlying brain injury is an exception. For this type of injury and in other head injuries that do not require surgical intervention, total restriction from contact and collision sports is not warranted. Many authors have recommended that return to these categories of sport can occur at least 1 full year after the recovery from the injury is complete (35).

Diagnostic imaging may not detect structural abnormalities in athletes who have cognitive dysfunction clinically (34). Specifically, MRI and CT scans, as well as EEG, do not always identify abnormalities in an athlete who has difficulty remembering his or her name, how the injury occurred, or the events up to and around the injury. In these situations, determining precisely when the athlete has returned to his or her neurologic baseline and, consequently, when the risk for a recurrent or a disproportionately severe head injury is no longer increased is difficult. If the athlete's reaction time, attention span, or concentration is impaired, the sports medicine physician should be concerned that the athlete may be at additional risk for a subsequent head injury. Unlike with an ankle sprain, an injury in which sports medicine physicians may allow an athlete to return to play if the athlete has recovered 80% of full function, partial recovery may be inappropriate in the athlete who is recovering from a head injury. If sophisticated neuropsychiatric testing that provides information regarding an athletes' cognitive function is unavailable, return-to-play decisions become even more problematic.

Many sports medicine physicians advocate adhering to the following three return-to-play guidelines in considering resumption of activity for the athlete with a head injury:

1. No athlete should be allowed to participate if he or she has *any* symptoms at rest or with exercise. These symptoms can include a mild headache or "feeling slowed."
2. Some form of "exercise challenge" should be initiated as the first step in allowing an athlete to return to practice or competition. This allows the athlete to be stressed with a cardiovascular challenge to determine if exertion precipitates any symptoms. This procedure also gives the athlete confidence that he or she is progressing in a setting that does not increase the risk of a second concussive impact. In addition, if symptoms recur, the athlete and coach will understand that a return to full competitive status is not yet warranted.
3. Individualizing treatment protocols and discussing return-to-play constraints and issues with the athlete, parent, coach, and athletic training staff is important.

Communication is imperative in avoiding misunderstandings regarding the athlete's disposition and the activities that are allowable. A concussed athlete has a greater risk (four to six times) of subsequent injury than does the nonconcussed athlete (9,63). The risk for recurrent head injury is difficult to predict; however, many sports medicine physicians feel that the risk diminishes with time. Explaining the importance of avoiding "SIS" and recurrent head injury to the athlete, the athlete's parents, and the coaching staff can often make the difference with regard to compliance with medical treatment and return-to-play protocols. Assessing whether the athlete is apprehensive about returning to activity is also crucial. The medical staff should not assume that the athlete wants to return to full competitive status. The athlete should be given the opportunity to discuss fears or concerns about return to play in a confidential setting. If the athlete has significant reservations regarding the resumption of full competitive activity, these concerns should be considered by the medical staff in the process of individualizing the athlete's return-to-play protocol.

The athlete, the athlete's parents, and the coaching staff should also understand that protocols that include progression of activity under close supervision and medical staff observation can allow an athlete to return to the practice setting earlier than the previous protocols that were based exclusively on the number of head injuries, the proximity of previous head injuries, and the classification of the previous head injuries.

Neuropsychologic Testing in Athletes

The use of NP testing in the assessment of and recovery from head injury is well established (64–66). NP testing has been used specifically in athletes who have sustained a head injury, and success in achieving good outcomes has been documented (32,34,67–71). Consequently, NP testing has gained attention in recent years in the athletic setting, and it increasingly may become an integral component of the preparticipation physical examination (PPE) for athletes who are involved in contact and collision sports. NP testing may also modify the manner in which athletes are evaluated, both prior to and following a head injury. Research studies now in progress are attempting to determine which of these NP tests are the most sensitive and specific for the deficits seen in athletes with head injuries.

NP testing examines brain behavior relationships and provides a reliable assessment and quantification of brain function. NP tests can be used to assess a broad range of cognitive functions, including the speed of information processing, attention, concentration, reaction time, visual scanning and visual tracking abilities, memory recall, and problem solving abilities (32,64–66,70,72,73). Both acute and chronic head injuries can be assessed by NP tests, and these tests may be more sensitive in assessing cognitive function than is classic medical testing (34,67–69,71).

The Penn State Concussion Program, initiated in 1995, prospectively assesses athletes at risk for head injury using a battery of NP tests. Preliminary results of this ongoing program indicate that NP testing is a useful tool for assessing MTBI in college athletes and that it can be extremely useful for making return-to-play decisions (71). The hope is that further testing with prospective controlled studies will provide even more information in this area.

Additional findings from the Penn State program include the following:

- The severity of the head injury correlates with the frequency of abnormalities in a number of tests.
- The length of time that an abnormality persists increases as the severity of the injury increases.
- A significant difference exists among athletes in terms of their scores for various tests. These data underscore the need for an individual baseline battery of tests.
- Symptoms do not always correlate with NP findings. Most mild injuries tend to be associated with mild deficits in cognitive function as assessed by NP testing, and they generally return to baseline measures between 5 and 10 days after injury.

Specific Sports: Implications and Debates

For many sports, the evaluation, treatment, and return-to-play decisions of MTBI are the same. The return-to-play decisions the sports medicine staff makes should be individualized based on consideration of the severity of injury, the presence of concurrent injuries, the age of the athlete, the level of play, the athlete's "readiness" to return, and the sport in which the athlete participates, as well as its inherent risks for injury. Boxing and soccer have received special attention with regard to MTBI because of the prevalence of certain mechanisms of injury.

Boxing

Boxing is a unique sport in which the intent is to render the opponent unconscious by multiple blows to the head. The "punch drunk" syndrome, which was first described by Martland in 1928, is also known as dementia pugilista or chronic progressive traumatic encephalopathy (73a). It is estimated to occur in 9% to 25% of professional boxers, with the incidence correlating to the number of fights and the length of the boxer's career (73b).

Abnormalities in cerebellar, pyramidal, extrapyramidal, and cognitive function, as well as personality impairments, have been described; these generally occur after an average of 16 years, with progressive deterioration (73c). The chronic effects of boxing on brain function are reviewed elsewhere and will not be covered here (73c). Several imaging techniques may be used to demonstrate these abnormalities in boxers (25).

Attempts have been made to decrease the number of deaths that occur in boxing, and several states have adopted guidelines that mandate time away from boxing after MTBI has occurred. The New York State Boxing Commission mandates a 45-day suspension from the sport for mild concussions and a 60-day suspension for moderate concussions; a 90-day suspension and normal results on CT and EEG testing are required for return to sport when the athlete has suffered a severe concussion. The hope is that these changes will ultimately decrease the number of athletes that sustain significant or recurrent injury.

Soccer

In soccer, the sport-specific skill of "heading" the ball is used to control, or redirect, the ball. Recently, significant debate has occurred about whether the abnormalities in neurologic function that are seen in boxers also develop in soccer players. Early data showed that soccer players demonstrated cortical atrophy on CT scans and abnormalities on EEG, as well as defects in cognitive function (27). More recent reports have reported abnormalities on neuropsychologic testing of soccer players in comparison to swimmers and track athletes (73d). Although these studies have gained media attention, they have significant flaws in methodology, including a lack of proper control groups, a lack of control for athletes who have sustained acute head injuries, and a lack of screening for other problems (e.g., motor vehicle accidents and alcohol use). In addition, much of the early data assesses players who participated with a leather ball that often was water-logged, which increases the weight by as much as 20%. These players also often continued to participate in the sport despite sustaining MTBI.

In a study of boxers in which track and soccer athletes were used as controls, no differences among any of the groups were demonstrated on assessment by MRI, CT scanning, and EEG (73c). A well-controlled study that compared national team players to track athletes did not show any difference on MRI evaluation (73e). In the only prospective research that has been done to assess the effect of heading on cognitive function, no effect from heading was demonstrated using a battery of neuropsychologic tests (73f).

Controversy exists regarding whether cognitive dysfunction actually occurs in soccer players, as well as about which factors are the etiologies of the damage. The assumption has been that the repetitive process of heading the ball is analogous to the blows that a boxer sustains. However, significant differences from the mechanism of injury that occurs in boxing are seen in the biomechanics of heading the ball. In soccer, the forces generally are linear (Fig. 28.8), whereas in boxing, the most danger arises from the rotational forces that occur when the competitor administers a left hook (Fig. 28.9). Moreover, in soccer, the head is used to strike the ball while the neck muscles contract to maintain the head and neck in a rigid or semi-rigid position. This increased stability decreases the forces incurred by the skull (according to Newton's second law of motion, which says that force = mass × acceleration). The risk of head injury in the sport of soccer actually is from repetitive or severe MTBI. Concussions are fairly common in soccer, although the mechanism generally is a blow from another opponent's body, the ground, or the goalpost. Purposeful heading, however, has not been reported as a mechanism for concussion in soccer. At this point in time, no convincing data demonstrates that soccer and, more particularly, heading causes changes similar to those seen in boxers. Additional research is needed in this area.

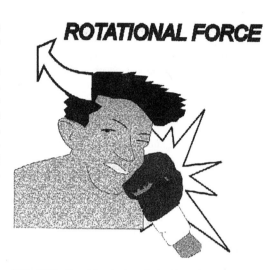

FIG. 28.9. Punching impact in boxing often produces rotational force. (From Garrett WE, Kirkendall DT, Squire DL, eds. *Principles & practice of primary care sports medicine.* New York: Lippincott Williams & Wilkins, 2001, with permission.)

Conclusions

MTBI is common in sport, and it can be associated with significant complications and sequelae, especially if these injuries are not recognized and treated appropriately. A significant spectrum of injury is found. Head injuries may vary in severity from a situation in which an athlete sustains a mild head injury, is observed for 20 minutes, then is allowed to return to play to the scenario in which a more severe head injury precludes a return to collision or contact sports. In this latter case, injury occurs, and the athlete is disqualified from further participation in contact or collision sports. Each instance must be individually evaluated, with a consideration of the injury, its severity, previous injuries, the sport, and the athlete's emotional state and support services. The healthcare team must maintain a high index of suspicion for injury and must use a systematic approach in treating these injuries. Early recognition of associated cervical spine and focal injuries is essential, and careful and close evaluation and follow-up of the injured athlete are crucial. Additional diagnostic testing or evaluation and the individualization of treatment in making sport-specific return-to-play decisions may be necessary.

New techniques for evaluating and assessing the athlete with MTBI will likely change the PPE of athletes at risk for head injury. These may include the use of NP tests as part of a preseason baseline assessment. More long-term prospective studies are necessary in order to delineate the natural history of MTBI. Prospective studies are also needed in order to define the utility of using these new tools in the return-to-

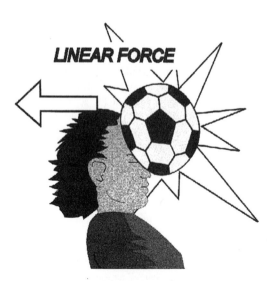

FIG. 28.8. Soccer heading typically produces linear force to the head. (From Garrett WE, Kirkendall DT, Squire DL, eds. *Principles & practice of primary care sports medicine.* New York: Lippincott Williams & Wilkins, 2001, with permission.)

play decision-making process. As additional information is obtained, the quality of care provided to the head-injured athlete is certain to improve.

OROFACIAL INJURIES

Facial Injuries

Determining the prevalence of orofacial injuries in sports is exceedingly difficult. These injuries are common, but the statistics may not accurately depict the extent and prevalence of real injury. Although many injuries happen in organized sports, most organizations do not keep detailed injury data on dental or facial injuries. Moreover, while injuries in organized sports are common, many more may occur in recreational settings, such as neighborhood play or recreational sports (e.g., biking or roller blading).

The use of facemasks, eye protection, and mouthguards has reduced the number and severity of orofacial injuries, but, in many sports, their use is optional (74). Physicians should be aware of the potential for injury and should encourage mouth and eye protection for any at-risk activity.

Dental Injuries

Anterior teeth, especially the maxillary central incisors, are the most frequently injured orofacial structures in sports-related orofacial trauma. This may be especially true in children whose the anterior teeth are disproportionately large and protrude farther over the mandible. In general, when a young athlete sustains trauma to the teeth, the quicker the patient is treated by a dentist, the higher the likelihood is of a favorable outcome. Tooth injuries include fractures, displacements, and avulsions.

Crown Fractures

Fractures of the tooth crown are common, and they are of variable severity. Fractures involving the enamel only are primarily a cosmetic problem that can be repaired at a convenient time. Sports medicine physicians can identify fractures that involve the dentin by noticing the presence of cream-colored or yellow-colored dentin under the outer enamel. These fractures produce more discomfort than the chips do, and they can compromise the pulp underneath. Pulp fractures, which are identified by the exposed pink or bleeding pulp, require immediate attention. Exposed pulp can become infected and can lead to the destruction of the tooth (75). If an athlete has an injury that includes a minor enamel or dentin fracture, one can allow sports participation if the athlete is reasonably comfortable (Fig. 28.10).

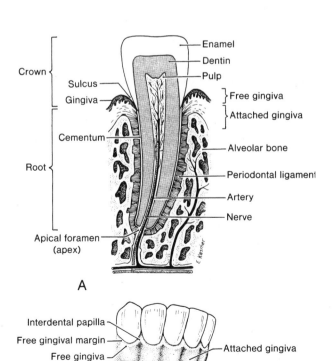

FIG. 28.10. Structure of normal teeth and gingiva. **A:** A tooth and its parts. **B:** Teeth and gingiva. (From Barker LR, Burton J, Zieve P, eds. *Principles of ambulatory medicine*, 4th ed. Baltimore: Williams & Wilkins, 1998, with permission.)

Tooth Displacement

Loosening of teeth, especially the front teeth, secondary to sports trauma is common in children. If the tooth moves less than 1 mm, it usually heals within 7 to 10 days with proper protection. A dentist should fashion a splint to promote healing. Teeth that move more than 1 mm or that are impacted may require more extensive treatment. The child should be seen by a dentist as soon as possible as teeth that are repositioned within 90 minutes of injury are more likely to recover (75).

Tooth Avulsion

Avulsions are not uncommon injuries, particularly in younger athletes, because the periodontal ligament is loosely structured to accommodate the erupting teeth. Avulsed teeth should be replanted as soon as possible. The avulsed tooth should be handled by the crown, not the root; and care should be taken not to harm the root surface. Except for removing very superficial contaminants, the root should not be cleaned. The tooth should be transported in commercially available tooth-preserving medium, sterile saline, milk, or the athlete's own saliva (i.e., tucked between the athlete's gums). Chances for successful replantation are correlated to expedited dental care (76).

Prevention

Mouthguards prevent the teeth and gums from injury, they protect the jaws from fractures and dislocations, and they may decrease the incidence of concussion and other types of injury. For a mouthguard to prevent injury, however, it must be worn (77). In some sports, mouthguards are mandatory; however, in sports where their use is not mandated, sports medicine physicians may be able to reduce the risk of dental trauma by encouraging the use of this protective equipment.

Mouthguards are either preformed, mouth formed ("boil and bite"), or custom made (see Chapter 8). Mouth-formed mouthguards are relatively inexpensive, and they offer good protection. For high-risk sports or for athletes with preexisting problems, a custom mouthguard may be more appropriate.

Nasal Injuries

Epistaxis

Trauma to the nose often causes bleeding. Most often, the bleeding is from an area in the anterior nares called Kisselbach's plexus, within which a collection of superficial vessels is located. Usually bleeding can be stopped with continuous pressure for 5 to 10 minutes to the soft cartilaginous part of the nose. The athlete should tilt his or her head forward to decrease the amount of blood that flows into the posterior pharynx.

If direct pressure is ineffective, a vasoconstricting spray or a nasal pledget soaked with vasoconstrictor can be used. Lidocaine with epinephrine is readily available and effective. If the area that is bleeding can be well visualized, chemical cautery with silver nitrate sticks can be employed. If these procedures are unsuccessful, anterior nasal packing should be attempted. If the athlete's nose is still bleeding despite anterior nasal packing, he or she may have a posterior bleed and may require referral to an otolaryngologist (78).

Nasal Fracture

The nasal bones are the most commonly fractured bones of the face, and the diagnosis is primarily clinical. The literature does not support the use of nasal x-rays (79). On examination, swelling, tenderness, crepitance, ecchymoses, or deformity may be found. Initial examination should also document patency of the nares. The nares may be occluded by septal deformity secondary to the fracture or by septal hematoma. If the athlete is seen before significant swelling develops and gross deformity is present, lateral pressure can substantially correct the deformity (80). These athletes should follow-up with a specialist. If any deformity remains or if reduction has not been attempted, the athlete should be seen by a specialist to perform a definitive reduction. Many otolaryngologists recommend that children should be seen 3 to 4 days after the trauma occurs to be evaluated and considered for reduction and that adults should be reexamined within 10 to 12 days for the same.

Treatment protocols for the management of a simple, nondisplaced nasal fracture include ice to prevent and reduce swelling and analgesia, mild oral analgesics, and protection from reinjury. The type of protection required after a nasal fracture varies by the sport. Commercially available facemasks or existing equipment can be modified to protect the nasal bones.

Septal Hematoma

Septal hematomas can result from hemorrhage that occurs between the two layers of mucosa that cover the septum. The athlete may notice that he or she has difficulty breathing through the affected nostril, increased pain, or fever. On examination, a red or bluish cherry-like structure is visualized. This structure should be evacuated immediately in order to prevent a possible infection or pressure necrosis of the nasal septum.

Ear Injuries

Lacerations

The external structures of the ear are highly vascular tissues, and they often bleed profusely when cut.

Lacerations should be repaired using anesthetic without epinephrine in order to avoid ischemia of the tissues. Only tissue that is obviously necrotic should be debrided.

Otohematomas

Otohematomas are injuries that result from sheering forces across tissue planes. These injuries are most frequently seen in wrestling and boxing. Blood and serum accumulate between the perichondrium and skin. This accumulation of fluid can lead to pressure necrosis of the cartilage or to secondary infection. If they are not treated appropriately, granulation, fibrosis, and irregular growth of new cartilage occur over time, causing deformation of the ear ("cauliflower ear") (81).

Initial treatment of an otohematoma should consist of aspiration of the accumulated fluid, followed by compression of the pinna to prevent reaccumulation. Compression can be accomplished in a variety of different ways. One of the simplest is using an over-the-counter swimmers' nose plug to compress gauze tightly against the area where the hematoma was drained. Gauze pads soaked in flexible colloidion or plaster cast material can also be molded to the shape of the ear and used for compression. In addition, bolsters can be sutured on both sides of the wound to achieve compression (78).

The cartilage of the ear is relatively avascular, and some clinicians recommend using appropriate antibiotics for prophylaxis against secondary infection. Compression should be maintained for 7 to 14 days, with repeat aspiration if fluid reaccumulates.

Eye Injuries

In 1997, an estimated 32,789 sports-related and recreation-related eye injuries were treated in hospital emergency rooms. The American Academy of Ophthalmology and American Academy of Pediatrics strongly recommend eye protection for all sports and recreational activity (81a). If protective eyewear were used consistently, the risk of significant eye injury has been estimated as being reduced by at least 90% (82). Children, in addition, may be more prone to eye injury as they learn a new sport. Increased risk for eye injury in young athletes may also be related to relatively decreased coordination and slower reaction times, when compared to the adult athlete.

In all eye injuries in young athletes, the initial physical examination should include an assessment of visual acuity. The athlete should also be questioned about his or her use of glasses or contacts. Pupil reactivity and eye movement should be evaluated before a more directed examination proceeds (Fig. 28.11).

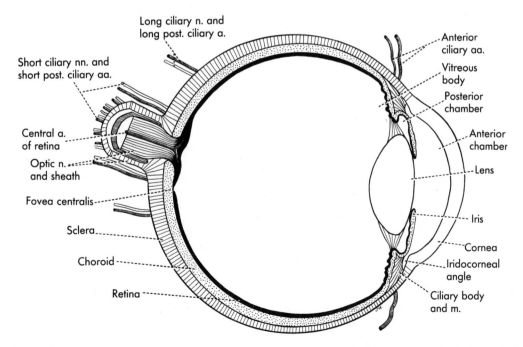

FIG. 28.11. Schema of the eyeball in horizontal section. (From Rosse C, Gaddum-Rosse P. *Hollinshead's textbook of anatomy*, 5th ed. Philadelphia: Lippincott-Raven Publishers, 1997, with permission.)

Lid Laceration

An ophthalmologist or facial and/or plastic surgeon should repair lid lacerations. Each anatomic layer must be approximated and meticulously repaired. Injuries may be complicated by trauma that involves the nasolacrimal system (medial lid and eye) or the levator muscle (upper lid).

Cornea

Corneal injuries are commonly encountered by primary care sports medicine physicians. Typical symptoms of an abrasion or foreign body include a sensation of something in the eye or behind the eyelid, pain, and, if the abrasion or foreign body is located over the central cornea, blurred vision. A topical anesthetic should be used to facilitate the examination. The eye should first be examined with white light and should then be stained with fluorescein. A cobalt blue light should then be used to fluoresce the areas of injury. After the fluorescein examination has been completed, irrigation of the eye, which removes the residual fluorescein, can help reduce subsequent eye irritation. The eye should be reexamined after the fluorescein has been removed. The upper eyelid should be everted in order to confirm the absence of foreign bodies. The use of topical anesthetics to aid in examination is helpful, but they should not be used for more than one or two doses in order to avoid irreversible corneal damage (78). The use of ophthalmologic preparations that include steroid drops should be avoided in athletes who have sustained corneal injuries.

When treating corneal foreign bodies or abrasions, the primary care physician should inform the patient and his or her parents that antibiotic ointment and cycloplegics blur vision and that they may prevent an athlete from returning to play. Athletes who have small abrasions and minimal discomfort and who do not have significant vision impairment may return to play.

Foreign Bodies

Small foreign bodies may be removed with a moistened tip of a cotton swab or the tip of a sterile hypodermic needle. A slit lamp, if the equipment is available, may facilitate removal. Metallic foreign bodies may leave a rust ring that must be treated by an ophthalmologist. After the removal of any foreign body, ophthalmic antibiotic eye ointment should be applied for 3 to 4 days. For comfort, the eye can be patched with gentle pressure for 24 to 36 hours. In young children, the use of eye patches is not indicated, unless the child is cooperative with this intervention. If the young athlete begins rubbing the patch into the affected orbit, the severity of the injury may be increased rather than decreased (83).

Abrasions

Abrasions appear as a bright patch following fluorescein staining under cobalt blue light. Ophthalmic antibiotic eye drops or ointment should be instilled after the fluorescein has been irrigated and the examination has been completed. The eye can be patched for comfort for 24 to 36 hours in older children. If pain and photophobia are severe, a topical cycloplegic can be used to dilate the pupil and to relieve pain caused by ciliary body spasm. Young athletes with corneal abrasions should be followed on a daily basis to ensure that the abrasion is healing and that a secondary infection is not developing.

Subconjunctival Hemorrhage

Subconjunctival hemorrhage is caused by the rupture of a blood vessel in the conjunctival or episcleral blood vessels. This type of injury to the eye is caused by trauma and by any condition that is associated with a forced Valsalva maneuver. Isolated subconjunctival hemorrhages are not associated with vision impairment or pain. Treatment of a subconjunctival hemorrhage is entirely symptomatic. Resolution of the lesion may require several weeks, and the hemorrhage may progress through color changes similar to contusions in musculoskeletal soft tissue. Subconjunctival hemorrhages do not require restriction from competition. Primary care physicians should be aware that subconjunctival hemorrhage may obscure the diagnosis of a ruptured globe. If the athlete has any disturbance in visual acuity or if he or she fails to make significant progress in recovery after trauma to the orbit, referral to an ophthalmologist should be considered.

Hyphema

A hyphema is a hemorrhage in the anterior chamber of the eye that results from the rupture of the ciliary or iris blood vessels. If the amount of bleeding is small, the athlete's visual acuity may be unaffected. More significant hemorrhage may cause blurred vision, pain, and photophobia. In athletes who have sustained an eye injury that results in a significant hemorrhage in the anterior chamber, the primary care physician may note a layer of blood in the anterior chamber. All hyphemas should be referred to an ophthalmologist. The goal of treatment protocols is to prevent rebleeding while the hyphema resorbs. In severe cases, the athlete may be admitted to the hospital. In the in-patient setting, activity is limited, the head of the bed is elevated to 45 degrees, and the eye is patched with a protective shield. The athlete should be advised that restrictions upon return to play may be prolonged, and he or she should be managed in conjunction with an ophthalmologist (81).

Iris

Traumatic Iridocyclitis

Blunt injury to the eye can contuse the ciliary body, leading to spasm and inflammation. This type of injury presents with a deep aching pain, photophobia, and blurred vision. Examination of the affected pupil will often document pupillary constriction secondary to papillary muscle spasm, in addition to perilimbal conjunctival injection (ciliary flush). Treatment for this type of injury consists of mydriatic and cycloplegic ophthalmic drops and close monitoring of intraocular pressure. Steroid ophthalmic drops also may be used, if the presence of corneal abrasions has been ruled out, to help resolve inflammation (80).

Traumatic Miosis or Mydriasis

Blunt injury may cause persistent pupil constriction or dilation. In contrast to eye trauma in athletes that results in traumatic iridocyclitis, these patients are relatively asymptomatic and no ciliary flush is observed. Pupil asymmetry may require additional neuroimaging studies and a thorough neurologic examination to rule out significant intracranial pathology. Traumatic miosis and/or mydriasis usually resolves spontaneously in a few days, but it can be permanent if a radial tear of the pupillary muscle has occurred (80).

In order to expedite the care of a young athlete who has sustained head, facial, or eye trauma, any preexisting pupil asymmetry should be documented at the PPE. The patient should be also be informed of this finding so that he or she can provide an accurate history to an examining physician who is not aware of this normal variant.

Iridodialysis

Iridodialysis is a separation of the iris from the ciliary body that creates an "accessory pupil." The injury is permanent, and it is often accompanied by a hyphema. Ophthalmologic consultation should be obtained.

Lens Subluxation and/or Dislocation

Blunt trauma to the eye may also cause lens subluxation or dislocation. Partial dislocation may produce visual disturbances that range from minimal visual disruption to monocular diplopia and blurred vision. Complete lens dislocation causes significant visual distortion. When the physician examines the eye, quivering of the iris with eye movement may be noted. Iritis, traumatic cataract formation, and acute angle closure glaucoma may be seen following injuries that cause lens dislocation. Ophthalmologic referral is indicated for management of this type of eye trauma.

Ruptured Globe

A ruptured globe occurs when an abrupt rise in intraocular pressure occurs secondary to trauma to the eye. When intraocular contents are visualized, the diagnosis is obvious and the injury must be managed as an ophthalmologic emergency. Less severe cases cause eye pain, decreased light perception, or severe compromise of visual acuity. A "tear drop" shaped pupil is a classic finding in a patient who has sustained an injury that has resulted in a ruptured globe. Any manipulation of the eye should be avoided. The affected eye should be patched, without pressure, using a metal eye shield. If a metal eye shield is unavailable, the closed end of a small cup can be fashioned into a makeshift eye shield. The patient should be transported immediately to an eye trauma center (80).

Facial Fractures

Orbit

Fractures of the orbit typically result from direct trauma to the periorbital structures of the face. The highest risk of this type of injury results from a small ball that has a curvature of 5 cm or less that makes direct contact with the orbit. A "blow-out" fracture occurs when the weakest part of the orbit—the orbital floor—fractures. The orbital contents may herniate through the floor of the orbit at the site of the fracture and may penetrate the maxillary sinus. The athlete typically presents with a periorbital hematoma and/or a protruding or sunken eye. The athlete may have diplopia with upward gaze secondary to entrapment of the inferior rectus muscle in the fracture line. The patient may also have decreased sensation on the maxillary surface. Radiographic studies may detect the fracture line or maxillary sinus clouding. A definitive diagnosis of orbital blow-out fracture is confirmed with CT of the orbit. All young athletes who have sustained an orbital fracture should be thoroughly evaluated for the possible presence of a ruptured globe. Antibiotic therapy should be started immediately, and referral should be made to an ophthalmologist (76). The decision to repair these fractures may be delayed 10 to 14 days because many of these injuries resolve without surgical intervention (Fig. 28.12) (84).

Zygoma

Fracture to the zygoma is caused by a direct blow to the cheek. Immediately following the injury, the sports medicine physician may note swelling and bruising, with a flattened appearance of the cheek or a palpable defect. The athlete should be examined closely for accompanying maxillary or orbital fractures. Treatment protocols for zygoma fractures consist of either closed or open reduction.

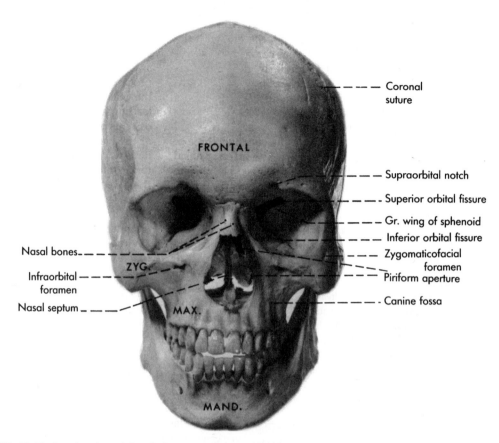

FIG. 28.12. Anterior view of the skull: zygomatic bone (*ZYG.*), maxilla (*MAX.*), and mandible (*MAND.*). (From Rosse C, Gaddum-Rosse P. *Hollinshead's textbook of anatomy*, 5th ed. Philadelphia: Lippincott-Raven Publishers, 1997, with permission.)

Maxilla

Fractures of the maxilla most commonly occur secondary to a direct blow to the middle portion of the face. They are classified as Le Fort I, II, and III. Physical examination of the affected area may include an observation that the face appears lengthened, and the midface may be mobile. Typically, malocclusion of the bite is found. CSF rhinnorhea or obstruction of the nasal airway may exist. If a maxillary fracture is suspected, the patient should be transferred immediately to the nearest trauma center for definitive diagnostic evaluation and management. This type of injury requires close monitoring of the athlete's airway. If the patient is conscious, he or she should be kept sitting up and leaning forward.

Mandible

In children, the emerging permanent teeth are proportionately larger than the other facial structures; this developmental characteristic predisposes them to contact injuries of the lower jaw (75). Consequently, any young

athlete with malocclusion of the jaw after trauma should be suspected of having a mandibular fracture. The mandible typically breaks in more than one place on opposite sides of the midline. On examination, the patient may have malocclusion, swelling, tenderness, palpable step-off defects, parasthesia or anesthesia of the lower lip or chin, or bruising on the floor of the mouth. Nondisplaced fractures are treated conservatively. Displaced fractures require close observation and maintenance of the young athlete's airway. During transport to a trauma center, the conscious patient should remain sitting up, and the jaw should be supported (80).

Conclusion

Facial and dental trauma is common in sports. Children may be more likely to sustain some injuries because of their developing coordination and slower reaction times. When these types of injuries occur, treatment protocols are similar to the interventions that are used in the adult athlete who has sustained facial trauma. Many orofacial injuries in young athletes can be prevented with the use of proper protective gear. Primary care physicians should ask young athletes about their use of protective gear, and the importance of these products should be reinforced at the PPE.

REFERENCES

1. Saunders RL, Harbaugh RE. The second impact in catastrophic contact-sports head trauma. *JAMA* 1984;252: 538–539.
2. Cantu RC. Second-impact syndrome. *Clin Sports Med* 1998;17:37–44.
3. Mortimer JA. Epidemiology of post-traumatic encephalopathy in boxers. *Minn Med* 1985;68:299–300.
4. Spear J. Are footballers at risk for developing dementia? *Int J Geriatr Psychiatry* 1995;10:1011–1014.
5. Mayeux R, Ottman R, Tang MX, et al. Genetic susceptibility and head injury as risk factors for Alzheimer's disease among community-dwelling elderly persons and their first degree relatives. *Ann Neurol* 1993;33:494–501.
6. McLatchie G, Jennett B. ABC of sports medicine. Head injury in sport. *BMJ* 1994;308:1620–1624.
7. Wojtys EM, Hovda D, Landry G, et al. Concussion in sports. *Am J Sports Med* 1999;27:676–688.
8. Kraus JF. Epidemiology of head injury. In: Cooper PR, ed. *Head injury*, 2nd ed. Baltimore: Williams & Wilkins, 1987:1–19.
9. Gerberich SG, Priest JD, Boen JR, et al. Concussion incidence and severity in secondary school varsity football players. *Am J Public Health* 1983;73:1370–1375.
10. Garrick JG, Requa RK. Medical care and injury surveillance in the high school setting. *The Physician and Sports Medicine* 1981;9:115.
11. Zariczny B, Shattuck LJ, Mast TA, et al. Sports related injuries in school age children. *Am J Sports Med* 1980;8: 318–324.
12. Bruce DA, Schut L, Sutton LN. Brain and cervical spine injuries in children and adolescents. *Prim Care* 1984;11: 175–194.
13. Hodgson VR. National operating committee on standards for athletic equipment. Football helmet certification program. *Med Sci Sports* 1975;7:225–232.
14. Bishop PJ. Impact performance of ice hockey helmets. *Safety Res* 1978;10:123–129.
15. Cantu RC, Mueller F. Catastrophic spine injury in football 1977–1989. *J Spinal Dis* 1990;3:227.
16. Pforringer W, Smasal V. Aspects of traumatology in ice hockey. *J Sports Sci* 1987;5:327–336.
17. National Collegiate Athletic Association. *Injury surveillance system*. Overland Park, KS: National Collegiate Athletic Association, 1991.
18. Greensher J. Non-automotive vehicle injuries in adolescents. *Pediatr Ann* 1988;17:114–121.
19. Thompson RS, Rivara FP, Thompson DC. A case-control study of the effectiveness of bicycle safety helmets. *N Engl J Med* 1989;320:1361–1367.
20. Bruno LA, Gennarelli TA, Torg JS. Management guidelines for head injuries in athletics. *Clin Sports Med* 1987;6:1.
21. Warren WL, Bailes JE. On the field evaluation of athletic head injuries. *Clin Sports Med* 1998;17:13–26.
22. Borczuk P. Predictors of intracranial injury in patients with mild head injury. *Ann Emerg Med* 1995;25:731–736.
23. Davis RL, Mullen N, Makela M, et al. Cranial computed tomography scans in children after minimal head injury with loss of consciousness. *Ann Emerg Med* 1994;24:640–645.
24. Hoffman JR. CT for head trauma in children. *Ann Emerg Med* 1995;24:713–715.
25. Jordan B, Zimmerman R. Computed tomography and magnetic resonance imaging comparisons in boxers. *JAMA* 1990;263:1670–1674.
26. Lampert PW, Hardman JM. Morphological changes in brains of boxers. *JAMA* 1984;251:2676–2679.
27. Tysvaer AT, Storli OV, Bachen NI. Soccer injuries to the brain: a neurologic and electroencephalographic study of former players. *Acta Neurol Scand* 1989;80:151–156.
28. Levin HS, Williams D, Crofford MJ, et al. Relationship of depth of brain lesions to consciousness and outcome after closed head injury. *J Neurosurg* 1988;69:861–866.
29. Mittl RL, Grossman RI, Heihle JF, et al. Prevalence of MR evidence of diffuse axonal injury in patients with mild head injury and normal CT findings. *Am J Neuroradiol* 1994;15:1583–1589.
30. Gentry LR, Godersky JC, Thompson B, et al. Prospective comparative study of intermediate field MR and CT in the evaluation of closed head trauma. *Am J Neuroradiol* 1988;150:673–682.
31. Jenkins A, Teasdale G, Hadley DM, et al. Brain lesions detected by magnetic resonance imaging in mild and severe head injuries. *Lancet* 1986;3:445–446.
32. Levin HS, Amparo E, Eisenberg JM, et al. Magnetic resonance imaging and computerized tomography in relation to the neurobehavioral sequelae of mild and moderate head injuries. *J Neurosurg* 1987;66:706–713.
33. Graham DI. Neuropathology of head injury. In: Narayan RK, Wilberger JE Jr, Povlishock JT, eds. *Neurotrauma*. New York: McGraw-Hill, 1996:46–47.
34. Putukian M, Echemendia RJ. Managing successive minor head injuries; which tests guide return to play? *The Physician and Sports Medicine* 1996;24:25–38.
35. Cantu RC. Return to play guidelines after a head injury. *Clin Sports Med* 1998;17:45–60.
36. Katayama Y, Becker DP, Tamura T, et al. Massive increases in extracellular potassium and the indiscriminate release of glutamate following concussive brain injury. *J Neurosurg* 1990;73:889–900.
37. Katayama Y, Cheung MK, Alves A, et al. Ion fluxes and cell swelling in experimental traumatic brain injury: the role of excitatory amino acids. In: Hoff JT, Betz AL, eds. *Intracranial Pressure VII*. Berlin: Springer, 1989:584–588.
38. Yoshino A, Hovda DA, Katayama Y, et al. Hippocampal CA3 lesion prevents the post-concussive metabolic derangement in CA1. *J Cereb Blood Flow Metab* 1991;11: S343.
39. Yoshino A, Hovda DA, Kawamata T, et al. Dynamic changes in local cerebral glucose utilization following cerebral concussion in rats: evidence of a hyper- and subsequent hypometabolic state. *Brain Res* 1991;561:106–119.
40. Kawamata T, Katayama Y, Hovda DA, et al. Administration of excitatory amino acid antagonists via microdialysis attenuates the increase in glucose utilization seen following concussive brain injury. *J Cereb Blood Flow Metab* 1992;12:12–24.
41. Yamakami I, McIntosh TK. Alterations in regional cerebral blood flow following brain injury in the rat. *J Cereb Blood Flow Metab* 1991;11:655–660.
42. Jenkins LW, Moszynski, Lyeth BG, et al. Increased vulnerability of the mildly traumatized rat brain to cerebral ischemia: the use of controlled secondary ischemia as a research tool to identify common or different mechanisms contributing to mechanical and ischemic brain injury. *Brain Res* 1989;477:211–224.
43. Hovda DA, Lee SM, Smith ML, et al. The neurochemical and metabolic cascade following brain injury: moving from animal models to man. *J Neurotrauma* 1995;12:143–146.
44. Bergsneider M, Hovda DA, Shalmon E, et al. Cerebral hyperglycolysis following severe traumatic brain injury in humans: a positron emission tomography study. *J Neurosurg* 1997;86:241–251.
45. Henderson JM, Browning DG. Head trauma in young athletes. *Med Clin North Am* 1994;78:289–303.

45a. Kushner DS. Concussion in sports: minimizing the risk for complications. *Am Fam Physician* 2001;64:1007–1014.

46. Kleiner DM, Cantu RC. *Football helmet removal (current comment)*. Indianapolis, IN: American College of Sports Medicine, 1996.

47. Cantu RC. Epilepsy and athletics. *Clin Sports Med* 1998; 17:61–69.

48. Edna TH. Acute traumatic intracranial hematoma and skull fracture. *Acta Chir Scand* 1983;149:449–451.

49. Marion DW. Head injuries. In: Fu FH, Stone DA, eds. *Sports injuries: mechanisms, prevention, treatment*. Baltimore: Williams & Wilkins, 1994:813–831.

50. Bornstein RA, Miller HB, van Schoor JT. Neuropsychological deficit and emotional disturbance in head-injured patients. *J Neurosurg* 1989;70:509–513.

51. Brown SJ, Fann JR, Grant I. Postconcussional disorder: time to acknowledge a common source of neurobehavioral morbidity. *J Neuropsychiatry Clin Neurosci* 1994;6:15–22.

52. Packard RC, Ham LP. Pathogenesis of post traumatic headache and migraine: a common headache pathway? *Headache* 1997;37:142–152.

53. Rizzo M, Tranel D. Overview of head injury and postconcussive syndrome. In: Rizzo M, Tranel D, eds. *Head injury and postconcussive syndrome*. New York: Churchill Livingstone, 1996:1–18.

54. Troncoso JC, Gordon B. Neuropathology of closed head injury. In: Rizzo M, Tranel D, eds. *Head injury and postconcussive syndrome*. New York: Churchill Livingstone, 1996: 47–56.

55. Barcellos S, Rizzo M. Post-traumatic headaches. In: Rizzo M, Tranel D, eds. *Head injury and postconcussive syndrome*. New York: Churchill Livingstone, 1996:139–176.

56. McCrory PR. Second impact syndrome. *Neurology* 1998; 50:677–683.

57. American Academy of Neurology Quality Standards Subcommittee. Practice parameter: the management of concussion in sports [Summary statement]. *Neurology* 1997;48: 581–585.

58. Colorado Medical Society Sports Medicine Committee. *Guidelines for the management of concussion in sports*. Revised May 1991. Denver, CO: Colorado Medical Society, 1990.

59. Nelson WE, Jane JA, Gieck JH. Minor head injury in sports: a new classification and management. *The Physician and Sports Medicine* 1984;12:103–107.

60. Torg JS. *Athletic injuries to the head, neck, and face*. St. Louis: Mosby-Year Book, 1991.

61. Kelly JP, Rosenburg JH. Diagnosis and management of concussion in sport. *Neurology* 1997;48:575–580.

62. Lovell MR, Iverson GL, Collins MW, et al. Does loss of consciousness predict neuropsychological decrements after concussion? *Clin J Sport Med* 1999;9:193–198.

63. Zemper E. Analysis of cerebral concussion frequency with the most commonly used models of football helmets. *J Athletic Training* 1994;29:44–50.

64. Abreau F, Templer DI, Schuyler BA, et al. Neuropsychological assessment of soccer players. *Neuropsychology* 1990;4:175–181.

65. Rimel RW, Giordani B, Barth JT, et al. Disability caused by minor head injury. *Neurosurgery* 1981;9:221–228.

66. Rimel RW, Giordani B, Barth JT, et al. Moderate head injury: completing the clinical spectrum of brain trauma. *Neurosurgery* 1982;11:344–351.

67. Alves WM, Rimel RW, Nelson WE. University of Virginia prospective study of football-induced minor head injury: status report. *Clin Sports Med* 1987;6:211–218.

68. Collins MW, Grindel SH, Lovell MR, et al. Relationship between concussion and neuropsychological performance in college football players. *JAMA* 1999;282:964–970.

69. Lovell MR, Collins MW. Neuropsychological assessment of the college football player. *J Head Trauma Rehabil* 1998;13:9–26.

70. Tysvaer AT, Lochen EA. Soccer injuries to the brain; a neuropsychologic study of former soccer players. *Am J Sports Med* 1991;19:56–60.

71. Echemendia RJ, Putukian M, Mackin RS, et al. Neuropsychological test performance prior to and following sports-related mild traumatic brain injury. *Clin J Sports Med* 2001;11:23–31.

72. McLatchie G, Brooks N, Galbraith S, et al. Clinical neurological examination, neuropsychology, electroencephalography and computed tomographic head scanning in active amateur boxers. *J Neurol Neurosurg Psychiatry* 1987;50: 96–99.

73. Porter MD, Fricker PA. Controlled prospective neuropsychological assessment of active experienced amateur boxers. *Clin J Sports Med* 1996;6:90–96.

73a. Critchley M. Medical aspects of boxing, particularly from a neurological stand point. *Br Med J* 1957;1:357–362.

73b. Mortimer JA. Epidemiology of posttraumatic encephalopathy in boxers. *Minn Med* 1985;68:299–300.

73c. Haglund Y, Eriksson E. Does amateur boxing lead to chronic brain damage? A review of some recent investigations. *Am J Sports Med* 1993;21:97–109.

73d. Matser EJT, Kessels AG, Lezak MD, et al. Neuropsychological impairment in amateur soccer players. *JAMA* 1999;282:971–973.

73e. Jordan SH, Green GA, Galanty HL, et al. Acute and chronic brain injury in United States National Team soccer players. *Am J Sports Med* 1996;24:205–210.

73f. Putukian M, Echemendia RJ, Evans TA, Bruce J. *Effects of heading contacts in collegiate soccer players on cognitive function. Prospective neuropsyhological assessment over a season*. Presented at American Medical Society for Sports Medicine annual meeting, April 9, San Antonio, TX, 2001.

74. Tesini DA, Soporowski NJ. Epidemiology of orofacial sports-related injuries. *Dent Clin North Am* 2000;44:1–18.

75. Sullivan SM. Maxillofacial injuries. In: Sullivan JA, Anderson SJ, eds. *Care of the year-round athlete*. Rosemont, IL: American Academy of Orthopaedic Surgeons and American Academy of Pediatrics, 2000:187–196.

76. Brukner P, Khan K. Facial injuries. In: *Clinical sports medicine*. Sydney: McGraw-Hill, 1993:169–180.

77. Ranalli DN. Prevention of sports-related traumatic dental injuries. *Dent Clin North Am* 2000;44:35–52.

78. Weaver EM, Czibulka A, Sasaki CT. Acute epistaxis: a step-by-step guide to controlling hemorrhage. *Consultant* 1999;39:901–916.

79. Rubinstein B, Strong EB. Management of nasal fractures. *Arch Fam Med* 2000;9:738–742.

80. In: Rosen P, Barkin R, Danzl DF, eds. *Emergency medicine: concepts and clinical practice*, 4th ed. New York: Mosby-Year Book, 1998:457–461.

81. Rubin A, Cheng J. Office management of facial trauma. *Clin Fam Pract* 2000;2:565–580.

81a. American Academy of Pediatrics and American Academy of Ophthalmology. Protective eyewear for younger athletes [Policy statement]. *Pediatrics* 1996;98:311–313.

82. Jeffers JB. Eye injuries. In: Sullivan JA, Anderson SJ, eds. *Care of the year-round athlete*. Rosemont, IL: American Academy of Orthopaedic Surgeons and American Academy of Pediatrics, 2000:179–185.

83. Fowler GC. Corneal abrasions and removal of corneal or conjunctival foreign bodies. In: Pfenninger JL, Fowler GC, eds. *Procedures for primary care physicians*. New York: Mosby, 1994:221–230.

84. Kaufman BR, Heckler FR. Sports-related facial injuries. *Clin Sports Med* 16:543–562.

29

Cervical Spine Injuries

Beverly C. Land and Mark S. Williams

Few injuries in children concern medical personnel and parents more than cervical spine (c-spine) injuries. Children are highly inquisitive and extremely active during childhood, but they often lack the fine motor control and neck strength that possibly could prevent a c-spine injury in an accident. Over the last several decades, playtime for children has rapidly become competitive team practice time. Consequently, the behavior generally is more aggressive, repetitive, and structured in content. As the psychologic demands on the child change, simultaneous development in his or her bones and ligaments is also seen. Musculoskeletal changes in the spine from birth to the age of 18 years are continuous and progressive, which factors significantly in the mechanism and type of injury sustained by the athlete at a particular age.

Spinal injuries to children under 8 years of age involve the c-spine in 75% of cases. In one spinal rehabilitation center, spinal cord injuries in 10% to 20% of patients were due to sports involvement (1). Football produces the highest percentage of spine injuries in sports. Other sports that have reported a high incidence of neck injuries include diving, wrestling, rugby, gymnastics, and ice hockey. In recreational diving, neck injuries comprise 4% to 14% of spine injuries reported in the literature (2). Fifty percent of these neck injuries cause complete quadriplegia (3).

This chapter covers the anatomy of the c-spine, the common mechanisms of injury, and proper stabilization and management of c-spine injuries on the field. The latter portion of the chapter highlights some of the more common pediatric neck injuries, ranging from sprains and strains, fractures, cervical instability, stingers, and neurologic injuries to transient quadriparesis and permanent quadriplegia. The chapter closes with a brief discussion of the crucial role of prevention.

ANATOMY

The c-spine in the pediatric population is a unique entity with regard to its flexibility, growth, ossification, and strength. The immature pediatric c-spine,

unfortunately, lends itself to increased motion and risk of injury. In early childhood, much of the c-spine is nonossified. Under the age of 1 year, the anterior ring of C-1 shows little evidence of ossification, which leads to difficulty in assessing any instability in the interpretation of the spine on plain radiographs. From the ages of 3 to 8 years, progressive ossification can be seen, beginning with the posterior aspect of the vertebrae and moving anteriorly. The internal diameter of the spinal canal, which encases the spinal cord, reaches its adult diameter by the age of 6 years. These changes support the assertion that spinal injury patterns differ between preadolescents and older children (4). As the child matures, further growth and ossification of the vertebral bodies can be followed chronologically with lateral radiographs.

Another structural change that can be identified on film is the progressive increase in angulation of the facet joint, from 30 to 70 degrees. Facets of the lower c-spine undergo the least change in angulation—from 55 degrees to the 70 degrees seen in the adult. Facets of the upper c-spine, however, change the greatest over time, from 30 degrees at birth to 70 degrees at maturity. In children, the upper spine is a relatively flat 30 degrees, but facet changes over time result in a more upright 70 degrees, which provides the spine with significantly more stability. This facet angulation contributes to the pseudosubluxation that is often reported at C-2 to C-3 and C-3 to C-4 in early childhood. This is a common, but generally not a pathologic, finding that can be seen on routine radiographs.

In children, ligamentous structures in the c-spine are extremely extensible. They can stretch up to 5 cm without disruption. This characteristic also contributes to the appearance of subluxation in the upper spine. The spinal cord, however, exhibits little extensibility, as the cord often stretches only 0.64 cm before injury occurs. Thus, the cord is often severely injured when the spine is placed in a hyperflexed position because the extreme range of motion stretches the cord beyond its extensible safe range. In addition to the relative ligamentous laxity seen in the spine, the main axis of cervical spinal motion moves more caudad as the child matures. Under the age of 8 years, the predominant motion of flexion in the c-spine is seen in the C-1 to C-3 region. As the child continues to age and the spinal structures mature, the majority of flexion occurs at the C-3 to C-5 levels. After the age of 12 years, the flexion axis of the c-spine is similar to the adult pattern, occurring at the C-5 to C-6 level.

The most vulnerable area of the c-spine in children is the spinal cord and its individual cervical nerve roots. Sprains and strains of the spine usually heal with minimal residual disability, but injuries to the neural structures are more likely to result in long-term morbidity.

Anatomically, the neural complex of the c-spine generally includes the spinal cord and the nerve roots exiting bilaterally from C-1 through C-8. These nerves are named for the vertebrae that comprise the lower segment of the foramen—for example, C-5 exits through the foramen formed by C-4 and C-5. In general, cervical nerves above C-4 are injured less frequently; injury to the cord at this level, however, can be catastrophic.

Spinal cord lesions below C-4 generally do not impair respiration, but they can involve motor and sensory function for all four limbs. The nerve root of C-4, along with the phrenic nerve, provides partial innervation to the diaphragm, so injury at this level can cause respiratory dysfunction. Transection or injury to the cord itself can effect bilateral motor and sensory dysfunction. Lesions of individual nerves produce unilateral deficits that can be motor, sensory, or mixed. These deficits are evident in the region of the c-spine proximally and down the upper extremity distally. Collectively, the nerves of C-5 through T-1 combine to form the brachial plexus. This complex is often injured in athletes, and the ability to determine the location of sensory deficits and the motor weakness in specific muscles specifically identifies at what level the injury has occurred.

The sensory pattern exhibited by the brachial plexus includes the distribution from C-5 to T-1. Comparison to the uninvolved side with light touch and a determination of the quality of sensation can help the clinician assess the function of that cervical level. C-5 is involved in sensation to the lateral aspect of the upper arm. The axillary nerve is the primary nerve providing sensation in this area. C-6 supplies sensation to the lower lateral arm and the hand as it innervates the thumb, the index finger, and the radial portion of the middle finger. This sensatory pattern stems from the sensory branches of the musculocuta-neous nerve. C-7 provides sensation to the middle finger by way of the radial nerve. The viability of C-8 can be tested with sensation to the ring and little fingers and up the medial aspect of the arm to the elbow. The medial antebrachial–cutaneous nerve is responsible for this sensory pattern. Finally, T-1 innervates the uppermost portion of the medial arm by way of the medial brachial cutaneous nerve.

Motor testing of the neck, shoulder, and upper extremity is extremely important for determining the injury level in the spine. Specific discussions of each muscle action and how to test each muscle are provided in detail in other texts. The deltoid and biceps are the main muscles innervated at the C-5 level. The biceps can also receive innervation from C-6. The primary nerve that can be tested at the C-5 level is the musculocutaneous nerve. At C-6, the biceps and the wrist extensors are the significant muscle groups supplied. The musculocutaneous nerve innervates the biceps, and the radial nerve provides most of the innervation to the wrist extensors. C-7 can be tested with the triceps, wrist flexors, and finger extension. Several nerves are tested at this level, including the radial, median, and ulnar nerves. C-8 may be tested by stressing the small interossei muscles and finger flexors. In finger flexion, innervation is shared by the median and ulnar nerves. T-1 tests finger abduction, with innervation from the ulnar nerve.

Vertebral disks in children have a high water content, and, compared to their counterparts in adults, they are extremely effective in absorbing and transmitting force down the length of the spine. Changes in the disk as the child matures include a decrease in the total water content and an increase in collagen deposition throughout the disk. This change may explain the higher incidence of endplate fractures and the increased rate of Schmorl's nodules in children and adolescents, compared to that of osseous injuries in older age groups (5).

PATHOMECHANICS

Normal range of motion of the c-spine consists of movement in flexion, extension, rotation, and side bending. Combinations of these motions are commonplace, and they can be significant factors in the mechanism of injury to the spine. Injury to the neck or c-spine is the result of external forces causing flexion, extension, rotation, or compression (6). When the neck or c-spine is forced beyond its normal physiologic limits, each of the above, alone or in combination, will lead to dysfunction and injury. Hyperflexion is the most common mechanism of injury seen in children. Hyperflexion injuries, which are caused by a sudden deceleration from frontal forces, may cause anterior elements of the neck to compress. The resulting damage to the anterior aspect of the spine may be a wedge fracture of the vertebral body, a chip fracture, or an anterior dislocation of the vertebrae. The most common site of injury is C-5 to C-6, especially in older children. Posterior spinal elements—namely, the posterior longitudinal ligament, as well as the ligamentum flavum—may rupture. In rare cases, even the posterior aspect of the disk may be torn. Anterior motion is limited by contact of the chin with the sternum. Hyperflexion injuries often occur in football as a result of improper technique when tackling an opponent. Head-first contact with an opponent with the top of the helmet ("butt blocking") causes the neck to hyperflex. Damage to the cord can be variable. The degree of injury may be as mild as a sprain, with no restriction in range of motion, to immediate and permanent quadriplegia.

Hyperextension type injuries were fairly common in football in the past, when the use of the top of the helmet for the initial point of contact when tackling or "spearing" was a commonly accepted technique. Due to the number of c-spine injuries resulting from this technique, spearing in football is now illegal at all levels of play. Whiplash, or forced extension of the neck, causes posterior compression and anterior disruption injuries (4). This injury may occur with forced forward acceleration that is caused by a block or tackle from the back. The spinous processes, facets, and arches may be injured posteriorly. Anterior disruption of the disk and anterior longitudinal ligament may result, as well as disruption of the vertebral arteries and nerves. As posterior muscles are stronger than anterior muscles and no other limitation to extension exists, extension injuries are potentially far more serious than flexion injuries. Fractures and dislocations are relatively common with the extension type of injury, and they often result in serious neurologic damage. Hyperextension injuries have also been reported in rugby, wrestling, and boxing.

Axial or vertical loading of the spine can be the cause of compression or burst injuries. In a normal head-up posture, the c-spine has a gentle lordotic curve, so forces are dissipated throughout the cervical musculature. Forward flexion of the spine of as little as 20 to 30 degrees causes straightening of the spine, with the vertebrae lining up directly one on top of one other. Increased axial forces on a straightened spine are distributed directly through the vertebral bodies and the intervertebral discs. As the discs become maximally compressed, the force creates a fracture or dislocation of the bony vertebrae. Dislocated or fractured vertebrae may compress or crush the spinal cord, resulting in severe neurologic abnormalities. The spinal artery may also be disrupted. This type of fracture often causes neurologic impairment by causing damage to both the motor and sensory nerve pathways below the level of the fracture. The deficit with burst fractures is usually bilateral, involving all four extremities, and it is often permanent in nature. In addition, neck fractures without head trauma may occur with sudden acceleration of the lower torso or buttocks cranially (7).

In athletics, a pure rotational injury is an unusual occurrence. However, subluxation of vertebrae may result from rotational forces that are cumulative to flexion or extension forces. Subluxation is more likely to occur in the presence of rotation with flexion, than that with extension. Most injuries are the result of combinations of the above mechanisms (8).

STABILIZATION AND EVALUATION

Current recommendations for pediatric c-spine protection have been based on extremely limited clinical information (9). Additional information regarding stabilization of the injured athlete can be found in Chapter 27. Evaluation of a child with a potential c-spine injury is difficult, even under the best of conditions. Often these children are frightened, and they do not understand why they cannot move or why they have been restrained. This situation is made even more difficult if the child is unconscious or if he or she is also suspected to have sustained a head injury.

Stabilization of a young athlete's c-spine is the first action that must be taken during assessment for a possible c-spine injury. Stabilization of the c-spine should be considered in any child who has sustained a severe blow to the head, shoulder, or neck. Children who show any evidence of a neurologic deficit or who complain of neck or back pain should be treated in a similar fashion, despite the lack of documented, significant trauma.

Basic resuscitative protocols should be used to assess the patient's airway, breathing, and circulatory status. The athlete should be then stabilized on a full-length spine board with a neck collar in place. A spine board can be modified for the child's relatively larger head (in proportion to the body) by the use of a recess for the occiput to lower the head or via a double mattress pad to raise the chest (10). On the football field or hockey ice, the face mask may be cut away for better access to the airway; the helmet and chin strap, however, should be left in place, unless their removal is absolutely required in order to maintain an open airway. Current recommendations indicate that the facemask should be removed completely as quickly as possible, even if the athlete is conscious (11). The shoulder pads should remain in place if the helmet remains on the injured athlete. An appropriate-sized cervical collar should be placed on the athlete. Adult-sized collars should not be used for the smaller athlete, even if they are the only available alternative (unless at the high school level—some adolescents have reached adult proportions). In general, collars of rigid plastic construction perform better than do the foam types (3). If a collar is not available, towels, intravenous (IV) bags, sandbags, padding, and/or manual restraint can be used to limit motion of the spine. The child should be placed on a full-length spine board using the log roll technique, with the help of four to six trained persons. C-spine stabilization must be maintained during this transfer. Once the athlete is stabilized on the backboard, a reassessment of the ABCs of resuscitation must be performed, followed by a thorough neurologic examination to document any deficits. Because the head of a child is proportionately larger than the body, padding under the shoulders may be required to maintain a coronal plane in the c-spine if the child is not wearing shoulder pads or a helmet. All children require elevation of the back to achieve a correct neutral position. Children who are younger than 4 years of age require more elevation (11). Asking the child to move specific joints of the upper and lower extremities while they are stabilized can be used to assess motor function grossly. Pin prick, pinching, stroking, or tickling the skin are methods for evaluating sensory function. These appraisals must be performed bilaterally. Once the evaluation is complete and documented, the athlete may then be removed carefully from the field of play, and he or she should be transported to the nearest medical facility that has the capability to evaluate and treat pediatric c-spine injuries.

Identification and location of the injured child's parents or guardian is important in the overall medical care of the child. Parents can help calm the child and can provide some comfort and familiarity to the child in a traumatic and frightening situation. The parent or guardian also is able to provide permission for the evaluation and treatment of the child upon arrival at the medical facility, thus expediting care. However, the parent should be kept away from the patient's side during the initial stabilization process.

During this initial evaluation, having the proper equipment is vital to the stabilization of the injured athlete. Full-length spine boards are highly recommended in order to accommodate the various sizes of children that are involved in sports. Recent innovations for spinal stabilization include the use of a Miller full body splint and vacuum mattress. Rigid cervical collars should be placed around the child's neck before he or she is placed on the spine board. Medical personnel at the site should have various sizes available for use, especially if they provide routine medical coverage for this age group. Sheets and blankets can be used under the shoulders for support, and they can provide the neutral position for the spine of children, if shoulder pads and a helmet are not being worn. Bolt cutters, a "trainer's angel," Dura shears, PVC pipe cutters, pruning shears, or some other type of cutting device must be present when covering sports that incorporate the use of helmets. These devices must be capable of cutting through the retaining clips of the face mask quickly and smoothly if access to the airway becomes necessary in an emergency. Care must be taken to prevent movement of the head or spine during face mask removal. Emergency medical service personnel who are present at a contest should also be equipped with pediatric laryngoscopes and blades, oral airways, IV equipment, and endotracheal tubes in case of emergency. Pediatric drug dosages should be reviewed regularly, and a reference sheet or card should be available at all times for quick referral. Finally, the most important factor in the care of the injured child is having a plan, rehearsing that plan, and ensuring that everyone involved knows his or her designated responsibilities.

RADIOGRAPHIC STUDIES

Radiographic evaluation is required for a child who is suspected of having an injury to the c-spine. Physicians who follow athletes must be aware of which radiographic evaluations are necessary for identifying c-spine injuries. No method for determining the presence of an unstable fracture at the time of injury is now available. However, cervical cord injury is usually accompanied by rigid cervical muscle spasm and pain (Fig. 29.1) (8). Patients who have been evaluated at a location other than a medical facility and who have been transported to the emergency department generally have been secured on a spine board with a cervical collar in place for stabilization. Definitive treatment must be deferred until the appropriate radiographs are obtained. The preferred initial radiographs are the cross table lateral, anterior–posterior (AP), and open mouth odontoid views (12); these are the minimal initial radiographical studies that should be ob-

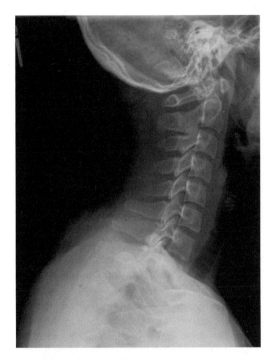

FIG. 29.1. Loss of normal cervical lordosis.

tained. These views are obtained while the athlete is still secured on the spine board with all equipment and restraints in place. Visualization of all seven cervical vertebrae, including the C-7 to T-1 vertebral segment, is required. When the clinician is evaluating an injured pediatric patient with a complaint of neck pain, a significant history of force that would cause a c-spine injury in a child or evidence of any neurologic deficit should direct the clinician to make the proper assessment and to direct specific radiographs to be done.

On the cross table lateral view, four lordotic curve lines should be evaluated for abnormalities. The first line that should be followed is that of the anterior vertebral bodies from C-2 to C-7. The second reference line examined is that of the posterior vertebral bodies. The third line of interest is the spinolaminar line, which should be uniform in alignment. A gentle lordotic curve should be formed by the tips of the spinous processes, which constitute the fourth line used as an evaluation tool. A disruption of any of these alignments should be considered a serious injury to the ligaments of the spine, and further evaluation and imaging studies should be undertaken.

Another measurement that can indicate significant pathology is the predental space of C-2. If the distance is greater than 4 to 5 mm (the normal distance is 3 mm on a pediatric film), the radiograph is considered abnormal. Disk spaces should be uniform in depth throughout the c-spine. The last evaluation for abnormal findings that can be routinely made on a cross table view is that of the Swischuk line. This line may help differentiate a C-2 to C-3 fracture (the hangman's fracture) from a normal finding of pseudosubluxation, which is commonly seen at this level in pediatrics. A line is drawn from the anterior spinous process of C-1 to C-3, and the finding is considered normal if it intersects or is within 1 mm anteriorly of the C-2 cortex (13). If the posterior cervical line is anterior to the posterior arch at C-2 by more than 2 mm, a true dislocation of C-2 must be considered, and the athlete should be evaluated further.

With any suspicion or documented pathology on the above plain films or any neurologic deficit in the athlete, further studies must be undertaken. For suspected or definite fractures, computerized tomography (CT) is the recommended study of choice. Sensitivity for a bony injury using this imaging format is greater than 97% in most studies (12).

Many clinicians regard magnetic resonance imaging (MRI) as the most definitive imagery study of soft tissue injury in and around the c-spine. Neurologic deficits resulting from fractures can also be appropriately imaged using this format. Use of this in examination is also the recommended study for obtunded patients with suspected c-spine injuries, as well as for patients who are suspected of having spinal cord injury without radiographic abnormalities (SCIWORA), a phenomenon that is seen more frequently among pediatric patients. The reported incidence of this entity ranges from 5% to 55% (13), with most studies reporting a rate of nearly 20% for all pediatric spinal injuries (2). By having additional information about swelling in and around the cord, identification of SCIWORA situations is more likely. The condition is thought to be a result of the momentary displacement of the spine and cord without an accompanying disruption of the bones or ligaments. Hyperextension, flexion, distraction, and lack of an adequate blood supply to the area can all be factors in this injury.

CT scans of the c-spine are the best method of delineating bony abnormalities, in addition to being the imaging modality of choice with obtunded patients and patients who have metal implants. This study is initially performed without contrast.

Soft tissue injuries, such as sprains and strains, and disc pathology can be isolated, or they can be present in conjunction with fractures; MRI is the diagnostic study of choice in these instances. This examination provides excellent detail of the status of the cord, injury to the disk, and impingement on the nerves as they exit the spinal column. Upper cord lesions are more likely to cause more serious deficits. MRI, however, does not always show the transection to or injury of the cord. Myelograms may be the follow-up study that is used to clarify any suspicious findings.

Additional views can be performed when the above examinations are negative, if suspicion remains as to the extent of injury, or following the guidance of the consultant. Oblique views of the spine offer a more precise visualization of the posterior elements of the vertebral body, but they are technically difficult to perform if the patient is still secured to the spine board. In an attempt to discern any subtle instability of the spine, secondary examinations can include the patient's active flexion and extension views within the limit of the patient's pain tolerance. Other specialized views occur at the direction of the consultant.

CONSULTATION

Consultation with specialists regarding the evaluation and treatment of c-spine injuries is extremely important. Depending on the degree of injury sustained by the athlete, enlisting the professional expertise of colleagues in radiology, orthopedics, neurosurgery, and physical medicine and rehabilitation early in the care can be of tremendous benefit to the athlete.

Initial radiographic studies of the injured athlete are fairly standardized for identifying significant disruptions of the bone of the c-spine. Obvious fractures, such as an odontoid fracture, hangman's fracture, and burst fractures, and dislocation of the vertebral column clearly require immediate consultation with the appropriate orthopedic or neurosurgical specialist. Often, these specialists recommend further imaging to facilitate the early stabilization and treatment of the injury.

Neurologic deficits, whether with or without surgical intervention, may benefit from evaluation by a physiatrist. The best timing for this consultant's initial evaluation remains somewhat unclear in the acute setting. The evaluation conducted by this specialist can provide documentation of the extent and location of a nerve injury, and it can assist in long term follow-up and management.

SOFT INJURIES

Injuries to the c-spine may involve isolated injuries to the muscles, ligaments, discs, fascia, or bone. More commonly, however, several structures are involved, with injury ranging in severity from simple contusions to permanent quadriplegia or death.

Contusions

Contusions to the anterior structures of the neck, such as the larynx, strap muscles, cricoid, and thyroid, can occur from blows from objects such as a baseball, a baseball bat, sticks, and other implements. Actions, such as being "clotheslined" across the neck by an opponent's arm while being tackled in football, can also cause a contusion anteriorly. Direct injury to the larynx or other structures, which is seen in sports such as hockey, lacrosse, martial arts, and boxing, causes significant edema and hemorrhage in the anterior aspect of the neck, which may compromise the athlete's airway. Immediate assessment and stabilization of the airway is critical in this injury scenario.

Blows to the posterior aspect of the neck can occur between players, but they often result in more serious injury if equipment, such as shoulder pads, neck rolls, and helmets, is not properly fitted. Cord concussion can result in patients who receive blows in this area; despite its alarming nature, however, recovery is common (9). Bony tenderness should be evaluated first, and, if it is present, the athlete should be treated as though he or she has sustained a fracture. Soft tissue tenderness, with no bony pain and no neurologic deficit, usually can be treated conservatively. Poorly fitted equipment must be corrected to preclude further injury to the athlete when he or she returns to play.

Strains and Sprains

Sprains and strains of the c-spine are the most common types of c-spine injuries seen in athletes. In the pediatric population, a larger head size in proportion to the body, weak cervical muscle strength, and improper tackling techniques are often causative factors in sprains and strains of the spine. Frequently, the posterior cervical muscles are injured when the neck is forced into hyperflexion or is placed into a position where the posterior muscles are forced into extension against resistance, which is commonly seen in wrestling. These soft tissue injuries tend to be less severe than the other injuries discussed in this chapter. However, recovery time with proper rehabilitation can take up to 6 weeks in many cases. Many different muscle groups in the neck can be the source of strain injuries. The diagnosis of a strain is actually one of exclusion, after more serious potential injury has been ruled out. The site of strain injuries generally appears to be the musculotendinous junction. Hemorrhage at this junction caused by shearing leads to inflammation, muscle spasm, and pain, which leaves the athlete with a decreased range of motion. The healing process with fibrous tissue takes over 6 weeks; however, an athlete usually can return to play when his or her range of motion and strength have returned to normal. As was discussed previously, the soft tissue of the c-spine helps to dissipate the high-energy forces, thus reducing the potential for spinal cord damage. Therefore, recovery of full range of motion of the c-spine and of strength is an important safety consideration in return-to-play decisions.

Grade I sprains and strains, in which the disruption of fibers is less than 30%, respond well to conservative therapy. Radiographic evaluation should be negative, and the physical examination should reveal only minimal discomfort, no bony tenderness, no neurologic deficit, and minimal decrease in the range of motion. The use of ice, heat, analgesics, and antiinflammatories can assist in decreasing discomfort and can help in regaining pain-free range of motion. Resistive exercises, which are initiated when the pain has decreased, help to strengthen the neck for the prevention of reoccurrences.

The presence of grade II injuries (30% to 70% of fibers are involved) is of much more concern, and these injuries should be extensively evaluated and thoroughly rehabilitated before return to play is considered. Marked tenderness is often present over the injured soft tissue area, with a generalized soreness that is referred to the muscles around the injured area. Moderate restriction of motion of the spine will be seen in all directions. The athlete may also complain of headaches, shoulder pain, and vertigo. Radiographic examinations including all seven cervical vertebrae in the AP, lateral, and oblique views may be necessary in order to be able to rule out a fracture (Fig. 29.1). Treatment of these athletes requires a much longer course of physical therapy, often includes c-spine support in a collar, and mandates the use of strengthening exercises prior to the resumption of activity. Modification in equipment should be considered when the athlete is allowed to return to practice; this should include the use of items such as a "cowboy" collar, a neck roll or restraining strap affixed to a helmet, and shoulder pads to restrict hyperflexion of the neck (see Chapter 8). Cervical sprains tend not to be isolated injuries, as the forces required to cause ligamentous or muscle–tendon injury also cause damage in other structures. If any question exists as to the severity of an injury, radiographs should be taken. Younger athletes have more instability in the c-spine, compared to older athletes. If a question regarding any instability is present, follow-up comparison x-rays at 2 to 4 weeks postinjury should be obtained to look for progression of any defect. Until

then, the athlete must be protected, and he or she is prohibited from returning to sports participation.

For an athlete who sustains a grade III sprain or strain that disrupts 70% or more of the fibers to the c-spine, evaluation with an orthopedist and neurosurgeon is recommended; pending that evaluation, protection with a hard cervical collar is also appropriate. The symptoms of a grade III injury include severe neck pain, with or without neurologic involvement; marked limitation in motion; and the presence of other associated symptoms, such as headache, nausea, lightheadedness, and dizziness. In addition to plain radiographs, an MRI may be considered in order to evaluate the soft tissues in and around the spine and cord further.

SCIWORA can be catastrophic. Athletes suffering from SCIWORA should receive bracing or possibly casting, analgesics, and nonsteroidal antiinflammatory agents. Studies have shown that many of these children are at higher risk for a more extensive injury if they return to activity less than 10 weeks from the date of the original injury (14). Long-term follow-up—often more than 3 months postinjury—is required with these athletes. Criteria for return to play must include the return of full range of motion, a significant recovery of the strength of the c-spine, no evidence of a neurologic deficit, and a stable spine on flexion and extension views. The last consideration for return to play must be the athlete's desire to return to activity. Any hesitation or apprehension about returning to sports participation should disqualify the athlete, until his or her confidence returns or until he or she decides not to resume that activity again.

FRACTURES AND DISLOCATIONS

Upper Cervical Spine

Injuries to the to the upper c-spine are seldom the cause of neurologic defect because the space available in the canal can accommodate some displacement. However, if a neurologic injury does occur in the upper c-spine, it can be fatal because of its effect on respiratory muscles. In the pediatric population, the clinician must remember that a child has much more mobility in the upper c-spine than an adult does. Pediatric patients also have a greater atlantodental space (up to 4.5 mm is normal), when compared to that of an adult (15).

In the Special Olympic population, the clinician should note that children with Down syndrome have an increased risk of subluxation at both the atlantoaxial and atlantooccipital regions. As part of the preparticipation physical examination (PPE), these children

TABLE 29.1. *Cervical spine fractures*

Upper
  Odontoid
  Wedge
  Hangman's
Lower
  Clay shoveler's
  Teardrop
  Jefferson
  Burst

must be radiographically evaluated prior to being allowed to start training (see Chapters 2 and 25). The following three common fractures occur in the upper c-spine: the odontoid fracture, the hangman's fracture, and the Jefferson fracture (Table 29.1).

Odontoid Fracture

Odontoid fractures are the most common injuries to the c-spine in children (13). Hyperextension of the neck may lead to a fracture of the odontoid process of C-2, creating an unstable joint in the upper c-spine. These are actually physeal fractures of the synchondrosis, and they usually are Salter–Harris type 1 fractures (13). The mechanism of injury generally is that the ring of C-1 strikes the odontoid process of the atlas, causing a shearing fracture, usually at the base of the dens. Three types of odontoid fractures, which are based on the location of the fracture, occur. Type 1 is the avulsion of the tip of the odontoid process. Type 2 is a fracture that occurs at the base of the process. Type 3 is a fracture of the process that extends into the body of C-2. Of these fractures, type 2 generally

is the most unstable fracture; type 3 is less unstable than type 2, and type 1 is generally extremely stable. Type 2 fractures, because of the inherent instability of the ability of C-1 to shift, are quite difficult to stabilize, and they often progress to nonunion. The open-mouth odontoid radiograph is the best initial film for demonstrating these fractures. Types 1 and 3 often heal well without further problems, but type 2, because of the problems mentioned above, often requires surgical intervention (16). Table 29.2 provides a summary of the basic fracture and dislocation types and their stability and/or complications. Neurologic deficits are rare if these fractures are identified early and as long as fracture fragments do not displace.

Hangman's Fracture

Hangman's fracture is a bilateral pars interarticularis fracture of C-2 that is produced by hyperextension of the neck. This type of fracture is rare in children, and, despite its historical name, it rarely produces death or even neurologic injury. This injury occurs most commonly in football and recreational diving. It is best identified with lateral radiograph. The treatment is usually nonoperative in nature, employing immobilization in a Minerva cast or a halo vest after positioning the spine into a neutral and stable position.

Jefferson Fracture

Compared to the above fractures, the Jefferson fracture is more difficult to identify, and, many times, CT is required for adequate visualization. However, the open mouth odontoid view can provide some

TABLE 29.2. *Cervical-spine fractures and dislocations*

	Stability and complications
Fractures	
Jefferson fracture (C-1 in four places)	Unstable; cast immobilization unless unstable in flexion and extension; neurosurgical intervention required if unstable
Odontoid fracture (C-2)	Unstable; type 2 requires surgery
Hangman's fracture (C-2 bilateral pars)	Unstable; immobilize in Minerva or halo vest usually nonoperative
C-5 fracture	Generally profound neurologic damage; neurosurgery consult
Clay shoveler's fracture (C-7)	Stable; symptomatic treatment
Wedge fracture	Stable; conservative treatment
Teardrop fracture	Variable; conservative treatment
Burst fracture	Variable; may require surgery
Dislocations	
Atlantooccipital dislocations	Typically fatal; requires neurosurgery to stabilize
Atlantoaxial rotary dislocations	Unstable; neurosurgery consult necessary
Bilateral facet dislocations	Unstable; neurosurgical consult
Unilateral facet dislocations	Variable; may require surgery

clues to help with diagnosis. The Jefferson fracture is a fracture of C-1 in four places—two anterior fractures and two posterior fractures—about the ring. It is most commonly caused by axial loading forces to the occipital condyles, which then result in the fracture of the ring. On radiographs, the lateral masses of C-1 should line up with the lateral masses of C-2. If a step-off laterally is observed, with overhangs on both sides of the atlas that cumulatively add up to more than 7 mm of the axis, then a fracture should be suspected. In these cases, disruption of the transverse ligament is probable. This interval may be increased up to 10 to 12 mm if the ligament is ruptured (17). Normally, this fracture can be treated conservatively, without surgical intervention, unless flexion and extension views subsequently show evidence of instability; in these cases, fusion should be considered. CT scans are useful in both the diagnosis of this injury and in the assessment of healing (13).

Upper Cervical Spine Dislocations

Dislocation or subluxation at the atlantooccipital joint is typically a fatal injury. Atlanooccipital dislocation (AOD) is the general term that is used to describe upper c-spine dislocations. Three types of AOD have been described. Type I is described as the anterior movement of the cranium with respect to the atlas. Type II, the most common among children, is caused by a longitudinal distraction of the occiput from the atlas. A type III dislocation results from the posterior movement of the cranium with respect to the atlas. If the patient survives the initial trauma, proper stabilization, transport, and advanced trauma life support are necessary. Definitive stabilization is obtained through neurosurgical intervention for unstable injuries.

Atlantoaxial rotary dislocation is a less threatening injury that occurs with forced flexion of the c-spine. In this injury, the alar ligaments are disrupted as the result of significant trauma. This can cause a rotational dislocation of C-1 on C-2. Again, stabilization with immobilization must occur, and neurosurgical consultation should be obtained.

Midcervical Spine Fractures

Fractures of the midcervical region are rare. Most often, they are seen as either unilateral or bilateral disk injuries and dislocations of the articular processes. Transient quadriplegia is common following rupture of the C-3 to C-4 disk. Surgical fusion of this level, accompanied by discectomy, may be the treatment of choice.

Lower Cervical Spine Fractures

Due to the dimensions of the pediatric spinal cord in the lower c-spine segments, fractures in the area are more likely to be associated with profound neurologic injury, although it is usually not catastrophic. Multiple fracture patterns, based on the type of force applied to the spine, can occur in the lower c-spine. Lateral radiographs, with cross table lateral film as the initial study, are critical for making the diagnosis of the majority of these fractures. C-5 is the most common fractured cervical vertebrae, and C-5/C-6 is the most common site for subluxation (18). In nearly 10% of all lower c-spine fractures, a second associated fracture may also be present. Injuries to the subaxial or lower c-spine can be caused by a combination of flexion, extension, rotation, and compression injury forces, or they occur in isolation. Some of the more common injuries that affect the pediatric athlete in this portion of the spine are mentioned below.

Clay Shoveler's Fracture

The clay shoveler's fracture commonly occurs at C-7. It is an avulsion fracture of the spinous process, and it is considered a highly stable fracture that requires only symptomatic treatment for pain and spasm (1). Vigorous exertion with neck extension is often the inciting event. AP and lateral radiographs generally are the only studies required for identification of this fracture (Fig. 29.2).

Wedge Fracture

Wedge fracture is a compression fracture that results from a hyperflexion force that causes impaction of the anterior portion of one vertebra onto another. Most of the force is concentrated over the anterior aspect of the spine, thus resulting in a crush or compression injury of the anterior aspect of the vertebral body. On radiographic evaluation, the defect is a wedge-shaped vertebral body with increased density on the anterior, superior, and inferior surfaces. The prevertebral soft tissue often swells, but this injury is a stable fracture that rarely results in neurologic abnormality. Therefore, treatment is conservative, and surgical intervention is usually not required for stabilization.

Teardrop Fracture

This fracture, named for its specific appearance on radiograph, has a good prognosis. A small teardrop-

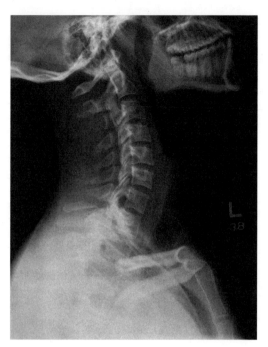

FIG. 29.2. Cervical spine fracture. Clay shoveler's type at C-7.

shaped fragment from the anterior–inferior corner of one of the vertebral bodies is seen. The force that causes this fracture is a significant flexion force on an axially loaded, hyperflexed spine. Contrary to the disruption seen of most flexion injuries, neither the posterior ligaments nor the intervertebral disc are disrupted. In teardrop fractures, the larger the fragment is, the more significant the injury is. Displacement of the fragment, however, rarely causes a spinal cord injury. This type of fracture is relatively stable, and, like the wedge fracture, it rarely requires reduction and surgical intervention.

Burst Fracture

As with most fractures, burst fracture is also the result of an axial load. The c-spine is moved into flexion to an angle of approximately 30 degrees, which causes the loss of the normal lordodic curve. Axially loading of the spine then occurs. As was discussed earlier, this force vector causes maximum energy absorption in the skeletal spine. A burst fracture commonly results from such forces. On lateral radiographs, the vertebral body may appear to be only slightly enlarged, and evidence of trabecular pattern disruption may be found. In many cases, by the time the radiograph is taken, fragments may

have been pulled back into alignment by their ligamentous attachments. Awareness of the pathomechanics of such a fracture expedites the diagnosis. Normally, this fracture is stable posteriorly because of the ligamentous pull, but displacement into the spinal canal can occur. Nonsurgical treatment may require reduction with immobilization. More often, however, surgical intervention is recommended if the fracture is unstable.

Lower Cervical Spine Dislocations

Bilateral Facet Dislocations

Bilateral c-spine facet dislocations are considered extremely unstable. This injury is characterized by a superior vertebral body translation over the inferior segment in excess of 50%, and it is often accompanied by severe spinal cord damage. Radiographs are usually sufficient to diagnose the extent of injury. Closed reduction and neurosurgical stabilization are usually necessary.

Unilateral Facet Dislocation

Unilateral facet dislocation is caused by a combination of axial loading, flexion, and rotational forces. The dislocated facet is often wedged in the intervertebral foramen. Less than a 50% shift of the superior vertebra on the lower segment is observed. A facet fracture may or may not be associated with this dislocation. Physical findings vary from no neurologic deficit to complete cord transection. The severity is also based on the presence or absence of an associated fracture of the facet. Treatment of this dislocation ranges from skeletal traction to reduce the dislocation to surgical stabilization; the choice of treatment often depends on whether an associated fracture of the facet is present and the extent of neurologic damage that has been caused by the dislocation. Consultation with neurosurgery or orthopedics is recommended early in the course of evaluation and treatment.

NEUROLOGIC INJURIES

Nerve injuries, excluding injury to the spinal cord, are generally classified into three broad stages based on the historical data and clinical examination findings (Table 29.3).

First-degree injury to a nerve, or neuropraxia, is the least severe injury. This reversible injury occurs at the site of the trauma to the nerve. Generally, the in-

TABLE 29.3. *Neurologic injuries*

Spinal cord injury
  Complete
  Partial
  Brown–Sequard
Spinal shock—transient
Quadraplegia
Spear tackler's spine
Burners/stingers

jury affects the motor and the large myelinated fibers of the nerve. Full recovery occurs within 2 to 3 weeks.

Second-degree injury is axonotmesis. Severe disruption of the axon of the nerve occurs and includes the surrounding myelin. A temporary loss of motor and sensory function usually exists. Within 72 hours, the ability to innervate the nerve distal to the injury is lost. The prognosis depends on the severity and location of the injury. The rate of reinnervation of the nerve in children has not been definitely determined, but it is thought to be similar to that seen in the adult (1 mm per day).

The most severe form of nerve injury is neurotmesis. This injury is thought to be irreversible, due to the disruption of the endoneurium, the area of functional regeneration of the nerve. The degrees of this injury indicate how many layers of the structure of the nerve have been involved. The worst prognosis is associated with complete disruption of the endoneurium, perineurium, and epineurium. The most severe injuries in this classification are usually surgically repaired with nerve grafts.

Spinal Cord Injury

Complete spinal cord injury is defined as the total loss of sensory or motor function below a certain vertebral level. This injury is one of the most feared injuries in athletics due to its devastating morbidity. Complete cord transections have an extremely poor prognosis. However, partial spinal cord injuries have demonstrated some capacity for functional improvement. Partial cord lesions are injuries to the cord in which some degree of motor or sensory function is maintained. The area of cord that sustains the trauma usually is the major determinant of the resultant clinical picture. If the cord lesion is more anterior, which is seen most often as a result hyperflexion injuries, the injured athlete tends to display more motor weakness, with some degree of sensory sparing. A central lesion to the cord involves more upper than lower extremity paralysis, and it is caused by forced hyperextension of the spine. Posterior lesions, although rare, are primarily sensory paralytic injuries. A mixed presentation is often observed with the Brown–Sequard syndrome, a variant of a central cord and posterior lesion that is characterized by ipsilateral motor paralysis and a contralateral sensory deficit. Overall, anterior, partial cord lesions have the poorest prognosis of all partial cord injuries (18).

Spinal Shock or Transient Quadriplegia

This injury is a "concussion," or transient impairment, of the spinal cord, and symptoms may last up to 48 hours. The reported incidence of paresthesia with transient quadriplegia was reported as 1.3 per 100,000 athletes in one football study (13). Spinal shock manifests most often as flaccidity and the loss of reflexes. During the "shock" phase, no prognosis for long-term recovery can be given. A patient may recover fully, or a complete spinal cord injury may be present. Spinal shock is said to exist as long as the bulbocavernosus reflex is absent, and the return of the reflex indicates the end of the "shock" period (19). Spinal cord shock may be more prone to occur in athletes with spinal cord stenosis, and a complete workup, including x-rays, MRI, and a CT myelogram, is mandated in cases of transient quadriplegia to search for stenosis and instability. However, Torg et al. (17) found that the occurrence of transient neuropraxia and injury associated with permanent catastrophic neurologic sequelae are unrelated. Moreover, cervical cord neuropraxia, whether with or without transient quadriplegia, does not predispose the athlete to permanent neurologic injury (17).

Spear Tackler's Spine

This condition was first described in 1993 after a careful review of data from the National Football Head and Neck Injury Registry (1). By definition, spear tackler's spine is the narrowing or stenosis of a cervical segment so that one or more vertebra have a canal to vertebral body ratio of 0.8 or less (17). This entity was reported in the literature for football players, but it does have the potential to occur in other sports that use the head as a battering ram for striking an unyielding object. The condition was first described as permanent neurologic damage that was sustained by four football players who demonstrated highly similar characteristics on plain c-spine radiographs. These findings were (a) developmental narrowing of the cervical spinal canal, (b) straightening or reversal of normal cervical lordotic curve at the time of injury, and (c) preexisting minor posttraumatic radiographic evidence of bony or ligamentous injury. Each of the players used spear tackling techniques (10).

No firm consensus exists on whether athletes with the above characteristics should be precluded from further participation in sports. The presence of a canal to vertebral body ratio of less that 0.8 is not necessarily a contraindication for participation in asymptomatic individuals (17). Some specialists recommend complete removal from contact or collision sports, while others propose that restoration of normal lordosis and abstinence from spear tackling are adequate for allowing participation (1,10,13).

Burners or Stingers

Burners (also called stingers or "pinched nerve") are the most common brachial plexus injuries reported in North America. These terms, which are used by athletes, coaches, and trainers, describe symptoms, including pain, burning, or tingling that radiates down the arm, that result from some trauma to the spine and shoulder (8). The symptoms usually last for only a few seconds to minutes; however, occasionally some players will experience symptoms for days or even longer.

Stingers may be caused by one of two mechanisms—a stretching or traction on the brachial plexus or a nerve root compression and/or impingement within the cervical neural foramen from forced lateral flexion of the spine. Younger players are more likely to sustain the traction type injury (8). The symptoms typically are purely sensory in nature, and they most commonly affect the C-5 and C-6 dermatomes. The numbness often lasts longer than the weakness. When muscular weakness does present, it usually affects the biceps, deltoids, supraspinatus, and infraspinatus.

Stingers are always unilateral, and they do not involve the lower extremities to any degree. If symptoms are bilateral and/or the lower extremities are involved, the presence of other types of injury must be considered.

Brachial plexus symptoms that last only a few seconds to minutes or those that clear completely (i.e., no evidence of neck pain, no restriction of range of motion, and strength has fully returned) permit the athlete to return to play. If any residual symptoms persist, participation in practice and competition should be restricted until further workup has been conducted and complete resolution of symptoms has occurred. Reports indicate that over half of all football players will have a stinger at least once in their career (7). An athlete who has recurrent stingers that occur within a short period of time during a single season should also be considered for further workup, and activity restrictions should be imposed pending the evaluation.

Neurologic evaluation for stingers should include c-spine radiographs initially and a MRI as indicated, and it should be conducted if symptoms have not resolved in a timely fashion or if a chronic problem develops. If any neurologic symptom persists for more than 2 weeks, electromyography should be performed to assess the extent of injury (8).

VASCULAR INJURIES

Injuries to the vertebral and carotid arteries are extremely rare, but they can occur in sports. These injuries are usually associated with neck motion at its physiologic extreme (e.g., that caused by a sharp blow), which initiates damage in the inner linings of the arteries. This can lead to clot formation, which results in an emboli, occlusion of the artery, and a resultant stroke. With fracture dislocations, injuries to the vertebral artery may occur, leading to a brainstem stroke (8).

DISK INJURIES

The location of disk herniation will dictate whether return to play is contraindicated. Most often, MRI is the imaging modality used to identify this injury. In general, athletes with healed anterior and lateral herniations can return to play. If surgery, (i.e., a diskectomy or fusion), is required on a lateral or central lesion, the following criteria must be considered before these athletes can return to competition: solid fusion at the site; pain-free, full range of motion; and no evidence of neurologic deficit on examination. Absolute contraindications to return to play include acute central disk herniation (17), symptomatic neck pain, and decreased range of motion or hardening of the disk that is associated with spinal stenosis.

SPECIAL CONSIDERATIONS

Congenital or Structural Abnormalities

Chapter 25 presents an in-depth discussion of abnormalities in the special athlete. These abnormalities generally are rare in the normal population of pediatric athletes, and they often are an incidental finding that is noted on plain film when an injury has occurred. Normally, by 8 years of age, the pediatric c-spine approaches the adult configuration. However, in the Special Olympic population, c-spine abnormalities have a much greater prevalence. Some of the disorders that have an increased risk of congenital and developmental alterations of the spine include Down syndrome, Kippel–Feil syndrome, and osteochondrodysplasias. Each of these conditions incorporates a potential for specific injuries. Currently, the governing body of the Special Olympics requires neck radiographs prior to participation in athletic competitions for all athletes with Down syndrome. The validity of preparticipation radiographs is discussed by the American Academy of Pediatrics (AAP) statement on atlantoaxial instability in Down syndrome (17a). Physicians who perform PPEs for Special Olympians must be mindful of these rules so that opportunities for full participation at all levels can be accomplished safely within the guidelines.

Klippel–Feil syndrome is a spectrum of congenital osseous anomalies of the c-spine. The most common physical finding is decreased cervical motion that is more prominent in side bending and rotation. Cervical radiculopathy or myelopathy are other common clinical findings found in the neurologic examination. These patients often are noted to have short necks, a low posterior hairline, and congenital cervical fusion. Radiographs of the c-spine, including flexion and extension views, are indicated. Findings often associated with Klippel–Feil syndrome are congenital scoliosis, the Sprengel deformity (congenital elevation of the scapula), hearing impairments, synkinesia, and congenital heart disease (Fig. 29.3). Renal pathology is also associated with this syndrome. Restriction of activities and cervical orthoses may be indicated for symptomatic treatment of these patients (15). The level of athletic involvement allowed is dependent on the amount of cervical motion and stability present in the athlete. If the patient has an active, full range of motion, without radiographic cervical anomalies, instability, disc disease, or degenerative changes, no contraindications for athletic participation are present (13).

Osteochondrodysplasias are heterogeneous, genetic disorders with intrinsic abnormalities of bone and cartilage growth and remodeling. Cervical instability occurs in a large percentage of these patients. The diagnosis is usually made after the child begins to drop below the 5th percentile for his or her height within the first year of life. A skeletal survey is helpful in establishing the diagnosis (15). Sports participation will be limited by skeletal deformities. If participation is desired, thorough c-spine and orthopedic evaluation is necessary.

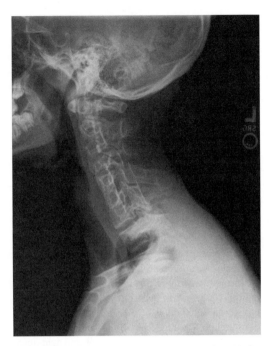

FIG. 29.3. Lateral spine hemivertebral body with fusion.

Other disorders that can affect the c-spine and, in so doing, influence athletic participation are achondroplasia, spondyloepiphyseal dysplasia, and the mucopolysaccharidoses. Patients with these disorders need to be evaluated thoroughly with radiographs and complete skeletal examination prior to participation in any sporting activities.

RETURN TO PLAY

The question most often asked of the physician by the athlete, parents, coaches, and trainers is "When can the athlete return to competition?" This question can come surprisingly quickly after a severe injury. The primary care physician must educate the athlete, the family, and the coaches regarding the potential severity of a c-spine injury. Everyone involved in the return-to-play decision process should appreciate that a conservative well-designed treatment plan for return to play is the best strategy.

As was previously discussed, soft tissue contusions and most strains and sprains of the spine require the return of pain-free normal range of motion and full muscular strength as the criteria for returning to the playing field. These criteria should not be compromised. The criteria for stingers and spear tackler's spine were also discussed in the context of these injuries. However, returning to participation is more complicated with this condition when neurologic or radiographic abnormalities have been noted. Athletes with c-spine fractures and dislocations may have undergone varying treatments, ranging from no treatment other than physical therapy to halo vest immobilization and open surgical correction. Most fractures require surgical stabilization. Obviously, athletes with permanent neurologic injury should be prohibited from further competition. Furthermore, athletes whose fractures require halo vest or surgical stabilization are considered to have insufficient spinal strength to return to contact sports safely. However, athletes with stable fractures that have healed completely can return to competition by the next season if normal strength and pain-free, normal range of motion have returned. Any athlete who has suffered a cervical fracture must be given proper warnings against participating in any contact or collision sports until the fracture is completely healed. Of course, proper documentation of all patient–doctor interactions and the warnings issued must be recorded.

Athletes who sustain an episode of transient quadriplegia are in a unique situation. These patients must have many factors evaluated prior to return to play, including spinal stenosis, functional stenosis, and functional reserve. Evaluation of these athletes requires more than a lateral radiograph in order to make a proper determination. To obtain all of the pertinent information needed to make a return-to-play decision, a myelogram, CT, or MRI is needed. These athletes represent a spectrum for return-to-play decisions in contact or collision sports (10). Torg et al. (17) recommended the following guidelines for managing athletes with developmental narrowing of the c-spine that is associated with cervical cord neurapraxia:

1. Canal to vertebral body ratio of 0.8 or less in asymptomatic individuals—no contraindications.
2. Ratio of 0.8 or less, with one episode of cervical cord neurapraxia—relative contraindication.
3. Documented episodes of cervical cord neurapraxia associated with intravertebral disc disease and/or degenerative changes—relative contraindication.
4. Documented episode of cervical cord neurapraxia associated with MRI evidence of cord defect or cord edema—relative or absolute contraindication.
5. Documented episode of cervical cord neurapraxia associated with ligamentous instability, symptoms of neurologic findings lasting more than 36 hours, and/or multiple episodes—absolute contraindication.

A combination of proper radiographic and consultative information is required to create an individualized plan for the injured athlete.

PREVENTION

Much time and effort is spent in practicing how to care for the athlete after he or she has been injured; however, too often, injury prevention is not emphasized enough. The process of prevention begins quite early with the proper competitive placement of children so that they are playing against others who are generally equal in size, strength, and coordination. Healthcare providers must evaluate the spine for strength and range of motion during the PPE, and they should determine if the child can safely wear the equipment that is required by the sport. Equipment managers must know the proper fit of all equipment that is issued and must ensure that it is worn correctly and that the child and the supervising adult know how to maintain it properly.

A major factor in injury prevention is the coaching staff. Coaches who teach and enforce correct techniques in all skills have a tremendous impact on decreasing injury rates. Teaching proper tackling techniques in football alone has decreased the rate of spinal cord quadriplegia. By making the face mask part of the helmet by rule, the injury rate dramatically dropped to only one case of quadriplegia in 1991 (19). Mandatory strength training of neck muscles should be monitored by coaches and trainers, as this is extremely important for protecting the athlete from injury. Along with the coach's daily enforcement of proper skill techniques in practice, referees and umpires can decrease illegal and dangerous play by enforcing application of the rules and by providing constant reminders about safe play throughout the game.

All of these actions provide a safe framework within which a child can compete safely. Although all risk of c-spine injury cannot be eliminated, an environment that is as safe as possible can be provided by attempting to address the above recommendations. Clinicians have a general understanding of how c-spine injuries occur, but no absolute guidelines can be devised with respect to an athlete's return to full athletic competition (5). However, through efforts to provide the safest environment possible, children can safely enjoy sports participation.

REFERENCES

1. Pizzutillo PD. The cervical spine. In: Stanitski CL, DeLee JC, Drez D, ed. *Pediatric and adolescent sports medicine*, Vol. 3. Philadelphia: WB Saunders, 1994.

2. Luke A, Micheli L. Sports injuries: emergency assessment and field-side care. *Pediatr Rev* 1999;20:291–301.

3. Birrer RB, Brecher DB. *Common sports injuries in youngsters*. Boca Raton, FL: CRC Press, 1987:35–42.

4. Birrer RB. Common injuries of the head and neck. In: Birrer RB, ed. *Sports medicine for the primary care physician*. Boca Raton, FL: CRC Press, 1994:165–170.

5. Wilberger JE. Athletic spinal cord and spine injuries, guidelines for initial management. *Clin Sports Med* 1998;17:111–120.

6. Huerta C, Griffith R, Joyce SM. Cervical spine stabilization in pediatric patients: evaluation of current techniques. *Ann Emerg Med* 1987;16:1121–1126.

7. Cantu RC, Micheli K. Head and spine injuries in youth sports. The young athlete. *Clin Sports Med* 1995;14:517–532.

8. Curran C, Dietrich AM, Bowman MJ, et al. Pediatric cervical-spine immobilization: achieving neutral position? *J Trauma* 1995;39:729–732.

9. Birrer RB. Special considerations in the injured child. In: Birrer RB, ed. *Sports medicine for the primary care physician*. Boca Raton: CRC Press, 1994:249–251.

10. Herzenberg JE, Hensinger RN, Dedrick DK, et al. Emergency transport and positioning of young children who have an injury of the cervical spine. The standard backboard may be hazardous. *J Bone Joint Surg* 1989;71:15–22.

11. Kleiner DM, Almquist JL, Bailes J, et al. *Prehospital care of the spine-injured athlete: a document from the inter-association task force for appropriate care of the spine-injured athlete*. Dallas: National Athletic Trainers Association, 2001.

12. Della-Guistina KD, Della-Guistina DA. Emergency department evaluation and treatment of pediatric orthopedic injuries. *Emerg Med Clin North Am* 1999;17:895–920.

13. Loder RT. The cervical spine. In: Morrissy RT, Weinstein SL, ed. *Lovell and Winter's pediatric orthopedics*, 4th ed. Vol. 2. Philadelphia: Lippincott-Raven Publishers, 1996.

14. Osenbach RK. Pediatric spinal cord and vertebral column injury. *Neurosurgery* 1992;30:385–390.

15. Nypaver M, Treloar D. Neutral cervical spine positioning in children. *Ann Emerg Med* 1994;23:208–211.

16. Akbarnia BA. Pediatric spine fractures. disorders of the pediatric and adolescent spine. *Orthop Clin North Am* 1999;30:521–536.

17. Torg JS, Gennarelli TA. Intracranial and cervical spine injuries. In: Garrett WE, Speer KP, Kirkendall DT, ed. *Principles and practice of orthopedic sports medicine*. Philadelphia: Lippincott Williams &Wilkins, 2000.

17a. Committee on Sports Medicine and Fitness. Atlantoaxial instability in Down syndrome. Policy statement. *Pediatrics* 1995;96:151–154.

18. Hall DE, Boydston W. Pediatric neck injuries. *Pediatr Rev* 1999;20:13–19.

19. Clarke KS. Epidemiology of athletic neck injury. *Clin Sports Med* 1998;17:83–97.

30

Back Pain and Injuries

Lauren M. Simon, William Jih, and J.C. Buller

Back pain can occur in children and adolescents, particularly when they have begun new or strenuous physical activities. It also is seen after long periods of inactivity, such as after summer vacation, when the athlete returns to sports. In order to understand low back pain in pediatric athletes, a review of the anatomy of the pediatric spine and the differential diagnosis of pediatric back pain is helpful.

ANATOMY OF THE PEDIATRIC SPINE

In most adults, the vertebral column (backbone) consists of 33 bones (vertebrae), which support the trunk (7 cervical, 12 thoracic, 5 lumbar, 5 sacral, and 4 coccygeal). In adults, the sacral vertebrae are fused to form the sacrum, and the coccygeal vertebrae form the coccyx. However, in children, fusion has not yet occurred; at birth, the sacral and coccygeal vertebrae are cartilaginous, and they begin to ossify during infancy. At birth, the vertebrae consist of three bony parts that are connected by hyaline cartilage. Fusion of the vertebral arch usually occurs by the 6 or 7 years of age. During puberty, five secondary centers of ossification develop in each vertebra, and these usually fuse by the age of 25 years. The age of fusion varies, so one must not confuse an open epiphysis with a fracture on a radiograph of the spine.

The typical vertebral parts are the body, the vertebral arch (which has two pedicles, two laminae, and one spinous process and which encloses the vertebral foramen through which the spinal cord passes), and the vertebral processes that extend from the vertebral arch. The vertebral processes are the spinous process, the transverse processes, and the four articular processes. The articular processes have articular facets; each joint between a superior and an inferior facet is called a zygapophyseal joint. Adjacent vertebrae are connected by fibrocartilaginous intervertebral discs and strong anterior and posterior longitudinal ligaments. The anterior longitudinal ligament extends from C-1 to the sacrum along the anterior surface of the vertebral bodies. Its fibers, which are attached to the intervertebral discs and the vertebral bodies, prevent hyperextension of the spine. The posterior longitudinal ligament extends along the posterior aspect of the vertebral bodies inside of the vertebral canal. Its fibers, which are also attached to the intervertebral discs and vertebral bodies, prevent hyperflexion of the spine. The intervertebral discs are fibrocartilaginous plates that are composed of an annulus fibrosus surrounding a gelatinous nucleus pulposus, and they play a role in weight bearing. When the nucleus pulposus protrudes through the annulus fibrosis, it is called a herniated or a ruptured disc (1). Discs may be damaged—they either protrude or are herniated—by forceful flexion and rotation of the spine. Sports that involve twisting of the spine or axial loading (downward pressure) of the spine, such as football, running, gymnastics, hockey, tennis, and weightlifting, can predispose an athlete to disc herniations.

The muscles that are used to produce flexion of the thoracic and lumbar intervertebral joints are the rectus abdominus and psoas major; extension is generated by the erector spinae and multifidus. The synovial joints between the articular processes of adjacent vertebra are called zygapophyseal (facet) joints. The facet joints, along with the intervertebral discs, participate in weight bearing. They also serve a role in rotation, flexion, and extension of the spine, and they allow gliding movement between adjacent vertebrae. Other ligaments in the spine are the ligamentum flavum, which connects the laminae of adjacent vertebral arches; interspinous ligaments and supraspinous ligaments, which connect adjacent spinous processes; and intertransverse ligaments, which connect the adjacent transverse processes.

The three groups of back muscles are described as superficial, intermediate, and deep. The superficial muscles, such as the trapezius and latissimus dorsi, connect the limbs to the trunk. The intermediate muscles and the serratus posterior are respiratory muscles. The deep muscles of the back are responsible for motion of the vertebral column. The superficial splenius muscles extend from the spinous processes of T-1 through T-6, and they insert on the base of the skull. The intermediate group of deep back muscles is the erector spinae muscles, which are arranged in lateral, intermediate, and medial columns. The common tendon of these three columns originates at the posterior part of the iliac crest, the sacrum, the sacroiliac ligament, and some of the lumbar and sacral spinous processes. The erector spinae muscles (e.g., iliocostalis, longissimus, and spinalis) are the main extensors of the spine. These muscles are the most frequently strained muscles in sports. The deep layer of the intrinsic deep back muscles is composed of small muscles (e.g., semispinalis, multifidus, and rotatores muscles).

The spinal cord is located in the vertebral canal from the occiput to the L-2 vertebra, and it is protected by the meninges, the vertebrae, and associated muscles and ligaments. It has an enlarged area at the cervical level, as well as one at the lumbosacral level that extends from the body of T-11 to the body of the L-1 level. Below L-2, the nerve roots continue as the cauda equina.

HISTORY AND PHYSICAL EXAMINATION FOR PEDIATRIC BACK PAIN

The following history should be obtained for back pain: the age of the young athlete; the timing of the onset of pain; the duration, location, radiation, and intensity of symptoms; the aggravating and relieving factors; and associated neurologic or medical conditions. Children may not remember specific dates, but they might remember whether the onset of pain occurred before or after special events (e.g., birthdays and holidays). The child should be questioned as to whether the pain occurred after a traumatic episode, such as a fall or an occurrence in a contact sport, or if it occurred insidiously over time. If pain occurs at night and it does not improve during the day, the possibility of a neoplasm should be considered. Pain located in the lumbar spine that is worsened by activities that require repetitive twisting or extension of the back may indicate spondylolysis. Diffuse generalized pain may indicate an inflammatory disorder. Pain radiating into the buttocks or lower extremity, with or without associated tingling weakness or numbness, may indicate a disc problem. Low back pain occurring several days after a viral upper respiratory infection may indicate the presence of a disc space infection. Change in gait, stumbling, bowel or bladder dysfunction, or weakness can indicate lumbosacral nerve root compression. Coordination or balance problems can indicate spinal cord pathology.

If a child has back pain associated with fever, chills, lethargy, bruising, or weight loss, the clinician should consider malignancy or infection. A child requires immediate attention if he or she has persistent pain that is unrelieved by medication, rest, or immobilization or if associated weight loss, fever, bowel or bladder dysfunction is observed. Pain that is increasing in intensity or duration also requires further evaluation.

During the in-office physical examination, the child should be examined barefoot, while wearing an examination gown that opens in the back. If the screening is conducted in the setting of a mass preparticipation physical examination (PPE) setting, such as at a school, the female child can wear a swimsuit or tank top as long as the entire back can be visualized. The examiner should perform a screening examination of the head, neck, and upper and lower extremities, before specifically examining the back. The clinician should specifically check for skin dimpling, hemangiomas, or café au lait spots, which may indicate spinal pathology. He or she should observe the patient's gait, watching for ataxia, antalgic gait, Trendelenburg gait, or a limp. The patient should be observed from behind and from the side to watch for kyphosis, scoliosis, excess lordosis, pelvic obliquity (2), or evidence of leg length discrepancy. The clinician should also look for other abnormalities on physical examination, such as foot deformities (e.g., cavus foot) or tight hamstrings. The patient should also perform a forward bending test (Fig. 30.1). In

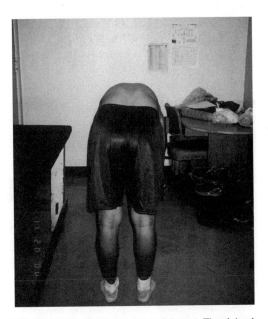

FIG. 30.1. Adam's forward bending test. The Adam's forward bending test is performed with the patient leaning forward, with his or her arms hanging down. The examiner stands behind the patient and looks for spinal abnormalities.

this procedure, the examiner stands behind a child who stands leaning forward with his or her arms hanging down and looks for spinal abnormalities, such as a rib hump. The range of motion of the spine in flexion, extension, rotation, and side bending should be assessed. Tight hamstrings noted on forward flexion in children with low back pain can be an indication of spondylolysis. The clinician must check for guarding or stiffness and palpate for tenderness over the spine and sacroiliac joints and for tenderness or spasm of the paraspinal muscles.

The neurologic examination should be used to assess for motor strength, sensory function, deep tendon reflexes, ankle clonus, or Babinski sign. The clinician should evaluate the athlete for the presence of referred pain from the sacroiliac joints or the hips. When the patient is in the supine position, he or she can be checked for sciatic nerve or nerve root irritation using the straight leg test. A figure four test, which is also known in the literature as FABERE (**f**lexion, **ab**duction, **e**xternal **r**otation, **e**xtension) or FABER (**f**lexion, **ab**duction, **e**xternal **r**otation) (Fig. 30.2), can be performed to check for sacroiliac joint disorder.

The straight leg test, which places the L-5 vertebra, the S-1 nerve root, and the sciatic nerve under tension, is performed with the patient supine. The examiner elevates one leg until the patient reports severe pain in the buttock or back or until the knee begins to bend, and the degree at which this occurs is recorded. The examiner then dorsiflexes the patient's ankle to see if this motion increases the pain. The FABERE test is performed with the patient supine. The exam-

iner places the patient's hip in flexion, abduction, and external rotation. The examiner then presses that hip into extension by placing the patient's foot against the opposite tibia and pushes the knee posterior toward the examination table (Fig. 30.2). In this position, a tensile force is transmitted to the sacroiliac joint, which will be painful if it is positive.

DIFFERENTIAL DIAGNOSIS OF BACK PAIN IN CHILDREN AND ADOLESCENTS

When a child complains of back pain, the differential diagnosis is quite extensive. The sources of back pain can be categorized by developmental, inflammatory, infectious, mechanical, traumatic, neoplastic, visceral, or metabolic disorders (Table 30.1) (3–20). The most important method for narrowing the differential diagnosis is by obtaining a detailed history. A complaint of night pain that is relieved with nonsteroidal antiinflammatory drugs (NSAIDs) can indicate osteoid osteoma or osteoblastoma. Pain associated with fever, chills, lethargy, weight loss, or bruising may indicate malignancy or infection. Back pain that occurs several days after ear infection or upper respiratory infection may originate from discitis. If back pain is associated with hyperextension (e.g., back hamstring is affected from maneuvers in gymnastics, butterfly stroke in swimming, or the top spin serve in tennis), spondylolysis may be present (2). Radicular pain or bowel or bladder dysfunction indicates nerve root irritation and potential disc protrusion. Joint pain in the morning that improves later in the day or associated eye problems, such as uveitis, direct the differential diagnosis toward arthritis or arthropathies, such as juvenile ankylosing spondylitis or juvenile rheumatoid arthritis.

DEVELOPMENTAL STRUCTURAL DISORDERS

Scheuermann Disease

Scheuermann disease is a common cause of structural kyphosis in the thoracic, thoracolumbar, and lumbar spine. Scheuermann disease is a structural kyphosis of unknown cause in which wedging of the vertebra is the major characteristic. The radiographic diagnostic criteria of Scheuermann disease are three or more consecutive vertebrae that are wedged more than 5 degrees (Fig. 30.3). The kyphosis is thought to be a growth disorder of the vertebral endplates, and it was first described by Scheuermann in the 1920s. This disorder occurs in either the thoracic, the thoracolumbar, or the lumbar spine.

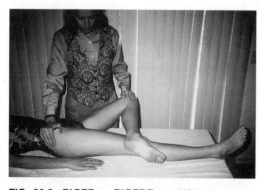

FIG. 30.2. *FABER or FABERE test.* With the patient supine, the hip joint is *f*lexed, *ab*ducted, and *e*xternally *r*otated. The examiner then presses the affected hip into extension by placing the patient's ipsilateral foot against the contralateral tibia in a figure four position and then pressing the affected hip posteriorly into the examination table. Elicited pain may suggest sacroiliac pathology.

TABLE 30.1. *Differential diagnosis of pediatric back pain*

Developmental
    Spondylolysis and/or spondylolisthesis
    Scheuermann disease
    Iliac apophysitis
    Lumbar epiphysitis
    Scoliosis (rarely painful)
Inflammatory
    Juvenile rheumatoid arthritis
Ankylosing spondylitis
Disc space calcification
Enteropathic arthritis
Infectious
    Discitis
    Vertebral osteomyelitis
    Tuberculous spondylitis
    Sacroiliac joint infection
    Epidural abscess
Mechanical and/or traumatic
    Disc degeneration
    Herniated nucleus pulposus
    Fractures
    Facet syndrome
    Spondylolysis and/or spondylolisthesis
Slipped vertebral apophysis
Musculoligamentous injury
Overuse syndromes
Neoplastic Disorders
    Benign
        Osteoid osteoma
        Osteoblastoma
        Histiocytosis
        Aneurysmal bone cyst
    Malignant
        Leukemia
        Lymphoma
        Wilm tumor
        Ewing sarcoma
        Osteosarcoma
        Rhabdomyosarcoma
        Spinal cord tumor
            Neuroblastoma
            Astrocytoma
Visceral disorders
    Retrocecal appendicitis
    Pneumonia
    Pyelonephritis and/or hydronephrosis
    Renal calculi
    Pleuritis
    Psoas abscess
    Retroperitoneal mass
Psychogenic
    Conversion reaction

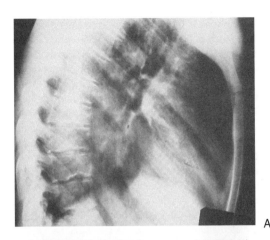

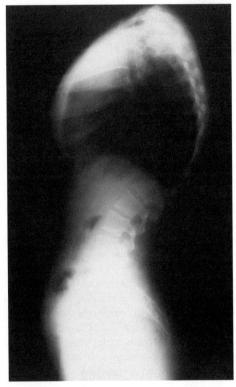

FIG. 30.3. *Scheuermann disease.* **A:** Lateral radiographic view of the spine in a patient with Scheuermann disease. Radiographic criteria include three or more consecutive vertebrae, each of which is wedged 5 degrees or more. Irregularities in the vertebral endplates are also seen. **B:** Kyphotic appearance of the spine in a standing lateral radiograph in a patient with Scheuermann disease, showing narrowed intervertebral disc spaces and irregular vertebral endplates.

Classification

    Scheuermann disease is subclassified as typical or atypical. Atypical Scheuermann disease is observed in the lumbar spine or thoracolumbar junction. Typical Scheuermann disease consists of rigid thoracic kyphosis in an adolescent or juvenile spine, with the apex of the kyphosis at T-7 to T-9. It is more common in males than females. Onset occurs at about 10 years of age. Before 10 years of age, visualizing Scheuermann disease is difficult because vertebral endplate abnormalities and wedging are not detectable until the ring apophysis ossifies (2). Spondylolysis and scoliosis have been reported in patients with Scheuermann disease (2). The typical presentation of Scheuermann disease in an adolescent is back pain over the kyphosis and poor posture. The kyphosis becomes more noticeable during the adolescent growth spurt. The patient has a round back deformity with increased lumbar lordosis when he or she is standing. The compensatory lumbar lordosis can cause low back pain. Usually, associated tight lumbodorsal fascia, tight hamstrings, and hip flexors are present. The child may complain of activity-related pain or of pain with prolonged sitting or standing. After the end of the growth spurt, the pain from Scheuermann generally resolves.

Clinical Evaluation

Scheuermann disease differs from postural scoliosis by a rigid, not flexible, kyphosis in the thoracic or thoracolumbar spine. Patients with typical Scheuermann disease have "thoracic kyphosis, a compensatory lumbar lordosis, anterior protrusion of the head, and rotation of the pelvis" (2). To visualize kyphosis, the clinician should stand to the side of the patient and should have him or her bend forward. A child with an "egg on side" appearance on lateral viewing of the forward bent spine probably has postural kyphosis. A child with an "egg on end" appearance on forward bending (i.e., acute angular deformity) probably has Scheuermann disease. After checking forward bending, the clinician should evaluate the patient for the commonly associated tight hamstrings and hip flexors. Additionally, he or she should conduct a neurologic examination, since Scheuermann disease may, in rare cases, display an associated spinal cord compression.

Radiographic Evaluation

Scheuermann disease is seen radiographically on the anterior-posterior (AP) and lateral views of the spine. By definition, at least 5 degrees of wedging on a minimum of three adjacent vertebrae must be seen for the condition to be termed Scheuermann disease. In addition to the anterior wedging of the vertebrae, the vertebral endplates are irregular. Associated disc space narrowing is observed. Schmorl nodes may be seen. If abnormal neurologic findings are observed

on examination, magnetic resonance imaging (MRI) or computerized tomography (CT) scans may be needed for evaluation.

Treatment of Typical Scheuermann Disease

Treatment of Scheuermann disease can include observation, nonoperative methods (e.g., exercise, physical therapy, bracing, or serial casting), or surgery, depending on the severity. Observation includes lateral radiographs every 6 months to verify that the condition is not progressing. Flexibility exercises and physical therapy are usually advised in order to correct tight hamstrings, to lessen the lumbar hyperlordosis, to strengthen the extensor muscles of the spine, and to stretch the pectoralis muscles. Abdominal strengthening exercises are part of the exercise regimen. If the thoracic kyphosis progresses to an angle greater than 50 degrees, bracing is indicated. Serial casting methods may be used, but bracing is preferable. The brace can be adjusted as the curve is corrected. The recommended brace for kyphosis correction is a Milwaukee brace, which is worn full time for 1 to 1.5 years. After this time period, the patient is weaned from the brace as long as no progression of the curve occurs. The Milwaukee brace is a dynamic three-point orthosis that promotes extension of the thoracic spine. In contrast to idiopathic scoliosis, in which the brace prevents curve progression, brace management can permanently normalize the deformity of the sagittal spine. Progression of thoracic kyphosis beyond 70 degrees indicates the need for spinal fusion surgery. If fusion surgery is performed, the athlete must be restricted from sports, except for swimming, for approximately 1 year postoperatively. Once the athlete has undergone spinal fusion, contact sports should be avoided.

Atypical Scheuermann Disease

Although typical thoracic Scheuermann disease is usually not seen disproportionately in athletes, atypical Scheuermann may be seen in athletes who are involved in sports that require repetitive flexion–extension of the spine, such as rowing, diving, or gymnastics. The peak incidence is between the ages of 15 to 17 years, and it is more common in males. Atypical Scheuermann is usually seen at the thoracolumbar junction or the lumbar spine. It may be caused by repetitive microtrauma, with resultant growth plate fractures and possible anterior disc herniation through the anterior apophyseal ring, which can lead to a subsequent deformation of the vertebrae (3). The athlete usually presents with a history of several months of pain with forward bending, which is relieved when he or she is at rest. He or she usually has tight hamstrings and tight thoracolumbar fascia. Radiographically, wedging and irregular vertebral endplates with disc space narrowing are seen. An apophyseal fragment at the anterior margin of the vertebral body rarely heals. In cases of persistent pain or vertebral wedging, the treatment consists of back bracing and abdominal strengthening and flexibility exercises. The back brace typically is worn for 23 hours per day for about 1 year (3).

Other types of kyphosis that may be seen in the pediatric population are spinal deformities, such as Marfan syndrome, achondroplasia pseudoachondroplasia, diastrophic dwarfism, neurofibromatosis, mucopolysaccharidosis, and childhood tuberculosis. In Marfan syndrome, which is a connective tissue disease, the common types of skeletal deformities are, in order of frequency, scoliosis, thoracic lordosis, and lumbar kyphosis.

Spondylolysis and Spondylolisthesis

Spondylolysis refers to a bilateral or unilateral defect in the vertebral pars interarticularis. It may be significant that is sufficient enough to allow forward translation of the vertebra in relation to the most adjacent caudal vertebra. This latter movement is termed spondylolisthesis and is derived from the Greek root "spondylos," meaning vertebra. "Lysis," moreover, means to break or sever, and "listhesis" means to slip or slide.

Beyond the age of 10 years, spondylolysis is the most common cause of back pain in the pediatric population (21,22). Although the exact cause of spondylolysis is controversial, spondylolysis seems to occur as a result of repetitive stress to the pars of L-5 (23–25). In the growing child, this stress is accentuated by flexion contractures of the hip joint and it is more prominent during growth. The child may feel pain when the back is extended (Fig. 30.4). Sports, such as diving, wrestling, gymnastics, football (Fig. 30.5), dance, and weightlifting, that create repetitive loading while in lumbar lordotic extension have been found to have a higher incidence of spondylolysis (26–30). Furthermore, a strong hereditary association appears to exist between spondylolysis and spondylolisthesis (31–35). Also, the incidence of spondylolysis appears to be increased in those with spina bifida of S-1 (35). The incidence of spondylolisthesis is greater during growth spurts (36–38). In their adolescent population with spondylolysis, Steiner and

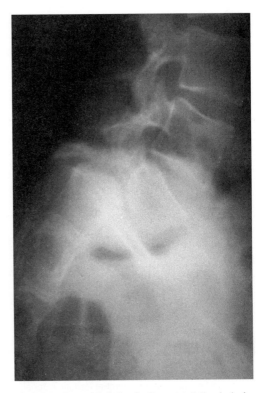

FIG. 30.4. *Spondylolisthesis.* Spondylolisthesis is forward displacement of one vertebral body on another. Note forward displacement of L-5 on S-1.

Micheli (39) found that the L-5 vertebra was affected 88.6% of the time, while Morita (40) showed a 96% involvement of L-4 or L-5 in a similar population.

Reports indicate that between 50% and 81% of those with spondylolysis have spondylolisthesis (23,41–44). However, no large population-based studies have examined the relationship of spondylolysis to listhesis (45). Therefore, the true incidence of listhesis in those with spondylolysis is unknown. Most patients with spondylolisthesis present with either pain or neurologic symptoms. However, the initial slippage is believed to be painless. In fact, studies have shown that 90% of patients with spondylolysis already have listhesis at presentation (41,42). Slippage of more than 30% to 50% is uncommon (45). A large majority of patients with spondylolysis are misdiagnosed as having lumbar strain. Some young athletes with spondylolisthesis do not experience pain or neurologic symptoms and therefore they do not seek medical care. Progression occurs in 4% to 5% of cases (44,46). Factors that have been associated with progression include adolescence, disc degeneration (36–38), the female gender, initial listhesis of more

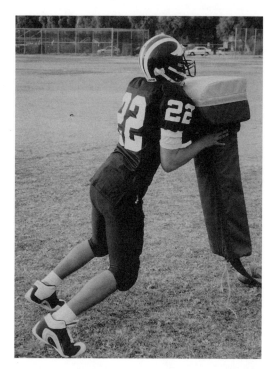

FIG. 30.5. *Extension mechanism.* Football player demonstrating the loading in lumbar lordotic extension.

than 50% (47), growth spurts, the amount of lumbosacral kyphosis, and the slippage angle (45).

Clinical Evaluation

Early diagnosis of spondylolysis is important, and this has been shown to affect outcome with conservative treatment. Blanda et al. (48) and Ciullo and Jackson (49) found, in separate studies, that longstanding symptoms were associated with the necessity for surgical intervention. Ikata et al. (50) found that the early detection of pars stress was essential for the success of conservative treatment. Although many patients with spondylolysis or listhesis have no symptoms, the common initial presenting complaint is pain. This pain appears to be brought on by certain activities and to be relieved by rest. It is usually described as dull and midline, and it can appear either unilaterally or bilaterally. The symptoms seem to worsen with extension or twisting of the lumbar spine. This action may cause pain to radiate down the buttock and/or thigh. The magnitude of pain does not appear to correlate with the amount of listhesis. Those who have a preexisting asymptomatic pars lysis or vertebral listhesis may become symptomatic af-

ter a minor event. In cases of severe listhesis, radicular symptoms and bowel or bladder control symptoms may signal the existence of neural injury.

The physical examination should always begin with careful observation of the patient's posture and gait; palpation and provocative tests should follow. The classic Phalen–Dickson gait can often be observed, especially in those patients who have a high degree of slippage (51). This gait is characterized by a flexed knee and hip. The mechanism for this is believed to result from a more vertical sacrum, which appears to flex the pelvis and to make flexing the knees necessary in order to remain upright (52). The clinician should also carefully look for dimpling of the skin, as is seen in spina bifida occulta or in vertebral listhesis. Palpation along the lumbar spine should then follow. Pain over the affected vertebra, along with paraspinal muscle spasm, is common. A notable step-off can sometimes be felt, and, in high-degree listhesis, a lumbosacral kyphosis, in which the bottom of the ribcage approaches the iliac crest, can be seen. Up to 70% of patients will have tight hamstrings (48,53–55). Provocative testing should include flexion, extension, and rotation of the lumbar spine. Pain with these tests, as well as in the standing one-legged lumbar extension test, is extremely common in spondylolysis or listhesis (Fig. 30.6). Neurovascular testing that includes evaluation of reflexes, strength, and sensory perception, should be performed.

Radiographic Evaluation

Imaging studies are essential in the evaluation and diagnosis of spondylolysis and spondylolisthesis. X-rays of the lumbosacral spine should include AP, lateral, and oblique views (Fig. 30.7). Libson et al. (56) reported that 20% of patients with spondylolysis can be missed without oblique views. Pierce (56a) found the sensitivity of AP, lateral, and oblique views for detecting spondylolysis to be 32%, 75%, and 77%, respectively. On oblique views, one should look for the classic "pearl necklace" or the broken neck of Lachapele's "scotty dog" (Fig. 30.8). For those patients with elongated but intact pars (57), Hensinger et al. (55) described the "greyhound sign," which refers to the elongated look of the pars on oblique radiographs. If the x-rays are normal or equivocal, a bone scan or single-photon emission computed tomography (SPECT) can be useful. SPECT has been found to be more sensitive for finding early lesions than either x-rays or bone scans are (58,59), but it is not very useful in detecting spondylolysis in patients who have had symptoms for longer than 3 months (60). CT, with or without con-

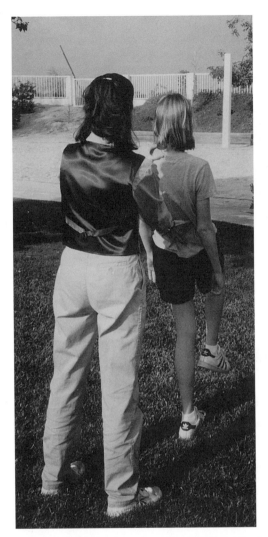

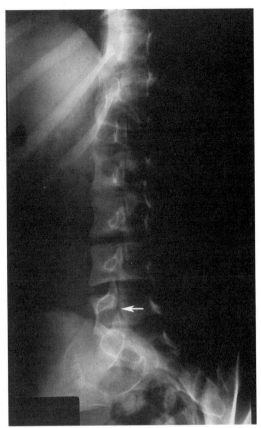

FIG. 30.7. *Spondylolysis.* An oblique radiograph of the lumbar spine shows a radiolucent defect in the pars interarticularis at L-5, indicating spondylolysis, which shows up as a "collar" on the "scotty dog."

FIG. 30.6. *Single leg hyperextension test.* The patient stands on one leg and hyperextends the spine. This maneuver is repeated on the other leg. Reproduction of the patient's pain symptoms with this maneuver indicates spondylolysis until proven otherwise.

trast; myelography; and MRI are useful in differentiating spondylolysis from other pathologic conditions and in evaluating nerve root compression (61).

Treatment

The focus of treatment for both spondylolysis and spondylolisthesis is symptom relief, healing of bone lesions, and the prevention of further slippage. Most patients with the mild to moderate form can be treated successfully with a conservative regimen.

Conservative treatment includes restriction from activities or movements of the lumbosacral spine, analgesia, and removal of the athlete from competitive sports for several months. Physical therapy for the conservatively treated patient should focus on strengthening the abdominal musculature, stretching out the hamstrings and hip flexor muscles, stretching the lumbodorsal fascia, using pelvic tilts and Williams' flexion exercises, and employing dynamic lumbar spine stabilization. Immobilization of the lower back often is used in the moderate patient, and this usually is accomplished with a brace. The different types of braces advocated in the literature focus primarily on the lower back, and they can be referred to as either a lumbosacral orthosis (48), an antilordotic brace (31,62), or a thoracolumbosacral orthosis (63). The success rate for treating symptomatic patients who have less than a 50% listhesis with a brace

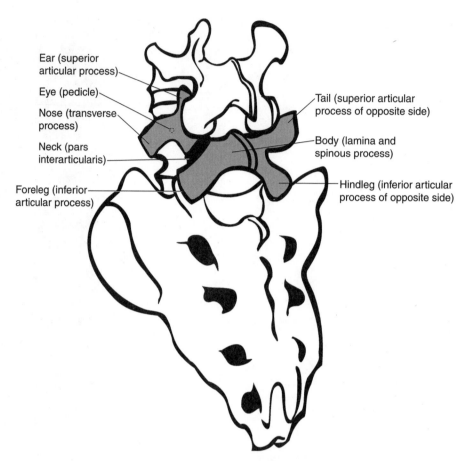

Ear (superior articular process)

Eye (pedicle)

Nose (transverse process)

Neck (pars interarticularis)

Foreleg (inferior articular process)

Tail (superior articular process of opposite side)

Body (lamina and spinous process)

Hindleg (inferior articular process of opposite side)

FIG. 30.8. *Scotty dog.* This is a drawing of the "scotty dog" view in a patient with spondylolysis in which the defect in the pars interarticularis of the facet joint resembles the "broken neck or pearl necklace" of Lachapele's "scotty dog" or a "collar" on the scotty dog's neck. (Illustration from DeEtte DeVille, M.D., with permission.)

and other conservative modalities has been reported as being between 40% and 100% (31,48,62,63). In these studies, the brace was worn at least 23 hours per day and was used continually for between 2 and 25 months.

Various algorithms can be followed when making a decision to treat a patient with spondylolisthesis. Wiltse (64) and Wiltse and Jackson (65) described a treatment protocol that has been used most often in the literature. Based on degree of listhesis and clinical symptoms, patients can be categorized as mild, moderate, or severe. The mild patient is asymptomatic, and he or she has listhesis of less than 50% of. For children up to 10 years of age, these patients can be treated with observation and x-rays on initial evaluation, followed by standing lateral lumbosacral radiographs periodically every 4 to 6 months; these are

conducted twice a year for children between 10 and 15 years of age and then once a year until the child stops growing. For mild patients with grade I listhesis (less than 25%), repetitive heavy lifting should be avoided. For the mild patient with grade II listhesis (25% to 50%), the clinician should also warn the patient regarding the risk of participation in contact sports and in sports that require repeated lumbosacral hyperextension. Patients in the moderate category are those who are symptomatic, with slippage of less than 50% and no neurologic deficits. These patients should be treated with the conservative approaches previously mentioned. Finally, patients considered severe are growing children whose listhesis is greater than 50%, mature adolescent patients with greater than 75% listhesis, and those who display significant persistent neurologic deficits.

Surgery should be considered in patients with severe cases of spondylolisthesis and in those for whom conservative treatment has failed to relieve symptoms. In addition, patients whose prolonged pain significantly limits them in the activities of daily living or for those with significant gait and postural deformities should be considered for surgery as well. Several different surgical procedures can be utilized for the stabilization of spondylolisthesis (45). The most common surgery is bilateral fusion of the transverse process to the sacral alae. An autologous iliac bone graft is used in this procedure. Patients with motor weakness, bowel or bladder dysfunction, or significant radicular symptoms may benefit from decompression of the nerve roots, as well as posterolateral *in situ* fusion (31,66–69). Those who advocate reduction of the spondylolisthesis focus on issues that may develop after normal fusion, such as pseudoarthrosis, the postoperative progression of listhesis, uncorrected deformity, loss of motion, and cauda equina syndrome (45). In cases of severe slippage, anterior fusion can be useful (66,70,71). In those cases of spondyloptosis, in which complete slippage of the vertebra off of the next caudal vertebra is observed, L-5 vertebrectomy has been used (72,73). However, the use of immobilization after surgery varies greatly in the literature (45).

Surgical intervention for spondylolisthesis carries a significant risk of complications. Pseudoarthrosis rates after fusion have been reported as being between 8% and 30% (74–76). The progression of slippage in patients with high-slip angles is relatively frequent, even after fusion (77,78). Iatrogenic neurologic injury after surgery is a moderate risk that occurs in 6% of patients after fusion (79) and in 25% to 30% after reduction surgery (80,81).

Return to Sports

Variation is found in the literature regarding recommendations on activity restriction with spondylolysis and spondylolisthesis. In general, children with symptomatic spondylolysis (i.e., those who have pain with activity) should be restricted from sports and should be placed on abdominal and spinal muscle strengthening exercises (82). In the symptomatic child with spondylolysis in which SPECT demonstrates an acute pars defect and for which a brace or cast is used for immobilization, the child may resume sports when he or she becomes asymptomatic following the cessation of immobilization. The average time for an athlete with symptomatic spondylolysis to achieve pain-free, full range of motion is 4 to 6 weeks (18). Some authors recommend a brace protocol in

which an athlete with symptomatic spondylolysis remains out of sports and participates in physical therapy for abdominal and antilordotic strengthening during the first month. He or she may return to sports after 1 month in the brace if pain free (82a). Other clinicians treat spondylolysis without bracing. In cases of asymptomatic spondylolysis in which a growing child is being followed by serial observation, the child may participate in all sports without restrictions (82).

In a growing child who has spondylolisthesis and slippage of less than 30% to 50% and low back pain, exercise and sports should be limited until the symptoms have resolved. If an orthosis is used, sports participation is restricted for 2 to 3 months; and, when the athlete is asymptomatic, he or she may return to sports (82). Each case should be individualized, and consultation with a spine specialist should occur with athletes who display a higher grade of slippage.

INFECTIOUS CAUSES OF PEDIATRIC BACK PAIN

Discitis

Discitis is an inflammatory condition of the intervertebral disk. It can also be referred to as infectious spondylitis. The exact etiology of discitis is still speculative. However, the cause is generally accepted to be infectious (20,82–84). In children, the source of infection is believed to arise hematogenously from the rich vascular supply of the adjacent vertebral bodies. As the athlete matures, the amount of disk penetration from these vessels decreases, which decreases the risk of hematogenous spread of infection. In the older population, infection is introduced by direct inoculation during surgery or with intraspinal or paraspinal injections. Children are most commonly affected between the ages of 2 and 7 years. Although much rarer, presentations in teenagers and young adults must not be overlooked or discounted.

Clinical Evaluation

Symptoms of discitis are variable and insidious, and they may include nonspecific back or abdominal pain. Three different patterns of clinical presentation are as follows: (a) the young child who presents with difficulty walking, a limp, or refusal to walk; (b) the 7-year-old to 15-year-old child with vague abdominal pain that is possibly associated with listlessness and an absence of abdominal findings; and (c) the child with nonspecific back pain associated with the loss of lumbar lordosis and a painful lumbar area on percussion (82). These symptoms may overlap. Occasionally, fever and generalized weakness can be associated with discitis. Teenagers and adults are more likely to present with more specific back complaints and even with pain that is radiating to the legs.

On physical examination, only paravertebral spasms may be evident. Many patients will exhibit some degree of back stiffness and a decreased range of motion. Flexion of the spine is limited and painful. Straight leg raising may elicit pain and spasms; however, neurologic deficits are characteristically absent.

Radiographic Evaluation

Clinical suspicion should prompt radiographic evaluation. Plain radiographs may show a narrowing of the intervertebral space with slight irregularity. Vertebral body sclerosis or endplate resorption may also be seen. Radiographs are usually normal in the first 3 weeks of the infection. A bone scan may show increased uptake at the affected disc space. Unlike other parts of the body in which joint aspiration is considered standard for diagnosis, disc and vertebral infections are usually treated without aspiration, due to potential morbidity of the procedure (82). Blood cultures, sedimentation rate, complete blood count, and a tuberculin test (purified protein derivative of tuberculin [PPD]) should always be obtained. Blood cultures are usually negative, and often the white blood cell count is not elevated. The sedimentation rate is usually elevated, and this finding should prompt a bone scan evaluation. The bone scan is usually diagnostic; however, in cases in which the bone scan is equivocal, an MRI can be obtained. An MRI is particularly useful in differentiating between discitis and vertebral osteomyelitis. MRI often shows involvement of the adjacent vertebrae (82). The differential diagnosis of discitis includes vertebral osteomyelitis, tuberculosis, spondylitis, Scheuermann kyphosis, spinal trauma, and a spinal abscess.

Treatment

Treatment should include a combination of rest and antibiotics. In more severe cases, intravenous antibiotics are indicated until symptoms are adequately controlled and the sedimentation rates approach normal. Antibiotics are generally selected to provide empirical coverage for *Staphylococcus aureus*; they are administered intravenously for approximately 7 days, followed by 3 to 5 weeks of oral antibiotics (82). Older patients with milder symptoms may be treated with oral antibiotics. Young children may be placed in a cast for 6 to 8

weeks, although the current trend is away from immobilization (82). If the disc infection is in the lumbar spine, a cast or orthosis may be used. If the discitis is in the lumbosacral region, a cast, rather than an orthosis, to the knees is used. Rest is indicated for 4 to 6 weeks. Patients typically respond rapidly to antibiotics and bed rest. They may return to previous levels of activity, if no associated complications, such as osteomyelitis, have occurred. In such cases, more prolonged treatment, and possibly surgery followed by physical therapy, may be needed before an athlete return to sports. Other complications that may occur are paraspinal or vertebral abscesses, which require surgical drainage. In athletes with more prolonged symptoms, orthotic spine support may be needed. Patients are routinely followed with serial radiographs for approximately 1 year to screen for further disc space narrowing.

Return to Sport

Athletes treated nonsurgically may return to walking after 4 to 6 weeks if they are pain free, and they may slowly resume an exercise program if they are symptom free for 4 to 6 weeks. Young children who had been casted for discitis may swim after the cast has been removed.

MECHANICAL OR TRAUMATIC INJURIES

Apophyseal Injuries

In addition to the atypical Scheuermann disease apophyseal injury that was discussed above, other apophyseal injuries can occur in the pediatric spine. Children involved with activities that require repetitive flexion and extension of the spine can sustain traction apophyseal injuries on the apophyses of the spinous processes. These painful injuries usually occur in the lower thoracic or the thoracolumbar junction of the spine. Treatment includes rest, NSAIDs, and activity modification until the patient is pain free. When the pain subsides, flexibility exercises and abdominal strengthening exercises can be performed, and the athlete can return to sports.

Apophyseal Avulsion Fracture

An apophyseal avulsion fracture of the vertebral body, which is also known as a slipped vertebral apophysis, is the fracture of the cartilaginous apophyseal ring, accompanied by posterior displacement into the spinal canal. This type of fracture is almost always associated with central disc herniation. This condition predominantly affects children and teens, as the immature spine of children and adolescents is predisposed to this condition. Between the vertebral bodies, cartilaginous rings separate the intervertebral discs and the bony vertebral body. These rings begin to ossify at about the age of 12 years, and they usually are completely fused to the vertebral body by the age of 18 years. Ossification is usually multifocal. The intervertebral disc is attached to this ring by fibers that are known as Sharpey's fibers. Repetitive motions, extreme flexion, and/or twisting motions subject this intervertebral unit to extreme stresses. The weakest point is the junction between the cartilage ring and the bony vertebral body. Either the stress of these movements is thought to produce a chip fragment that displaces posteriorly into the spinal canal, pulling the associated portion of the intervertebral disc with it, or *vice versa*. Commonly, the ligaments remain intact.

Clinical Evaluation

An apophyseal avulsion injury occurs from a specific mechanism of injury. This type of injury has been associated with adolescent athletes participating in sports with repetitive lumbar motions, such as wrestling, gymnastics, weightlifting, and volleyball. The majority of cases involve the lower lumbosacral intervertebral levels. Males appear to be more frequently affected than females, probably because boys reach skeletal maturity at a later age than girls do. Thus, the immature male skeleton is exposed to competitive sports for a longer period of time.

Athletes with this condition typically report symptoms of disc herniation. Limitation of flexion and extension of the spine and of the lower extremities is reported by the young athlete. Pain and spasm are frequently noted. Usually, no numbness or paresthesia is present. On physical examination, areas of paraspinal muscle spasm may be found, along with a decreased range of motion. Neurologic findings are typically absent.

Radiographic Evaluation

The diagnosis is usually made with plain radiographs, although a CT scan is the diagnostic test of choice. AP radiographs of the spine may not show any defect, so obtaining lateral radiographs is important. The lateral radiograph may show a fragment of ossified bone in the canal. The CT scan, however, is more sensitive and specific for demonstrating the pathology. A myelogram may also be of benefit in demonstrating the presence and extent of spinal cord com-

pression. Although an MRI is extremely useful in the evaluation of pure central soft disc herniation, it may miss an associated avulsion apophyseal fracture. Differentiating between the two is crucial because surgical treatment of the two conditions is different.

Treatment

Treatment of this condition is similar to that of simple disc herniation. Rest, heat, analgesia, and massage can sufficiently manage the symptomatic pain. Patients without any significant compromise of the spinal canal maybe treated nonsurgically. In patients with significant neural compression and symptoms, surgery to remove the bony fragments from the spinal canal is performed. In postsurgery rehabilitation or in athletes who are being managed nonsurgically, athletes are required to undergo back strengthening and stretching exercises as soon as their pain tolerance allows. Back braces or corsets may be useful for immobilizing certain patients. When full pain-free mobility and strength are regained, an athlete may return to full sports participation.

Mechanical Back Pain

Mechanical back pain may occur secondary to acute or chronic musculoligamentous sprain or strain or from overuse injuries to muscle–tendon units, ligaments, joint capsules, or facets. It occurs in older children (>10 years of age), and it is more common in older adolescents. In contrast to the adult population, mechanical back pain in children is a diagnosis of exclusion.

When an athlete has pain on extension of the spine, with tenderness over the posterior aspect of the spine and tight hamstrings, tight lumbodorsal fascia, and spondylolysis have been ruled out, other causes of mechanical back pain should be considered (84–86). Injury to the posterior elements of the spine, such as muscles, tendons, facet joints, ligaments, and joint capsules, has been given various names, including facet syndrome, posterior element overuse syndrome, hyperlordotic back pain syndrome, and mechanical low back pain (84).

Hyperlordotic Back Pain

Hyperlordotic back pain is a type of mechanical low back pain that is usually caused by mechanical strain of the ligaments and facet joints of the lumbar spine. It can also occur from acute or chronic muscle strain (86). This condition is usually associated with hyperlordosis of the lumbar spine. Poor posture in the pediatric population may predispose them to low back pain. Symptoms usually include an aching low back that is associated with activities that involve long periods of standing. The physical examination reveals functional hyperlordosis of the lumbar spine in the standing position that is associated with tight hamstrings, tight lumbodorsal fascia and musculature, and decreased flexibility. No neurologic deficits are seen normally. Treatment includes abdominal and pelvic strengthening exercises and antilordotic exercises, plus flexibility exercise of the spine and upper and lower extremities. Some children with persistent pain may benefit from antilordotic braces and antiinflammatory medications.

Facet Syndrome

The facet joint is a synovial type joint between the vertebrae. Although not commonly thought of as a source of pain, the joint is a richly innervated site. Mechanical irritation from facet arthritis of the adjacent nerve root that produces a synovitis may be an etiology of the pain. Inflammatory mediators from synovial damage may also irritate nerve fibers.

Clinical Evaluation

Facet syndrome remains a diagnosis of exclusion. It usually occurs in older adults, rather than children (3). Athletes typically complain of low back pain, which may radiate to the lower legs (20). The pain characteristically does not follow a radicular pattern. Patients may complain of stiffness in the morning, and usually the pain may be relieved with walking. Generally, the neurologic examination is also normal. Straight leg testing is usually negative; however, hyperextension of the leg typically produces pain. Pressure over the facet joints may elicit pain.

Radiographic Evaluation

Plain radiographs may show sclerosis, foramina encroachment, or arthritic changes. CT scans may be able to confirm the diagnosis earlier than radiographs would.

Treatment

Treatment is largely accomplished through mobilization and stabilization of the supporting musculature. Exercise programs should be tailored to strengthen the paraspinous muscles. Pain control is initially mediated through use of NSAIDs. Intrafacet steroid injections under fluoroscopy should be reserved for severe cases in which the pain may limit the athlete from undertaking an exercise regimen; they are not recommended in the pediatric age group (20). Truly refractory cases may benefit from surgical spinal fusion or facet denervation surgery.

Soft Tissue Injuries

Musculoligamentous injuries in children are a diagnosis of exclusion. In children, back pain as a chief complaint is suspicious for a pathologic cause, whereas adolescents complain of occasional nonspecific backache that is not pathologic, particularly with prolonged sitting or standing. Symptoms that are worrisome for serious causes of back pain may be constitutional (fever, chills, weight loss, bruising, and/or lethargy), neurologic (radicular pain, numbness, tingling, and/or bowel or bladder dysfunction), and pain quality (constant pain, increasing pain, and/or night pain). Athletic activity-related pain may indicate the presence of a stress fracture, whereas constant or night pain may indicate a neoplastic process. Pain can come from acute injury or as a result of an overuse injury to the muscles, ligaments, and joints of the back. A factor that predisposes athletes to back injury is the adolescent growth spurt, in which the soft tissues fail to keep up with the rapid bone growth, which results in decreased flexibility that predisposes these athletes to musculoligamentous and apophyseal injuries of the spine. Sports that involve repetitive bending and twisting of the spine, such as football, gymnastics, and racquet sports, have a higher incidence of overuse back injuries (3). In pediatric patients with back pain, the pain may be referred to the thighs or buttocks, and this does not always indicate the existence of a herniated disc. Muscle strains often occur with a known mechanism of injury, and the resultant pain is aggravated by activity and improved with rest. Muscle strains are a diagnosis of exclusion in the young athlete. Usually, localized pain with range of motion is observed. On physical examination, tenderness and sometimes palpable muscle spasm of the affected muscles (e.g., the paraspinous muscles) are often present, along with asymmetrical trunk motion, tight hamstrings, and tight lumbodorsal fascia.

Radiographic Evaluation

Evaluation should include plain lumbosacral radiographs to look for osseus injury, especially in the athlete whose symptoms begin with trauma or other structural causes of pain. If a known mechanism of injury consistent with muscle strain has occurred, radiographs can be delayed; they are then ordered only if the symptoms do not resolve within 3 to 6 weeks (3,7,86).

Treatment

Relative rest and ice massage of the affected area are used to treat for the acute injury. NSAIDs may also be used. Once the acute pain has resolved, the athlete may begin a stretching and strengthening program for rehabilitation, and he or she can then resume regular athletic activities. The symptoms usually occur briefly, and they are self-limited. Failure to resolve symptoms with a 4 to 6 week back-strengthening program warrants workup for other etiologies of the pain.

Herniated Nucleus Pulposus

In young athletes, lumbar disc herniation symptoms have an appearance similar to that of muscle strain, with spasm, limited range of motion, and pain. Disc herniations rarely occur in children, but they may be seen in adolescents (Fig. 30.9). The true incidence of disc herniation in adolescents is unknown, but it is much less common than in adults. Most reports indicate that between 0.8% and 3.8% of all disc herniations occur in the pediatric population (3). The diagnosis of disc herniation in the young athlete can be difficult to make because they usually do not present with the classic radicular symptoms of adults.

When the nucleus pulposus protrudes through the annulus fibrosis, the condition is referred to as a herniated or ruptured disc. Young people have strong intervertebral discs that are firmly attached to the cartilaginous vertebral endplates. In some injuries, the vertebra may fracture before the disc ruptures (1). Discs may be damaged—either protruded or herniated—by forceful flexing and rotation of the spine. Sports that involve repetitive twisting of the spine or axial loading (downward pressure) of the spine, such as football, basketball, soccer, running, gymnastics, ice hockey, tennis, and weightlifting, have been implicated in disc herniations in the pediatric population. Nucleus pulposus protrusions usually occur posterolaterally where the annulus is thinnest and strong

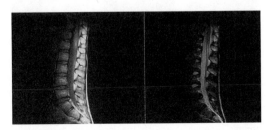

FIG. 30.9. *Disc herniation.* Magnetic resonance imaging of disc bulging or dessication at L-4 to L-5 level, without foraminal or canal compromise.

support by the posterior longitudinal ligament is lacking. This lack of support is most commonly seen at the L-5 to S-1 or the L-4 to L-5 level. Herniations of the nucleus pulposus may press on the spinal nerve roots, thus resulting in back or leg pain. When a disc protrusion presses on a nerve root, the nerve root affected is usually one inferior to the disc. When present, radicular pain and numbness from nerve root compression usually follow the corresponding dermatome. Concommitant loss of bowel and bladder control in a patient with a ruptured disc indicates cauda equina syndrome from a large central disc herniation and requires emergent surgical consultation and surgical decompression.

Clinical Evaluation

The most common complaint in an adolescent with a ruptured disc is low back pain or pain located in the buttocks or hip. A young athlete with disc herniation can also present with only mild pain and an asymmetrical gait or running pattern. The pain with a herniated disc may occur after vigorous activity or it may have a slow onset. The pain is usually aggravated by increased activity or Valsalva maneuvers, such as sneezing or coughing. The athlete or coach may notice asymmetry of hamstring flexibility or paravertebral spasm. Limited range of motion of the lumbar spine and lumbar scoliosis from paravertebral muscle spasm are usually noted. The athlete may be crouched forward somewhat, or he or she may lean away from the side of the herniated disc to relieve pressure on the nerve root. Although the following are rarely seen in pediatric disc injuries, foot, knee, or ankle weakness; diminished Achilles and patellar reflexes; and, depending upon the level of the injury, decreased sensation in parts of the lower extremities may be seen. Radicular leg pain may or may not be observed. The child may demonstrate a stiff lumbar spine with limitation of forward bending and straight leg raising.

Radiographic Evaluation

Evaluation should include plain radiographs so that one can look for osseous injury, especially in the athlete whose symptoms began with trauma, or narrowed disc space. Plain radiographs are usually normal in the young athlete with a herniated disc, and they rarely show a narrowed disc space. If the symptoms fail to resolve with conservative treatment of rest and analgesics, further radiologic evaluation with MRI or noncontrast CT, noninvasive studies that can show a neurocompressive lesion, are indicated. These studies have replaced myelography in many centers. Additional tests that can be used to localize the level of nerve root compression are electromyography and nerve conduction study.

Treatment

Conservative therapy is the main treatment for pediatric disc injury. Initial treatment involves rest from impact load or flexion and extension activities and resting the back in a neutral position. Due to the deconditioning effect, complete bed rest is contraindicated in athletes, except in severe disc disease (85). A relative rest period, involving pain-free activities, should be used for the first few weeks instead. Ice and NSAIDs are used for pain control. In cases of severe muscle spasm, muscle relaxants may be used. The relative rest period is followed by gradual mobilization and an exercise program. The back rehabilitation program is designed to relieve pain and spasm and to maintain a neutral spine position. As the pain is reduced, flexibility exercises of the trunk, hamstrings, quadriceps, hip rotators, and abdominal and paravertebral muscles can be advanced. Strengthening both the paravertebral and abdominal musculature is important for maintaining a neutral spine. Aerobic conditioning, such as stationary bike workouts, walking, and swimming, can be advanced when the pain has been reduced.

If conservative measures do not alleviate pain in an adolescent athlete with discogenic back pain, a flexible polyethylene brace with 15 degrees of lumbar lordosis may help the adolescent athlete resume daily activities (3). If the symptoms persist despite conservative management or if cauda equina syndrome with bowel or bladder dysfunction or severe motor loss is present, surgical intervention is indicated.

Return to Sport

When the athlete who does not require surgical intervention has achieved full pain-free mobility and strength, usually after several months, most orthopedists allow a full return to sports activities. Recovery from a disc rupture may take months. Therefore, a return to vigorous sports activities should be avoided for 6 to12 months after documented discogenic back pain in a child (3). If neural element irritations are prolonged, the child may have difficulty returning to his or her previous performance level.

For those athletes who require surgical intervention, the orthopedist or neurosurgeon should have a thorough discussion with the athlete and his or her parents about the theoretical risks of degenerative changes in the spine with contact sports before the decision about a return to sports is made. The athlete may have to change sports or the position played in his or her sport to a less demanding position in order to avoid exacerbating the symptoms.

Sacroiliac Sprain Syndrome

Sacroiliac joints have a synovial membrane and strong anterior and posterior ligaments, and these structures may be a cause of low back pain. Pain occurs over the sacroiliac joints, and it is usually unilateral. It may occur from trauma, or it may be secondary to another injury, such as a herniated disc, which creates guarding of the low back and resultant impaired back mechanics.

Clinical Evaluation

The athlete may have tenderness over the sacroiliac joint, buttock, or posterior superior iliac spine. The FABER test (Fig. 30.2), the knee to chest maneuver, or Gaenslen test may produce pain. Gaenslen extension test (Fig. 30.10) is performed with the athlete supine, while the leg of the affected side hangs over the edge of the table. The examiner presses down on the thigh to hyperextend the hip while putting the unaffected leg in the knee–chest position. A positive test produces pain in the affected sacroiliac joint.

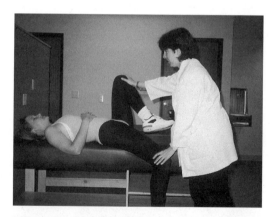

FIG. 30.10. *Gaenslen extension test.* Gaenslen extension test is performed with the athlete supine and the leg on the affected side hanging over the table. The examiner presses down on the ipsilateral thigh, while placing the contralateral leg in knee–chest position. A positive test—pain in the ipsilateral sacroiliac joint—may indicate sacroiliac pathology.

Treatment

Sacroiliac joint mobilization exercises and antiin-flammatory agents are used for treatment. The athlete may return to all sports when he or she is pain free.

Fractures

Fractures of the pediatric spine are uncommon. Sports-related catastrophic injuries to the thoracic or lumbar spine are rare, and acute catastrophic fractures to the spine are beyond the scope of this chapter. They may occur during contact sports, or they can result from a fall. When an acute fracture is suspected, spinal immobilization on a backboard should be accomplished by trained personnel, and the child should be transported to the hospital for definitive diagnosis and treatment (see Chapter 27).

Noncatastrophic thoracolumbar spine injuries include spinous and transverse process fractures and compression fractures. Spinous and transverse process fractures usually result from a direct blow, and are associated with pain and swelling. The treatment is symptomatic. Athletes usually can return to sports within 3 to 6 weeks.

Visceral Causes of Pediatric Back Pain

When the clinician is evaluating a child with back pain, referred pain from visceral disorders is part of the differential diagnosis. When symptoms warrant the consideration of visceral causes of back pain (e.g., retrocecal appendicitis), pyelonephritis, kidney stones, or pneumonia should be considered.

DIAGNOSTIC STUDIES FOR PEDIATRIC BACK PAIN

Radiologic Evaluation

In many cases of back pain in the pediatric athlete, a thorough history and the physical examination pinpoint the cause of the pain. Additional diagnostic studies for back pain include AP and lateral plain radiographs of the spine. If the mechanism of injury (e.g., muscle strain with localized symptoms that resolve spontaneously within 2 to 3 weeks) is evident in the history and physical examination (4,18), the use of radiographs can be delayed (7). In nonmuscular causes of back pain in children, radiographs should be taken at the time of initial evaluation. Imaging is also indicated if pain persists despite the initiation of an exercise program; if fever or other constitutional symptoms, neurologic symptoms, severe low back stiffness, or hamstring tightness is present; if scoliosis or kyphosis is found; or if back pain is acutely severe or night pain is observed (4).

Plain radiographs can be used for diagnosis of many of the disorders (e.g., Scheuermann kyphosis or fractures) that lead to pediatric back pain. A few weeks after a disc space infection ensues, disc space narrowing may be seen, along with destruction of the vertebral endplates, on plain film. Spondylolysis may be seen on oblique radiograph of the lumbar spine, and spondylolisthesis may be seen on the lateral radiograph. Tumors also may be seen on plain radiographs.

Other diagnostic imaging studies can be helpful when clinical suspicion of an abnormality is high, but the plain radiographs are negative. A technetium-99 bone scan is sensitive for detecting spinal abnormalities, such as an occult fracture, infection, or a neoplasm, but it is not specific. SPECT may localize an abnormality when a bone scan is equivocal. SPECT scans are very useful for identifying spondylolysis when plain radiographs are negative, but the clinical index of suspicion remains high. The SPECT scan will show increased activity in the region of the pars interarticularis.

If the neurologic examination of the athlete is abnormal, imaging of the spinal cord and spinal canal is warranted to look for bone tumors, spinal cord tumors, herniated discs, syringomyelia, and other lesions. MRI has supplanted the use of CT myelography for assessing the neural or disc pathology. MRI or bone scan can also identify discitis. CT is the imaging study of choice for evaluating further bone lesions that are seen on plain radiograph or bone scan. Even though bone tumors and stress fractures may be seen on MRI, soft tissue edema can interfere with the interpretation of bony abnormalities (7). CT scans can also distinguish between a herniated disc and a slipped vertebral apophysis.

Laboratory Evaluation

In addition to the imaging modalities discussed above for the evaluation of back pain in the pediatric athlete, additional diagnostic studies may be helpful in making a definitive diagnosis. When inflammatory disease or a connective tissue disorder is suspected, laboratory studies, such as complete blood count (CBC), erythrocyte sedimentation rate (ESR), rheumatoid factor, antinuclear antibody (ANA), and HLA-B27 (tissue typing) studies, may be used. When the presence of an infection is suspected, the CBC, ESR, and C-reactive protein may be helpful.

TREATMENT AND REHABILITATION OF PEDIATRIC BACK PAIN

The goal of treatment for back pain and injuries in the athlete is to reduce pain, to restore range of motion, and to regain and improve strength so that the athlete can return safely to sports participation. The specific treatments have been outlined in the back pain disorder sections above, and they include relative rest, icing, NSAIDs, rehabilitation exercises, and, in some cases, immobilization or surgery. In musculoligamentous injury, supervised rehabilitation can be started once the pain has been controlled. The athlete must be supervised, at least initially, to ensure the use of proper technique with rehabilitation exercises. Although a variety of back rehabilitation protocols exist, trunk and lumbar stabilization exercises are the mainstay of back injury rehabilita-

tion. Supine pelvic tilts, supine single or double knee to chest maneuvers, supine straight leg raises and lowering, (Fig. 30.11A–30.11C),and standing wall slides (with the back against wall and feet about 12 in. from the wall) are some of the exercises used for back rehabilitation. Exercises that use an exercise ball (Fig. 30.11D and 30.11E) are frequently used for trunk and lumbar stabilization. The patient should be monitored for any increase in pain or symptoms that occurs during or after rehabilitation. If the athlete remains symptom free, rehabilitation can progress to include gentle flexibility and aerobic conditioning. After range of motion, strength, and flexibility improve, sport-specific proprioceptive activities can be added to prepare the athlete for return to his or her sport. In cases in which the athlete is not permitted to return to his or her preinjury sport (e.g., athletes with high-grade spondylolisthesis who played foot-

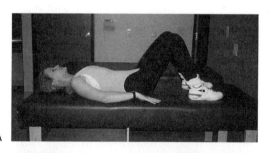

A

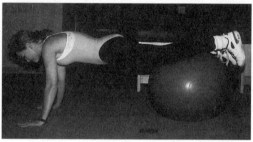

B

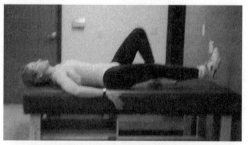

C

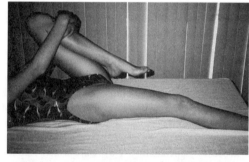

D

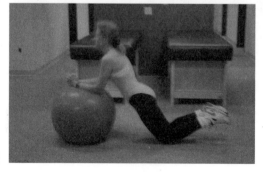

E

FIG. 30.11. *Back rehabilitation exercises.* **A:** Pelvic tilt. **B:** Supine knee to chest stretch. **C:** Straight leg raise and lowering. **D,E:** Exercise ball used for trunk and lumbar stabilization exercises.

ball), instructions on techniques for performing other permitted activities can be provided. The psychologic loss that such athletes may feel should also be addressed (see Chapter 9).

Considering the psychologic impact of the injury and rehabilitation phase on the athlete, such as the loss of socialization while he or she is away from his or her teammates, is important. Addressing the athlete's (and parents') hopes and expectations and the athlete's interest level in returning to his or her sport is another crucial component. A child who is being pressured to play a sport may not be as motivated to progress in rehabilitation as the athlete who has a great desire to return to sports is.

RETURN TO SPORT

Decisions on when an athlete can return to sport participation should be individualized. Some factors involved in this decision are the injury type, the needs of the patient, the extent and success of treatment, and the type of sport involved. Specific recommendations are discussed under the pertinent diagnostic subheadings above. In general, however, in athletes who had surgical intervention, return-to-play decisions should be guided by the orthopedic surgeon. If an athlete who required surgical correction of a spinal deformity, such as scoliosis, the athlete may return to noncontact sports about 6 months after becoming pain free; contact sports, however, are not recommended because of the risk of fracture of the surgical rod. Similarly, an athlete with spondylolisthesis who required surgical intervention should not return to contact sports, such as football. In cases of spondylolysis, an athlete may return to contact sports after becoming symptom free if he or she has regained muscle strength and flexibility; this may take from weeks to several months. In contrast, athletes with musculoligamentous injuries can return to sports participation much more quickly; they can be cleared when they are pain free and have regained a normal range of motion.

PREVENTION

In order to prevent injuries, the primary care physician must understand the specific physical requirements of a particular sport and the potential acute, chronic, or overuse injuries of that sport. The American College of Sports Medicine (87) has estimated that 50% of the overuse injuries in children and adolescents are preventable. Some factors related to improper training techniques, such as changes in the intensity and duration of participation or in equipment, predispose ath-

letes to spinal injuries. Disparities between the size and strength of athletes also can lead to injury. Growth considerations also affect the athlete's tendency to injury. During rapid growth, joint tightness can occur when bones lengthen faster than muscle–tendon units, thus producing inflexibility and dynamic muscle imbalances that can lead to injuries (87). If these findings are noted, preventive changes in training regimens and techniques can be instituted to reduce the risk of injury. One example of a training modification is emphasizing flexibility training in adolescent athletes who are particularly at risk for injury during the adolescent growth spurt. Another prevention strategy to help children avoid injury from weak or inflexible musculoskeletal structures is participation in general strength and fitness conditioning activities prior to participation in specific sports programs.

SUMMARY

Most cases of back pain in children and adolescents can be evaluated and treated by the primary care physician. The diagnosis usually can be made from a detailed history and a physical examination with radiographic evaluation if the pain is persistent or if associated suspicious history or physical examination findings are present. Careful note of the mode of onset, the nature and severity of pain, and recent changes in symptoms or associated systemic symptoms should be elicited by the history, followed by the performance of a physical examination to localize the findings (15). If organic pathology is absent, nonspecific treatment, such as relative rest and NSAIDs, can be used for pediatric back pain. If symptoms persist after several weeks of treatment, a detailed search for the cause of the back pain, including specialized radiographic studies (e.g., MRI, CT, or bone scan), is warranted, and laboratory studies should be performed. In cases of severe or progressive scoliosis, spondylolisthesis, disc space narrowing, fracture, or tumor, referral to an orthopedic specialist is advised. With early identification of the cause of pediatric back pain, treatment can be individualized and monitored to maximize the chances for an athlete's safe return to his or her sport.

REFERENCES

1. Moore KL. *Clinically oriented anatomy*, 3rd ed. Baltimore: Williams & Wilkins, 1992.
2. Morissy RT, Weinstein SL, eds. *Lovell and Winter's pediatric orthopaedics*, 4th ed. Philadelphia: Lippincott-Raven Publishers, 1996.
3. Stanitski CL, DeLee JC, Drez D, eds. *Pediatric and adolescent sports medicine*. Philadelphia: WB Saunders, 1994.

4. Sponseller PD. Evaluating the child with back pain. *Am Fam Physician* 1996;54:1933–1941.

5. Payne WK, Ogilvie JW. Back pain in children and adolescents. *Pediatr Clin North Am* 1996;43:899–917.

6. King H. Evaluating the child with back pain. *Pediatr Clin North Am* 1986;33:1489–1493.

7. Richards BS. Clinical assessment of back pain in children. *J Musculoskeletal Med* 1998; 15:31–40.

8. Acute Low Back Problems Guidelines Panel. Acute low back problems in adults: assessment and treatment. *Am Fam Physician* 1995;51:469–934.

9. Gillette RD. A practical approach to the patient with back pain. *Am Fam Physician* 1996;53:670–676.

10. Wheeler AH. Diagnosis and management of low back Pain and sciatica. *Am Fam Physician* 1995;52:1333–1341.

11. Johnson RJ. Low back pain in sports. Managing spondylolysis in young patients. *The Physician and Sports Medicine* 1993;21:53–59.

12. Krengel WF, King HA. Scoliosis: diagnostic basics and therapeutic choices. *J Musculoskeletal Med* 1995;12:54–66.

13. Lonstein JE. Scoliosis: updates managing school screening referrals. *J Musculoskeletal Med* 1999;16:593–605.

14. Bunnell WP. Spinal deformity. *Pediatr Clin North Am* 1986;33:1475–1487.

15. Bunnell WP, Shook JE. Orthopaedics in the pediatric office. *Curr Probl Pediatr* 1992;22:13–47.

16. Boachie-Adjei O, Lonner B. Spinal deformity. *Pediatr Clin North Am* 1996;43:883–897.

17. Emans JB. Diagnosis of childhood and adolescent scoliosis. *J Musculoskeletal Med* 1985;2:11–24.

18. Congeni J. Evaluating spondylolysis in adolescent athletes. *J Musculoskeletal Med* 2000;17:123–129.

19. Weinstein SL, ed. *The pediatric spine: principles and practice.* New York: Raven Press, 1994.

20. Nicholas JA, Hershman ED, eds. *The lower extremity and spine in sports medicine*, 2nd ed. St. Louis: Mosby, 1995.

21. King HA. Back pain in children. *Pediatr Clin North Am* 1984;31:1083–1095.

22. Turner PG, Hancock PG, Green JH, et al. Back pain in childhood. *Spine* 1979;60:100–108.

23. Wiltse LL, Widell E Jr, Jackson DW. Fatigue fracture: the basic lesion in isthmic spondylolisthesis. *J Bone Joint Surg Am* 1975;57:17–22.

24. Farfan HF, Osteria V, Lamy C. The mechanical etiology of spondylolysis and spondylolisthesis. *Clin Orthop* 1976;117:40–55.

25. Jackson DW, Wiltse LL, Dingeman RD, et al. Stress reactions involving the pars interarticularis in young athletes. *Am J Sports Med* 1981;9:304–312.

26. Ferguson RJ, McMasters MC, Stanitski CL. Low back pain in college football linemen. *J Bone Joint Surg Am* 1974;56:1300.

27. McCarroll J, Ritter M. Lumbar spondylolysis and spondylolisthesis in college football players. *Am J Sports Med* 1986;14:404–406.

28. Sward L, Hellstrom M, Jacobsson B, et al. Spondylolysis and the sacrohorizontal angle in athletes. *Acta Radiol* 1989;30:359–364.

29. Letts M, Smallman T, Afanasiev R, et al. Fracture of the pars interarticularis in adolescent athletes: a clinical-biomechanical analysis. *J Pediatr Orthop* 1986;6:40–46.

30. Teitz CC. Sports medicine concern in dance and gymnastics. *Pediatr Clin North Am* 1982;29:1399–1421.

31. Turner RH, Bianco A Jr. Spondylolysis and spondylolisthesis in children and teen-agers. *J Bone Joint Surg Am* 1971;53:1298–1306.

32. Friberg S. Studies on spondylolisthesis. *Acta Chir Scand* 1939;82:56.

33. Albanese M, Pizzutillo PD. Family study of spondylolysis and spondylolisthesis. *J Pediatr Orthop* 1982;2:496–499.

34. Laurent L. Spondylolisthesis in children and adolescents. *Acta Orthop Scand* 1961;31:45–64.

35. Wynne-Davies R, Scott JH. Inheritance and spondylolisthesis: a radiographic family survey. *J Bone Joint Surg Br* 1979;61B:301–305.

36. Schlenzka D, Poussa M, Seitsalo S, et al. Intervertebral disc changes in adolescents with isthmic spondylolisthesis. *J Spinal Disord* 1991;4:344–352.

37. Szypryt EP, Twining P, Mulholland RC, et al. The prevalence of disc degeneration associated with neural arch defects of the lumbar spine assessed by magnetic resonance imaging. *Spine* 1989;14:977–981.

38. Henson J, McCall IW, O'Brien JP. Disc damage above a spondylolisthesis. *Br J Radiol* 1987;60:69–72.

39. Steiner ME, Micheli LJ. Treatment of symptomatic spondylolysis and spondylolisthesis with the modified Boston brace. *Spine* 1985;10:932–943.

40. Morita T, Ikata T, Katoh S, Miyake R. Lumbar spondylolysis in children and adolescents. *J Bone Joint Surg Br* 1995;77:620–625.

41. Fredrickson B, Baker K, Mcholick W, et al. The natural history of spondylolysis and spondylolisthesis. *J Bone Joint Surg Am* 1984;66:699–707.

42. Osterman K, Schlenzka D, Poussa M, et al. Isthmic spondylolisthesis in symptomatic and asymptomatic subjects, epidemiology, and natural history with special reference to disk abnormality and mode of treatment. *Clin Orthop* 1993;297:65–70.

43. Blackburne JS, Velikas EP. Spondylolisthesis in children and adolescents. *J Bone Joint Surg Br* 1977;59:490–494.

44. Saraste H. Long-term clinical and radiological follow-up of spondylolysis and spondylolisthesis. *J Pediatr Orthop* 1987;7:631–638.

45. Lostein JE. Spondylolisthesis in children. Cause, natural history, and management. *Spine* 1999;24:2640–2648.

46. Frennered AK, Danielson BI, Nachemson AL. Natural history of symptomatic isthmic low-grade spondylolisthesis in children and adolescents: a seven-year follow-up study. *J Pediatr Orthop* 1991;11:209–213.

47. Speck GR, McCall IW, O'Brien JP. Spondylolisthesis: the angle of kyphosis. *Spine* 1984;9:659–660.

48. Blanda J, Bethem D, Moats W, Lew M. Defects of pars interarticularis in athletes: a protocol for nonoperative treatment. *J Spinal Disord* 1993;6:406–411.

49. Ciullo JV, Jackson DW. Pars interarticularis stress reaction, spondylolysis, and spondylolisthesis in gymnasts. *Clin Sports Med* 1985;4:95–110.

50. Ikata T, Miyake R, Katoh S, et al. Pathogenesis of sports-related spondylolisthesis in adolescents. *Am J Sports Med* 1996;24:94–98.

51. Phalen G, Dickson J. Spondylolisthesis and tight hamstrings. *J Bone Joint Surg Am* 1961;43:505–512.

52. Newman P. The etiology of spondylolisthesis. *J Bone Joint Surg Br* 1963;45:39–59.

53. Hensinger RN. Spondylolysis and spondylolisthesis in children and adolescents. *J Bone Joint Surg Am* 1989; 71:1098–1107.

54. Bell DF, Ehrlich MG, Zaleske DJ. Brace treatment for symptomatic spondylolisthesis. *Clin Orthop* 1988;236: 192–198.

55. Hensinger RN, Lang JR, MacEwin GD. Surgical management of spondylolisthesis in children and adolescents. *Spine* 1976;1:207–216.

56. Libson E, Bloom RA, Dinari G, Robin GC. Oblique lumbar spine radiographs: importance in young patients. *Radiology* 1984;151:89–90.

56a. Pierce ME. Spondylolysis: what does this mean? A review. *Australas Radiol* 1987;31:391–394.

57. Krenz J, Troup J. The structure of the pars interarticularis of the lower lumbar vertebra and its relationship to the etiology of spondylolysis. *J Bone Joint Surg Br* 1973;55:735–741.

58. Bellah RD, Summerville DA, Treves ST, Micheli LJ. Low-back pain in adolescent athletes: detection of stress injury to the pars interarticularis with SPECT. *Radiology* 1991;180:509–512.

59. Bodner RJ, Heyman S, Drummond DS, et al. The use of single photon emission computed tomography (SPECT) in the diagnosis of low-back pain in young patients. *Spine* 1988;13:1155–1160.

60. Lusins JO, Elting JJ, Cicoria AD, et al. SPECT evaluation of lumbar spondylolysis and spondylolisthesis. *Spine* 1994;19:608–612.

61. Smith JA, Hu SS. Management of spondylolysis and spondylolisthesis in the pediatric and adolescent population. *Orthop Clin North Am* 1999;30:387–399.

62. Bell DF, Ehrlich MG, Zaleske DJ. Brace treatment for symptomatic spondylolisthesis. *Clin Orthop* 1988;236: 192–198.

63. Pizzutillo PD, Hummer CD. Nonoperative treatment for painful adolescent spondylolysis or spondylolisthesis. *J Pediatr Orthop* 1989;9:538–540.

64. Wiltse L. Spondylolisthesis in children. *Clin Orthop* 1961;21:156–163.

65. Wiltse LL, Jackson DW. Treatment of spondylolisthesis and spondylolysis in children. *Clin Orthop* 1976;117:92–100.

66. Bohlman HH, Cook SS. One-stage decompression and posterolateral and interbody fusion for lumbosacral spondyloptosis through a posterior approach: report of two cases. *J Bone Joint Surg Am* 1982;64:415–418.

67. DeWald RL, Faut MM, Taddonio RF, et al. Severe lumbosacral spondylolisthesis in adolescents and children: reduction and staged circumferential fusion. *J Bone Joint Surg Am* 1981;63:619–626.

68. Laurent LE, Osterman K. Operative treatment of spondylolisthesis in young patients. *Clin Orthop* 1976; 117:85–91.

69. Velikas EP, Blackburne JS. Surgical treatment of spondylolisthesis in children and adolescents. *J Bone Joint Surg Br* 1981;63:67–70.

70. Bradford DS. Treatment of severe spondylolisthesis. A combined approach for reduction and stabilization. *Spine* 1979;4:423–429.

71. Freebody D, Bendall R, Taylor RD. Anterior transperitoneal lumbar fusion. *J Bone Joint Surg Br* 1971;53: 617–627.

72. Gaines R, Nichols W. Treatment of spondyloptosis by two stage L5 vertebrectomy and reduction of L4 onto S1. *Spine* 1985;10:680–686.

73. Lehmer S, Steffee A, Gaines R. Treatment of L5-S1 spondyloptosis by staged L5 resection with reduction and fusion of L4 onto S1. *Spine* 1994;19:1916–1925.

74. Saraste H. Spondylolysis and spondylolisthesis. *Acta Orthop Scand Suppl* 1993;251:84–86.

75. Van Rens TJ, van Horn JR. Long-term results in lumbosacral interbody fusion for spondylolisthesis. *Acta Orthop Scand* 1982;53:383–392.

76. Muschik M, Sippel H, Perka C. Surgical management of severe spondylolisthesis in children and adults: anterior fusion *in situ* versus anterior spondylodesis with posterior transpedicular instrumentation and reduction. *Spine* 1997;22:2036–2042.

77. Dandy D, Shannon M. Lumbo-sacral subluxation. *J Bone Joint Surg Br* 1971;53:578–595.

78. Boxall D, Bradford DS, Winter RB, et al. Management of severe spondylolisthesis in children and adolescents. *J Bone Joint Surg Am* 1979;61:479–495.

79. Schoenecker P, Cole HO, Herring JA, et al. Cauda equina syndrome after *in situ* arthrodesis for severe spondylolisthesis at the lumbosacral junction. *J Bone Joint Surg Am* 1990;72:369–377.

80. Dick W, Schnebel B. Severe spondylolisthesis: reduction and internal fixation. *Clin Orthop* 1988;232: 70–79.

81. Bradford D, Gotfried Y. Staged salvage reconstruction of grade-IV and V spondylolisthesis. *J Bone Joint Surg Am* 1987;69:191–202.

82. Morrissy RT, Wenstein SL, eds. *Lovell and Winter's pediatric orthopaedics* 5th ed. Philadelphia: Lippincott Williams & Wilkins, 2001.

82a. d'Hemecourt PA, Gerbino PG, Micheli LJ. Back injuries in the young athlete. *Clin Sports Med* 2000;19: 663–679.

83. Price CT, Moon BS. The limping child: an age-based approach to evaluation. *J Musculoskeletal Med* 1977; 14:32.

84. Zetaruk MN. The young gymnast. *Clin Sports Med* 2000;19:757–780.

85. Mellion MB, Walsh WM, Shelton, GL, eds. *The team physician's handbook*, 2nd ed. Philadelphia: Lippincott Williams & Wilkins, .

86. Oski FA, DeAngelis CD, Feigin RD, Warshaw JB, eds. *Principles and practice of pediatrics*, 2nd ed. Philadelphia: JB Lippincott Co, 1994.

87. DiFiori JP. Overuse injuries in children and adolescents. *The Physician and Sports Medicine* 1999;27:75–89.

31

Chest and Abdominal Trauma

Bernard A. Griesemer

Professionals who care for young athletes encounter episodes of chest and abdominal trauma less frequently than they encounter musculoskeletal injuries that involve the extremities. Chest and abdominal injury represent 7% (1) to 11% (2) of sports-related injuries that present to emergency care facilities. However, with head and neck injuries, injuries that involve chest and abdominal trauma represent a disproportionate risk of severe life-threatening injuries to all athletes, including those in the pediatric age range. These injuries (chest, abdominal, head, and neck) are more likely to require in-patient hospital care and critical care services.

The acuity and severity of these injuries demand a level of care and skill from healthcare providers that requires initial training in trauma management and ongoing education and recertification in order to maintain clinical skills. The knowledge and technical skills acquired in the Pediatric Advanced Life Support (PALS) program and the Advanced Trauma Life Support (ATLS) program are of major importance when a sports medicine physician encounters chest and/or abdominal trauma during competition or practice. This chapter includes an overview of the recommended procedures that are included in these emergency management protocols.

The relative risk of thoracoabdominal injuries varies widely from one sport to another. In general, the risk is higher in collision and contact sports (e.g., football and rugby), in sports in which a projectile is involved in the competition (e.g., javelin and baseball), and in those where the potential exists for high-velocity contact either with objects on or surrounding the field of play (e.g., skiing, snowboarding, and cycling) or with equipment or other items integral to the competition (e.g., motocross, equestrian, or shooting events). Statistics also may indicate an increased risk within certain categories or combinations of competitive scenarios (e.g., collision sports in older adolescent males) (3).

Regardless of the relative statistical risk of injury for a particular event, physicians who provide medical care at athletic events should be aware of the fact that serious chest and abdominal trauma to competitors, staff, and spectators could occur in a wide variety of competitive situations.

Blunt trauma, as opposed to penetrating trauma, is the most common type of trauma to the chest and abdomen in athletic practice and competition. Blunt trauma can result from an athlete's contact with another player, the ground, barriers surrounding the field of play, or equipment. The risk of injury from many of these threats, especially those resulting from contact with the barriers surrounding the field of play or equipment, can be reduced. A team physician can provide an important component of preventive medicine by doing a "walk around" prior to practice or competition. Delaying or canceling competition or practice because of an unsatisfactory playing surface, such as wet or icy conditions, irregularities in the natural or artificial turf, or poor lighting, are appropriate interventions from the team physician. In the pediatric-aged athlete, competition venues that exceed the skill level or age level of the competitor (e.g., downhill skiing courses) also may require intervention on the part of the team physician. Securing goals and field of play barriers can prevent many episodes of severe, and even fatal, trauma to the chest and abdomen (4). Removing nonessential equipment, such as equipment lockers, training tables, and field of play maintenance equipment, from the area of competition also reduces the risk of trauma to the athlete. Likewise, during practice or competition, moving nonessential spectators, sideline players, and support personnel away from the field of play eliminates yet another possible contact point that could result in trauma to the chest and abdomen for the competitors. Moreover, these noncompeting individuals also are at risk for blunt trauma to the chest and abdomen as a result of a collision with players and from trauma that is caused by equipment used in the competitive event (e.g., a thrown baseball).

Although less frequent than cases involving blunt trauma, more serious episodes of trauma to the chest and abdomen are seen with penetrating trauma. In sports that involve projectile objects, such as archery, shooting sports, and field events where the competition involves projectiles (e.g., javelin), the team physician can and should assist the competition managers in removing spectators and noncompeting athletes from the field of play.

Many cases of sports-related trauma in the pediatric-aged athlete involve simultaneous trauma to the chest and abdomen. Trauma to the chest and abdomen during athletic competition frequently involves multiple organ systems. For example, injuries to the superficial soft tissue structures (skin, muscle, and breast) or the skeletal structures (rib) are often not life threatening if they are an isolated injury. Injuries to these structures, however, may herald significant life-threatening injuries to the underlying vital organ systems. The extent of injury to underlying organs may not be apparent immediately. The cardiovascular, pulmonary, and central nervous systems are all at risk in sports-related injuries to the trunk that present initially as superficial injuries.

CHEST INJURIES

As was noted above, injuries to the thorax can range from common minor injuries that involve superficial structures to less common life-threatening conditions to the underlying vital organs. Abrasions and minor lacerations to the skin usually require only on-site wound cleansing and protection from additional injury. However, because these minor injuries may be associated with a more significant underlying organ injury, the athlete should remain under close observation. This period of close observation is especially warranted if the athlete returns immediately to practice or competition. If the athlete is leaving the practice or competition area following injury or if he or she has completed the practice or competition, follow-up instructions should be provided to the parent or caregiver. These instructions should include information regarding the signs and symptoms of a more serious underlying injury and instructions for immediate follow-up care if the athlete's condition deteriorates.

Minor Injuries

Primary care physicians often encounter young athletes who experience chafing injuries to the skin surrounding the breast tissue. Not only is this frequently seen in young female athletes, but it is also observed in the young male athlete who is experiencing the physiologic breast tissue hypertrophy associated with pubertal development. The use of moistur-

izing creams and padding to reduce further irritation from jerseys or equipment should resolve the irritation. If the area of inflammation increases in severity, providing appropriate topical or systemic antibiotic coverage may be indicated.

Blunt trauma may also result in contusions and hematomas to mammary tissue. In young female athletes who sustain these injuries, firm support during the healing stage, cool compresses to the injured area, and protection from subsequent injuries are the main interventions. Modification in protective equipment (e.g., chest protectors similar to those used in youth baseball) or in playing technique (e.g., allowing the use of cross-chest folded arms in a soccer penalty kick) may provide additional protection for breast tissue. The young athlete may return to play when the signs and symptoms of tissue damage have resolved. More serious injuries may require close monitoring of symptoms during a graduated return to activity.

Musculoskeletal Injuries

Injuries to skeletal structures of the thorax may result from blunt trauma, penetrating trauma, or overuse injury. A direct blow to the sternum that results in a sternal fracture is a relatively unusual injury in pediatric and adolescents sports. Sports that have the potential for high velocity or increased force (e.g., rodeo, motocross, and skiing) can cause a sternal fracture. If a sternal fracture occurs, the force required to fracture the sternum is of such a degree that the most immediate and serious concern is damage to the underlying mediastinal structures. Severe blows to the sternum should prompt immediate and close observation of the athlete and rapid intervention if cardiopulmonary compromise occurs. Management of an isolated sternal fracture is usually conservative, and it focuses on the relief of symptoms with analgesics, as well as on protection from additional injuries.

The sternum, especially the interface between the sternum and the ribs, commonly is the site of acute discomfort in a young active adolescent. Costochondritis commonly affects young adolescents, and it is seen following viral illnesses, with overuse of the upper extremities, with rapid changes in intensity of exercise or competition profiles, or with a combination of all of these factors. Differentiating sternal discomfort from underlying medical conditions requires close attention to the medical history, especially as it relates to the onset or worsening of the symptoms with physical activity, the presence or absence of a history of trauma, and the presence or absence of fever and other evidence of an infectious process.

Significant substernal or costochondral chest pain coincident with activity, especially if it is associated with other signs of neurologic or cardiovascular compromise, warrants immediate and thorough evaluation. Sternal pain associated with fever in a toxic-appearing young athlete should prompt an immediate evaluation for a myocardial or pericardial infection. Chronic, recurring substernal pain associated with activity also may be seen in the individual who is predisposed to gastroesophageal reflux, and this condition may require a modification of preevent and postevent meal planning in addition to medication.

Acute, isolated traumatic rib fractures associated with blunt trauma are managed conservatively with analgesics and protective equipment. As with fractures of the sternum, if signs and symptoms of underlying organ injury become apparent, close observation and further diagnostic studies are indicated. Return-to-play considerations for both sternal and rib fractures are related to the disappearance of symptoms, the absence of underlying organ damage, and evidence of adequate healing on radiograph. Stress fractures of the ribs are seen in rowing sports, weightlifting, and weight training, as well as other sports that require repetitive stress on the musculoskeletal thoracic cage at the insertion of the muscle groups that stabilize and control shoulder dynamics. Persistent, localized chest wall pain with respiratory excursion, direct pressure, or shoulder movement may require radionucleotide imaging studies in order to confirm the diagnosis. Conservative management for stress fractures includes rest, analgesics, and, possibly, the modification of technique to prevent recurrences. Return-to-play considerations are similar to those in acute traumatic rib fractures—resolution of symptoms and evidence of healing on imaging studies.

Types of activity that may result in acute or subacute injuries to the ribs are also those that are likely to cause acute and subacute muscle injury in the supporting structure of the thorax. Direct blows to the chest wall may result in muscle hematoma. In the absence of rib fracture, the use of conservative management regimen that includes gentle compression to the site of injury and protective equipment to prevent additional injury is appropriate. Rehabilitation of the injured muscle group with stretching, modalities (e.g., ice, ultrasound, or muscle stimulation), and graduated strengthening exercises may expedite the athlete's return to play and may reduce the risk of reinjury.

Repetitive movement that requires prolonged or forceful exertions with the shoulders abducted greater than 90 degrees may cause or may exacerbate thoracic outlet pathology. Activity that results in compression of the neural or vascular tissue at the thoracic outlet may result in the initial presentation or the further exacerbation of the typical paresthesias and the vascular compromise to the upper extremities that is associated with this syndrome. The configuration of a specific athlete's first and second ribs and the surrounding supporting musculature may predispose the athlete to significant neurovascular compromise with certain types of activity. Modification of training and competitive techniques, rest, and analgesics will assist in minimizing the symptoms of this condition, but complete elimination of thoracic outlet symptoms with the resumption of activity may be problematic.

Cardiac Complications

With a direct blow to the anterior chest, especially in the young athlete whose chest wall compliance is greater than that of a more physically mature adult athlete, the risk of sustaining a life-threatening injury is significant. Commotio cordis, or "cardiac concussion," is most commonly reported in sports, such as youth baseball, in which a thrown object impacts the sternum and results in the development of life-threatening arrhythmias or asystole. Rapid recognition of the severity of this type of injury and the prompt initiation of cardiopulmonary resuscitation procedures are critical for the patient's survival. The use of chest protectors in youth sports in which participants have higher risks for projectile impact on the anterior chest may reduce the risk of this type of injury. Blunt trauma to the anterior chest can result in a wide variety of traumatic lesions to the heart, including damage to the coronary arteries, which leads to ischemic changes and subsequent myocardial infarction (5). Young athletes who sustain blunt trauma to the anterior chest should be observed closely for signs and symptoms of cardiac ischemia and/or arrhythmias immediately after such an injury. The athlete also should be considered a candidate for aggressive evaluation in the days and weeks following the injury if signs and symptoms subsequently develop.

Both blunt trauma and penetrating trauma to the anterior chest may result in hemorrhaging that progresses to cardiac tamponade. As in cases of commotio cordis, rapid recognition of the serious progression of the cardiovascular compromise, the quick initiation of cardiopulmonary resuscitation, and the immediate activation of emergency medical transport are critical for reducing the risk of mortality or severe morbidity.

Respiratory Complications

The medical literature documents a wide range of trauma to the lungs associated with athletic activity.

Blunt trauma to the anterior or posterior chest wall may result in a localized contusion to the lung surface. These lesions, which are often associated with traumatic rib fracture and pleuritic inflammation, resolve with conservative management. Close observation for the possible complications of pulmonary contusions, such as infection, embolic events, or atelectasis, may require close observation for days to weeks. Return-to-play considerations are based upon the resolution of symptoms and, if indicated, a return to baseline in pulmonary function studies.

Barotrauma to the lungs is a risk for athletes who participate in diving. Close attention to ascent and descent technique, especially in the younger, less experienced diver is critical in preventing this type of injury.

Blunt trauma, penetrating trauma, and barotrauma may all lead to pneumothorax or hemothorax. Close observation of the injured athlete for signs of progressively severe dyspnea should prompt immediate evaluation of the symmetry of breath sounds and institution of appropriate medical and surgical interventions.

Spontaneous pneumothorax also has been found in young athletes during practice or competition. As in cases of pneumothorax associated with trauma to the chest, the rapid and thorough evaluation of athletes who are experiencing progressively severe dyspnea is critical.

Vascular Injuries

Trauma to the thorax also may cause damage to the major vessels of the heart, resulting in an immediate catastrophic rupture or more slowly progressing dissecting lesions of the vessel walls. Traumatic injury to other vascular structures in the thorax, such as the coronary arteries, the intercostal vessels, and the subclavian vessels, has been reported in the medical literature. An accurate history of the mechanism of injury and the point of impact in the traumatic event may provide valuable information for assisting the team physician to differentiate serious underlying vascular damage from a less serious injury to superficial structures. Close observation of the cardiovascular stability of the athlete is a key component in the management of these injuries.

Neurologic Damage

Trauma to the upper chest may result in damage to the neurologic plexus, and this finding may become more evident as the cardiovascular status of the injured athlete is stabilized. Stabilization of injuries to the skeletal, vascular, and pulmonary structures surrounding these neural structures minimizes the compounding effect of compression or ischemic damage to a plexus that has sustained a traction, compression, or direct laceration injury.

Trauma to the back of the upper trunk may result in damage to the structures of the thoracic spine and posterior rami. In addition, team physicians may encounter injuries to a young athlete's posterior chest that result in damage to the long thoracic nerve. After the initial inflammation and pain have subsided, the physician will note a subsequent scapular winging that may respond poorly to rehabilitation and restrengthening efforts. Stabilization of injured tissue in the vicinity of the damaged neural system, protection from additional injury, and aggressive rehabilitation will hasten the athlete's safe return to physical activity.

Return-to-play considerations in these cases may require the team physician to take the lead in coordinating an entire medical team in order to present the athlete with the best, most coordinated, and cost-effective care. This team approach is often the most successful care program for leading to a planned progression of increased physical activity and a return to safe competition.

When a team physician encounters an episode of acute chest trauma during an athletic practice or competition, assessment of the severity of the injury should progress in a systematic manner that has been well documented in trauma life support programs. The current ATLS manual for physicians (6) emphasizes that the majority of cases of both blunt and penetrating chest trauma do not require thoracotomy and that they can be adequately managed by physicians who have kept their ATLS skills current.

ABDOMINAL INJURIES

Sports-related injuries are reported to cause 10% of all abdominal injuries (7). Similar to the statistics seen in sports-related chest trauma, abdominal injuries are disproportionately likely to result in severe injuries that require hospitalization, intensive care observation, and surgical intervention. Injuries to the abdomen may be more likely than episodes of chest trauma to present with subacute signs and symptoms of internal organ damage. Close observation of the athlete with an abdominal injury may extend for many days following the traumatic incident.

Mechanisms of blunt and penetrating trauma to the abdomen are similar to those seen in injuries to the chest. As noted in the introduction, abdominal trauma is often seen concurrent with chest trauma. Significant trauma to one area of the trunk in athletic competition or practice should prompt immediate, close, and ongoing observation of the less involved area.

Abdominal trauma can be viewed in terms of the type of organ that is injured. The abdominal cavity contains both solid internal organs and hollow organs, each of which may be more sensitive to certain types of insult. Injury to the neural structures that are contained in the abdomen also may be affected by both blunt and penetrating trauma. Finally, injury to the supporting structures of the abdomen will be considered.

Organ Injuries

One of the more commonly injured solid organs in the abdominal cavity is the spleen. Blunt trauma to the left upper quadrant of the abdomen is frequently seen when a player collides with another player, field of play barriers, equipment, and spectators. Many physicians who care for athletes frequently have seen splenic injury in skiing, snowboarding, and sledding accidents when the young athlete has collided with a tree or other natural object. If the blunt or penetrating trauma results in a fracture to the pedicle of the spleen, the young athlete will rapidly become hemodynamically unstable. Trauma that results in a contusion to the body of the spleen or in a subcapsular hematoma may present with left upper quadrant abdominal pain that becomes progressively more severe over a period of minutes to hours. In these less severe injuries, the patient may remain hemodynamically stable. Many athletes with splenic trauma present with left shoulder pain (Kerr sign) that may make the delineation of isolated abdominal and chest injuries more complicated for the examiner. Imaging studies to determine the extent of the injury and the clinical stability of the patient allow the surgical team to determine whether conservative management or more aggressive surgical intervention is appropriate. Subsequent to the phase of acute injury management, these same factors also assist the team physician in planning progressive return to activity and competition.

Trauma to the right upper quadrant of the abdomen may result in damage to the liver and its adjacent organs. Penetrating trauma in this area can result in catastrophic bleeding and subsequent hemodynamic collapse. Blunt trauma can result in damage similar to types seen in trauma to the spleen. Laceration to the body of the liver, depending on the severity, may present with a variety of signs and symptoms, ranging from upper quadrant abdominal pain to hemodynamic shock. Localized areas of damage to the surface of the liver may result in a subcapsular hematoma that can be managed conservatively if the patient's clinical condition remains stable. More extensive damage may require surgical intervention in order to stabilize the athlete's bleeding.

Trauma to the right upper quadrant also may result in damage to the gall bladder, the common duct, and associated support structures. As in cases of liver trauma, the signs and symptoms of the damage may progress to immediate shock in the more severe cases or to a subacute presentation over a period of hours or days. Following upper abdominal trauma, an athlete with progressively severe right upper quadrant abdominal pain, chest pain and dyspnea, or evidence of hemodynamic instability requires immediate and aggressive management. Imaging studies to determine the extent of the damage will assist the medical and surgical team in determining appropriate care and return to activity and competition.

Team physicians are more likely to see renal injuries than injuries to other solid abdominal organs. Damage to renal and adrenal tissue can be seen with trauma to the anterior, lateral, and posterior aspects of the abdomen. Both blunt and penetrating trauma can result in life-threatening injury due to the disruption of the vascular supply at the renal pelvis or a severe fracture or laceration to the renal body with disruption of the capsule. Rapid hemodynamic instability will necessitate immediate stabilization of the patient and transport to an emergency medical facility. When a fracture or laceration to the body of the kidney is limited to a segment of the renal body and hemorrhage is confined to the subcapsular space, the athlete will usually present with flank pain and gross hematuria, but he or she may remain hemodynamically stable. In limited lacerations or contusions to the renal parenchyma, close observation, adequate hydration, rest, and protection from further injury are appropriate interventions. Imaging studies to determine the extent of injury will help guide intervention strategies and return-to-play considerations in the stable patient. The team physician also may be asked to assist in follow-up monitoring of blood pressure and urinalysis to document the resolution of hematuria.

Trauma to the epigastric area of the abdomen may result in damage to the pancreas. Lacerations, fractures, and contusions to the pancreas and its supporting structures may result in immediate hemodynamic instability and may require emergent shock management. Less severe lesions may present with localized abdominal pain, elevation of enzyme levels, and progressive signs of peritonitis over a period of hours to days. Fluid management, rest, protection from further injury, and close observation for an extended period of time may be required.

In the female athlete, trauma to the abdomen also may result in trauma to the ovaries and adjacent structures. An athlete may be predisposed to injury in this system because of the presence of ovarian cysts. An athlete who is experiencing clinical symptoms that may be related to cyst formation may benefit from imaging studies to determine the level of activity restrictions or the appropriate use of additional protective equipment to minimize the risk of significant trauma. Abdominal trauma to the hollow organ, the uterus, also has been reported in the sports medicine literature. Contusions to the uterine body and damage to adjacent supporting structures require close observation, especially as return to activity and competition progresses. Barotrauma in water skiing and wake boarding events has also been observed. Team physicians must remain acutely aware of the increased risk of both blunt trauma and repetitive ballistic movement in the young female athlete who is pregnant. Finding an appropriate time and place that accommodates the need to ask the athlete sensitive questions about the possibility of pregnancy may be difficult for the team physician. Although this task may be complicated, it is a necessary component of abdominal injury management in the young female athlete.

Abdominal trauma also may involve the hollow abdominal organs of the gastrointestinal tract. Barotrauma to the stomach has been reported in cases of blunt trauma to the epigastric area, but it also has been reported in diving without the athlete sustaining a direct blow to the abdomen. Rupture of the stomach wall, with release of stomach contents into the peritoneal space, results in rapid development of peritonitis and hemodynamic instability. Barotrauma from diving is less likely to result in damage to the small and large intestine. Blunt abdominal trauma or penetrating trauma to the abdomen is highly likely to result in intestinal damage because of the large area that the bowel represents. Bowel wall contusion may present with initial abdominal tenderness and few other symptoms. Progressive abdominal discomfort and clinical signs of a bowel obstructive pattern will warrant further evaluation and possible surgical intervention. Similarly, trauma to the mesentery may present as initial nonspecific discomfort following blunt abdominal trauma and may then progress over a period of hours or days to increasing abdominal discomfort, distention, and other obstructive symptoms. When trauma to the mesentery is a component of blunt abdominal trauma, hematoma formation may result. This may progress to vascular compromise of extensive sections of the bowel, and it involves a serious risk of mortality and morbidity. Close observation of the athlete for a period of days to weeks may be warranted.

In addition to the possibility of traumatic insult to the kidney, the hollow organ of the genitourinary system that is susceptible to injury with trauma to the abdomen is the urinary bladder. Lower abdominal trauma, especially to a distended bladder, may result in injury ranging from vesicular wall contusion or hematoma formation and consequent hematuria to urinary bladder rupture with subsequent hemodynamic instability and progressive signs of peritonitis.

Neurologic Injuries

A common neurologic injury that is the result of epigastric abdominal trauma is seen with trauma to the solar plexus. Having the "wind knocked out of you" is usually a transient phenomenon with little or no residual effect. Prolonged spasm of the diaphragm or persistent dyspnea beyond 1 to 2 minutes should prompt immediate and thorough evaluation. Consequently, when this injury mechanism is suspected, removal of the athlete from competition is warranted until signs and symptoms resolve. Subsequently, close observation of the athlete who is reentering practice or competition following this injury is also advisable.

Structural Injuries

As in chest injuries in sports, injuries to the abdominal wall also are frequently seen in young athletes. Superficial skin abrasions and minor lacerations are managed with local cleansing and protection from further injury. Contusion to subcutaneous structures, including superficial muscular tissue, may require a longer healing time and a more gradual return to competition. Trauma to the posterior aspect of the trunk may result in contusion and hematoma formation in the paraspinal musculature. Ice, compression, and stretching of the affected muscle after the acute phase of the injury may be helpful in facilitating the return to physical activity. In both anterior and posterior lower trunk injuries, the clinical challenge is to determine the absence of underlying tissue damage. Spasm of the paraspinal musculature may be alleviated with stretching, ice, ultrasound, and muscle stimulation. Return-to-play decisions are made on the basis of absence of underlying organ damage and the resolution of symptoms.

Crush Injuries

Sports injuries that may involve a crush injury to the pelvis (e.g., equestrian or motocross sports) may result in a fracture to the pelvis. Management of the actual fracture is usually conservative, involving rest, analgesics, and protection from further injury. The force involved in a fracture to the pelvis is of such intensity that the presence of significant damage to underlying soft tissue organs should be strongly suspected. Close observation for hemodynamic instability and close monitoring of the genitourinary system are required. Damage to the insertion points of the muscle groups that stabilize the trunk and lower extremity also is a concern in incidents that result in crush injuries of the pelvis. Injuries of this severity also are associated with damage to the major vessels in the abdomen and pelvis, including the descending aorta and iliac vessels. Rapid, accurate assessment of the severity of the injury, appropriate on-field emergency stabilization, and immediate transport to a trauma facility are required.

IMMEDIATE MANAGEMENT OF CHEST AND ABDOMINAL TRAUMA IN THE ATHLETE

Sports-related trauma to the chest and abdomen, along with injuries to the head and neck, are more likely to result in life-threatening injuries than are injuries to the extremities. The risk of morbidity and mortality in these injuries is significantly higher than that of the more commonly occurring musculoskeletal injuries. Preventive strategies, proper training, and the availability of the appropriate equipment are extremely important, given the poor prognosis in many instances where sports-related injury involves trauma to the chest, abdomen, or both (see chapter 27).

A major component, both in prevention and in management of this category of injury, is the preparticipation physical examination (PPE). The identification of preexisting conditions, such as absence of a paired organ or prior injury to a vital organ system, is relevant to preventive interventions. Appropriate modification of protective equipment may be indicated in athletes who have preexisting structural lesions, either congenitally or as a result of prior surgery. Infectious disease processes, such as mononucleosis, increase the risk of splenic injury with abdominal trauma and require restrictions on physical activity and competition until sufficient time (usually 4 to 6 weeks) has passed to allow resolution of organ inflammation and enlargement. Physiologic conditions, such as pregnancy, also are important to consider for a young athlete who is engaging in sports that have a higher risk not only of hyperthermic conditions but also of repetitive ballistic trauma or direct blows to the lower abdomen.

The challenge for many medical teams who care for athletes is facilitating communication between the physician who performed the PPE and the athlete, the athlete's family, and the medical team covering the athletic event. As part of the team physician walk around prior to an event or practice, asking the coaching staff, the trainer, or school administrative personnel whether any athletes on the teams have preexisting health problems is appropriate.

Team physicians also can assist the nonmedical staff in preventing episodes of chest and abdominal trauma by paying close attention to hazardous field conditions and to natural objects that may pose a threat to the athlete during the preevent survey. As has been mentioned previously, delays in practice or competition may be warranted while waiting for field conditions to improve or hazardous areas to be repaired. In some competitive events, such as cross country or equestrian events, changing the route of the competition can reduce the risk of blunt or penetrating chest and abdominal injuries. Permanently installed equipment, such as goalposts and barriers surrounding the field of play, should be adequately secured and padded. Nonpermanent equipment should be removed from the field of play or practice area, or it should be secured behind field of play barriers. If this is not practical, adequate padding of equipment lockers and related equipment is appropriate.

Spectators at athletic practice or competition may represent an injury risk to athletes, and they may also be at risk of injury from the athlete. Removing nonparticipating players, support staff, and spectators from the field of play will reduce the dual risk of injury.

In severe cases of abdominal and chest trauma, the risk of mortality and morbidity is closely related to the ability of the medical team to expedite care and transport of the injured athlete to a trauma center. Preparation for practice or competition should involve a review of emergency procedures, equipment, and supplies. Review and even rehearsal of emergency medical service notification should include communication systems and access route security. Problems in accessing the field of play because of parking and spectator congestion may cause significant delays in transport at a time when every minute is critical.

When an incident of chest or abdominal trauma occurs, on-field assessment of the injury by the medical team should occur quickly. The importance of basic life support procedures cannot be overemphasized. Determination of the mechanism of injury, the force generated, the presence of penetrating versus blunt trauma, and the possible organ systems involved are important initial steps in assessing the injured athlete.

Especially in cases involving chest trauma, hypoxia is the most significant factor in morbidity. Consequently, assessment of airway, breathing, and circulation should be the initial component of the on-field assessment (see chapter 27). This primary survey begins with the assessment of the integrity of the athlete's airway. The team physician should listen immediately for the movement of air from the athlete's mouth and nose. The volume of air movement and the presence or absence of stridor will provide an immediate indication of the severity of the injury. If the initial survey determines that the athlete's airway is unstable, the emergency medical system (EMS) should be activated immediately. Management of the airway in an unconscious athlete should include an assumption that the athlete has sustained a catastrophic neck injury. Airway maintenance is established with jaw thrust maneuvers in which the neck remains immobilized. Head tilt maneuvers are inappropriate in an unconscious athlete. If the airway cannot be maintained with these basic maneuvers, progressively more aggressive interventions, including provisions for endotracheal intubation, should be initiated.

Further assessment of an athlete's respiratory status consists of ongoing observation of the breathing pattern. The severity of the injury can be determined by the amount of work that the athlete must expend to maintain adequate respiratory functions. The use of accessory sternal and abdominal muscles, an increasingly rapid respiratory rate, and progressively more shallow breaths are all indicators of deterioration in the athlete's breathing status.

The third basic component of the primary survey of the athlete who has sustained chest of abdominal injury is to assess the stability of the circulatory system. The athlete's pulse should be assessed with regard to pulse rate, quality, and regularity of rhythm. In determining the severity of any hemodynamic instability, utilizing examination techniques that include assessment of peripheral capillary refill is important. Deterioration in peripheral capillary refill is a much earlier and more valuable indicator of the athlete's circulatory status than is measurement of the blood pressure. Late indicators of shock, such as hypotension, may not be present in the early stages.

Immediately after a determination of the integrity of these vital systems, determining the absence of serious injury to the head and neck should follow.

If the initial assessment of the athlete with chest or abdominal trauma shows that he or she is hemodynamically stable and that no associated neurologic damage is present, a conservative approach is appropriate. The athlete should be removed from play and should be observed for any delayed or progressing signs of cardiorespiratory compromise or for any new or progressively severe chest or abdominal symptoms. The athlete should be maintained NPO (non per oral [nothing by mouth]) during this initial assessment period. If the athlete becomes or remains asymptomatic, he or she may be considered for immediate return to play as long as further close observation can be maintained. Communication with the athlete, parent, and medical and surgical support staff regarding the details of the injury and the importance of further observation is extremely crucial. Specifically, any deterioration in the athlete's cardiorespiratory or neurologic status should prompt immediate transport to an emergency medical facility. Any emesis; localized abdominal pain; progressive abdominal distention; or progressively severe back, shoulder, or chest pain should be considered warning signs of worsening or unsuspected internal injury. Over a period of days to weeks following an abdominal injury, the presence of fever, hematuria, vaginal bleeding or discharge, or compromise of the neurovascular status of the lower extremities should be thoroughly investigated.

If the initial on-field assessment of the injured athlete shows that the athlete's hemodynamic status is unstable, the EMS system should be activated. The athlete's craniovertebral integrity should be secured, and, immediately thereafter, his or her airway integrity should be assured. The athlete should remain NPO, and, if possible, vascular access should be obtained. The athlete with chest and/or abdominal trauma who is assessed as being hemodynamically unstable should be transported immediately to an emergency care facility, unless sophisticated medical care is available on site.

If the athlete has sustained penetrating trauma to the chest or abdomen, the EMS system should be activated immediately, and basic life support assessment and procedures should be initiated. In addition to maintaining the integrity of the athlete's airway and his or her craniovertebral stability, the athlete should remain NPO and should be kept as immobile as possible. In most cases of penetrating trauma in which an object is still present in the wound, current recommendations usually call for leaving the object in place. Parts of the object that are external to the wound can be shortened or removed as necessary to facilitate transport. Segments of the foreign object that remain in the wound should be secured firmly enough to prevent further tissue damage with movement.

Chest and abdominal trauma, in addition to head and neck trauma, require the highest degree of skill from a sports medicine team. The members of the medical team must be aware of the anatomy and the potential organs at risk in each incident of injury.

SUMMARY

Recognition of the risk of injury for a particular sport and the evaluation of the mechanism of injury should be included in a medical team's preparation for event coverage. Also, prior to an event, the team physician can provide valuable preventive medical care by assessing and modifying the risk of trauma from the field of play by examining field conditions and looking for potential objects of collision. Controlling the field of play in sports that use projectile objects reduces the risk of penetrating trauma. Also, prior to an event, the team physician should determine that all necessary equipment and support personnel, including EMS availability, are in place. If an injury occurs, the team physician should ensure that all basic life support emergency procedures are fol-

lowed and that craniovertebral integrity is maintained. Finally, communication with the athlete, the athlete's family, and other medical professionals is critical in assuring that appropriate follow-up is a component of the medical management plan.

REFERENCES

1. Sandelin J. Acute sports injuries requiring hospital care. *Br J Sports Med* 1986;20:99–102.
2. Davis J, Kuppermann N, Fleisher G. Serious sports injuries requiring hospitalization in a pediatric emergency department. *American Journal of Diseases of Children* 1993;147:1001–1004.
3. Watson A. Sports injuries during one academic year in 6799 Irish school children. *Am J Sports Med* 1984;12: 65–71.
4. United States Consumer Product Safety Commission. Injuries associated with soccer goalposts: United States, 1979–1993. *Mor Mortal Wkly Rep* 1994;43:153–155.
5. Atalar E, Acil T, Aytemir K, et al. Acute anterior myocardial infarction following a mild nonpenetrating chest trauma—a case report. *Angiology* 2001;52: 279–282.
6. American College of Surgeons. *Advanced trauma life support*, 6th ed. Chicago: American College of Surgeons, 1997.
7. Berqvist D, Hedelin H, Karlsson G, et al. Abdominal trauma during thirty years: analysis of a large case series. *Injury* 1981;13:93–99.

32

Shoulder Injuries

Robert Sallis and Ken Honsik

The upper extremity is the most commonly involved area for pediatric injury. This is even more true for throwing athletes.

This chapter discusses characteristics specific to pediatric shoulder injury, as well as essential components of the physical examination. Diagnosis and treatment of specific shoulder injuries, including pertinent radiologic findings, also are discussed.

BIOMECHANICS OF THROWING

Shoulder injuries commonly occur in sports that require throwing or other overhead motions.

The kinetic energy of the throwing motion is generated mainly in the legs and torso, and it is transferred through the arm to the ball. Injuries to the shoulder can occur with improper muscular generation of kinetic energy, incorrect transfer of energy through the shoulder and elbow to the ball, or inappropriate dissipation of energy that remains following release of the ball.

Four distinct phases in the throwing motion exist, and the pain occurring at each phase has a specific etiology (Fig. 32.1).

Cocking is the first phase of the throwing motion. In this phase, the shoulder is abducted to 90 degrees, hyperextended, and maximally externally rotated. Anterior subluxation may occur as the humeral head is forced forward during this phase. Anterior cuff tendinitis may occur secondary to irritation by the humeral head. Symptoms of dead arm syndrome typically occur during this phase, and they are often associated with anterior labral tear.

The acceleration phase occurs when the body strides forward and transfers its energy to the throwing arm. During this phase, the shoulder is rapidly internally rotated. Muscle strains involving the internal rotators (i.e., the subscapularis, latissimus, and pectoralis major) are commonly seen during this phase. Impingement syndrome resulting from the acceleration phase often produces symptoms as the supraspinatus rubs against the undersurface of the coracoacromial arch.

Release and deceleration constitute the third phase of the throwing motion. During this phase, posterior subluxation can occur as the humeral head is forced backwards via contraction of the rotator cuff muscles. Posterior cuff tendinitis may occur secondary to irritation by the humeral head. Additionally, the posterior

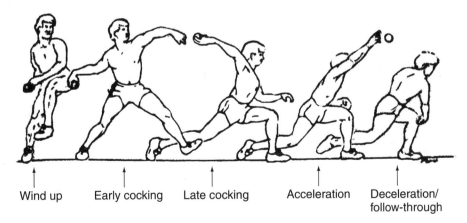

| Wind up | Early cocking | Late cocking | Acceleration | Deceleration/follow-through |

FIG. 32.1. Phases of the throw. (From Glousman R, Jobe F, Tibone J, et al. Dynamic EMG analysis of the throwing shoulder in glenohumeral instability. *J Bone Joint Surg Am* 1988;70:220, with permission.)

labrum and capsule may be damaged by repeated traction in this area.

The follow-through phase dissipates the remaining kinetic energy from the arm by sending it back through the body to the trailing leg. Muscle strains may occur with repeated concentric stress to the posterior shoulder. The teres minor and the long head of the triceps are most commonly involved.

CHARACTERISTICS UNIQUE TO THE YOUNG ATHLETE

For the purpose of this chapter, the pediatric population will be defined as those athletes who are skeletally immature. The presence of epiphyseal plates about the shoulder provides regions of lesser strength of the bone when compared to the adjacent capsule and ligaments. Therefore, injury is more likely to occur at the bony physis than at the ligament or capsule. Chronic microtrauma can also result in a stress-related injury to the growth plate. Injury of either type carries the risk of growth disturbance. Immature bone is more vascular and porous, and it has less mineral content than the mature bone. This plasticity allows for unique fracture patterns, such as greenstick fractures. Fortunately, the same characteristics that make immature bone more susceptible to injury also allow it to mend and remodel more quickly (2).

PHYSICAL EXAMINATION REVIEW

A good shoulder examination is essential for making the correct diagnosis in young athletes with shoulder injuries. Radiographs should be obtained before a thorough physical exam is conducted for any child who is reluctant to move his or her shoulder.

Observation

The physician should examine the athlete with both shoulders exposed. Useful information can be obtained by looking for asymmetry between the shoulders, atrophy, position, and swelling. This is an excellent technique for detecting fractures, dislocations, acromioclavicular separation, and rare congenital anomalies.

Range of Motion

Range of motion (ROM) should be assessed both actively and passively. It should include forward flexion, extension, abduction, external rotation, and internal rotation (Fig. 32.2). Decreased active ROM suggests a muscle, tendon, or nerve injury. Reduction of both active and passive ROM suggests a mechanical block, such as a labrum tear, adhesive capsulitis, or severe impingement.

Strength

Resisted strength testing should always be performed in comparison to the uninjured side. True weakness is suggestive of a rotator cuff tear. Pain with resisted rotator cuff testing is suggestive of tendonitis, while true weakness suggests a tear. The main mus-

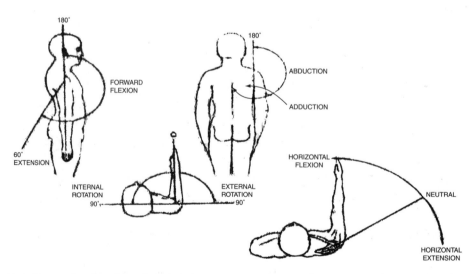

FIG. 32.2. Range of motion. (From Reid DC. *Sports injury assessment and rehabilitation.* London: Churchill Livingstone, 1992:897, with permission.)

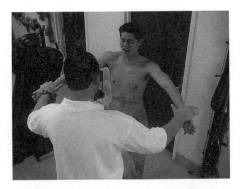

FIG. 32.3. Supraspinatus strength testing.

cles that should be assessed include the rotator cuff and biceps muscles. These are evaluated using the following tests:

- The *supraspinatus* is isolated by resisted abduction, with the arms positioned at 90 degrees abduction, slight forward flexion, and the thumbs pointing downward (Fig. 32.3).
- The *drop arm test* is useful for detecting a complete rotator cuff tear. It is performed by having the athlete attempt to lower his or her arm slowly from a fully abducted position. If the athlete's arm drops, a significant loss of rotator cuff function is likely.
- The *infraspinatus and teres minor* are external rotators. The patient should resist external rotation both with elbows at his or her sides and at 90 degrees of flexion for evaluation (Fig. 32.4).
- The *subscapularis* is responsible for internal rotation, and it can be isolated by instructing the athlete to resist internal rotation with elbows at 90 degrees of flexion (Fig. 32.5) or by having him or her attempt to push the hand away from the lower back against resistance. The second test is called the *push-off test* (Fig. 32.6).

- Biceps strength is assessed by asking the athlete to resist forward flexion with the shoulder at 90 degrees and the elbows extended. This is called the *Speed test*, and it can also be used to help detect biceps tendonitis (Fig. 32.7).

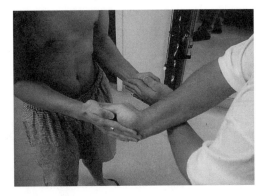

FIG. 32.5. Resisted internal rotation for subscapularis strength testing.

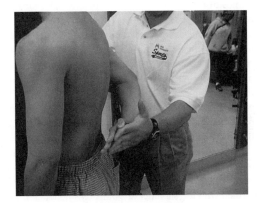

FIG. 32.6. Push-off test.

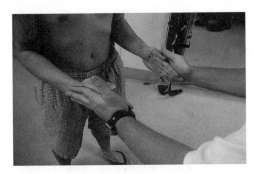

FIG. 32.4. Infraspinatus/teres minor strength testing.

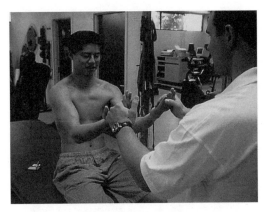

FIG. 32.7. Speed test.

Palpation

The shoulder joint and girdle (e.g., the clavicle, acromioclavicular joint, sternoclavicular joint, scapula, bicipital groove, proximal humerus, and subacromial space) should be palpated for areas of tenderness or deformity. Any step-off, deformity, or bony point tenderness should be evaluated radiographically.

Specific Tests

Numerous tests are of use for detecting specific pathology, such as impingement, acromioclavicular dysfunction, instability, labrum tears, and scapular dyskinesis.

With the *Neer sign*, the shoulder is forward flexed (up to 180 degrees) by the examiner (Fig. 32.8) . If the patient experiences discomfort at the upper ROM, the test is considered positive for impingement.

The *Hawkins impingement sign* is performed at 90 degrees abduction, 45 degrees forward flexion and the elbow flexed at 90 degrees. The examiner then internally and externally rotates shoulder to the extremes of motion (Fig. 32.9). A positive test for impingement is eliciting pain at either extreme.

The *impingement test* is an extremely useful diagnostic tool for determining if a limited ROM is mechanical or secondary to pain resulting from impingement. Lidocaine without epinephrine is injected into the subacromial bursa. If ROM and strength significantly improve following the injection, impingement or rotator cuff tendonitis is more likely to be the cause of the symptoms (Fig. 32.10).

The *crossover test* can be used to detect impingement, but it is most useful in determining whether acromioclavicular pathology is present. The test is performed with the shoulder at 90 degrees abduction, inclding horizontal adduction. The elbow is then pushed

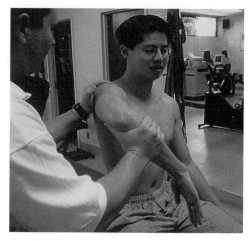

FIG. 32.9. Hawkins impingement sign.

medially toward the chin (Fig. 32.11). The test is positive if pain is elicited. If other signs of impingement are negative and crossover is positive, the clinician should consider the possibility of injury to the acromioclavicular (AC) joint.

Instability tests include the apprehension sign, relocation test, load and shift test, and sulcus sign.

The *apprehension sign* places the patient's shoulder at 90 degrees abduction and 90 degrees external rotation. The examiner places forward pressure behind the shoulder and rearward pressure on the elbow and forearm (Fig. 32.12). If the athlete feels as if his or her shoulder is going to dislocate or "pop out," then the test is positive.

During the *relocation test* (Fowler sign), the patient's arm is placed in the same position as the apprehension test, except the patient is supine. Down-

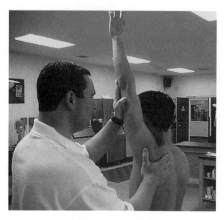

FIG. 32.8. Neer sign.

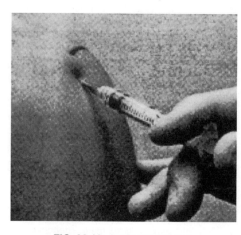

FIG. 32.10. Impingement test.

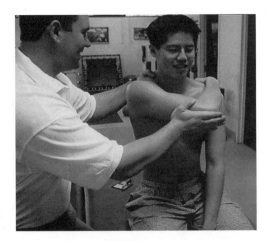

FIG. 32.11. Crossover test.

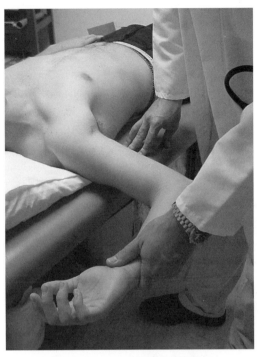

FIG. 32.13. Relocation test (step 1).

ward force (external rotation) is applied on the forearm until apprehension is achieved (Fig. 32.13). Downward pressure is then simultaneously applied to the anterior shoulder and humeral head (Fig. 32.14) . If the patient's apprehension is alleviated, the test is positive for anterior instability.

In performing the *load and shift test*, the examiner grasps the proximal humeral head and exerts alternating anterior and posterior force while stabilizing the scapula (Fig. 32.15). Laxity is present if increased anterior and/or posterior translation of the humeral head occurs in comparison to the opposite shoulder. In cases of extreme laxity, the examiner may be able to sublux the humeral head anteriorly.

To execute a *sulcus sign*, the examiner grasps both wrists or elbows of the athlete and pulls down while simultaneously observing for an asymmetric sulcus or divot below the acromion above the lateral deltoid (Fig. 32.16). These suggest inferior laxity of the joint capsule.

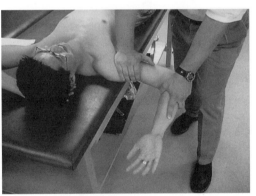

FIG. 32.14. Relocation test (step 2).

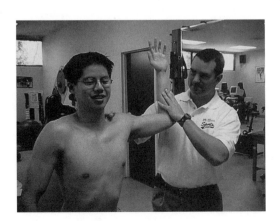

FIG. 32.12. Apprehension test.

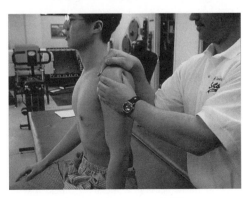

FIG. 32.15. Load and shift.

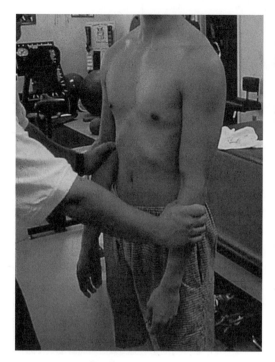

FIG. 32.16. Sulcus sign.

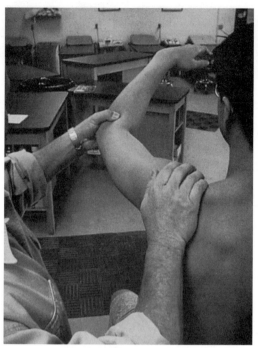

FIG. 32.17. Clunk test.

The *clunk test* is commonly used to determine *labrum* injury. Gentle axial compression is applied to the humerus by placing one hand posterior to the humeral head and using the other hand to apply pressure and keep the elbow at 90 degrees of flexion. The humerus is slowly brought through a full circumduction (Fig. 32.17). A clunk or mechanical stop may indicate a labral tear. The presence or absence of a physical finding should be compared to the opposite shoulder.

Proper *scapular motion* is of particular importance to throwing athletes, in whom it should be evaluated.

Scapular winging is demonstrated by having the athlete push against a wall with his or her arms extended (Fig. 32.18). If one scapula is more prominent, weak serratus anterior and scapular stabilizer muscles should be suspected. This may be related to long thoracic nerve injury.

Scapular excursion measurements are made from each scapular apex to the spine. They are first done with the scapula at rest (Fig. 32.19) and then in abduction (Fig. 32.20). Greater scapular excursion, when compared to the other side, may indicate poor scapular stability. This is important to the biomechanics of the throw because scapular weakness may lead to other more distal arm problems.

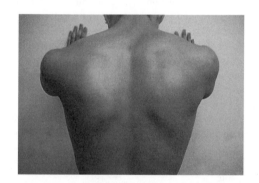

FIG. 32.18. Test for scapular winging (normal example).

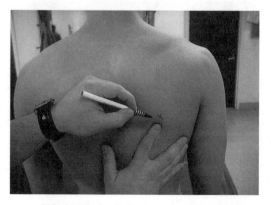

FIG. 32.19. Scapular excursion (at rest).

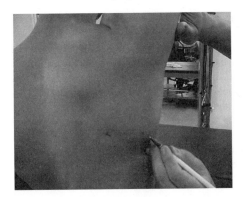

FIG. 32.20. Scapular excursion (in abduction).

Radiographs

Because of the presence of growth plates, obtaining comparison views is useful if a fracture is suspected. The most commonly useful views include the following:

True anterior–posterior (AP) view: useful for evaluating growth plates and for viewing humeral neck fractures.

Y-view (Fig. 32.21): excellent for determining position of the humeral head in relation to the glenoid. this view is useful if traumatic dislocation is suspected.

Outlet view (Fig. 32.22): similar to the Y-view, but useful in cases of chronic impingement to detect subacromial spurring or to characterize acromion

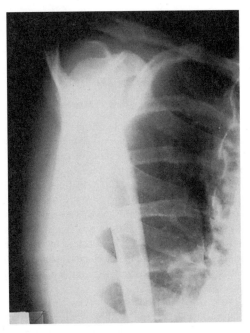

FIG. 32.22. Normal outlet view.

shape. A hooked or beaked acromion will increase the likelihood of impingement.

Axillary view (Fig. 32.23): useful for detecting acute dislocation and evidence of chronic recurrent dislocation (i.e., Hill–Sacks lesion and bony Bankart lesion). The Hill–Sacks lesion appears as a divot in the posterior humerus. This is formed by the repetitive impact of the posterior humerus onto the anterior glenoid during dislocation. The bony Bankart lesion is an avulsion or chip fracture of the anterior glenoid, created when the humeral head initially displaces anteriorly or when the posterior humeral head recoils back upon the anterior glenoid, as described above for the Hill–Sacks lesion.

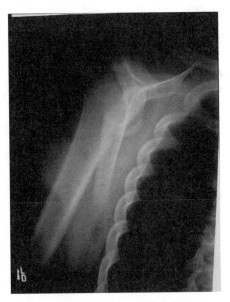

FIG. 32.21. Normal Y-view.

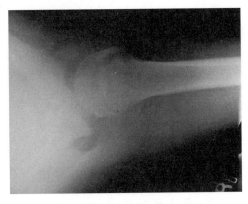

FIG. 32.23. Normal axillary view.

Clavicle views (*if injury is suspected*): taken at a cephalad angle. Recent studies suggest that weighted views rarely direct a change in management (3).

CLAVICLE INJURIES

Clavicular Shaft Fractures

The most common clavicle fracture is through the midshaft (diaphysis) of the bone. The majority of these injuries were commonly thought to be caused by indirect trauma (fall on outstretched hand), but recent reports suggest direct trauma as the chief mechanism of injury (4,5). The clavicle forms an S-shaped curve that is convex anterior proximally and concave anterior distally. The junction between these two curves is a relatively weak spot, particularly to axial loading. This may explain why fractures are more common at this site (6). Indirect trauma is more likely to result in a greenstick fracture to the midshaft.

If any athlete has fractured the clavicle, he or she will present with pain and swelling over the midportion of the clavicle and reluctance to move the affected shoulder. If a fracture is suspected, clavicle views should be obtained. In a complete fracture (Fig. 32.24), the distal end of the clavicle will more likely be displaced inferiorly, secondary to the weight of the arm, while the proximal clavicle can be displaced superiorly by the strong pull of the sternocleidomastoid muscle.

Initially, the clinician should examine the skin over the clavicle closely for neurovascular compromise or evidence of open fracture. Radiographs should then be obtained. If a fracture is present, the patient should be placed in a figure-of-eight brace or arm sling.

The figure-of-eight brace or sling should be continued for 3 to 6 weeks to allow healing in children and for 6 to 12 weeks in older adolescents. Follow-up should occur every 2 to 3 weeks, and the radiograph should be repeated at 6 weeks or once the clavicle is clinically healed. The athlete may use his or her arm for daily activities, as pain permits. The parents should be informed about the likelihood of a bump or bony deformity, which may take 6 to 12 months to remodel or which can be permanent. Athletes should avoid contact sports for at least 6 months after clinical and radiographic healing. A return may be considered in 2 to 4 months for sports like basketball, baseball, and soccer.

Orthopedic consults should be obtained for open fractures, neurovascular compromise of soft tissues, nonunion after 12 weeks, or improved cosmetic result (elective).

Distal Clavicle Injuries

Distal clavicle fractures are difficult to distinguish from true acromioclavicular separations. These injuries are most commonly caused by a fall on the point of the shoulder (common in horseback riding). Children who are less than 13 years old are more likely to fracture the distal end of the clavicle because of the comparatively high strength of the acromiocoracoid clavicular ligament complex. The ligament complex typically remains intact, while the distal clavicle herniates through the superior potion of the periosteal sheath. Curtis (5) and Rockwood and Green (7) have described six types of distal clavicle fractures and/or pseudodislocations (Fig. 32.25).

Types I to III can be treated conservatively with good results and full return of function. Types IV to VI

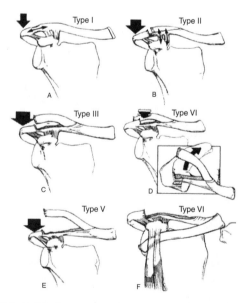

FIG. 32.25. Distal clavicle fracture and/or dislocations. (From Rockwood CA, Green DP, eds. *Fractures in children*, 2nd ed. Philadelphia: JB Lippincott Co, 1984, with permission.)

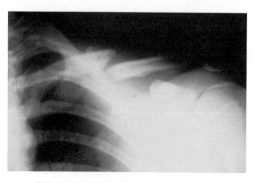

FIG. 32.24. Midshaft clavicular fracture.

are typically treated surgically with open reduction and fixation for increased stability and cosmetic results. Conservative management consists of initial immobilization with a shoulder sling, followed by progressive ROM exercises and strengthening. These injuries take 4 to 6 weeks to heal and return to full function. The athlete is allowed to return to sports once his or her strength and full and painless ROM have returned.

True acromioclavicular dislocation or separations may occur in children older than 13 years. These injuries are classified in a manner similar to the Rockwood and Green diagram (Fig. 32.25), but they often represent disruption of the AC-coracoacromial (CC) ligament complex rather than fracture. Types I to III are managed conservatively over 4 to 6 weeks, while Types IV to VI usually require an orthopedic consult for possible surgical management.

Proximal Clavicle Injuries

Injuries to the medial end of the clavicle are rare. The typical force causing this injury is indirect. The epiphysis usually does not ossify until 18 years of age, and it does not fuse until 25 years of age. For this reason, these injuries mimic lateral clavicular fracture and dislocations. The shaft will usually rip through the periosteal sheath, migrate superior, and deviate either anterior or posterior. The athlete will present with pain and swelling over the sternoclavicular joint. A cephalad and/or apical radiographic view may detect asymmetry in position (the serendipity view). The best test for detection and description is a computerized tomography scan.

Anterior displacement is unstable initially, but it usually heals well by callus and modeling. Posterior displacement may require open reduction under general anesthesia for possible impingement upon the trachea. Both injuries are treated for approximately 4 to 6 weeks with a figure-of-eight brace (8). Because of instability and the potential for complication, an orthopedic surgeon manages most medial clavicle fractures or dislocations.

PROXIMAL HUMERAL HEAD FRACTURES

In the pediatric population, shoulder trauma will likely result in a fracture of the proximal humeral head before it causes glenohumeral dislocation. The following three main types of fractures occur in children at distinct age groupings:

Salter I fractures occur predominantly in children 5 years old and younger. In these patients, the possibility of abuse also should be considered, and a thorough exam should be performed. Because 80%

of growth is provided by the proximal physis, excellent healing is rapidly achieved with 2 to 3 weeks of immobilization.

Metaphyseal fractures typically occur in children between the ages of 5 to 10 years, presumably due to thinning of the metaphyseal cortex from rapid growth. Most fractures do not require reduction. Because of the large amount of remodeling that occurs at this age, even a bayonet apposition—complete displacement of the fracture fragments with overlap (Fig. 32.26)—is expected to heal well in children up to 10 to 12 years old. Closed reduction is required if the distal fragment of the humerus is embedded in the deltoid, if angulation deformity is greater than 50 degrees, or if a bayonet apposition occurs in a patient older than 12 years of age (9).

Salter II fractures are generally not seen until after 11 years of age. The fracture displaces anteriorly because of the anterior periosteum, which is thin in comparison to the relatively dense and strong posterior sheath. These fractures heal well without reduction if angulation is less than 35 degrees and if displacement is less than 50%. If greater deformity exists in a child older than 11 years of age, closed reduction with possible percutaneous pin fixation is recommended (Fig. 32.27) (9).

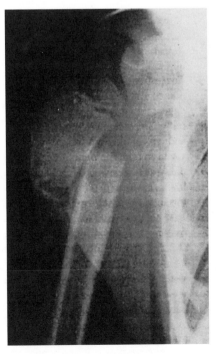

FIG. 32.26. Proximal humeral head fracture (metaphyseal–bayonet type).

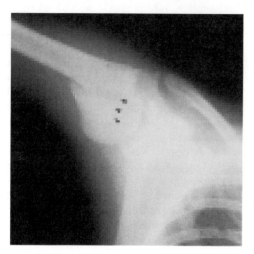

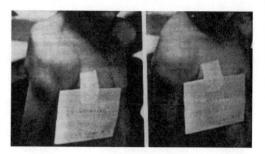

FIG. 32.28. Glenohumeral dislocation. (From Curtis RJ Jr. Anatomy, biomechanics and physiology: shoulder injuries. In: Stanitski CL, ed. *Pediatric and adolescent sports medicine*. Philadelphia: WB Saunders, 1994:183–190, with permission.)

FIG. 32.27. Salter II fracture of the proximal humeral head. (From Ryu RKN, Fan RSP. Adolescent and pediatric sports injuries: pediatric surgery for the primary care pediatrician (part 2). *Pediatr Clin North Am* 1998;45:1601–1635, with permission.)

PROXIMAL HUMERAL EPIPHYSITIS ("LITTLE LEAGUER SHOULDER")

Proximal humeral epiphysitis, or "Little Leaguer shoulder," which is seen in adolescents involved in overhead throwing sports—most commonly in high performance male pitchers (11 to 13 years old)—is a stress injury to the growth plate of the proximal humerus (rotational stress). The athlete presents with complaints of pain localized to the proximal humerus during the act of throwing or serving. Weakness, swelling, and limited ROM are usually absent. Widening of the proximal physis compared to the unaffected side on external and internal rotation views helps to confirm the diagnosis. The treatment for this injury is rest from activity for at least 3 months. Physical therapy and strengthening exercises during this time are not suggested, as they may worsen symptoms. If the athlete is asymptomatic after 3 months of rest, he or she may begin an extremely gradual, supervised return-to-throwing program. Radiographic healing may lag behind clinical healing, and it should not be used as a criteria for return to play (2,10). The early development of proper fundamentals and control, rather than stressing the importance of velocity, is preventive.

GLENOHUMERAL DISLOCATION

Shoulder dislocations can occur in the young athlete involved in contact or collision sports, and they result from a collision with an opponent that forces the shoulder into abduction and external rotation or from a fall on an outstretched hand. The majority of shoulder dislocations are anterior. With an anterior dislocation, the humeral head is forced anteriorly and inferiorly to the glenoid (Fig. 32.28).

Symptoms include pain and the sensation of the shoulder being "out of joint." On examination, an obvious deformity will be seen at the glenohumeral joint, with the shoulder appearing flattened, instead of rounded, in the deltoid area. The arm is generally held slightly abducted and internally rotated, and it is often supported by the opposite hand. Limited ROM prevents touching the uninvolved shoulder with the finger of the involved arm. The physical examination incorporates a check of neurovascular status, including pulses in the wrist and sensation in the deltoid area (i.e., axillary nerve injury).

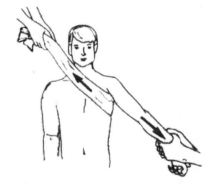

FIG. 32.29. Traction–countertraction technique. (From Curtis RJ Jr. Anatomy, biomechanics and physiology: shoulder injuries. In: Stanitski CL, ed. *Pediatric and adolescent sports medicine*. Philadelphia: WB Saunders, 1994:183–190, with permission.)

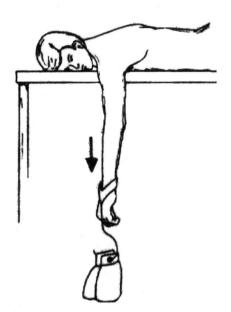

FIG. 32.30. Stimson technique (From Curtis RJ Jr. Anatomy, biomechanics and physiology: shoulder injuries. In: Stanitski CL, ed. *Pediatric and adolescent sports medicine.* Philadelphia: WB Saunders, 1994:183–190, with permission.)

Glenohumeral instability is a frequent cause of shoulder problems, and it often coexists with rotator cuff injury, impingement, and glenoid labrum injury.

The pathophysiology of shoulder instability that leads to shoulder pain typically follows a stepwise pattern. Repeated overhead motions can stretch the static restraints (capsule and glenohumeral ligaments). The dynamic stabilizers (rotator cuff muscles) are then forced to increase activity to compensate for the loss of stability provided by the static stabilizers. As the dynamic stabilizers fatigue, subluxation occurs, leading to increased translation of the humeral head, which, in turn, irritates the rotator cuff tendons, labrum, and glenoid.

Shoulder laxity can be caused by repetitive microtrauma, as noted above, or following a macrotraumatic event, such as shoulder dislocation. "TUBS" and "AMBRI," which are defined below, are useful mnemonics for describing the characteristics of traumatic and atraumatic shoulder dislocations.

TUBS	AMBRI
*T*rauma	*A*traumatic
*U*nilateral	*M*ultidirectional
*B*ankart	*B*ilateral
*S*urgery	*R*ehabilitation
	*I*nferior capsular tightening

Treatment begins with closed reduction, which is usually easily achieved in young athletes. A variety of maneuvers can be used to relocate a dislocated shoulder (e.g., traction–countertraction [Fig. 32.29] and Stimson [Fig. 32.30]). Postreduction care is relatively controversial. Most clinicians agree that, with a first time anterior dislocation, a 3-week to 4-week period of immobilization, followed by an aggressive rehabilitation program, is appropriate. Recurrence is extremely common (approaching 90%). For this reason, surgical treatment is commonly recommended for first time dislocators who are active in sports. Athletes who have a second dislocation should be considered for surgical treatment to prevent recurrence.

SHOULDER INSTABILITY

The shoulder is a highly mobile joint with a delicate balance that must be maintained between the tremendous mobility and adequate stability. The normal degree of glenohumeral translation typically is increased in young athletes (e.g., throwers or swimmers) who use repetitive overhead motions. Occasionally, this laxity may be increased to the point where these athletes develop instability, which is defined as symptomatic translation (i.e., subluxation or dislocation).

Patients with shoulder instability often present with extremely subtle symptoms. They may describe their shoulder feeling "loose" or may say that it feels as though it "slips out." More commonly, patients with shoulder instability present with other problems, such as rotator cuff or labrum injuries. Examination findings in a patient with shoulder instability include a positive apprehension sign and relocation test. Patients who have very lax shoulders may develop inferior instability, which is demonstrated by the presence of a sulcus sign. Improvement in patient discomfort during the relocation test suggests anterior instability, while worsening may suggest the presence of primary impingement.

Treatment of shoulder instability begins with managing any associated tendinitis, impingement, or labrum injury. The rehabilitation program focuses on strengthening the rotator cuff, as well as on flexibility exercises. In general, those who demonstrate anterior subluxation tend to have weakness of the internal rotators and a loss of external rotational flexibility. Those with posterior subluxation tend toward weakness of the external rotators and a loss of internal rotational flexibility. Rehabilitation should focus on correcting these deficits in patients with shoulder instability.

ROTATOR CUFF INJURIES

Rotator Cuff Tendinitis

In the young athlete, rotator cuff tendonitis typically is related to overuse. The presence of glenohumeral instability and certain anatomic factors (e.g., the shape of the acromion or prior injuries to the bone or soft tissue) can contribute to the development of this condition. Radiographs (e.g., outlet or Y-view) may be done to help confirm this. Athletes with type III acromions are at higher risk for developing rotator cuff problems (Fig. 32.31).

Symptoms of rotator cuff tendinitis typically begin with pain that occurs while the athlete is throwing or is involved in other repetitive overhead activities. This pain tends to improve with rest and to worsen with increased activity. Athletes also may complain of early fatigue or a loss of pitching control. Resisted rotator cuff motion, which most commonly includes the supraspinatus tendon, produces pain. The infraspinatus, teres minor, subscapularis, and biceps tendons may also be involved. Rotator cuff tendonitis generally responds well to conservative management, most importantly rest. The throwing athlete should consider having his or her technique reevaluated by an experienced coach as minor adjustments might help prevent reoccurrence.

Impingement Syndrome

Impingement occurs when the rotator cuff and biceps tendons are pinched underneath the acromion and coracoacromial ligament. Trauma to the acromion or AC joint can also narrow the space that accommodates the rotator cuff tendons.

Pain that worsens with overhead activity (e.g., combing hair) is a symptom of impingement. Furthermore, patients will have symptoms suggestive of rotator cuff and/or biceps tendinitis. On examination, these patients will have a painful arc, typically between 80 and 120 degrees of abduction, and pain with resisted rotator cuff motion, most commonly with supraspinatus and biceps motions. Impingement signs (e.g., Neer's test, Hawkins test, and the crossover test) help confirm the diagnosis. The **impingement test** is rarely used in the pediatric athlete secondary to the rarity of significant injury, and it should be considered only in the older adolescent.

In the young athlete (< 25 years of age), stage I impingement is by far the most common, and stages II and III are rarely seen. Edema, hemorrhage, and inflammation in the rotator cuff tendons, all of which are reversible with rest and conservative management, are present with stage I. Stages II and III involve irreversible changes to the tendons and surrounding tissues, and they are rarely seen in athletes who are less than 25 years of age.

Rotator cuff tendonitis and stage I impingement are quite difficult to differentiate in the young athlete. Fortunately, they both respond equally well to conservative management, including rest, a modification of the throwing technique, and a correction of underlying instability, if present.

Rotator Cuff Tear

Rotator cuff tears are rarely seen in the young athlete. Tears are most commonly related to chronic rotator cuff tendinitis and impingement seen in adult athletes. In the young athlete, a tear may be related to a specific traumatic episode or dislocation. On examination, patients with a rotator cuff tear exhibit true weakness of the rotator cuff.

The treatment of rotator cuff injuries is accomplished in a stepwise fashion. The cornerstone of treatment is rest from repetitive overhead shoulder motion, which aggravates the injury, and a restriction of ROM to below the horizontal plane of motion. Icing and nonsteroidal antiinflammatory medications can help relieve the symptoms. Once the pain has resolved, a ROM program should be started. Flexibility exercises should be used to help the athlete regain full ROM. Once full motion is achieved, a strengthening program that focuses on the rotator cuff muscles can be started. Following restoration of strength and flexibility, a graduated throwing program that gradually increases the intensity and frequency of throwing motions until the patient has returned to full throwing, can be initiated as Fig. 32.32 demonstrates. In a nonthrowing athlete, a similar graduated progression to full activity can be used. Corticosteroids can be injected into the subacromial bursa if patients are not responding to conservative measures after 1 to 2 months. Surgery should be considered only for chronic impingement or large rotator cuff tears.

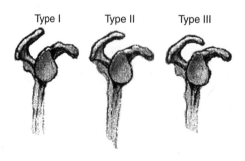

Type I   Type II   Type III

FIG. 32.31. Acromion types.

Return to Throwing Program

Returning to throwing after an injury or surgery requires correct rehabilitation of the shoulder including stretching and strengthening. Throwing requires the transfer of energy from the body though the shoulder, elbow, wrist, and hand to the ball. The entire body must be prepared to throw.

Mechanics of throwing must be evaluated by a coach or trainer to aid in return to throwing and decrease chance of reinjury.

Step	Warm up	25 throws	Rest/Warm up	25 throws	Rest/Warm up	25 throws
1	30 ft toss	45 ft	15 min/30 ft toss	45 ft		
2	30 ft toss	45 ft	10 min/30 ft toss	45 ft	10 min/30 ft toss	45 ft
3	30 ft toss	60 ft	15 min/toss	60 ft		
4	30 ft toss	60 ft	10 min/toss	60 ft	10 min	60 ft
5	30 ft toss	90 ft	15 min/toss	90 ft		
6	30 ft toss	90 ft	10 min/toss	90 ft	10 min/toss	90 ft
7	30 ft toss	120 ft	15 min/toss	120 ft		
8	30 ft toss	120 ft	10 min/toss	120 ft	10 min/toss	120 ft
9	30 ft toss	150 ft	15 min/toss	150 ft		
10	30 ft toss	150 ft	10 min/toss	150 ft	10 min/toss	150 ft
11	30 ft toss	180 ft	15 min/toss	150 ft		
12	30 ft toss	180 ft	10 min/toss	180 ft	10 min/toss	180 ft
13	30 ft toss	180 ft	10 min/toss	180 ft	10 min/toss	180 ft (repeat)
14	toss	Return to mound or position				

Pitcher off the mound Program

Stage 1 – Fastball only

Step 1   Interval throw (120 ft phase above)
15 throws at 50%

Step 2   Interval throw (120 ft phase above)
30 throws at 50%

Step 3   Warm up
45 throws at 50%

Step 4   Interval throw (120 ft phase above)
60 throws at 50%

Step 5   Interval throw (120 ft phase above)
30 throws at 75%

Step 6   30 throws at 75%
45 throws at 50%

Step 7   45 throws at 75%
15 throws at 50%

Step 8   60 throws at 75%

Step 9   45 throws at 75%
15 throws at batting practice

Step 10   45 throws at 75%
30 throws at batting practice

Step 11   45 throws at 75%
45 throws at batting practice

Stage 2

Step 12   30 throws at 75%
15 throws breaking balls
45 fast balls only at batting practice

Step 13   30 throws at 75%
30 breaking balls
30 batting practice

Step 14   Simulated game
progress by 15 throws per workout

FIG. 32.32. Program for returning to throwing.

GLENOID LABRUM INJURIES

Injury to the glenoid labrum is seen less commonly in young athletes. It typically occurs after direct or indirect trauma, as in the case of shoulder dislocation. Additionally, glenoid labrum injuries can occur following recurrent anterior and posterior humeral head translation during the throwing motion when instability is present.

Symptoms of a labrum injury include pain with overhead activity that is often associated with a painful clicking or snapping in the shoulder. Symptoms are often worse during the cocking or follow-through phases of a throwing motion. On examination, patients with glenoid labrum injuries often have tenderness over the glenohumeral joint line. A positive clunk test, which takes the shoulders through the full range of motion, suggests a torn labrum.

Treatment of glenoid labrum injuries begins with conservative measures, including rest, ice, and nonsteroidal antiinflammatory medications. Recurrent instability should be corrected with an appropriate rehabilitation program, as was outlined previously. Surgery (e.g., arthroscopic debridement) may be needed if the athlete does not respond to conservative treatment.

DEAD ARM SYNDROME

Dead arm syndrome is relatively rare in the younger athlete. Typically, it is associated with anterior instability and a torn anterior labrum, probably as the result of subluxation of the humeral head, which causes a transient stretch to the brachial plexus during a hard throw. Symptoms of dead arm syndrome include a sudden paralyzing pain and numbness that radiates down the arm and that is typically noted during the cocking phase of a hard throw. It is often followed by a lingering feeling of weakness about the shoulder. Examination findings suggest a labral tear and anterior cuff tendonitis, as were previously described. Treatment includes physical therapy similar to that outlined for shoulder instability and labrum injuries. Surgery may be needed to correct the instability, as well as to repair injuries to the glenoid labrum.

RETURN TO PLAY

Shoulder problems commonly recur when athletes return to play too quickly. An athlete should rest the shoulder from activity until it is pain free, and he or she may then begin rehabilitation exercises as pain allows. Emphasis should be placed first on the return of full ROM and flexibility before beginning strengthening exercises. Throwers begin a structured return-to-throw program once they are pain free. The program gradually increases both the number and intensity of throws. Progressions are made each day only if the athlete remains pain free. Pitchers may begin a return-to-mound program with increasing levels of intensity only after the basic return-to-throw program has been successfully completed. In general, the longer a player has had a painful shoulder, the longer the safe return to full competition will take.

PREVENTION

The best way to treat pediatric shoulder injuries is prevention. This is accomplished through solid coaching and through the promotion of healthy competitive attitudes. Providing an athlete with good fundamentals and mechanics before emphasizing speed, power, and aggressiveness will give him or her a solid base for allowing skills to mature in a controlled and effective manner. Emphasis should always be on a gradual progression of activities in order to avoid overuse injury. For instance, the early pitching emphasis should be on the mastery of proper throwing mechanics and control, followed by off-speed pitches (change-up) and, finally, by breaking pitches (curves, sliders, etc.). Protective gear, when appropriate, should be made available, its use should be encouraged, and a proper fit should be ensured. Coaches and parents should also consider preparticipation shoulder rehabilitation exercises (e.g., rotator cuff strengthening and flexibility) for highly competitive athletes, especially if the athlete has had a history of shoulder problems.

CONSULTATION

Primary care physicians can effectively diagnosis and manage the vast majority of pediatric shoulder problems. Referral for physical therapy is often helpful to guide rehabilitation, while orthopedic referral is needed for complicated fractures and surgical treatment in cases that have not responded to conservative measures.

SUMMARY

Pediatric shoulder injuries can be difficult to decipher, and the primary care physician is often faced with the daunting task of being the first provider to evaluate these problems. Fortunately, most injuries unfold into manageable scenarios when the clinician uses a systematic approach that combines a thorough history and physical examination with appropriate radiographic tests and provides a sports medicine or orthopedic referral when they are needed.

REFERENCES

1. Landin LA. Fracture patterns in children. Analysis of 8,682 fractures with special reference to incidence, etiology and secular changes in a Swedish urban population 1950-1979. *Acta Orthop Scand* 1983;202:1–109.
2. Paterson PD, Waters PM. Shoulder injuries in the childhood athlete: pediatric and adolescent sports injuries. *Clin Sports Med* 2000;19:681–692.
3. Yapp JJL, Curl LA, Kvitne RS. The value of weighted views of the acromioclavicular joint: results of a survey. *Am J Sports Med* 1999;27:806–809.
4. Stanley D, Trowbridge EA, Norris SH. The mechanism of clavicular fractures: a clinical and biomechanical analysis. *J Bone Joint Surg Br* 1998;70:461–464.
5. Curtis RJ Jr. Anatomy, biomechanics and physiology: shoulder injuries. In: Stanitski CL, ed. *Pediatric and adolescent sports medicine*. Philadelphia: WB Saunders, 1994:183–190.
6. Eiff MP. *Fracture management for primary care*. Philadelphia: WB Saunders, 1998:115–42,251–271.
7. Rockwood CA, Green DP, eds. *Fractures in children*, 2nd ed. Philadelphia: JB Lippincott Co, 1984.
8. Barnes DA. Fractures of the clavicle. In: Pizzutillo PD, ed. *Pediatric orthopaedics in primary practice*. New York: McGraw-Hill, 1997:3–7.
9. Devito D. Management of fractures and their complications. In: Morrissy RT, ed. *Lovell and Winter's pediatric orthopaedics*. Philadelphia: Lippincott-Raven, 1996: 1236–1240.
10. Carson WG Jr, Gasser SI. Little Leaguer's shoulder. A report on 23 cases. *Am J Sports Med* 1998;26:575–580.

33

Elbow Injuries

Joel L. Shaw and Francis G. O'Connor

As involvement in organized sports has increased in recent years, the frequency of sports-related injuries, including elbow injuries, has similarly increased. Unfortunately, the elbow tends to receive less attention in training than do the shoulder and hand. Because of its position in the axis of the central portion of the upper extremity, it is prone to and has the potential for multiple traumatic and overuse injuries (Tables 33.1 and 33.2). Elbow injuries are especially common in baseball players, but injuries to this structure can be seen in all types of athletic activity, including gymnastics, wrestling, and football. In one study that followed 172 baseball pitchers between the ages of 9 to 12 years, the incidence of elbow injuries requiring treatment over a 1-year period was about 40% (1). This chapter focuses on the diagnosis and management of common elbow injuries that are encountered by primary care physicians.

FUNCTIONAL ANATOMY

Osseous Anatomy

Three bones come together at the elbow to form the three articulations that provide both static and functional stability at the elbow joint (Fig. 33.1). The distal humerus is formed by two condyles, the trochlea and the capitellum, thus creating the articular surfaces of the humerus. The distal end of the humerus joins with the proximal ends of the radius and ulna to form the elbow joint. The trochlea, or medial condyle, is grooved, and it articulates with the semilunar notch of the ulna to form the humeroulnar joint. They form a modified hinge joint that remains in contact through all degrees of flexion but that is most stable at less than 20 degrees or greater than 120 degrees. This joint allows flexion and extension. The radial head articulates with the capitellum, or lateral condyle, which is spherical, to form a combination hinge and pivot joint, the humeroradial joint. This joint is responsible both for flexion and extension movement and for axial rotation of the forearm. Finally, the ra-

dial head articulates with the lesser sigmoid notch of the ulna to form the radioulnar joint, which also allows axial rotation or pronation and supination. With these joints, the elbow is able to move from 0 to 135 degrees of flexion and with 75 to 80 degrees of pronation and supination. The bony structures provide about 50% of elbow stability, with the ligamentous structures supplying the remainder (2).

Soft Tissue Anatomy

Four major muscle activities are performed by separate muscle groups at the elbow. The biceps brachii, brachioradialis, and brachialis muscles perform flexion. Extension utilizes the triceps and anconeus muscles. The supinator and biceps brachii perform supination. Finally, pronation combines the activities of the pronator quadratus, pronator teres, and flexor carpi radialis muscles (3).

Three main nerve branches pass through the elbow joint. The median nerve runs along the anterior side of the elbow just medial to the biceps tendon and the brachial artery. It travels between the two heads of the pronator teres, and, at this point, the nerve is at risk for entrapment injuries. It innervates the muscles responsible for pronation of the elbow. The ulnar nerve travels along the medial side of the arm posterior to the medial epicondyle and through the cubital tunnel, and it finally enters the flexor carpi ulnaris. The cubital tunnel is its most likely site for compression. The radial nerve travels along the lateral side of the elbow. It passes anterior to the lateral epicondyle and divides into the superficial branch (sensory) and the deep branch (motor) of the radial nerve. The proximal edge of the supinator muscle forms the arcade of Frohse, through which the deep branch travels and the site at which it is most likely to be injured (4).

The ligament complexes of the elbow serve to reinforce the osseous stability. The two main ligaments are the medial collateral ligament (MCL) complex and the lateral collateral ligament (LCL) complex

TABLE 33.1. *Traumatic injuries*

Medial	Lateral	Posterior
Medial epicondylar fracture Supracondylar fracture	Lateral epicondylar fracture Capitellum fracture Radial head fracture Radial head subluxation	Elbow dislocation Olecranon fracture

TABLE 33.2. *Overuse injuries*

Medial	Lateral	Posterior	Anterior
Medial epicondylar stress lesion	Radiocapitellar compression syndrome Osteochondritis dissecans Panner disease	Olecranon impingement syndrome Olecranon apophysitis Triceps tendinitis	Forearm splints

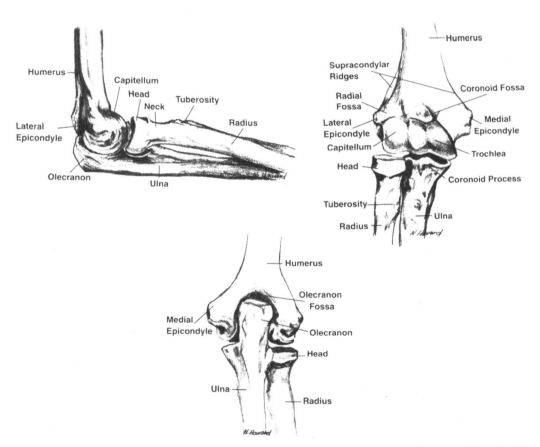

FIG. 33.1. Bones of the elbow. (From O'Connor FG, Olivierre CO, Nirschl RP. Elbow and forearm injuries. In: Lillegard WA, Butcher JD, Rucker KS, eds. *Handbook of sports medicine: a symptom-oriented approach*, 2nd ed. Boston: Butterworth-Heinemann, 1999:141–157, with permission.)

(Fig. 33.2). These ligaments are formed by thickenings of the elbow capsule.

The MCL complex is formed by the anterior MCL, the posterior MCL, and the transverse MCL. The anterior MCL starts from the inferior and most lateral portion of the medial epicondyle or apophysis, depending on maturity, and extends to the medial aspect of the coronoid process. This ligament remains tight throughout the entire range of elbow flexion and therefore provides about 70% of the elbow's valgus stability. The posterior MCL originates from the posterior portion of the medial epicondyle and attaches to the medial part of the semilunar notch of the ulna. This portion of the MCL becomes tight only past 90 degrees of flexion, and it is insignificant in the formation of valgus stability. The transverse does not appear to contribute in any way to valgus stability, and its anatomy varies significantly among individuals (2).

The LCL provides both rotational and varus stability of the elbow. In general, the LCL, or radial ligament, originates at the lateral epicondyle and inserts throughout the annular ligament (AL). The four components of the LCL are the radial collateral ligament (RCL), the lateral ulnar collateral ligament (LUCL), the accessory lateral collateral ligament (ALCL), and the AL. The RCL begins at the lateral epicondyle and inserts broadly into the AL. It remains tight throughout the range of flexion and extension of the elbow; therefore, it appears to provide the majority of varus stability of the elbow. It also forms a portion of the origin of the supinator muscle. The LUCL originates at the posterior fibers of the RCL, passes superficial to the AL, and inserts at the crista supinatoris of the ulna. It appears to provide inferior rotatory stability to the humeroulnar joint. The ALCL originates from the tubercle of the supinator muscle and inserts into the

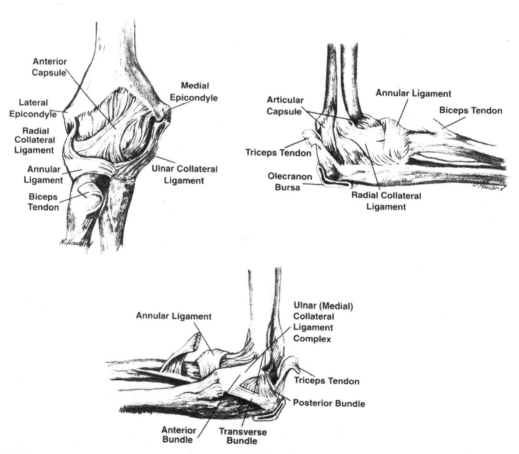

FIG. 33.2. Ligaments of the elbow. (From O'Connor FG, Olivierre CO, Nirschl RP. Elbow and forearm injuries. In: Lillegard WA, Butcher JD, Rucker KS, eds. *Handbook of sports medicine: a symptom-oriented approach*, 2nd ed. Boston: Butterworth-Heinemann, 1999:141–157, with permission.)

inferior margin of the AL. It only contracts during varus stress, and it remains relaxed during flexion, extension, pronation, and supination. The ligament provides additional support for the AL during varus stress. Finally, the AL is a tight band of tissue that extends from the anterior portion of the lesser sigmoid notch to the posterior portion of the same. It forms a circular band that wraps around the radial head to maintain its contact with the ulna, thus providing varus stability to the radius and preventing separation of the radius from the ulna (5).

Epiphyseal Development and Ossification Centers

In order to treat elbow injuries in pediatric patients, an understanding the development of bone and the timing of ossification centers in the average patient is paramount because these factors will affect both patterns of injury and appearance on radiographs. The pattern of ossification progresses in a predictable manner throughout childhood. The articular surfaces of the elbow do not begin the process of ossification at birth. This process begins during the first 6 months after birth. In general, the pattern of ossification occurs sooner in girls than in boys. For instance, the proximal radius appears in 50% of girls by 3.8 years of age, whereas the same extent is not achieved in boys until 4.5 years of age. An easy way to remember the timing of development of the specific ossification centers is to follow the mnemonic CRITOE. The Capitellum is the first center to develop, and it begins ossification within the first year of life. This is followed by the Radial head at 3 to 6 years of age, the Internal (medial) epicondyle at 4 to 7 years of age, the Trochlea at 6 to 10 years of age, the Olecranon at 9 to 10 years of age, and the External (lateral) epicondyle at 11 to 12 years of age (Fig. 33.3) (6).

After cessation of growth, the capitellum, trochlea, and lateral epicondyle join to form a common epiphyseal center. This humeral epiphyseal center is separated from the medial epicondyle by the metaphysis of the humerus. Between approximately 14 to 16 years of age, the metaphysis of the humerus and the humeral epiphyseal center join. At about the same time, the radial and ulnar epiphyseal centers fuse with their appropriate metaphyses. The medial epicondyle is the last center to fuse with its metaphysis; this occurs at 14 years of age or greater in girls and 17 years of age or greater in boys. Remembering the timing of fusion and the location of the medial epiphysis is important, due to its potential for dislocation. It is in close proximity to the trochlea, which does not ossify

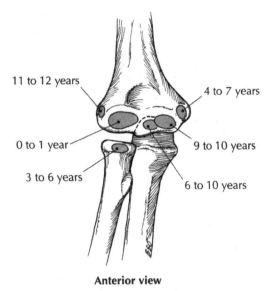

Anterior view

FIG. 33.3. Ossification centers of the elbow. Demonstrates the age when ossification centers first develop in the distal humerus, proximal radius, and proximal ulna. (From Fick DS, Lyons TA. Interpreting elbow radiographs in children. *Am Fam Physician* 1997;55: 1278–1282, with permission.)

until the medial epicondyle is already present. If a radiograph shows the presence of the trochlea without the presence of the medial epicondyle, the most likely cause is dislocation of the medial epicondyle into the normal position of the trochlea. Ossification centers appear as a single bony focus on radiograph. For this reason, without an adequate understanding of the timing of ossification centers, they may be misinterpreted as fractures, or, conversely, treatment of a fracture may be delayed.

CLINICAL ASSESSMENT

History

The history is extremely important for identifying the mechanism of injury to narrow the differential diagnosis. Initially, the physician should determine the recreational and occupational activities in which the patient was involved that could be associated with specific modes of injury. Determining when the symptoms first appeared can help to identify which type of activities, such as a fall, a collision, or repetitive trauma, may have caused the injury. This is often problematical in children who do not understand the significance of certain levels of pain. This can be most difficult to determine in young baseball players or other athletes who may continue to perform despite the initial pain because they assume that the soreness is normal with their type of activity. Whether the pain occurs after activity, during activity, or at rest, may give an idea of the severity of the injury. The location of the pain, along with its duration and character, can again help narrow the differential diagnosis. As with any injury that causes pain, knowing what makes the pain better or worse is important. The loss of function and the unwillingness to move the elbow can be other signs of severe injury. Symptoms that may be suggestive of nerve damage include the radiation of pain, weakness, or parasthesias. Combinations of symptoms should be used to form a differential diagnosis more accurately (3).

Physical Examination

The complete examination of the elbow should include inspection, palpation, range-of-motion (ROM) testing, neurologic assessment, examination of the associated areas, and special tests. A thorough review of the physical examination can be found in Hoppenfeld (7). Due to the position of the elbow in the central portion of the upper extremity, the elbow is a common site for referred pain from other injured areas. Specifically, the practitioner should look for concomitant cervical radiculopathy, shoulder injuries (e.g., rotator cuff injuries and traumatic dislocations of the shoulder), and wrist injuries (e.g., nerve entrapments). All of these injuries can result in elbow pain. Overuse injuries of the elbow frequently can be associated with injuries to the shoulder girdle (4).

With injuries to the elbow, assessing this joint for instability with regard to the complex ligamentous structures that were discussed in "Soft Tissue

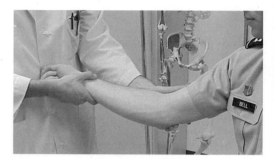

FIG. 33.5. Varus stress test. The forearm is placed in pronation. A positive test results in lateral pain and/or laxity.

Anatomy" above is crucial. The first tests for investigating instability of the ulnar and radial ligamentous structures involve placing the patient's forearm in 20 degrees of flexion. This position allows the olecranon to be released from its position within the olecranon fossa of the humerus. In this position, the practitioner applies both valgus stress (Fig. 33.4) and varus stress (Fig. 33.5) to the forearm to determine the presence of medial or lateral laxity, apprehension, pain, or decreased mobility (4). The posterolateral rotatory instability test, which is sometimes referred to as the lateral pivot–shift test, is specifically used to isolate the ulnar portion of the LCL for evidence of instability. In this test, the patient should be placed supine. The arm should be extended over the patient's head, while the shoulder is rotated externally (Fig. 33.6). At

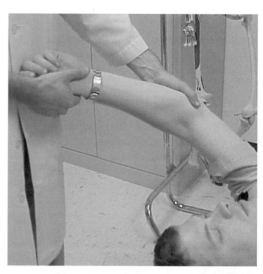

FIG. 33.6. The starting position of the posterolateral rotatory instability test. For this test, the shoulder is rotated externally.

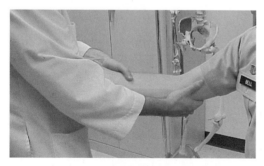

FIG. 33.4. Valgus stress test. The forearm is placed in supination. A positive test results in medial pain and/or laxity.

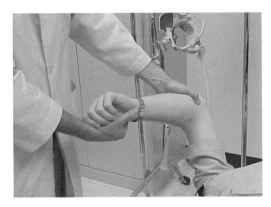

FIG. 33.7. Posterolateral rotatory instability test. In this test, forearm supination, valgus stress, axial loading, and flexion of the elbow are conducted simultaneously. In the awake patient, apprehension indicates a positive test.

this point, the practitioner should apply supination, valgus stress, axial loading, and flexion of the elbow simultaneously (Fig. 33.7). In an awake patient, any apprehension associated with this test should be considered a positive test. When a patient undergoes this procedure following the administration of general anesthesia, a positive test will result in the displacement of the ulna and the dislocation of the radial head (3).

Radiology

The appearance of the radiographs is dependent on the child's age and his or her development of bone tissue, as the section "Epiphyseal Development and Ossification Centers" demonstrated. In most injuries requiring radiographic evaluation, anterior–posterior (AP) and lateral projections are the views commonly utilized. Oblique views are sometimes employed to evaluate injuries of the radial head or distal humerus. Some doctors believe that comparison views can be helpful for differentiating between fractures and ossification centers, although this view has not been proved accurate in clinical studies.

As is true for reading all radiographs, the use of a systematic approach when evaluating radiographs of the elbow is crucial. In an adequate lateral view, the trochlea and capitellum should line up directly, and the ulna should be positioned directly below the radius. If the radiograph has been exposed properly, adipose tissue surrounding the muscle and fascia of the arm will appear as radiolucent shadows. On the lateral view, the anterior humeral line and the central radial line are used to evaluate for dislocation. The anterior humeral line, which is the plane that runs directly along the anterior cortex of the humerus, intersects through the middle third of the capitellum. The central radial line, which is a line directly through the middle of the radial cortex, should pass the anterior humeral line in the middle third of the capitellum. The surfaces of all three bones (humerus, radius, and ulna) should then be evaluated for any abnormalities.

In significant elbow trauma, production of joint effusions (fat pad sign) may occur in the elbow. These effusions may result in the development of fat pads along the surface of the elbow joint capsule. Fat pads appear as triangular-shaped radiolucencies that are anterior or posterior to the distal humerus. Anterior fat pads are often visible in a normal elbow, and they are only considered abnormal when they become significantly raised or if they are more perpendicular to the humeral cortex. The posterior fat pad is normally positioned in the olecranon fossa. It only becomes visible with significant injuries, such as an intraarticular fracture, a spontaneously reduced dislocation, or an infection that causes joint effusion (6).

SPORTS-SPECIFIC BIOMECHANICS

The Throwing Elbow

The elbow joint often is considered one of the most stable joints in the body due to the tight alignment of its surfaces. Its stability is related to the combination of congruent articular surfaces and supporting soft tissue. The articular surfaces, ligaments, and capsular structures provide static stability while the muscles and tendons confer dynamic stability. In general, the ligaments and capsule provide about 50% of the elbow's stability, and the osseous structures supply the other 50% of stability. The majority of ligament support is due to the anterior MCL. Primary bone support is due to the humeroulnar joint and the olecranon, although the radial head provides between 15% and 30% of the resistance to valgus stress.

Throwing is best understood by studying the process of throwing a baseball. The usual pattern is divided into five stages (Fig. 33.8). The first phase, or wind-up, continues until the ball leaves the glove hand. The second phase, early cocking, ends when the front foot hits the ground, and it involves abduction and internal rotation of the shoulder. The third phase, the late cocking phase, ends when the shoulder reaches maximum external rotation. Phase four, or acceleration, starts with internal rotation of the shoulder and ends when the ball is released. Phase five, or follow-through, involves all activity following the re-

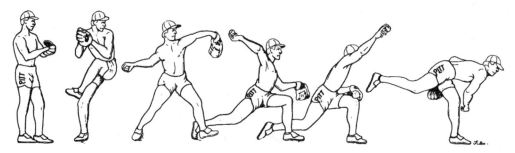

FIG. 33.8. Phases of the baseball pitch. The baseball pitch is divided into five stages: stance, windup, cocking (early and late), acceleration, and follow-through. (From Fu FH, Stone DA, eds. *Sports injuries: mechanisms, prevention, and treatment*, 2nd ed. Philadelphia: Lippincott Williams & Wilkins, 2001, with permission.)

lease of the ball. The muscles involved in this process include the extensor digitorum communis (EDC), the brachioradialis (BR), the flexor carpi radialis (FCR), the flexor digitorum superficialis (FDS), the extensor carpi radialis longus (ECRL), the extensor carpi radialis brevis (ECRB), the pronator teres (PT), and the supinator (S).

The wind-up phase involves flexion and pronation of the forearm and extension of the wrist. Low activity in all muscles is seen during this phase. No differences in muscle activity are noted for the fastball and curveball during this phase. The early cocking phase involves elbow flexion, wrist and metacarpophalangeal joint extension, and mild forearm pronation. This phase involves moderate activity of the ECRB, ECRL, EDC, BR, and PT when throwing the fastball. Throwing a curveball requires less activity of the BR, probably due to the lower need for elbow flexion. The late cocking phase requires wrist extension, elbow flexion, and pronation of the forearm to 90 degrees. Pronation is greater when the individual is throwing a fastball. Wrist extension and supination, however, are stronger when the pitcher is throwing a curveball. The acceleration phase requires extension of the elbow and flexion of the wrist and metacarpophalangeal joints to thrust the ball forward. The curveball requires much more activity of the ECRL and ECRB than does the fastball. Finally, the follow-through phase results from maximal pronation of the forearm and internal rotation of the humerus. In this phase, the curveball again requires increased activity of the wrist extensors. The major difference between the curveball and fastball is the increased activity of the ECRL and ECRB that is required to throw a curveball.

When one understands the phases of throwing as they relate to the elbow, the four potential mechanisms for injury become apparent, including tension on the medial aspect of the elbow, compression of the lateral articular surfaces, shear forces on the posterior articular surface, and extension overload on the lateral elbow complex. During early cocking and late cocking, tension is applied to the location on the medial epicondyle where the flexor muscles and ulnar collateral ligaments attach. Because the developing medial epicondylar ossification center is the weakest portion of this area during early development, injury or avulsion of this area is the most common result of this stress. Other possible injuries of the medial elbow may include traction spurs, ulnar nerve injury, or flexor muscle strain. Compression of the lateral elbow occurs mainly during early and late cocking. This injury can result in growth disturbances, osteochondritis dissecans, osteochondrosis, and abnormalities of the radial head. Posterior damage occurs during late cocking as a result of shear forces on the olecranon fossa, and during follow-through from hyperextension of the elbow. These forces may result in posterior medial spurs, olecranon spurs, triceps strain, and coronoid process spurs. Finally, lateral extension overload also occurs during the acceleration phase. Pronation of the forearm applies tension forces to the lateral ligaments and lateral epicondyle and potentially results in lateral epicondylitis. This group of injuries can all be included in overuse injuries due to repetitive throwing (8), and they are commonly referred to as "Little League Elbow."

Gymnastics and the Pediatric Elbow

Gymnastics is a very popular sport in the pediatric age group, particularly among young girls. Gymnastics, however, is a sport that has a high rate of injury (9). While lower extremity injuries predominate, with ankle sprain representing the most common injury, upper extremity injuries are also common (10). Garrick and Requa (11) reported that nearly one-third of women's gymnastics injuries involved the upper extremity, with 7% involving the elbow. Pettrone and Ricciardelli (12), in a study of 15 women's club gymnastics teams, found that the injury rate in gymnastics was exceeded only by football, wrestling, and softball.

Gymnastics routines place the elbow in positions and involve stresses that are unique to this athletic activity. Gymnastics, through handstands and tumbling, causes the upper extremity to act as a weight-bearing joint, which results in compressive force loads. The swinging apparatus (e.g., a high bar or uneven bars), however, subjects the pediatric elbow to considerable tensile loads. In addition, as gymnastics requires the athlete to "lock out" elbows for proper position stabilization, posterior elbow problems are not uncommon (5).

The combination of stresses encountered by the young gymnast subjects the pediatric elbow to an array of overuse and traumatic disorders. The most significant injury that the gymnast may encounter is an elbow dislocation, which may occur as the result of a hyperextension injury on the uneven or parallel bars or following a missed tumble or vault. Associated growth plate or epicondylar fractures or osteochondral injuries to the capitellum may complicate these dislocations.

Compressive and tensile load injuries can otherwise mirror those problems seen in the constellation of disorders known as Little League Elbow and thus include medial epicondylar stress lesions, capitellar osteochondritis, and olecranon fossitis. In addition, the unusual weight bearing in gymnastics predisposes to the injury termed forearm "splints," which is unique to gymnastics. This injury is somewhat analogous to leg "shin splints;" however, in the case of forearm splints, the ulna and its musculotendinous attachments are involved, and they should be considered in the differential of the young gymnast presenting with forearm and/or elbow pain of overuse origin.

TRAUMATIC ELBOW DISORDERS

Medial Epicondylar Fracture

In evaluating the medial epicondyle, the clinician must not underestimate the importance of remembering the timing of its development. It is first apparent by radiograph at about 4 years of age. It develops slowly, and it fuses with the humeral shaft after all of the other epiphyses have fused. This occurs between about 14 and 17 years of age. Therefore, looking for the normal appearance of this ossification center in radiographs of the elbow is important. Another potential area of confusion is its somewhat posterior, as well as medial, location in the alignment of the elbow. For this reason, comparison views of both elbows can be helpful in order to determine the normal position of the medial epicondyle (5).

Medial epicondylar fractures most commonly occur in children between the ages of 9 to 15 years. They represent about 10% of elbow injuries in the pediatric population. This injury is uncommon in younger age groups. It is usually caused by valgus stress along the elbow joint in which the flexor muscles apply tension to the medial epicondyle. Most of these fractures result in Salter–Harris type I or II injuries, although types III and IV also occur occasionally. The traction resulting from the flexor pronator origin causes inferior displacement of the fragment. In some instances, the fragment may also be trapped in the elbow joint. This fracture often occurs in conjunction with posterolateral dislocation of the elbow. Fifty percent of these fractures occur with partial or complete dislocation of the elbow (5).

The amount of displacement is used to determine the appropriate treatment. Fractures with less than 2 mm displacement should be treated initially with posterior splint immobilization. Within 1 to 2 weeks, the acute symptoms typically resolve and the splint may be removed temporarily to start active motion exercises. If no residual abnormality appears on radiograph at 6 weeks, the immobilization should be stopped. At this point, ROM exercises should become more aggressive, and strength exercises should be initiated. The patient may return to competitive activity, such as throwing, when he or she is able to show normal ROM, strength, and endurance in sports-specific activity (8).

Any fracture with a large fragment and displacement of the fragment by more than 2 mm should undergo open reduction with internal fixation. Two screws are used to fix the fragment. Initially, the patient should be placed in a posterior splint. ROM exercises should begin about 1 to 2 weeks after surgery with the aid of a functional orthosis. At 6 weeks, a radiograph should be taken for evaluation, and, if no sign of displacement is observed, the orthosis should be removed (8).

If only a small fragment is displaced, evaluating the elbow with a radiographic valgus stress test can be helpful; the clinician, however, must keep in mind that small *in situ* fragments usually resorb. In this test, the patient lies supine on the radiographic table. The arm should be placed in complete external rotation. The weight of the forearm will result in valgus stress on the elbow, while preventing the rest of the body from supporting the elbow. This allows a complete evaluation for stability of the elbow. A negative test permits conservative treatment of the elbow. A positive test requires excision of the fragment and correction of the attachments of the origins of the ligament and muscles to the medial epicondyle (8).

Early complications of a medial epicondylar fracture may include hypesthesia, parasthesia, or paralysis due to ulnar nerve entrapment in the area of the fracture. These symptoms may require open reduction of the fracture and decompression of the cubital tunnel. Displaced fractures of the medial epicondyle may result in malunion or nonunion of the joint at a later date if they are not appropriately treated. In some cases, even if the patient is symptom free with good ROM for years, the patient may develop ulnar palsy. Symptoms may include parasthesia (85%), atrophy (81%), paralysis (62%), pain (39%), and anesthesia (25%). Physical examination findings in one study found atrophy and weakness in 96% of patients and anesthesia in 77%. Surgical treatment, such as anterior intramuscular transplantation, approaches a success rate of 70% (5).

Lateral Epicondylar Fracture

The related ossification center first appears around 10 years of age. It fuses with the lateral condyle fairly early at about 14 years of age. It can easily be confused with a fracture because of its significant separation from the humerus during development and the fact that its distal portion fuses with the capitellum prior to the fusion of its proximal portion. Injury of the lateral epicondyle alone is an uncommon occurrence. At times, however, injury may occur in concordance with an elbow dislocation. Open reduction and internal fixation are rarely necessary for the following reasons. First, usually minimal displacement of the fracture fragment is seen. Second, this specific injury usually occurs in children close to the age of skeletal maturity; therefore, it rarely results in an arrest of growth. Appropriate treatment includes initial immobilization followed by an early return to ROM exercise and activity (5).

Supracondylar Fracture

Supracondylar fracture is common in children with immature skeletal systems. It is most commonly caused by falling on an outstretched arm or hyperextension of the elbow. It less commonly follows the application of a direct axial force to the forearm during elbow flexion. The diagnosis can be difficult when minimal displacement occurs. It is made by direct palpation of the bony make-up at the elbow joint and by careful radiographic evaluation. Oblique views are best for the detection of nondisplaced fractures.

Gartland's classification of supracondylar fractures provides a good basis for treatment of these injuries. Type I fractures are nondisplaced, type II are partially displaced fractures, and type III are completely displaced fractures. Type I fractures should be treated with either a sling or a collar and cuff for 3 weeks and should be followed by ROM exercises until full ROM is achieved. Treatment of type II fractures depends on the determination of the position of fracture fragments. Splinting or casting provides adequate treatment of properly positioned fragments. Reduction and splinting are needed to treat fragments that are significantly angulated. Type II fragments are preferably treated with closed reduction and percutaneous pinning. These fractures must be immobilized after the appropriate treatment.

The most significant complication that can be associated with these fractures is injury to the brachial artery, which constitutes an orthopedic emergency. This can be caused by laceration of the artery or with compression of the artery by the surrounding soft tissue. Volkmann ischemic contracture or compartment syndrome is an associated complication. Volkmann contracture can result in paralysis and permanent damage of the muscles of the forearm. Monitoring the peripheral pulses and capillary refill to watch for arterial injuries is important. Severe pain with passive extension of the fingers is the classic clinical finding that suggests compartment syndrome. Other findings that should make the clinician suspicious of this injury include intense pain, sensory symptoms, and muscle weakness. The clinician must remember that the presence of a pulse does not rule out the possibility of compartment syndrome because the absence of a pulse occurs late in the course of compartment syndrome. Surgical decompression of the compartment should be performed immediately after determining the presence of increased compartment pressures. The development of a cubitus varus deformity as a result of malunion of the fracture is another common complication that occurs in about 10% of these patients. Fortunately, the deformity is often cosmetic only, so it does not cause functional difficulties. These fractures also can result in damage to the ulnar nerve or entrapment of this nerve (4).

Elbow Dislocation

Elbow dislocations are the second most common major joint dislocations, and they are surpassed only by shoulder dislocations. They usually occur when a patient falls on an outstretched and extended arm. Usually, the dislocation occurs without an associated fracture. The most common dislocation is a posterior dislocation, which accounts for about 90% of dislocations. In these injuries, the coronoid process disengages from the trochlea and moves posteriorly. This can result in injuries to the anterior and posterior bands of the MCL, LCL, brachialis muscle, and flexor–pronator muscle group and to the articular cartilage.

The initial evaluation of a potential dislocation is important for improving the final outcome. The history should include a determination of the mechanism of injury. The clinician must evaluate the shoulder, wrist, and distal radial ulnar joint for other associated injuries. Examination of the elbow should involve an evaluation for associated elbow fractures. A complete neurovascular exam is necessary, and it should include pulses, capillary refill, and an examination for brachial artery and ulnar nerve injury.

Reduction is the next step in treatment. In the field, the determination of whether immediate reduction is necessary or whether the joint can be splinted and the patient can be transported to the emergency room is important. This decision should be based on a number of separate issues. If the injury occurs fieldside and the physician knows the correct technique, reduction without radiographs is appropriate. Radiographs therefore should not be the rate-limiting step. If sedation or analgesia appears to be necessary, reduction probably is best accomplished in an emergency department setting. Early reduction can be beneficial for pain relief and for an improvement of neurovascular status. Also, if reduction is delayed, swelling and muscle spasm can make reduction more difficult. Reduction should be performed by the following steps (Fig. 33.9). Place the patient prone on a flat surface. Flex the injured arm at about 90 degrees over the edge of the surface. Attempt to straighten the ulna at a central position. While grabbing the injured arm at the wrist, apply traction and supination to the forearm. This should effectively remove the coronoid process from its position in the olecranon fossa. Next, use the other hand to apply pressure to the olecranon, while pronating the forearm. This force should cause definitive reduction. Success can be confirmed by a "clunk" and a return of the joint to normal appearance. The elbow should be examined for stability by moving the elbow through its full ROM. Finally, the elbow should be splinted at 90 degrees with a complete evaluation of neurovascular stability. Postreduction films should be taken and checked for alignment of the radial head and the capitellum.

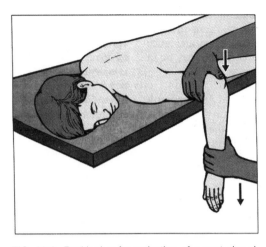

FIG. 33.9. Positioning for reduction of a posterior elbow dislocation. With the patient in a prone position and the elbow at 90 degrees, allow the forearm to hang over the end of the table. Apply downward traction to the forearm, while providing gentle pressure to the olecranon. (From Ross G. Acute elbow dislocation: on-site treatment. *The Physician and Sports Medicine* 1999; 27:121–122, with permission.)

As part of follow-up, the patient should be informed to watch for signs of neurovascular compromise, especially pain. The most common complication is residual stiffness. Chronic instability is uncommon, although the presence of associated ligament damage can result in instability. Splinting should be continued for 5 to 10 days. After this period, the patient should begin ROM exercises. ROM can begin within 1 to 2 days of injury, if it is appropriately supervised by medically trained staff. Appropriate and early treatment usually results in a good prognosis (13).

Radial Head Fracture

Fractures of the radial head most often occur with falls onto an outstretched arm while the elbow is extended. Common symptoms seen in these injuries include radial head tenderness, swelling of the elbow, and pain with flexion or rotation of the elbow. The Mason classification can be used to determine the appropriate treatment of these fractures. Type I fractures are nondisplaced fractures, type II are displaced fractures, and type III are comminuted fractures. A complex fracture, which is defined as fractures associated with other injuries, such as other fractures or ligamentous injuries, requires different management techniques.

Simple type I fractures respond extremely well to nonsurgical treatment. Treatment involves the use of a sling for pain control and early motion exercises. Extremely painful fractures, due to hemarthrosis, are best treated with aspiration, followed by injection of anesthetic into the posterolateral triangle of the elbow. Good results are achieved in about 95% of type I fractures. Rare associated complications can include nonunion, the loss of elbow extension, decreased rotation, and persistent pain with use of the elbow.

A number of ways to treat type II fractures are found, and the proper choice is best determined with examination of the elbow after injection of an anesthetic. If the elbow maintains 20 to 140 degrees of flexion and 70 percent of forearm rotation, a nonsurgical treatment is well accepted. Nonsurgical treatment involves immobilization for 3 weeks, followed by the initiation of active and active-assisted ROM exercises. Patients who present with inadequate ROM should be treated with early open reduction and internal fixation of the radial head. The former treatment of early radial head excision is now considered unacceptable due to the inconsistency of the results. Delayed radial head excision may be indicated in patients who present late after injury or in those with continued discomfort after initial nonsurgical treatment.

Type III fractures are best treated with early excision of the radial head within 48 hours. After excision of the radial head, the ligaments that remain maintain adequate stability of the elbow joint. If excision is delayed, the treatment results in poor functional results of the elbow joint.

Complex fractures are treated similarly to parallel simple fractures. The injury should be treated with surgical or nonsurgical stabilization of the associated injury prior to treatment of the fracture. In general, ligamentous injuries should not be surgically repaired when they are associated with dislocation of the elbow. In the treatment of unstable radial fractures, metal implants may be used to replace the radial head. In general, the prognosis for uncomplicated simple radial head fractures is good. However, if associated injuries are present, complications, such as chronic stiffness, chronic aching, and osteoarthritis, are fairly common (4).

Lateral Condyle Fracture

Lateral condyle fractures can be extremely serious, due to the disruption of the joint surface. Presenting symptoms include pain in the area of the capitellum and tenderness without noticeable deformity. AP and lateral films should be evaluated first to attempt to determine the amount of involvement of the articular surface. Oblique views and films of the normal elbow may be required to define the extent of the injury better. Any amount of displacement requires open reduction and internal fixation. Inaccurate reduction can result in arthritic changes, ulnar nerve neuropathy, cubitus valgus, and chronic instability. Other less common, but more significant, complications may include avascular necrosis and growth disturbances (4).

Radial Head Subluxation

Radial head subluxation, which is often referred to as "nursemaid's elbow," is common among preschool-aged children. It is usually caused by a sudden jerking of the forearm or wrist that is associated with the application of a longitudinal and pronation force to the elbow. The common scenario includes the situation in which the child and his or her attendant are walking in the grocery store or up stairs, the attendant is in a hurry, and the child is misbehaving. The injury occurs when the attendant pulls against the activity of the child. After the injury, the child will hold the affected arm close to his or her side, with the elbow flexed and pronated. The child reports significant pain, and he or she will not allow anyone to touch the elbow. In the sports arena, this injury may occur with trampoline exercises or in games of tug of war.

The cause of the injury is sudden tearing of the AL, which normally surrounds the radial head and keeps it in place. Damage to the AL results in temporary subluxation of the radial head so that it loses its contact with the capitellum. The proximal part of the AL becomes trapped between the surfaces of the joint when the tension is released. Because of this, after the release of tension, the radiographic examination will appear normal in this injury.

Treatment involves a return to normal anatomy. This is accomplished by applying quick supination to the forearm, while the elbow is held in flexion. A common scenario, which actually results in treatment, occurs when the technician taking the radiograph reduces the subluxation by positioning the elbow for an AP radiograph. Almost immediately after reduction, the child's pain resolves, and he or she returns to normal elbow and forearm function. Sometimes, placing the elbow in a splint for a short period of time is helpful to allow healing of the AL. The final step involves education of the caregiver. The physician should explain to the caregiver how the injury occurs and should encourage the caregiver to avoid these types of activity (14).

Olecranon Fractures

Olecranon fractures occur either as isolated injuries or in combination with elbow dislocation. Isolated fractures usually occur as a result of direct trauma. The most common presentation stems from an effusion. Effusions are common because the injury occurs intraarticularly. As a result of the effusion, the patient can have difficulty extending the elbow, and he or she may also exhibit ulnar nerve neuropathy. A posterior splint or elbow immobilizer in which the elbow is flexed at 90 degrees should be used in nondisplaced fractures. ROM therapy should begin within 2 to 3 days with pronation and supination exercises. Initial extension and flexion exercises should begin after approximately 2 weeks. Immobilization should be used until about 6 weeks, when the fracture appears to achieve union. Displaced fractures require treatment by an orthopedic surgeon. Most often, they are treated with reduction and internal fixation, followed by early motion to avoid residual stiffness. If the displacement is less than 30 degrees, treatment with surgical excision and reattachment of the triceps tendon may be possible (4).

OVERUSE DISORDERS

Little League Elbow

This disorder is due to overuse, and it is most common in children from 9 to 13 years of age who are baseball pitchers. The forces involved in pitching, which were discussed in "The Throwing Elbow" in this chapter, cause increased tension and stretching forces on the medial elbow and compression of the lateral side of the elbow. These forces can result in hypertrophy of the ulna and humerus. Hypertrophy of the olecranon process of the ulna may impinge on its adjacent fossa of the humerus, also resulting in posterior stresses in these patients. By far, the most common injury in these patients involves the medial side, although the lateral injuries that do occur can be much more detrimental with regard to long-term morbidity. All of these related injuries respond well to the cessation of the stressful activity if the limitations occur soon enough. For this reason, the most important therapy is prevention.

Prevention requires the cooperation of players, parents, and coaches. The player's responsibility includes his or her efforts to remain healthy and eagerness to be involved in appropriate training. Any workout or athletic activity should include appropriate stretching and conditioning. Both aerobic and anaerobic conditioning is needed to promote athletic fitness. Strength

training, which should organized so that it is age appropriate, is an important aspect of a throwing program. Strengthening the forearm muscles—both the flexors and extensors—prior to the start of the season is crucial. All of this preparation makes the athlete less prone to injury. In order for these programs to reach their maximum effectiveness, the training regimen must be structured so that it remains interesting to the young athlete. Training in moderation, instilling fun into the program, and including the parents in the program all help to maintain interest in the program.

Coaches play an extremely important part in preventing injuries. They are entrusted with the responsibility of teaching young athletes the fundamentals of the game. Part of this instruction should include teaching the correct mechanics of pitching and throwing. Suggestions for appropriate technique include not allowing the athlete to open his or her lead shoulder while throwing and preventing the athlete from lifting the back foot from the ground too early (15). Learning the proper technique at an early age can prevent acute and chronic injuries. Youth leagues already regulate the number of innings pitched per week to limit injuries, but incorporating limits on the number of pitches per outing can also be beneficial. Whiteside et al. (16) suggest 50 pitches per game, while Hall and Galea (15) suggest 90 to 100 pitches per game. In either case, this activity should be followed by 2 days of rest from pitching. Pitching is not safe for children under the age of 8 years.

The coach must also understand at what age an athlete should begin throwing specific pitches. The change-up is the first pitch after the fastball that is safe to learn. Because the change-up requires similar mechanics to the fastball, the pitch should not cause increased stress to the elbow. The curveball causes more stress because of the more forceful supination and the ulnar deviation of the forearm, which results in increased medial stress. Because of the difficult mechanics required to throw the curveball, it should not be thrown until the athlete is approximately 13 to 14 years of age. Finally, children should be educated to report any symptoms of elbow pain as soon as it occurs.

If prevention is not successful, the elbow injuries discussed below, including osteochondritis dissecans, medial epicondylar stress lesions, and posterior impingement injuries, may occur.

Osteochondritis Dissecans

Osteochondritis dissecans (OCD) is described as "a localized injury or condition affecting an articular surface that involves separation of a segment of cartilage and subchondral bone" (17). The anterolateral surface of the humeral capitellum is the most common area in the elbow that is affected. Although the incidence of OCD is not known, it is a rare disorder. It most commonly occurs in males who are from 9 to 15 years of age. The diagnosis often is made years after the initial injury. One study found that diagnosis commonly is made about 3 to 4 years after symptoms began, with the mean age of diagnosis between 17 to 20 years (18). Although this injury usually occurs in baseball players, it can also occur in athletes involved in wrestling, football, gymnastics, shooting, shot put, and golf. Some researchers and clinicians also believe that certain individuals may have a genetic predisposition to OCD (15).

The diagnosis of osteochondritis dissecans is made by a combination of clinical findings and imaging studies. Elbow pain is reported in 90% of patients, and 55% are noted to have decreased ROM. Symptoms generally include the intermittent occurrence of pain. Pain occurs with activity, and it tends to resolve with rest. Other symptoms may include clicking, stiffness, swelling, a loose body sensation, and locking. The symptoms often affect athletic performance. If a history of acute injury is present, the possibilty of an osteochondral fracture must be investigated. A plain radiograph should be obtained initially. Findings may include radiolucency of the capitellum, loose bodies, hypertrophy of the radial head, and osteophytes (Fig. 33.10). These findings may appear in only two-thirds of cases. A bone scan is a sensitive indicator of this injury, although it can also signal the existence of other injuries. Magnetic resonance imaging (MRI) is considered the most useful study for determining the presence and significance of OCD lesions. T2-weighted images can determine fragment detachment based on the fluid between separate surfaces. It also can aid in establishing the staging of OCD lesions, and it can facilitate early treatment by permitting the detection of contusions and stress lesions prior to fragmentation.

Understanding the staging prior to discussing the treatment of these lesions is important. OCD can be identified as types I through III. Type I lesions involve fragments that remain intact. In these lesions, no displacement of the fragment or fracture of the articular cartilage occurs. Type II lesions are associated with partial detachment of the fragment. Fracture of the articular surface also is present in these lesions. Type III lesions are associated with complete detachment of the fragment, which then lies free in the elbow joint. The appearance usually includes hypertrophy of the loose body, as well as fibrous tissue build-up in the capitellum (8).

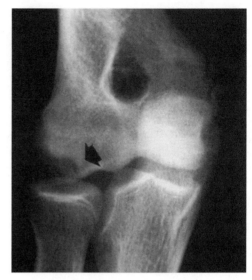

FIG. 33.10. Osteochondritis dissecans of the capitellum (*arrow*). (From Fu FH, Stone DA, eds. *Sports injuries: mechanisms, prevention, and treatment*, 2nd ed. Philadelphia: Lippincott Williams & Wilkins, 2001, with permission.)

Treatment can follow either a conservative or an operative route. The choice of which is used should be based on the size and site of the lesion, the presence of loose bodies, and the effect on the articular cartilage.

Lesions that are diagnosed early respond well to conservative therapy, especially in the younger athlete. When an athlete becomes symptomatic, he or she should quit throwing until the pain resolves. Early OCD lesions should be treated with a change in activity, nonsteroidal antiinflammatory drugs (NSAIDs), and ice. Changes in activity include the discontinuation of throwing and any other activities that cause stress to the elbow. Other therapy should include stretching and strengthening of both the flexor and extensor muscle groups. After the resolution of elbow pain, the patient should gradually increase his or her level of activity. Special emphasis should be placed on strengthening and on correcting technique. If symptoms do not resolve after 8 to 12 weeks of conservative therapy, operative treatment should be considered. Surgery usually involves debridement with curettage and drilling of the OCD lesion bed. Removal of the loose bodies should also be done, followed by slow return to activity after reconditioning (15).

Medial Epicondylar Stress Lesion

Most often, in young throwing athletes, a medial injury involves apophysitis of the elbow. Apophyseal injuries are associated with the immature skeleton. To understand these lesions, the clinician needs to understand the characteristics of the growing skeleton. Growth sites of the immature skeleton include the physeal plate, the joint surface, and the apophysis. The apophysis is the cartilage site where a major tendon is attached to a growing bone. The apophyseal growth plate is distinct from the physeal plate, and it grows at a slower rate than the epiphyseal plate. While the apophysis is still maturing, it has a much higher risk of injury. This area is associated with a significant amount of tension, due to the insertion of major muscles at this site.

According to Peck (19), "apophyseal injuries involve inflammation at the site of a major tendinous insertion onto a bony prominence that is undergoing active growth." Apophysitis is believed most likely to be due to repetitive microtrauma in the area of the apophysis, as is seen with pitching. This repetitive trauma seems to cause tiny avulsion fractures and eventually evolves into an inflammatory process. A macrotraumatic event possibly may also exacerbate the injury caused by repetitive microtrauma. Another related cause of apophysitis is associated with the immaturity and growth of the muscles and tendons. Growth spurts often are correlated with what is referred to as the musculotendinous imbalance—a phenomenon caused by the fact that muscle tends to develop more slowly than bone (19). As a result, the muscle can be tight and inflexible during periods of rapid growth, and this inflexibility results in increased tension at the apophysis. The combination of immaturity, increased tension, and repetitive microtrauma from sports activity culminates in injury and inflammation of the apophysis.

Medial apophysitis can occur in any athlete who uses a repetitive overhead arm motion, especially children who are from 9 to 13 years of age. Inflammation occurs in the area where the forearm flexor muscles originate at the medial epicondyle. This apophysis is the last growth plate in the elbow that closes. The symptoms include medial elbow pain, diminished throwing effectiveness, and decreased throwing distance. Examination demonstrates medial epicondylar tenderness and pain with resisted flexion of the wrist. Radiographs should be taken to look for medial epicondylar fragmentation. The initial treatment should include activity modification for 4 to 6 weeks, including restricted throwing and continued aerobic conditioning by running or biking. Almost all cases respond well to this period of initial rest when combined with the use of ice and NSAIDs. After the initial response, as in OCD, the athlete should begin rehabilitation with a slow return to throwing, in association with an extensive program that involves stretching and strengthening of the forearm muscles (19).

Ligament rupture, flexor tendinitis, and MCL sprain also should be considered in patients who present with medial elbow pain. These injuries are fairly uncommon in young throwing athletes, but they are much more common among young adults. Tenderness in the medial aspect of the elbow is usually present for months or years prior to ligament injury. Usually, ligament rupture is a sudden event that results in pain that is severe enough to prevent continued throwing. Medial elbow instability is noted on examination following these injuries and is accompanied by a positive radiographic medial stress test. These injuries require surgical reattachment of the injured ligament and a long rehabilitation. Tendinitis and MCL sprain respond well to rest, ice, and NSAIDs, followed by a course of conditioning, strengthening, and rehabilitation (8).

Posterior Impingement Injuries

Olecranon impingement syndrome occurs from repetitive trapping of the olecranon in the olecranon fossa that is caused by valgus stress at the elbow, such as that which occurs in throwing sports. This repetitive pressure causes stress to both articular surfaces that are in contact at the olecranon, and the continued overload can result in the formation of osteophytes and loose bodies. Throwing sports, racket sports, boxing, and basketball may cause this phenomenon. Associated symptoms include posterior elbow pain, clicking, and other indicators consistent with mechanical abnormalities. Physical examination shows that the pain appears to be worse with extension of the elbow. During ROM examination, the patient may demonstrate crepitus and limited extension as a result of mechanical abnormalities. He or she may also display a mild instability. Plain radiographs may show the presence of loose bodies or osteophytes, but a computed tomography or MRI may be necessary for an adequate evaluation of this injury. If no loose bodies are noted by radiography, the injury should be treated initially with conservative therapy. Conservative therapy should include modification of activity, NSAIDs, and therapeutic exercise to attempt to increase the strength and flexibility of the elbow. If the pain continues after an adequate course of conservative therapy or if the patient has loose bodies or signs of mechanical compromise, he or she should undergo surgical evaluation. Arthroscopic treatment may be needed to remove loose bodies or to excise the osteophytes (4).

Another possible cause of posterior elbow pain in an athlete with overuse injury may be triceps tendinitis that is caused by repetitive extension of the elbow, resulting in tendon overload. In these patients, posterior elbow pain usually worsens with forceful extension of the elbow. This injury may occur in weight lifting, boxing, gymnastics, racket sports, and throwing sports. On physical examination, the tenderness is found at or above the insertion of the triceps to the olecranon. Extension against resistance results in worsened elbow pain. Radiographs of this elbow injury are usually unremarkable. The initial therapy includes rest, ice, and NSAIDs. After improvement in the level of pain, exercise therapy should focus on strengthening the triceps. A program to improve flexibility should also be initiated. Steroid injections generally are not indicated due to the increased risk of tendon rupture. If tendon rupture is suspected, the patient should be referred immediately for surgical intervention. Rupture should be suspected in injuries associated with a fall onto an outstretched arm and in physical examination findings that show significant pain, swelling, and a depression proximal to the olecranon on palpation (4).

Olecranon apophysitis is another cause of posterior elbow pain that is associated with overuse. Similar to that which occurs in medial apophysitis, the combination of muscle–tendon imbalance and the growth process of the apophysis can result in stresses to the olecranon apophysis. This pattern can result in apophysitis at the olecranon. Athletes complain of increasing posterior elbow pain with this condition. These disorders are most common in throwing and racket sports as well. Tenderness normally is limited to the area of the olecranon, and it increases with extension against resistance. Separation of the apophysis can remain into adulthood. Persistent apophyseal damage can result in avulsion fractures and additional ossification at the insertion at the olecranon, which results in the inhibition of extension. Treatment of this condition is symptomatic. Rest is required to enhance the revascularization and to allow repair. Maintaining the muscle conditioning is also important. Immobilization of the elbow at 90 degrees for 4 to 6 weeks is required if radiography shows epiphyseal widening. These patients also should perform ROM exercises. Finally, these ath-

letes should begin resistance strengthening to promote their return to activity. If avulsion or nonunion is found, the patient requires an orthopedic consult and surgical repair (4).

Panner Disease

Panner disease, or osteochondrosis, is a disruption of the growth centers of a child, usually between the ages of 7 and 12 years, due to avascular necrosis and degeneration of the capitellum of the humerus. The necrosis is followed by recalcification of this area. These children complain of achy elbow pain that increases with activity and that often involves swelling of the elbow. In most cases, only minimal loss of motion is observed, and extension is less affected than in other overuse injuries. This injury tends to be distinguished from OCD by the lower age of occurrence— 7 to 12 years of age as opposed to 13 to 16 years— and the uncommon association of limited ROM. The lesion of Panner disease is focal, involving the subchondral bone of the capitellum and the overlying articular cartilage. The anterior central capitellum is the most common location of involvement because the head of the radius articulates with the capitellum in this area. Radiographs show irregularity that is a consequence of the alternating areas of sclerosis and osteopenia. Views of the opposite side may indicate that the epiphysis on the radial side is smaller and that, comparatively, it is irregular. Panner disease has a self-limiting course. As growth continues, the capitellar epiphysis will return to its normal architecture, size, and contour. Because it is self-limited, the treatment should include rest, restricted throwing, NSAIDs, and ice. Splinting may be helpful for limiting pain and tenderness in more significant cases. Radiographs should be conducted at a later date to monitor healing. Deformity and arthritis are extremely rare complications of this disorder (8).

Radiocapitellar Compression Syndrome

Radiocapitellar compression syndrome occurs as a result of repetitive valgus stress. Often, it is associated with chronic medial instability. Throwing causes repeated valgus stress to the elbow. This repetition inhibits healing of the MCL. As a result, the elbow develops MCL weakness due to microtrauma, posterior elbow compression, and radiocapitellar joint compression. This lateral compression causes the radial head to press against the capitellum. This pressure can result in osteophytes, loose bodies, and chondromalacia. In immature athletes, the physis is weaker than the ligaments, including the MCL; therefore, the lateral apophysis is injured much more quickly than is the MCL. For this reason, inflammation, irregular ossification, overgrowth, and pain often occur in the radiocapitellar region before injury to the MCL.

Because of potential injuries involving the medial, lateral, and posterior elbow in radiocapitellar compression syndrome, evaluating all of these areas on physical examination is important. Athletes may notice both medial and lateral pain while they are throwing with decreased velocity. The valgus stress test, as described in physical examination in "Clinical Assessment" above, generally shows instability in these patients. If MCL instability has developed along with radiocapitellar compression, the patient may notice symptoms consistent with ulnar neuritis. Although this condition should be diagnosed by clinical examination, radiographic tests may be helpful in some cases. AP and lateral radiographs may show osteophytes, loose bodies, olecranon hypertrophy, avulsion fractures, and ossification within the ligament. A gravity stress radiograph may be used to identify MCL instability.

Treatment of radiocapitellar compression syndrome in which involvement of the MCL is nonexistent or minimal, which is typical in young athletes with immature bones, can normally be addressed with conservative therapy. In most young patients, rest, ice, and NSAIDs will be effective. After resolution of symptoms, the athlete should begin a stretching and strengthening program to prevent reinjury. The strengthening program should be followed by a gradual increase in a throwing regimen. Patients with concomitant MCL injury may require more extensive treatment. If instability continues after a long period of rest, especially in older, more competitive, high-performance athletes, the patient may require surgical treatment, such as repair or reconstruction of the MCL. Athletes who undergo surgery have an extremely high success rate, with return to activity in less than 1 year in most patients (2).

Forearm Splints

Forearm or wrist splints are seen mostly in young gymnasts, especially in males, as a result of work on the pommel horse. The injury is believed to be similar to shin splints. According to Aronen (20), wrist splints are due to strain from overuse at the origin of the extensor carpi ulnaris. The typical patient with this injury has a history of forearm overuse associated with lateral forearm pain that increases with activity. Pain relief can be achieved with ice before and after

practice. Athletes are able to return to activity more quickly by wrapping the forearms and taping the wrists prior to activity. Prevention includes strengthening of the forearm, especially the wrist extensors, and improvements in technique. The gymnast and his or her coach should also be educated about the dangers of overtraining (4).

REFERRAL GUIDELINES

Primary care physicians can safely manage the majority of elbow disorders. However, several injuries, if not managed properly, can result in significant long-term patient morbidity. The primary care physician must always pay attention to the growth plates, and he or she should obtain films of both sides in order to compare bilateral growth plates. A few overuse injuries require comanagement with orthopedics, including a medial apophysis with a separation greater than 3 mm and lateral elbow pain that raises the concern of possible OCD. Any athlete with persistent or recurrent pain, persistent swelling, flexion contractures, and failure to respond to short-term conservative therapy or activity modification should also be evaluated by an orthopedist. A number of guidelines should also be followed for the treatment of traumatic injuries. If an x-ray is suspicious for fracture but not definitive, oblique and contralateral views should be included for further evaluation. All children with elbow fractures should be considered for orthopedic referral. Children with suspected supracondylar fractures should be referred as early as possible. Because of the severe morbidity of compartment syndrome, the clinician must maintain a high degree of suspicion for this complication. If these guidelines are followed, a primary care physician should be capable of properly managing elbow injuries.

RETURN TO PLAY

Return to play is a process in which the initial goals of the rehabilitative process are a return of normal and symmetric ROM, minimal pain on palpation, and 90% of strength as compared to the other extremity. After achieving these goals, the rehabilitation effort next focuses on returning the athlete to his or her sports-specific function. In baseball, for example, the athlete can start throwing in special controlled situations (i.e., in a training area with a sleeve). Rehabilitation then should progress slowly from the long toss to a short toss on the mound. If the patient has no difficulties with these activities, the next step is attempting some simulated games in a practice setting.

At this point, the athlete should be ready to pitch in a game setting with a limited pitch count, with a gradual progression to normal pitch counts, as tolerated. If the athlete reports mild pain that diminishes with activity, rehabilitation may continue to progress. If the mild pain increases with activity, rehabilitation should be decelerated. Specific injuries, including osteochondritis dissecans and fractures, should be discussed with the orthopedic surgeon prior to starting rehabilitation. The process of return to a sports-specific function should be highly individualized.

REFERENCES

1. Lyman SL, Fleisig GS, Osinski ED, et al. Incidence and determinants of arm injury in youth baseball pitchers: a pilot study [abstract]. *Med Sci Sports Exerc* 1998;30:S4.
2. Lee MJ, Rosenwasser MP. Elbow trauma and reconstruction: chronic elbow instability. *Orthop Clin North Am* 1999;30:81–89.
3. Chumbley EM, O'Connor FG, Nirschl RP. Evaluation of overuse elbow injuries. *Am Fam Physician* 2000;61:691–700.
4. O'Connor FG, Olivierre CO, Nirschl RP. Elbow and forearm injuries. In: Lillegard WA, Butcher JD, Rucker KS, eds. *Handbook of sports medicine: a symptom-oriented approach*. 2nd ed. Boston: Butterworth-Heinemann, 1999:141–157.
5. Morrey BF, ed. *The elbow and its disorders*, 2nd ed. Philadelphia: WB Saunders, 1993.
6. Fick DS, Lyons TA. Interpreting elbow radiographs in children. *Am Fam Physician* 1997;55:1278–1282.
7. Hoppenfeld S. *Physical examination of the spine and extremities*. New York: Appleton-Century-Crofts, 1976.
8. Bradley JP. Upper extremity: elbow injuries in children and adolescents. In: Stanitski CL, DeLee JC, Drez D, eds. *Pediatric and adolescent sports medicine*. Philadelphia: WB Saunders, 1994:242–261.
9. McAuley E, Hudash G, Shields K, et al. Injuries in women's gymnastics. *Am J Sports Med* 1987;15:558–565.
10. Snook GA. Injuries in women's gymnastics. a five-year study. *Am J Sports Med* 1979;7:242–244.
11. Garrick JG, Requa RK. Epidemiology of women's gymnastics injuries. *Am J Sports Med* 1980;8:261–264.
12. Pettrone FA, Ricciardelli E. Gymnastic injuries: the Virginia experience 1982–1983. *Am J Sports Med* 1987;15:59–62.
13. Ross G. Acute elbow dislocation: on-site treatment. *The Physician and Sports Medicine* 1999;27:121–122.
14. Renshaw TS. The upper extremity. In: Renshaw TS, ed. *Pediatric orthopedics*, 1st ed. Philadelphia: WB Saunders, 1986:23–29.
15. Hall TL, Galea AM. Osteochondritis dissecans of the elbow: diagnosis, treatment, and prevention. *The Physician and Sports Medicine* 1999;2:75–87.
16. Whiteside JA, Andrews JR, Fleisig GS. Elbow injuries in young baseball players. *The Physician and Sports Medicine* 1999;6:87–102.
17. Schenck RC Jr, Goodnight GM. Osteochondritis dissecans. *J Bone Joint Surg Am* 1996;79:439–456.
18. Mitsunaga MM, Adishian DA, Bianco AJ Jr. Osteochondritis dissecans of the capitellum. *Trauma* 1982;22:53–55.
19. Peck DM. Apophyseal injuries in the young athlete. *Am Fam Physician* 1995;51:1891–1895.
20. Aronen JG. Problems of the upper extremity in gymnastics. *Clin Sports Med* 1985;4:61–71.

34

Hand and Wrist Injuries

Eron Grant Manusov

An estimated 35 million children actively participate in sports in the United States (1,2). In the pediatric population, 15% to 60% of injuries involve the hand and wrist. Fifty percent of those injuries are a result of overuse. The incidence of hand and wrist injury, however, varies with the sport. The wrist and hand are most likely to be injured during basketball, football, boxing, softball, and skiing (3). Half of skateboarding injuries involve the wrist and hand. Upwards of 79% of injuries in gymnastics involve the hand and wrist. Hand and wrist injuries are rare in swimming and soccer.

Fortunately, serious limb-threatening injury in the pediatric athlete is rare. The magnitude of the injury, however, can be underestimated because of the generally non–weight-bearing nature of the wrist and the tendency to label these injuries as sprains and thus to pressure children to continue playing (1). *Physicians must remember that the diagnosis of pediatric wrist sprain does not exist*. The exact injury to the wrist and hand must be defined, and its severity must be determined, in order to minimize long-term disability. The complexity of the joints and the presence of growth plates (epiphysis) can complicate the diagnosis, management, and success of treatment. Misdiagnosis of a serious ligament or osseous injury as a sprain can lead to chronic instability or pain.

The primary care physician can greatly improve the outcome if the approach to the wrist and hand is organized and systematic and if he or she has a good understanding of the pertinent anatomy and function. The intercalated components of the wrist are such that injury to one component affects the entire function of the wrist. Normal motion may be compromised, which can result in pain and deformity. The specific injury patterns to the ligaments and bones of the hand and wrist follow the anatomy. Therefore, normal skeletal, motor, and nerve function must be reviewed in order to conduct a thorough examination of an injured young athlete. The diagnosis and management of both wrist and hand injuries are discussed separately because of the unique functioning of each and the ligamentous anatomic differences.

AN APPROACH TO PEDIATRIC WRIST INJURIES

The wrist is a complex joint with multiple articulations and ligaments (2,3). Evaluation begins with a careful history and physical examination. Problems unique to the pediatric patient can occur as a result of injury or with alteration of the growth plate (epiphysis), the apophysis, or the blood supply to rapidly growing bones. The incidence and severity of the problems are influenced by the age of the patient. First, the clinician must identify when, where, and how the injury or pain began. *When* did the injury occur or how long has the patient complained of pain? *Where* did the injury occur and under what conditions? *How* did the injury occur? What was the mechanism of injury and what was the exact position of the hand? What previous treatments have been tried? Exacerbating factors, such as pain only during a certain movement or swelling and ecchymoses, help with isolating the area that is involved. Knowledge of the specifics of the injury pattern and the exacerbating or alleviating factors will improve the diagnosis, treatment, and the prevention of further injury. Knowledge of the sport and its specific biomechanical demands will improve the diagnostic accuracy and management success.

The physical examination begins with an inspection of the shoulder, elbow, wrist, and hand. Assessment of active motion of the shoulder and elbow and of the extremity in both supination and pronation is essential. Motion of these joints is essential for the proper function of the wrist and hand. The wrist and hand can then be inspected for swelling, ecchymosis, and deformity. In general, the greater the extent of the injury is, the greater the swelling and ecchymosis. Surface anatomy consists of the distal wrist crease, the thenar eminence on the ulnar border and the hypothenar eminence on the radial border, and the distal and proximal palmar creases. Pain should be localized to the distal radius–ulna, the midcarpal joint, the proximal row, or the distal carpal row. The proximal row consists of the scaphoid, lunate, triquetrum, and pisiform carpal bones. The distal carpal row is composed of the trapezium, trapezoid, capitate, and hamate (Fig. 34.1). Each carpal bone and articulation should then be palpated. The distal wrist crease corresponds to the distal radial–ulnar joint. The examiner can palpate the joint and its syndesmosis for pain and motion by placing his or her thumb on the volar distal wrist crease and the forefinger on the dorsal distal wrist crease. The radial and ulnar styloid processes are prominent on the lateral and medial wrist, respectively. The pisiform is palpable on the volar surface of the wrist, within the tendon of the flexor carpi ulnaris (FCU), and on the scaphoid, in the anatomic snuffbox distal to the radial styloid process.

No tendons, except the sesmoid pisiform, originate from or insert onto the carpal bones. The function of the wrist is therefore passive, with carpal bones that act as an intercalated segment. The general tendency of the carpal bones is to rotate separately or as separate groups. For example, as the scaphoid rotates, the lunate or the triquetrum naturally rotates in a different direction. The ligaments between carpal bones and rows keep the intercalated bones moving in synchronization. The ligamentous configuration of the wrist is a double inverted V, which keeps the two rows from collapsing (Fig. 34.2). The proximal inverted V is formed by the radial–lunate and ulnolunate intracapsular extrinsic ligaments. The distal inverted V is formed by the two components of the deltoid ligament, the capitoscaphoid and capitotriquetral ligaments. The space of Poirier, which is located over the capitolunate articulation, is a potentially weak space that is devoid of ligaments, thus potentially allowing perilunate instability in hyperextension injuries (Fig. 34.3).

Motor nerve function and testing are listed in Table 34.1. The medial nerve provides sensation to the medial hand, thumb, second finger, and the medial half of the third finger. The ulnar nerve provides sensation to the lateral hand, the fifth and fourth fingers, and the lateral half of the third finger. The muscles of the hand are divided into extrinsic and intrinsic muscles. The extrinsic muscles have their bellies in the forearm and

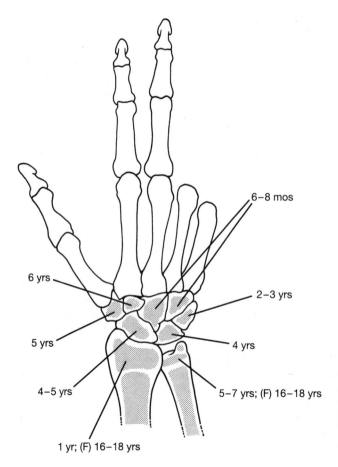

6–8 mos

6 yrs

2–3 yrs

5 yrs

4 yrs

4–5 yrs

5–7 yrs; (F) 16–18 yrs

1 yr; (F) 16–18 yrs

FIG. 34.1. Carpal bones and age at the time of appearance of the ossific nucleus. The pisiform is not shown, and the ossific nucleus appears between 6 and 8 years of age. (From Beaty JH, Kasser JR, eds. *Rockwood and Wilkins' fractures in children,* 5th ed. Philadelphia: Lippincott Williams & Wilkins, 2001, with permission.)

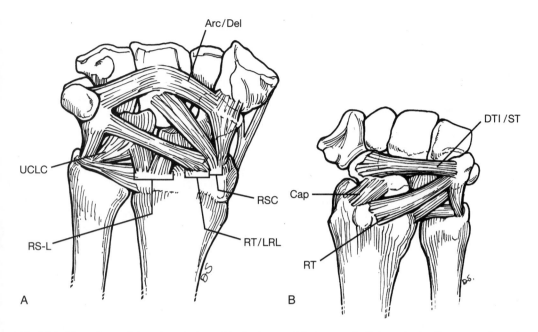

FIG. 34.2. The volar and dorsal extrinsic and intrinsic carpal ligaments. **A:** Selected volar ligaments about the wrist. Abbreviations: RS-L, radioscaphoid–lunate; RT/LRL, radiotriquetral/long radiolunate; RSC, radioscapho-capitate ligament; Arc/Del, arcuate or deltoid ligament; UCLC, ulnocarpal ligament complex, including ulnocarpal volar ligament, disc-triquetral, and disc-lunate ligaments. **B:** Dorsal ligaments about the wrist. Abbreviations: Cap, capsular attachments; RT, radiotriquetral ligament; DTI/ST, dorsal transverse intercarpal ligament or scapho-trapezial ligament. (From Beaty JH, Kasser JR, eds. *Rockwood and Wilkins' fractures in children*, 5th ed. Philadelphia: Lippincott Williams & Wilkins, 2001, with permission.)

their tendon insertions in the hand, and they are further divided into flexor and extensor muscles. The flexor pollicis longus (FPL) inserts on the volar phalanx of the thumb, and it can be evaluated by bending the tip of the thumb. The flexor digitorum profundus (FDP) is tested by flexing the tip of the finger while the distal joint is stabilized in extension. Each flexor digitorum superficialis (FDS) can be tested by flexing the finger at the proximal interphalangeal joint (PIP). The other fingers must be stabilized in extension in order to block profundus function.

The FCU, flexor carpi radialis (FCR), and palmaris longus (PL) are evaluated by flexing the wrist. The FCU inserts on the pisiform. The PL inserts into the palmar fascia, and the FCR inserts on the volar aspect of the index metacarpal. The tendons can be identified by flexing the wrist while simultaneously opposing the thumb and the small finger. The PL lies between the FCU on the ulnar side and the FCR on the radial side.

The extrinsic extensor muscle tendons pass over the dorsum of the wrist in six compartments to insert on the hand. The first dorsal compartment contains the tendons of the abductor pollicis longus (APL) and ex-

tensor pollicis brevis (EPB). They are evaluated by asking the patient to abduct the thumb with the wrist in the neutral position. The second dorsal compartment contains the tendons of the extensor carpi radialis longus and brevis. They are evaluated by having the patient close his or her fist and extend the wrist. The third dorsal compartment contains the tendon of the extensor pollicis longus that passes by the Lister tubercle of the radius. The fourth dorsal wrist compartment contains the metacarpalphalangeal (MCP) joint extensors of the fingers. The extensor digitorum communis (EDC) and the extensor indicis proprius (EIP) are evaluated by extending the fingers at the MCP joints. The EIP extends the pointer finger when the other fingers are bent in a fist. The fifth dorsal wrist compartment contains the tendon of the extensor digiti minimi (EDM), and it extends the fifth finger while the others are bent in a fist. The sixth dorsal wrist compartment contains the tendon of the extensor carpi ulnaris (ECU), which attaches to the dorsal base of the fifth metacarpal. The ECU tendon is evaluated by extending the wrist dorsally and abducting it.

The intrinsic muscles consist of the thenar muscle group; the adductor pollicis, lumbrical, and in-

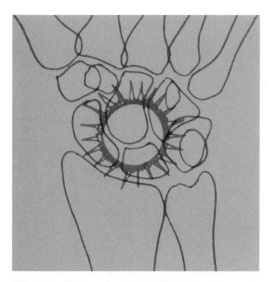

FIG. 34.3. The space of Poirier. This is an open area on the palmar side of the carpus that is defined by the paucity of the ligamentous support tissue that exists between the extrinsic and intrinsic ligaments of the medial and lateral sides of the wrist. Through the space of Poirier is where many wrist instability patterns manifest themselves. (From Watson HK, Weinzweig J, eds. *The wrist.* Philadelphia: Lippincott Williams & Wilkins, 2001, with permission.)

The adductor pollicis is innervated by the ulnar nerve, and it is tested by forcibly holding a piece of paper between the thumb and index finger. The thumb will flex at the interphalangeal (IP) joint (Froment sign) when this muscle is weak. The interosseous and lumbrical muscles flex the MCP joints, extend the IP joints, and abduct and adduct the fingers. The ulnar nerve innervates the interosseous muscles, which are tested by asking the patient to spread his or her fingers apart. Having the patient hyperextend the middle finger at the MCP, while moving the finger medially and laterally, will isolate the interosseous muscles and will prevent recruitment of the extrinsic extensor muscles. The hypothenar muscles include the abductor digiti minimi, the flexor digit minimi, and the opponens digiti minimi. They can be tested by abducting the fifth finger with the wrist in the neutral position.

A simple sketch of the wrist and hand is useful for documenting the range of motion (ROM) of each joint and the location of pain, swelling, ecchymosis, and neurologic deficits. Grip and pinch strength should also be recorded. Four roentgenographic views of the wrist—the posteroanterior (PA) in neutral position, the 45-degree pronated oblique, the PA with ulnar deviation, and the lateral view of the wrist in neutral position—can be obtained to visualize the musculoskeletal anatomy better (Fig. 34.4).

MEDICAL MALPRACTICE

Primary care physicians must make maintaining a high index of suspicion with injury to the hand and wrist imperative. Ligaments and tendons maintain a complex intercalation of multiple joints. A stretched or torn ligament could result in significant long-term morbidity. Repetitive injury to growing bones can result in growth arrest and subsequent deformity

terosseous muscles; and the hypothenar muscle group. These muscles have both their insertions and origins within the hand. The thenar muscle group includes the abductor pollicis brevis, the opponens pollicis, and the flexor pollicis brevis. These muscles oppose and abduct the thumb. To examine these muscles, the clinician should have the patient oppose his or her thumb and little finger so that the nails are parallel. Palpating the thenar muscles to ensure that they contract is important.

TABLE 34.1. *Motor nerve function and testing*

Nerve	Muscle function	Examination for function
Radial	Extensor carpi radialis, brevis, and ulnaris	Extension resistance
	Extensor pollicis brevis and longus	Push against extended thumb
	Abductor pollicis longus	Push against abducted thumb
	Extensor digitorum communis	Extend the metacarpal phalangeal with flexed proximal interphalangeal (PIP) with the wrist in neutral
Median	Extensor indicis and digiti minimi	Flex isolated PIP while the fingers are held in extension
	Flexor pollicis longus	Pull away a flexed thumb
	Abductor pollicis longus	Abduct thumb against resistance
	Opponens pollicis	Oppose the 5th finger and thumb

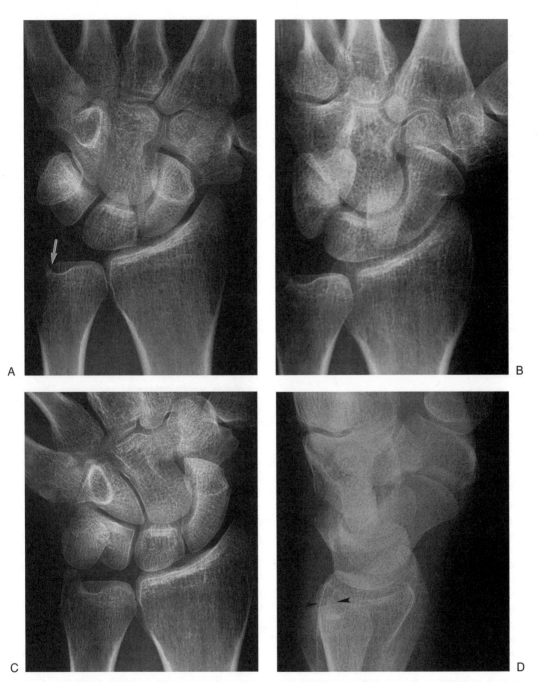

FIG. 34.4. Four views of the normal wrist. **A:** Posteroanterior (PA) in neutral position; ulnar styloid (*arrow*). **B:** Forty-five degree pronated oblique. **C:** PA with ulnar deviation. **D:** Lateral view of the left wrist in neutral position. (From Watson HK, Weinzweig J, eds. *The wrist*. Philadelphia: Lippincott Williams & Wilkins, 2001, with permission.)

and chronic pain. Damage to a growing epiphysis can cause angulation, misalignment, and growth differential.

Comparison of the injured and the opposite hand can be useful in determining what is "normal" for a particular patient. Comparison radiographs are necessary in all skeletally immature patients (Fig. 34.4). If a patient describes pain and the initial radiographs are normal, immobilizing the injured extremity and reevaluating in 1 week is always prudent. Physical therapy and hand occupational therapy often are helpful in the fashioning of splints and postimmobilization rehabilitation.

Documentation of the initial evaluation should include the ROM of all the joints involved, a neurosensory examination, and assessment of vascular flow. Frequent reevaluations during both the periods of immobilization and rehabilitation are necessary, and these should be documented. Parents must be informed of the complexity of the wrist and of the potential for long-term sequelae after injury. Discussion and education with both the parents and patient will improve the outcome and will often lessen the opportunity for misunderstanding and medical malpractice concerns.

DISTAL RADIUS AND ULNA INJURIES

Fractures

Forty-five percent of all long bone, acute fractures in children occur in the radius (4). Although fracture is common, morbidity is rare. The most common acute injury is caused by a fall on an outstretched hand, which is the so-named FOOSH injury. A buckle, or torus, fracture can occur when the tough periosteum remains intact but buckles circumferentially. The term "torus" refers to the thickened fortified base of a Greek column, which the fracture resembles. If only one side of periosteum bends and the opposite side breaks, the fracture resembles a break to a greenstick, and thus it is often called a "greenstick" fracture. Many clinicians advocate completing the fracture so that no differential bone growth or angulation occurs. Remodeling in the pediatric age group is rapid, so complete, full recovery is expected after simple immobilization. The distal radius, or "colles fracture," refers to a closed fracture in which the apex of the distal fragment points in the volar direction. The fracture type is common in older adults, but it rarely occurs in children due to the greater elasticity of young bone. Closed reduction to anatomical alignment may be necessary. Up to 20 degrees of angulation is acceptable because remodeling is often com-

plete in children. Management includes immobilization with a circumferential short-arm cast for 4 to 6 weeks in the position of function. During contact sports, the fracture site should be protected by a removable splint for an additional 2 weeks.

If the fracture involves the epiphysis, the prognosis and management is based on the Salter–Harris classification of physeal injury (see Fig. 26.3 in Chapter 26). A type I fracture occurs if the force of injury follows the physeal–epiphysis junction. If the force of the injury follows the junction but then crosses the metaphyses, the injury is labeled as a type II injury. Type I and II injuries are managed with 4 to 6 weeks of cast immobilization. When the fracture force follows the physeal junction and then crosses the more crucial epiphysis, potentially disrupting active cell growth (type III), or when it crosses both the epiphysis and metaphyses (type IV), long-term growth differential and angulation can occur. Orthopedic consultation should be obtained with types III and IV injuries and when 2 mm or more of displacement of the metaphyseal, or the Thurston Holland, fragment is observed (2). Up to 20 to 30 degrees of dorsal or volar angulation is acceptable as the majority of injuries will remodel. All type V, or crush injuries of the epiphyses, require orthopedic consultation. The major complications of distal radial–ulnar injury are growth plate arrest, angulation, and fracture redisplacement. Serial roentgenographs of arrested physes should be taken for monitoring until growth has ceased. If a deformity is still present after all remodeling has occurred, surgical corrective osteotomy can be attempted. Return to play after type I or II injuries may resume 2 weeks after the conclusion of immobilization and rehabilitation. A removable splint should be used for an additional 2 weeks for contact sports. Types III and IV epiphyseal injuries should not return to play for the remainder of the season, and they must complete appropriate rehabilitation.

Repetitive Injury and the Distal Radial Ulnar Joint

The extent of repetitive injury to the distal ulnar joint depends upon the sport involved, the patient's age, technique, and training schedules. Certain sports, especially gymnastics, have significant repetitive forces across the wrist that can result in stress injury to the distal radial and ulnar physes. With these injuries, athletes describe stiffness and pain with dorsiflexion of the wrist. Widened epiphyses, cystic changes, and beaking of the distal metaphysis may be demonstrated on radiographs (Figure 34.5). Treatment consists of rest, either with or without cast im-

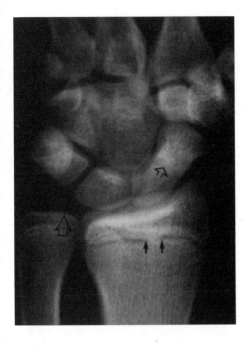

FIG. 34.5. Stress changes in a female gymnast. Early physeal arrest (*small arrows*) and positive ulnar variance (*large open arrow*) are present. A stress fracture of the body of the scaphoid (*small open arrow*) can also be seen. (Courtesy of Thomas J Graham. M.D.) (From Rockwood CA Jr, Wilkins KE, Beaty JH, eds. *Fractures in children*, 4th ed. Philadelphia: Lippincott-Raven, 1996, with permission.)

mobilization. Long-term sequelae are rare; however, the athletes and parents should be clearly informed of the potential for growth arrest of the affected joint.

Often referred to as "gymnast's wrist," growth arrest of the distal ulna or radius resulting from repetitive forceful dorsiflexion can cause chronic pain and subsequent ulnar variance. Arrest of radius growth results in positive ulnar variance. Arrest of ulna growth can result in negative variance (Fig. 34.6). Ulnar variance has been directly correlated with length of time an athlete has spent in gymnastics (5).

Up to 87% of elite gymnasts sustain radial physeal injuries and more than 80% of gymnasts complain of significant wrist pain during their careers (3,5–7). In addition to wrist pain, ulnar variance can result in impingement and deformity. Prevention is difficult because many gymnasts are required to perform wrist loading maneuvers. Early intervention when wrist pain occurs, with immobilization when necessary, training in the use of appropriate techniques, strengthening exercises, and rest, can decrease the morbidity of physeal injury.

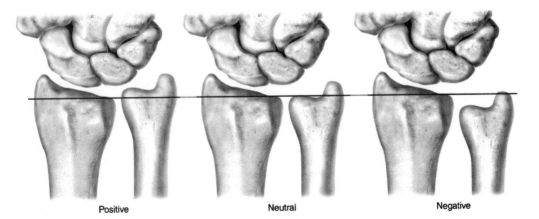

Positive   Neutral   Negative

FIG. 34.6. Ulnar variance. This is the distance in the coronal plane between two lines perpendicular to the axis of the radiuvariance. If the radius variance is larger, the distance is positive; if it is the same, then the distance is neutral; if it is shorter, then the distance is negative. (From Watson HK, Weinzweig J, eds. *The wrist*. Philadelphia: Lippincott Williams & Wilkins, 2001, with permission.)

TABLE 34.2. *The management of distal radial ulnar joint injury*

Acute trauma	
Volar dislocation	Long-arm cast in pronation for 6 wk
Dorsal dislocation	Long-arm cast in supination for 6 wk
Chronic repetitive injury	
Ulnar carpal impingement (no TFCC tear)	Ulnar shortening
TFCC perforation (negative ulnar variance)	Arthroscopic debridement
TFCC perforation (neutral ulnar variance)	Arthroscopic debridement and/or ulnar shortening
TFCC perforation (positive ulnar variance)	Ulnar shortening and TFCC debridement

Abbreviation: TFCC, triangular fibrocartilage complex.
From Stanitski CL, Delee JC, Drez D. *Pediatric and adolescent sports medicine*. Vol. 3. Philadelphia: WB Saunders, 1994:262–278, with permission.

Acute Distal Radial Ulnar Joint Injury

Acute distal radioulnar joint (DRUJ) injuries in children are rare (7,8). Their diagnosis and management are outlined in Table 34.2. The two major types of injuries are acute dislocations of the DRUJ and triangular fibrocartilage complex (TFCC) lesions (6). DRUJ dislocations occur with forced wrist extension or flexion, such as occurs in gymnastic floor exercises. Acute dorsal dislocations should be managed with 6 weeks in a long-arm cast with the forearm in full supination. Volar dislocations should be maintained in full pronation for the same amount of time. Return to full participation is possible after 6 to 8 weeks of adequate rehabilitation (1,3,8).

TFCC injuries can occur during ulnar loading, as is seen in the bench press. The TFCC is a ligamentous structure that stabilizes the DRUJ and that supports 18% of the compressive loads of the carpal bones at the wrist. The function of the TFCC can be readily understood if one has a clear appreciation of its anatomy (Fig. 34.7). It is shaped like an isosceles triangle, in which the base is found along the attachment to the sigmoid notch of the distal radius. The apex is at the insertion into the fovea and the base of the ulnar styloid. The sides of the triangle are free of attachment, and they are composed of the palmar and radioulnar ligaments. Between these borders stretches the free floating articular disc. Since it lies on, but is not attached to, the articular surface, the TFCC can rotate freely with pronation and supination of the radius. The ulnocarpal meniscus homologue sits within the most ulnar recess of the DRUJ. The ulnolunate and ulnotriquetral ligaments extend distally from the volar radioulnar ligaments. Dorsally, the ECU sheath lends support by blending with the dorsal radioulnar ligament and the dorsal DRUJ capsule.

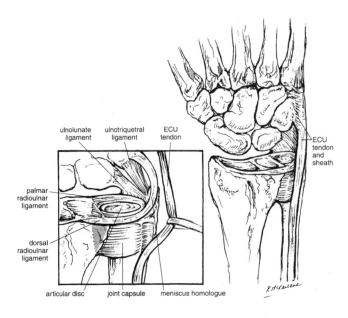

FIG. 34.7. Triangular fibrocartilage complex with meniscal homologue. Components include the articular disc, dorsal and palmar radioulnar ligaments, meniscus homologue, ulnolunate and ulnotriquetral ligaments, and extensor carpi ulnaris tendon and its sheath. (From Watson HK, Weinzweig J, eds. *The wrist*. Philadelphia: Lippincott Williams & Wilkins, 2001, with permission.)

TABLE 34.3. *Summary of ligamentous injuries*

Radial side ligamentous injuries	Ulnar side ligamentous injuries
Acute	Acute
Dorsal perilunar dislocation	Triquetrolunate instability
Lunate dislocation	Triquetrohamate instability
Scapholunate dissociation	Triangular fibrocartilage injury
	Acute extensor carpi ulnaris subluxation
Chronic	Chronic
Dequervain tenosynovitis	Extensor carpi ulnaris tendinitis
Extensor carpi radialis longus and brevis tenosynovitis	Subluxating extensor carpi tendon
Extensor pollicus longus tendinitis	Triquetrohamate impingement syndrome
Scaphoid impingement syndrome	Flexor carpi ulnaris and pisiform tendinitis
Radial styloid impingement syndrome	Ulnar nerve entrapment
Flexor carpi radialis tendinitis	Hypothenar hammer syndrome

ROM, including lateral and medial, as well as flexion and extension, and the point of maximal tenderness should be recorded. To localize TFCC tenderness, the clinician should palpate the hollow between the pisiform, FCU, and ulnar styloid. Performing the examination with the wrist in pronation keeps the dorsal radioulnar ligament and the extensor digiti quinti (EDQ) dorsal, thus allowing unobstructed palpation of the complex. In addition, forced ulnar deviation will impact the ulnar styloid and will result in pain, if the TFCC is involved. The supination test can also aid in identifying dorsal and peripheral TFCC tears. In a seated position, the athlete is asked to try to lift the underside of the table with the palms of his or her hand. Focal pain and an inability to lift are indicative of TFCC involvement.

The piano sign can demonstrate DRUJ laxity. To perform this test, the athlete places his or her palm flat on the table and exerts pressure in a downward direction. The downward pressure of the entire hand results in excessive volar motion of the ulna that is similar to that of a pianist. However, children are often hypermobile, and the DRUJ itself has a normal ROM. Comparison of the injured to the uninjured wrist will give a good indication of the patient's normal joint motion. The clinician must remember that tendonitis can coexist with TFCC pathology. Inflammation of nearby tendons can be discerned by careful palpation of each tendon; these are reviewed in Table 34.3 (9–11).

A true PA view of the wrist in the neutral position is important for assessing ulnar variance. A lateral view is required in order to assess carpal alignment and DRUJ position. If subluxation of the DRUJ is suspected, a lateral computerized tomography (CT) scan in which the DRUJ is in full pronation and supination and in the neutral position will demonstrate excessive motion. Comparison views with the uninjured wrist

will help the clinician discern between normal and excessive translation of the ulna on the radius. The use of the wrist arthrogram has been studied extensively but has, by and large, been replaced by magnetic resonance imaging (MRI) (12–14).

Removing the inciting force is the treatment of choice. Rest, ice, splint immobilization for 2 to 3 weeks, and subsequent physical therapy can be effective for TFCC lesions. The presence of ulnar deviation with TFCC tears are graded according to Palmer, and the appropriate surgical management is listed in Table 34.4. Surgical management should be postponed until skeletal maturity is complete. The decision to operate is influenced by the competition timetable, the level of performance, the degree of pain and of restriction of motion, and the failure of conservative management. The athlete's return to his or her previous level of performance (e.g., high school, collegiate, or international) after surgical correction is variable.

CARPAL INJURIES

Ligamentous Instabilities of the Wrist

Ligamentous injury resulting in instability is rare in the young athlete. As the child matures skeletally, however, the injury pattern parallels that of adult athletes; these parallels are shown in Table 34.3. The most common ligamentous carpal injury is scapholunate dissociation. The scapholunate ligament can be either acutely torn, or it may be worn by repetitive motion. The scaphoid normally moves out of the way, or becomes more vertical, by palmar flexing with radial deviation, and the lunate typically is forced to move with the scaphoid. If the scapholunate ligament is not intact, the scaphoid will palmar flex, but the lunate will follow its natural tendency to dorsiflex with

TABLE 34.4. *Diagnosis and management of carpal fractures*

Fractures	Radiograph	Treatment
Scaphoid	Scaphoid series	LAC thumb spica, 6 wk
Initial views normal	Scintography	SAC with serial radiographs until union
Proximal one-third,	—	Refer to orthopedic surgery
displaced or delayed		AVN risk
Lunate	PA and lateral, scintography, CT	Refer to orthopedic surgery
		AVN risk
Triquetrium body	Oblique wrist	SAC, 4–6 wk
	PA and lateral views	Refer to orthopedic surgery
Pisiform	Supinated oblique or carpal tunnel view	SAC, 4–6 wk
		Refer if comminuted or displaced
Hamate hook	Carpal tunnel view, CT	SAC, 6 wk repeat
Capitate	PA and lateral	Refer to orthopedic surgery
		AVN risk
Trapezoid	PA and lateral	SAC for 3–6 wk
		Suspect ligament instability
Trapezium	PA and lateral, carpal tunnel view	Nondisplaced; SAC, 6 wk
		Refer displaced fractures to
		orthopedic surgery

Abbreviations: AVN, avascular necrosis; CT, computerized tomography; LAC, long-arm cast; PA, posterior anterior; SAC, short-arm cast.

radial deviation. The result will be a vertical scaphoid (rotatory subluxation) and a dorsiflexed lunate (dorsal intercalated segment instability [DISI]) (Fig. 34.8). A Watson scaphoid test may be positive on physical examination. In this test, the patient's wrist is placed in ulnar deviation so that the scaphoid is in the neutral horizontal position. The examiner's thumb is then placed volar on the scaphoid tubercle, and the four fingers are placed on the dorsal distal radius. The patient's hand is deviated radially, while the thumb prevents the scaphoid from palmar flexing. If the scapholunate ligament is not intact, the proximal pole will be forced dorsally with a palpable click and pain.

PA roentgenographs may demonstrate a scapholunate space greater than 3 mm (called the Terry Thomas sign after a comedian with a gap between his front incisors) or a cortical ring sign (the scaphoid has a short appearance; end-on projection of the rotated scaphoid gives a ringed appearance). Lateral views demonstrate that the lunate is dorsiflexed, with a capitolunate angle greater than 15 degrees and a scapholunate angle greater than 65 degrees. The radial carpal arthrogram will demonstrate spillage, and MRI can further delineate the tear and edema.

Orthopedic consultation should be obtained in these cases. If the scapholunate alignment is normal, the arm should be immobilized for 6 weeks in a long-arm cast. If the alignment of the scapholunate is abnormal, surgical management is recommended. Surgical treatment of chronic scapholunate disassociation is controversial. The current recommendation is that surgical management be delayed until adulthood. Patients should be removed from play, and, after 6 to 8 weeks of adequate rehabilitation, they can be considered for return to play.

Perilunate and lunate dislocations occur with a hyperextension injury to the wrist that causes the scaphoid to extend and strike the dorsal lip of the radius. The volar radioscaphoid and scapholunate ligaments are ruptured, freeing the proximal pole of the scaphoid, while compressive forces wedge the capitate between the scaphoid and lunate. Continued dorsiflexion essentially causes the distal carpal row to come to rest in a position dorsal to the lunate and radius. Further force ruptures the dorsal restraining radiocarpal ligament, allowing the lunate to "flip" palmward (the spilled teacup sign), as the remaining carpal bones relocate. The physical examination should devote particular attention to the median nerve, which can be injured or compressed as a result of the injury. Radiographs demonstrate a dislocated lunate with the "spilled teacup sign." Lunate dislocations should be referred to orthopedic surgery for definitive therapy.

Triquetrolunate instability is a result of rupture of the triquetrolunate ligament. Normal ulnar deviation causes the triquetrum to dorsiflex, producing dorsiflexion in the lunate and scaphoid. If the triquetrolunate ligament is ruptured, the triquetrum will dorsiflex with ulnar deviation, but the lunate and scaphoid will follow their normal tendency to volar flex. This results in a volar intercalated segment instability

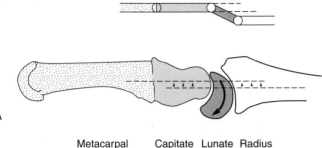

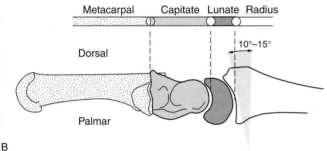

FIG. 34.8. A: In dorsal intercalated segment instability, the scaphoid has rotated into extension. **B:** In the neutral position, the longitudinal axes of the third metacarpal and the radius are collinear. The lunate is supported in a neutral attitude, as it is neither flexed nor extended. (From Watson HK, Weinzweig J, eds. *The wrist.* Philadelphia: Lippincott Williams & Wilkins, 2001, with permission.)

(VISI). A painful click is felt as the wrist is compressed and is moved from ulnar to radial deviation. Pain, laxity, and crepitus can be assessed with dorsal and/or volar motion of the pisiform and triquetrum. Roentgenographs are often normal. A VISI pattern with a dorsiflexed triquetrum, a volar-flexed scaphoid and lunate, and a scapholunate angle greater than 70 degrees can be demonstrated on lateral plain views. MRI is not accurate because of the relatively small ligament size, but, as the technology improves, it may become a diagnostic option (12). Pain without dislocation can be managed with 3 weeks of immobilization. Persistent pain and dislocations should be referred to orthopedic surgery. Surgical management, however, should be delayed until skeletal maturity.

Carpal Fractures

Scaphoid fractures account for more than 70% of wrist fractures. The peak incidence is between 12 and 15 years, and they are rarely reported in children under 10 years of age (2,14). The distribution of scaphoid injury in children is different from that of adults. Seventy-five percent of fractures occur at the distal pole, 20% are waist fractures, and 5% occur at the proximal scaphoid. A FOOSH injury can result in a scaphoid fracture if the wrist is simultaneously dorsiflexed. Scaphoid injury is more common in sports such as skating, skateboarding, and bicycling. Proper protective gear, such as wrist splints, can prevent scaphoid injuries.

The scaphoid is the only carpal bone to cross the midcarpal joint. The shape and position of the scaphoid prevents the proximal row from collapsing in a zigzag configuration under compressive loads. Although each carpal bone is susceptible to specific forces, the scaphoid's unique position, function, and blood supply predisposes it to injury. The entire scaphoid relies on an interosseous blood supply that enters the proximal pole and extends to the distal pole. Fracture disrupts the blood supply, and avascular necrosis of the distal pole can occur.

The physical examination may reveal pain that is centered in the anatomical snuffbox, as well as decreased ROM of the proximal wrist. Usually, however, the findings are subtle, including minimal swelling and tenderness in the snuffbox and a minimally reduced ROM. The clinician should grasp the scaphoid by both poles, while moving the wrist laterally and medially. Pain or instability and the normal motion of the scaphoid can be assessed more accurately in this manner than by relying on "snuffbox" tenderness alone. Examining the uninjured scaphoid can help the examiner accurately assess the normal motion and position of the scaphoid. The proximal pole can be palpated in the anatomical "snuffbox," the borders of which consist of the extensor pollicis longus, the abductor pollicis brevis, and extensor pollicis brevis on the dorsum of the hand. The distal pole or tubercle can be palpated on the volar surface. The differential diagnosis includes a nondisplaced Salter I fracture or a distal radius buckle fracture.

Most scaphoid fractures will heal with early immobilization. Plain radiographs that include a specialized scaphoid view may not demonstrate the presence of a fracture. If a high index of suspicion remains, the wrist should be immobilized in a short-arm thumb spica cast. If repeat radiographs in 2 weeks are negative and the pain is still present, bone scintiography can be conducted. A negative scan virtually rules out the presence of a fracture, and the scan will be positive within 72 hours of the injury (1). If the scan is negative and the physical examination still produces pain, a diagnosis of scapholunate dissociation should be considered (1,3,10). Athletes with nondisplaced distal pole and tubercle fractures can be managed with 6 weeks of immobilization. A padded cast, if its use is allowed by the sport, can be worn to allow the athlete to continue play. Compressive forces should be avoided, and treatment should be followed by appropriate rehabilitation. Fractures through the waist and proximal pole should be immobilized with a long-arm thumb spica cast for 4 weeks and should be followed by the application of a short-arm thumb spica cast until union is demonstrated or for 5 months. Contact sports are not allowed until union occurs. Established scaphoid nonunions and acute displaced fractures require orthopedic consultation (3,13).

Fractures of other carpal bones are extremely rare in children. Dorsal triquetral fractures resulting from either a direct blow or acute dorsiflexion can be managed with short-arm cast immobilization for 3 to 4 weeks; continued athletic participation is allowed. Hook of hamate fractures, although rare, do occur secondary to torque around a shafted object, such as a golf club, baseball bat, or tennis racquet. Pain is localized at the volar surface of the wrist. Carpal tunnel radiographs are usually adequate; however, if the anatomy is not clearly delineated with these, a CT scan can be obtained. Bone scintiography is highly sensitive, but it is not specific because of the poor anatomical definition of scintiography and the normally increased activity of the actively maturing growth plate. MRI is useful for the evaluation of wrist dislocations and many subluxations, and it may demonstrate occult fractures, edema, and tears. Recent evaluation of the wrist using kinematic MRI has improved the diagnosis of subtle ligament tears and instability. Kinematic MRI uses MRI technology and various joint positions to evaluate the interconnections with motion. The advantage of kinematic MRI over conventional MRI is the ability to evaluate complex joint motion. In addition, pain that occurs only with certain motions can be assessed, and specific information about joint abnormalities can be identified (14). Kinematic MRI requires additional training for radiologists and radiology technicians, and it currently is not readily available.

Avascular Necrosis and Lunate Injury

Kienböck disease, or avascular necrosis of the lunate, is another cause of wrist pain in the pediatric age group. The exact incidence is unknown; however, Kienböck disease is most common among white males between the ages of 18 to 38 years, although it has been reported at the extremes of ages (8 to 71 years of age), in women, and in all ethnic groups. It generally affects the dominant wrist, and it is unilateral. Only 3% to 7% of cases are bilateral. The precise etiology remains uncertain, but diminished blood supply to the lunate leads to pathologic necrosis of the lunate, the collapse of the bony architecture, and alteration of normal wrist mechanics, as described by Kienböck in 1910. The blood supply disruption may be due to either macrotrauma or microtrauma. Anatomic variations, such as abnormalities in blood supply and ulnar variance, that may predispose a patient to avascular necrosis have been identified.

The blood supply of the lunate has been extensively studied. Ninety percent of lunate bones have extensive extraosseous arterioles that enter from multiple lacunae on both the dorsal and ventral surface. The remaining 10% have lacunae on the dorsal or ventral surface only. The arteries form anastamoses in the shape of either an X, Y, or I. A lunate anastamosis that is I-shaped or lacunae that enter only one surface can predispose the bone to avascular necrosis if the vascular supply is compromised.

Vascular compromise of the lunate can occur from direct acute trauma, but it more commonly occurs as a result of repetitive trauma that causes microfractures and excessive stress to the microscopic architecture. In addition, the presence of ulnar variance may affect the incidence of Kienböck disease. Those individuals with a relatively short ulna place a greater amount of sheer stress on the radius and the radial side of the lunate (6). The result is greater mechanical sheer forces across the lunate during wrist motion. Clearly, those sports that require repetitive hand motion, such as tennis, handball, volleyball, golf, gymnastics, and martial arts, present the highest risk for Kienböck disease (8,15).

Often acute injuries to the wrist are mistakenly considered sprains. The severity of the initial injury is underestimated, and continued dorsal wrist pain may progressively worsen until wrist motion is compromised. Dorsal swelling and decreased flexion and extension can be found on the physical examination, and patients will describe weakened grasp. Supination and pronation are usually preserved.

Kienböck disease is staged according to radiographic findings, as described by Lichtman. Stage I is defined by dorsal lunate pain and restricted motion with normal roentgenographs. Increased lunate density is the hallmark of stage II Kienböck disease. Stage III is defined by the collapse of the lunate on AP views, in addition to proximal migration of the capitate, ulnar deviation of the triquetrium, and scapholunate disassociation. Severe alterations in carpal architecture with subchondral stenosis and diffuse osteophyte formation occur in stage IV Kienböck disease. This stage is a late finding, and it is rare in children.

The goals of treatment for Kienböck disease are the reduction of pain and the prevention of carpal collapse and secondary arthritis. No universally accepted approach exists for treatment, which can include lunate resection, with either silicone or tendon interposition arthroplasty; intercarpal arthrodesis; ulnar lengthening; radial shortening; wrist arthrodesis; proximal row carpectomy; fibrous arthroplasty; radial–carpal arthrodesis; and cast immobilization. Success rates have been extremely variable, and the patient's return to preinjury status is unpredictable. The management approach depends on the stage of the disease at diagnosis, and it varies among surgeons. Obviously, a high index of suspicion and early referral to a hand surgeon are recommended. Remember, the diagnosis of wrist sprain does not exist in children.

Finally, a common complaint involving the carpal bones is pain and enlargement of the pisiform sesamoid bone. This bone, which is connected to the FCU, is the only carpal bone to have an extrinsic ligament attachment. Due to the volar location and its ligamentous attachment, the pisiform can be either fractured or involved in a repetitive apophysitis. Fractures are managed with immobilization or surgery, if the bone is displaced. Apophysitis can result from constant traction and can cause pain and swelling. Many parents will be concerned about the possiblity of a tumor or abnormal growth and deformity, so both the parents and the athlete should be reassured. Conservative management with nonsteroidal antiinflammatory drugs (NSAIDs), ice, and padding, when appropriate, is the treatment of choice. The diagnosis and management of all carpal fractures are outlined in Table 34.4.

HAND AND FINGER INJURIES

The anatomic function of the hand and fingers is complicated, and it relies on a system of pulleys to enable complex finger motion (Fig. 34.9). Injuries that can appear to be minimal may actually be serious enough to require surgical repair. Because the anatomic principles can be confusing, a good reference book should be readily available (16). The physical examination is directed to each anatomic principle, and, because of the intricate system for motion, it is reviewed with each injury type.

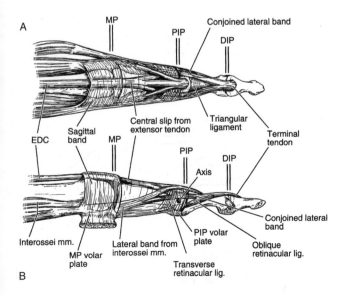

FIG. 34.9. Anteroposterior **(A)** and lateral **(B)** views of the extensor mechanism of the digit. Abbreviations: PIP, proximal interphalangeal joint; DIP, distal interphalangeal joint. (From Craig EV, ed. *Clinical orthopaedics.* Philadelphia: Lippincott Williams & Wilkins, 1999, with permission.)

Phalangeal and Interphalangeal Injuries

Jersey Finger

Jersey finger was first described in rugby players, but it can occur in any situation in which a player grabs the shirt of a moving opponent. The most common scenario is one player reaching out to tackle another player so that a finger catches the jersey and is pulled away. The injury is caused by the closed rupture of the FDP tendon from its insertion onto the distal phalanx. The mechanism of injury is the forced extension of the distal phalanx while the finger is maximally flexed. The injury can be restricted to the tendon, or a small piece of bone can be avulsed from the volar surface of the phalanx (Fig. 34.10).

Physical Examination

Tenderness on the volar surface of the distal phalanx may be the only finding on the initial examination. Permanent disability, however, can occur if this injury is not diagnosed properly. A tendon rupture will result in the inability to flex the distal phalanx while the PIP is blocked in extension. The tendon may retract into the palm, causing a complete disruption of the blood supply and scarring. If a bony fragment is present, it may be caught at the PIP or distal interphalangeal (DIP) joint. A lateral roentgenograph may identify the location of the avulsed fragment, but the practitioner should not underestimate the extent of injury because of the small size of the avulsed fragment (17).

Treatment

All flexor tendon ruptures and lacerations need surgical repair. The wrist and finger should be splinted in slight flexion, and referral should be made to an orthopedic surgeon within 7 to 10 days (18). Return to play can be allowed after immobilization and 2 weeks of appropriate rehabilitation. If the rules of the sport allow a splint to be worn, patients can wear a removable splint to protect the joint for an additional 2 months after initial immobilization.

Mallet Finger

Mallet finger is caused by forced flexion against active extension of the distal phalanx. Disruption of the extensor digitorum tendon from its insertion on the dorsal aspect of the distal phalanx will result in weakness or an inability to extend the distal phalanx.

Physical Examination

Three types of mallet finger injuries are seen. Type I is an incomplete disruption of the extensor tendon. The distal phalanx may drop, but weak active extension remains. Type II results in a 45-degree flexion deformity. The extensor tendon is completely disrupted, and no active extension occurs. The distal phalanx subluxes underneath the middle phalanx in the type III mallet finger injury. It is unable to flex or extend, and it may appear deformed. Mallet finger injury in children may involve the epiphyses. Figure 34.11 demonstrates two types of transepiphyseal fractures in children. Radiographically, four types of mallet-equivalent fractures are observed (Fig. 34.12). In type A equivalent fractures, the distal fragment involves the proximal third of the phalanx, and it remains in approximation to the distal phalanx. A type B

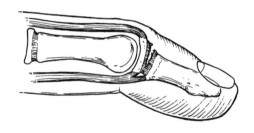

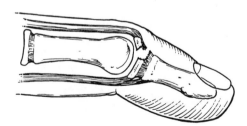

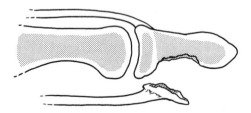

FIG. 34.10. A flexor digitorum profundus avulsion fracture of the distal phalanx, the jersey finger. (From Beaty JH, Kasser JR, eds. *Rockwood and Wilkins' fractures in children*, 5th ed. Philadelphia: Lippincott Williams & Wilkins, 2001, with permission.)

FIG. 34.11. Transepiphyseal fracture in children, resulting in a mallet finger. (From Craig EV, ed. *Clinical orthopaedics*. Philadelphia: Lippincott Williams & Wilkins, 1999, with permission.)

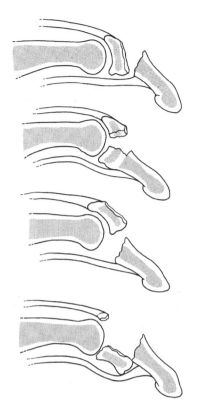

FIG. 34.12. The mallet fractures, type A to D. (From Beaty JH, Kasser JR, eds. *Rockwood and Wilkins' fractures in children*, 5th ed. Philadelphia: Lippincott Williams & Wilkins, 2001, with permission.)

equivalent fracture occurs when the fragment avulses from the phalanx, leaving the remaining distal phalanx to volar flex. A type C equivalent fracture is present if the fragment and the distal phalanx distract. Type D equivalent fractures consist of the lodging of the fragment in the joint.

Treatment

Most extensor digitorum ruptures can be managed nonoperatively. The distal phalanx is placed in full extension or even hyperextension, while the PIP remains unsplinted. Prefabricated mallet finger splints are effective, and these should not be removed for at least 6 to 8 weeks. Another 4 weeks of extension immobilization may be necessary if the distal phalanx continues to drop. Otherwise, 4 weeks of night splinting should be sufficient. Type III and type D injuries should be referred to an orthopedic surgeon. Patients can return to play after immobilization and appropriate rehabilitation. The use of a protective splint for an additional 4 weeks is advisable.

Boutonnière Deformity

Central extensor tendon rupture, or *boutonnière deformity*, is a result of disruption of the extensor mechanism at the PIP joint, and it can be caused by either a direct blow to the dorsum of the hand or forced flexion of the PIP joint.

Physical Examination

The injury is common in basketball and baseball. The central slip is ruptured from its insertion on the dorsal surface of the middle phalange. The lateral bands are allowed to slip in a volar direction, thus allowing the PIP joint to herniate dorsally through the central slip (Fig. 34.13).

Treatment

Boutonnière deformity is splinted in extension for 6 to 8 weeks, followed by protective splinting during play for an additional 2 months. Misdiagnosis and delayed treatment should be referred to an orthopedic surgeon.

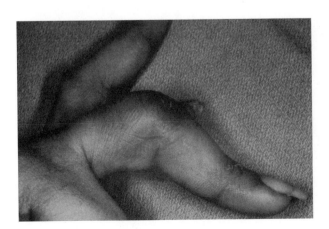

FIG. 34.13. Central extensor tendon or *boutonnière deformity* injury. (From Craig EV, ed. *Clinical orthopaedics*. Philadelphia: Lippincott Williams & Wilkins, 1999, with permission.)

Trigger Finger

Trigger finger is a nonspecific tenosynovitis of the flexor tendon sheath that results from repetitive use. The inflamed tendon and sheath catch on the closely applied pulley system.

Physical Examination

Patients complain of pain and a "snapping" sensation during extension and flexion. Trigger finger injuries are rare in children, but they can occur during sports with repetitive finger use, such as gymnastics and bowling,

Treatment

Night splinting and NSAIDs constitute the first line of treatment. A trigger finger, however, may require the injection of a steroid into the tendon sheath. Surgery may be necessary for recalcitrant cases. The timing of return to play depends on the sport in which the athlete is involved. Splinting to reduce motion and thereby inflammation is advisable if symptoms persist.

Volar Plate Injuries

Volar plate injuries occur from forced hyperextension or direct trauma to the interphalangeal joint. Injury to the volar plate is common in football, basketball, and baseball. The distal phalange dislocates either dorsally or laterally. Volar dislocations are rare, and they can be difficult to reduce. The volar plate is a fibrous plate that connects the proximal middle phalange with the distal proximal phalange. The effect is that it links both phalanges and prohibits subluxation.

Physical Examination

After a dislocation of the interphalangeal joint, the volar plate may rupture or avulse its insertion. If the injury is not appropriately treated, the result may be

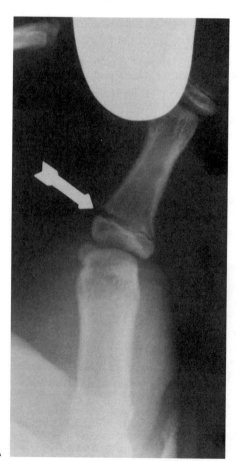

FIG. 34.14. The spectrum of presentations of ulnar collateral ligament injuries of the thumb. **A:** On stress examination, a widening of the physis (*arrow*) is seen. Instability is inferred, although no fracture is seen. **B,C:** Various fracture sizes. A Stener lesion is described when the avulsed fracture slips under the aponeurosis. (From Beaty JH, Kasser JR, eds. *Rockwood and Wilkins' fractures in children*, 5th ed. Philadelphia: Lippincott Williams & Wilkins, 2001, with permission.)

A

an unstable subluxating joint. In addition, the avulsed fragment may become caught in the pulley mechanism or joint. If the joint relocates immediately, the patient may complain only of pain and swelling of the joint. The persistent dislocated joint will appear deformed, and gentle traction with pressure over its dislocated base can reduce the joint. As with all dorsal dislocations, hyperextending and unlocking the involved joint may be necessary. The lateral collateral ligaments are often involved, and they also should be palpated and evaluated to determine the extent of damage. The avulsed fragment and the the extent of injury may be evident on radiograph.

Treatment

The joint should be immobilized with a dorsal block extension splint for 2 to 3 weeks. An aluminum splint can be initially angled at 90 to 110 degrees, and progressive degrees of extension can be allowed each week at the reevaluation appointment. The joint should be protectively splinted during play for an additional month. It will be stiff for 2 months; physical therapy to maximize the rehabilitation should be undertaken (18).

Thumb Injuries

Thumb injuries are more common than interphalangeal joint injuries, and they require an even more extensive evaluation. The *gamekeeper's or skier's thumb* is a result of forced abduction and hyperextension of the thumb. The injury can occur when a fixated ski pole is forced out of the grasped hand. The ulnar collateral ligament may be stretched, ruptured, or avulsed.

Physical Examination

A grade I sprain is diagnosed by pain with minimal swelling and no instability. A grade II sprain may be more tender, demonstrating some laxity and signifi-

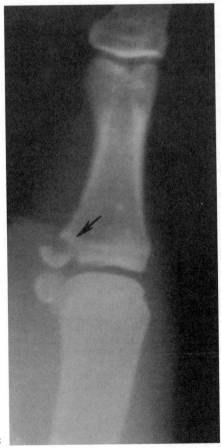
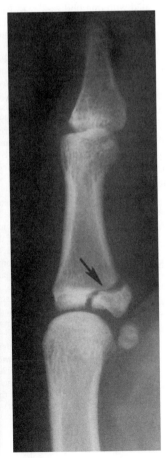

B, C

FIG. 34.14. (continued).

cant swelling. A grade III sprain presents with complete disruption of the supporting ligaments. Grade I and II sprains will heal with nonoperative treatment; however, complete tears often require surgical management. Diagnosis of a grade III sprain may be made by physical examination after roentgenographs are obtained. The thumb should be examined with the MCP fully flexed, in order to evaluate the ulnar and radial collateral ligaments. Many patient's thumbs allow considerable lateral motion, and therefore the affected thumb's motion should be compared to that of the non-involved thumb. A difference of 15 degrees or more of lateral laxity compared to the unaffected side or an absolute laxity of 35 degrees confirms the diagnosis. If the ulnar collateral ligament avulses from its phalangeal insertion, the bony fragment (the *Stener lesion*) can be caught in the adductor aponeurosis, and it will not heal without surgical intervention (Fig. 34.14). Diagnosis of a Stener lesion can be made by arthrography or, more commonly, at the time of surgery.

Treatment

Grade I and II lesions are treated with immobilization in a thumb spica cast or a splint for 2 to 4 weeks. Some grade II injuries may be painful despite adequate splinting. The joint should be further protected during play for an additional 4 weeks. The treatment of grade III repairs is controversial. In an absence of a Stener lesion, many orthopedic surgeons will initially attempt thumb spica immobilization. All grade III injuries, however, should be referred to an orthopedic specialist for further evaluation and management. Extensive rehabilitation and physical therapy improve joint motion and allow more effective use of the joint after treatment. Because of the potential morbidity of thumb injury, conservative management, with return to play dependent on the sport and the need to play, should be pursued.

CONCLUSION

The wrist and hand are extremely complicated, and they rely on the motion of the ligaments, the intrinsic and extrinsic tendon attachments, the variation of blood supply, and the intercalated bone motion. Definite weaknesses in design predispose them to certain injury patterns. In addition, additional predisposing factors in growing children complicate the management of these injuries. A systematic approach to the diagnosis can greatly facilitate management. Providers

need to maintain a high index of suspicion for injury in pediatric wrist and hands, and the management of injuries should be conservative. The approach can be summarized as follows: diagnose, immobilize, and return to play only after adequate rehabilitation. Because of the complex movement of the wrist, what appears to be only a minor injury in a child can result in chronic pain and disability in the adult.

REFERENCES

1. Lillegard WA, Butcher JD, Rucker KS. *Handbook of sports medicine: a symptom-oriented approach.* Boston: Butterworth-Heinemann, 1998.
2. Stanitski CL, Delee JC, Drez D, eds. *Pediatric and adolescent sports medicine.* Philadelphia: WB Saunders, 1994:262–277.
3. Honing EW. Wrist injuries pinpointing pathology in a complex joint. *The Physician and Sports Medicine* 1998;26:40–49.
4. Rettig AC. Epidemiology of hand and wrist injuries in sports. *Clin Sports Med* 1998;17:401–406.
5. Mandelbaum BR, Bartolozzi AR, Davis CA. Wrist pain syndrome in gymnasts. *Am J Sports Med* 1989;17:305–317.
6. Palmar AK. Triangular fibrocartilage complex lesions: a classification. *J Hand Surg* 1989;14A:594–606.
7. Mooney JF, Siegel DB, Korman AL. Ligamentous injuries of the wrist in athletes. *Clin Sports Med* 1992;11:129–140.
8. Huurman WW. Injuries to the hand and wrist. *Adolesc Med* 1998;9:611–625.
9. Ablolve RH, Moy OJ, Peimer CA. Pediatric hand disease. Diagnosis and treatment. *Pediatr Clin North Am* 1998;45:1507–1524.
10. Aronowitz ER, Leddy JP. Closed tendon injuries of the hand and wrist in athletes. *Clin Sports Med* 1998;17:449–467.
11. Wedderhopp N, Kaltoft M, Lundgaard B, et al. Injuries in young female players in European team hand ball. *Scand J Med Sci Sports* 1997;7:342–347.
12. Heuck A, Bonel H, Stabler A, et al. Imaging in sports medicine: hand and wrist. *Eur J Radiol* 1997;26:2–15.
13. Schreibman KL, Freeland A, Gilula LA, et al. Imaging of the hand and wrist. *Orthop Clin North Am* 1997;28:537–582.
14. Ton ER, Pattynama PM, Bloam JL, et al. Interosseous ligaments: device for applying stress in wrist MR imaging. *Radiology* 1995;196:863–864.
15. Katarincic JA. Fractures of the wrist and hand. *Occup Med* 1998;13:549–568.
16. Alexander AH, Lichtman DM. *The wrist and its disorders.* Philadephia: WB Saunders, 1988:329–343.
17. Idler RS. *The hand American society for surgery of the hand,* 3rd ed. New York: Churchill and Livingstone, 1990:5–96.
18. Snead DS, Rettig AC. Bone, joint, and tendon injuries of the hand in the athlete. *J Musculoskeletal Med* 2000;103–111.

35

Thigh, Hip, and Pelvis Injuries

Lauren M. Simon

HIP AND PELVIS INJURIES

Growth Considerations

Sports injuries of the hip and pelvis can be divided into acute, chronic, or overuse injuries, as well as other injuries that can affect the skeletal or soft tissues. In order to understand the injuries in the pediatric hip and pelvis, understanding the normal progression of skeletal growth can be helpful. The proximal femur has an epiphyseal plate at birth that later becomes the greater trochanteric and subcapital epiphyseal plate. Another epiphyseal plate develops at the lesser trochanter. The appearance and fusion of the secondary centers of ossification of the hip and pelvis occur in a predictable pattern (1). The ossific nucleus of the femoral head appears between the age of 4 and 6 months; that of the greater trochanter, between the ages of 2 to 5 years; and that of the lesser trochanter, between the ages of 8 to 12 years. The lesser and greater trochanteric epiphyses fuse between 16 and 18 years of age. The subcapital femoral epiphysis fuses at about 18 years of age. The primary ossification centers of the pubis, ilium, and ischium form the acetabulum of the pediatric pelvis. The iliac crest, the anterior superior iliac spine, and the anterior inferior iliac spine secondary ossification centers appear at about 13 to15 years of age, and they fuse at approximately 15 to17 years, 21 to 25 years, and 16 to18 years of age, respectively. The ischial tuberosity ossification center appears at about 15 to 17 years and fuses at about 19 to 25 years of age (1). The apophyseal areas of active growth cartilage where muscles attach to bones are particularly susceptible to acute and overuse injuries.

Traumatic Injuries

Apophyseal Avulsion Fractures

Avulsion fractures to the apophyses of the hip and pelvis are usually related to sports injuries in adolescents during the time between the appearance of and the fusion of these secondary ossification centers. The usual acute mechanism is a sudden forceful eccentric or concentric muscle contraction that occurs with rapid acceleration or deceleration forces. They can also occur with a sudden extreme stretch or passive muscle lengthening, such as those seen in gymnastics and cheerleading maneuvers that involve splits. In other types of avulsion injuries in which no specific causative event is known, the avulsion injury is thought to be from repetitive chronic traction that displaces the apophysis. The amount of displacement is related to the specific muscular attachments and to the extent of injury (2). Symptoms of apophyseal injury include localized pain and swelling over the affected area, muscle weakness, and limited range of motion (3). The potential apophyseal avulsion injury sites in the hip and pelvis are outlined below (Fig. 35.1), and they include the greater and lesser trochanter of the femur, the ischial tuberosity (Fig. 35.2), the anterior superior iliac spine, the anterior inferior iliac spine, the iliac crest, the acetabular rim, and the symphysis pubis adductor insertion.

Greater Trochanter

Greater and lesser trochanteric avulsions are rarely reported in the adolescent athlete. The hip external rotators, such as the obturators, the gemelli, and the gluteus minimus and medius, attach at the greater trochanteric apophysis. An avulsion fracture can occur from strong contraction of the hip abductors, such as is seen with cutting maneuvers. The pain is usually acute, it is localized to the greater trochanter, and the athlete cannot walk normally or bear weight solely on the affected leg. Pain can be reproduced by palpation, passive hip adduction, or active abduction. The athlete may hold the leg slightly flexed and abducted. A radiograph can confirm the diagnosis of avulsion of the greater trochanter.

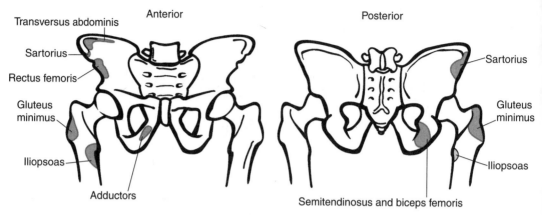

FIG. 35.1. Avulsions of the hip and pelvis. The following muscles of the hip and pelvis and their associated avulsion sites are depicted: gluteus minimus—greater trochanter; iliopsoas—lesser trochanter; hamstring muscles—ischium; sartorius—anterior superior iliac spine; rectus femoris—anterior inferior iliac spine; and the adductor group—pubis. (Drawn by DeEtte DeVille, M.D. Adapted from Ruane JJ, Rossi TA. When groin pain is more that 'just a strain': navigating a broad differential. *The Physician and Sports Medicine* 1998;26:78–93, with permission.)

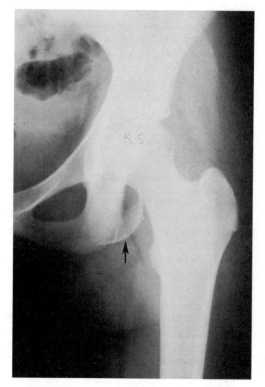

FIG. 35.2. Ischial apophysis avulsion (*arrow*).

Lesser Trochanter

The iliopsoas muscle attaches on the lesser trochanter, and a strong contraction during kicking, jumping, or sprinting sports can result in an avulsion fracture with the potential for displacement, since the iliopsoas muscle pull is relatively unopposed. Usually, the athlete has sudden pain in the anterior hip or groin, and he or she may experience a "pop" or snapping sensation in the groin. The athlete may hold the leg adducted and internally rotated. Pain is reproducible with palpation over the avulsion area and with resisted hip flexion. When the athlete is examined in the seated position, he or she will be unable to flex the affected hip actively (Ludloff sign) (1). A plain radiograph may not visualize the avulsion if the lesser trochanter is not well visualized.

Ischium

The hamstring muscles originate on the ischium. Strong, eccentric hamstring muscle contraction during sports, such as hurdling and long jumping, or with gymnastic split maneuvers (i.e., with the knee extended and the hip flexed) can cause avulsion of the ischial tuberosity. The athlete experiences acute pain, and he or she has difficulty walking or sitting after the injury. Tenderness and a palpable defect is felt at the ischial tuberosity. Pain is reproducible upon straight leg raise (hip flexion) and with hip extension. Radiographically, a crescent-shaped fragment of the apophysis is seen.

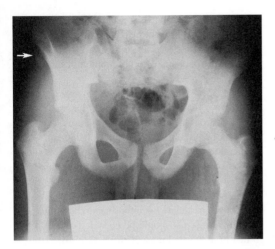

FIG. 35.3. Anterior superior iliac spine avulsion (*arrow*).

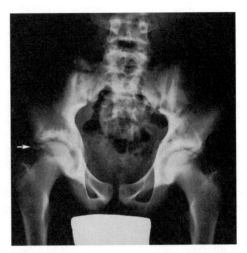

FIG. 35.4. Anterior inferior iliac spine avulsion (*arrow*).

Anterior Superior Iliac Spine

The sartorius muscle and some of the tensor fascia lata fibers attach on the anterior superior iliac spine (ASIS). Strong contraction of the sartorius during running, hurdling, or sprinting in which the hip is extended and the knee is flexed can avulse the ASIS. This is sometimes a bilateral injury. The athlete may notice a pop or snap, along with acute pain at the ASIS at the time of injury. The athlete experiences tenderness, and a defect may be felt on palpation of the ASIS area. Passive hip extension or active flexion reproduces the pain. A radiograph reveals the avulsed fragment (Fig. 35.3).

Anterior Inferior Iliac Spine

The direct head of the rectus femoris attaches to the anterior inferior iliac spine (AIIS). The direct head of the rectus femoris avulses the AIIS in runners or in kicking sports, such as football and soccer, when the hip is hyperextended and the knee is flexed (1). Migration of the avulsed fragment may be limited by the reflected head of the biceps femoris (2). Pain is present at the AIIS area, and it may be reproduced upon palpation or with active flexion or passive hyperextension of the hip. The radiograph may show variable displacement of the avulsed fragment (Fig. 35.4).

Iliac Crest

The abdominal and trunk muscles insert into the iliac crest apophysis. Anteriorly, the internal and external oblique, the tensor fascia lata, the gluteus medius, and the transverse abdominus muscles and, posteriorly,

the gluteus maximus and some of the latissimus attach to the iliac crest. Avulsion of the iliac crest, which is an uncommon injury, is suspected to occur from forceful abdominal muscle contraction in sports such as running (2). The athlete has tenderness over the iliac crest apophysis, and pain is reproduced upon trunk rotation, lateral bending, and resisted hip abduction. The radiograph demonstrates the avulsion fragment.

Acetabular Rim and Symphysis Pubis

In addition to the apophyseal avulsions injuries discussed above, Paletta and Andrish (1) reference case reports of acetabular rim avulsion in a rugby player and adductor avulsion at the symphysis pubis in young male sprinters.

Treatment

There is no universal agreement on the treatment of acute apophyseal avulsion fractures. A conservative nonsurgical treatment regimen of rest, ice, protected weight bearing, analgesics, and a gradual return to sport has been used, especially when the fracture fragment is minimally displaced or is nondisplaced. Wojtys (4) and DiFiori (5) refer to the program developed by Metzmaker and Pappas (6), which used a five-phase nonoperative rehabilitation program for apophyseal avulsion injuries to return athletes successfully to full participation within 4 months. Phase 1 consisted of rest, ice, and positioning to relax the involved muscle group in order to relieve tension on the avulsed fragment in the first 7 days after injury. Phase

2 included a gradual increase in excursion of the injured musculotendinous unit and limited crutch, partial weight bearing from 7 to 20 days postinjury. Phase 3 is comprised of a guided, comprehensive resisted exercise program to increase strength and range of motion from 14 to 30 days postinjury. After the patient has achieved 50% of the expected muscle strength, phase 4, which integrates the use of the injured musculotendinous unit with other muscles in the pelvis and lower extremity, is begun at 30 to 60 days postinjury. Limited athletic activity is allowed in this phase because risk of reinjury is great before normal strength is regained. In phase 5, after the athlete regains his or her full strength, range of motion, and integration of the musculotendinous unit with the other muscles, he or she may return to full sports participation (6). Other authors recommend surgical treatment of apophyseal avulsion injuries, particularly if wide displacement of the fragment is seen (1).

Imaging the Pediatric Hip

Plain radiography is the primary imaging modality that is used to evaluate apophyseal avulsion fractures of the hip and pelvis. Conventional radiographs also are quite useful for evaluating most clinical hip and pelvis disorders (1,6,7). Plain radiographs are inexpensive, they generally are readily available, and they are sensitive and specific for many hip and pelvis problems.

Additional imaging modalities, such as magnetic resonance imaging (MRI), computerized tomography (CT), bone scan, or ultrasound, are useful in special clinical situations after plain radiographs have been evaluated.

MRI shows marrow edema, contusions, soft tissue tumors, or abscesses. MRI is a good choice of study to evaluate Legg–Calvé–Perthes disease and iliac apophysitis. CT scans show greater bony detail than MRI. Bone scans can be used for imaging osteomyelitis. Ultrasound can visualize joint fluid, such as that seen in septic arthritis or toxic synovitis.

Acute Fractures and Dislocations

In addition to apophyseal avulsion fractures, other traumatic injuries to the hip and pelvis, such as fractures and dislocations, can be sustained by children and adolescents.

Femoral Neck Fractures

Acute fractures of the head and neck of the femur are uncommon in children. Most of these fractures are rare in sports, and they usually result from high velocity trauma (1). Subtrochanteric fractures are also rare in sports. The classic signs of a hip fracture are excruciating pain and external rotation of the hip (8).

Pelvic Fractures

In addition to the avulsion fractures discussed above, nonphyseal pelvic fractures, stable and unstable pelvic ring fractures, acetabular fractures, and iliac wing fractures can occur. These fractures are high-energy injuries that, although they are rarely seen in sports, may sometimes occur in collision sports. The presence of associated genitourinary, abdominal, and neurologic injuries should be considered, in addition to that of associated musculoskeletal injuries (9).

Hip Dislocation

Acute hip dislocations, which are more common than hip fractures in children, require emergent treatment. Most of hip dislocations are posterior, and the child's leg is held flexed, adducted, and internally rotated. Although posterior hip dislocation is most commonly described as a dashboard injury, these injuries are sometimes seen in athletes. In collision sports, such as football and ice hockey, a severe fall on the hip, in which the femur is driven backward while the hip is flexed and the leg is adducted, can cause a posterior hip dislocation (10). Of critical importance is the sports clinician's ability to identify this injury rapidly because of the high risk of avascular necrosis. Rapid reduction reduces the risk of avascular necrosis, which occurs with a rate of about 40% if reduction is delayed beyond 6 hours postinjury (10). The athlete with hip dislocation will have severe buttock pain, posterior thigh pain, hip or pelvic pain, and an inability to bear weight. The affected leg appears shortened, and the hip is flexed adducted and internally rotated (10). A radiograph should be taken before reduction is attempted so that the clinician can check for an associated acetabular or femoral head fractures (10). Usually, reduction of the dislocated hip is done under spinal or general anesthesia. When an associated fracture of the acetabulum or femoral head occurs, open reduction is often necessary. After reduction, initial bed rest for about 1 week, followed by 4 to 6 weeks of protected weight bearing on crutches and range of motion exercises (these progress to isometric and then isokinetic hip flexor and extensor exercises), should be instituted. A thorough discussion about the risks of complications from the injury and the potential risks from return to the involved sport should be undertaken before a return-to-play decision is made.

Stress Fractures

Stress fractures of the femoral neck, femoral shaft, or pelvis occur from repetitive microtrauma and overuse syndromes. Femoral neck stress fractures should be suspected in track and field athletes who have persistent groin pain, buttock or thigh pain, tenderness over the femoral neck, and limitation in hip flexion and internal rotation. Stress fractures may occur after changes in training, including the use of a new pair of running shoes, a change in the running surface, or an increase in the intensity or duration of training. Serious complications, such as nonunion or avascular necrosis of the femoral head, can occur if a femoral neck stress fracture is not identified (11). Duffey et al. (8) and Devas (12,13) have described two types of femoral neck stress fractures—a transverse stress fracture that is usually seen in adults and a compression type stress fracture that may be seen in children. The compression type stress fracture usually does not displace, and it can be treated with non-weight bearing or limited weight bearing, cross training, or nonimpact loading conditioning, such as swimming. Stress fractures in the femoral shaft also have been reported as a type of sports-related stress fracture. Femoral shaft stress fractures can be difficult to diagnosis because of the vague localization of pain in the thigh (14).

Stress fractures in the pelvis occur at the ischial and superior pubic rami and at the inferior ramus. The most common site for a stress fracture is at the junction of the inferior pubic ramus and the ischium (9), and this diagnosis may be considered in an athlete with inguinal, perineal, or adductor area pain with painful palpation of pubic ramus. Groin pain that is aggravated by activities, such as hopping or a single leg stance, is another common finding. These fractures are seen more frequently in female distance runners. When stress fractures are seen, particularly in the female athlete, the clinician should take a good nutritional and menstrual history to assess the athlete's risk for the female athlete triad (amenorrhea, disordered eating, and osteoporosis). Weight bearing as tolerated by pain symptoms is progressed in treatment. These fractures may require several months of healing before a complete return to running can be achieved.

Pathologic Fractures

When physical examination findings are more severe than the history of injury suggests or if an unusual skeletal injury is found, the prudent course for the clinician should include the consideration of the possibility of a pathologic fracture or another pathology. A pathologic fracture is defined as a fracture through abnormal bone. It may occur as an acute fracture, or its onset may be insidious. Some conditions that may present as pathologic injuries are malignant neoplasms, such as osteogenic sarcoma (Fig. 35.5) and Ewing sarcoma, and benign lesions, such as unicameral bone cysts, osteoid osteoma, and fibrous dysplasia (15). Other pathologic conditions, such as renal osteodystrophy and hypothyroidism, can predispose the athlete to injury.

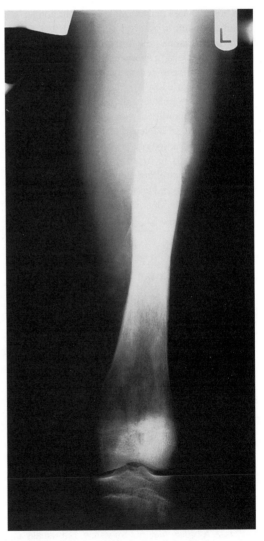

FIG. 35.5. Osteogenic sarcoma. Osteogenic sarcoma of the left femoral shaft in a 12-year-old boy.

Maintaining a high index of clinical suspicion if a sprain, strain, or overuse type injury does not improve is important because pathologic conditions may present with activity-related pain that is similar in appearance to these entities so that the condition is misdiagnosed. Some clinicians advocate early radiographic imaging of overuse type injuries in order to avoid missing a pathologic process (15).

Soft Tissue Injuries to the Hip

In addition to skeletal injuries in the pediatric athlete's hip, soft tissue injuries to the hip can occur, including hip pointers, contusions, abrasions, sprains, and strains. Soft tissue injuries are more common than bony injuries in these athletes. A hip pointer is a contusion to the iliac crest (Fig. 35.6) that results from direct trauma with formation of subperiosteal hematoma as seen in sports such as football, basketball, volleyball, and gymnastics (1,16). A hip pointer can also be caused by a violent muscle contraction when an athlete tries to avoid a blow (16). These injuries may be confused with apophyseal injuries to the iliac crest. In adolescent athletes, a radiograph should be taken to look for an avulsion fracture of the iliac crest. Goals of treatment include reducing the bleeding and controlling pain. Rest, icing, a gradual return to activity, and protective padding are used for treatment (Fig. 35.7).

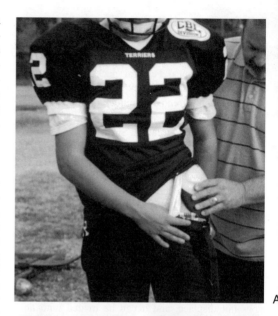

A

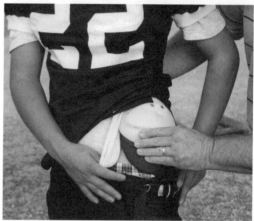

B

FIG. 35.7. Protective padding for hip pointer. After treatment of the hip pointer, the area should be protected from reinjury by a firm pad when the athlete is permitted to return to sport. Various types of padding can be used. **A,B:** The athletic trainer is using an old football shoulder pad (padded interiorly and hard exteriorly) to protect the iliac crest.

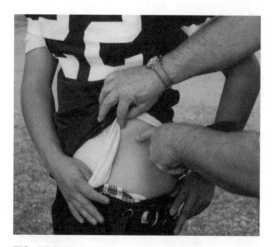

FIG. 35.6. Hip pointer. A hip pointer, which is often seen in sports such as football, is a contusion of the iliac crest. A bruise may not be visible, but usually extreme tenderness to palpation of the affected area is present.

Sprains and Strains

As an athlete nears skeletal maturity with fusion of epiphyses and apophyses, the physes no longer are the weak link, and the athlete is at greater risk for muscular, tendinous, and ligamentous injuries. Strains may be caused by excessive passive stretch, forceful contraction, or repetitive microtrauma to the musculotendinous units (9). Some of the disorders caused by these mechanisms are apophysitis, osteitis pubis, iliotibial band friction syndrome (tensor fascia latae syndrome), and piriformis syndrome.

Apophysitis

Apophysitis is inflammation of a bony outgrowth that may occur secondary to repetitive microtrauma and chronic traction stress at the attachment of tendon to bone. The myotendinous unit may avulse if it is traumatized, and this may cause acute, severe pain. The symptoms and physical examination findings localize pain to the apophyseal region in both acute injuries and long-standing apophysitis. Iliac apophysitis may be seen in adolescent distance runners; this condition is localized to the iliac crest apophysis, and it may occur bilaterally. The abdominal muscles attach from above and the hip abductors attach from below the iliac crest, resulting in traction from both directions (17). Stress on the abdominal oblique muscles with resisted trunk rotation will reproduce the pain (2). Apophysitis of the iliac crest is seen in sports that involve a lot of running (e.g., soccer, track, running, basketball, and dance), which exerts a pull on muscles about the hip, and in athletes who have tight hip flexors and abductors (18). Another site of apophysitis is the ischial tuberosity. The athlete may complain of chronic hip or buttock pain, with tenderness with palpation over the ischial tuberosity. Treatment of apophysitis includes relative rest, ice, training modifications, and a flexibility program to reduce the possibility of reinjury (17).

Osteitis Pubis

Osteitis pubis is an inflammation of the symphysis pubis that is thought to result from repetitive minor trauma. It is presumed to occur from traction stress on the symphysis that is caused by the adductors and gracilis, which is attached to the inferior aspect of the symphysis, from repetitive cutting or twisting motions (11) or from strenuous conditioning of the adductors or rectus abdominis. This condition is seen in long-distance running and in sports with sprinting that is associated with sudden directional changes, pivoting, or kicking, such as soccer, track, and basketball. Sports that involve swinging the arms across the body have been associated with this condition (19), and it may also be seen in postpartum patients.

An athlete with osteitis pubis may present with tenderness over the symphysis pubis or medial groin (19,20). The pain may radiate to the hip. Due to the sometimes diffuse nature of the pain, osteitis pubis may be confused with other disorders. The clinician must consider the possibility of a hernia or nerve irritation in the differential diagnosis. A sports hernia of the oblique aponeurosis presents with tenderness at the superficial inguinal ring. Obturator or inguinal nerve entrapment presents with tenderness and weakness of the adductors. Pain with resisted thigh adduction and limited hip rotation is usually present in osteitis pubis. Radiographs of the symphysis pubis may not detect any abnormalities for several weeks, and, if a nucleotide bone scan is clinically indicated, it may be useful in detecting inflammation at this site in the early course of the condition. Treatment consists of rest, ice, nonsteroidal antiinflammatory medication, and hip adductor and rotator stretching. These injuries may require months of treatment to become pain free. Prolonged rest (more than 6 months) may be mandated before the athlete becomes pain free and is able to resume athletics (3).

Iliotibial Band Syndrome

Iliotibial band syndrome also is referred to as tensor fascia latae syndrome. However, in rare cases, a muscle strain of the tensor fascia lata may be seen without tightness of the iliotibial band (ITB) (21).

The ITB is a fascial band composed of fibers from the tensor fasciae lata and the gluteus maximus. It crosses two joints as it extends from the hip to the lateral femoral epicondyle and inserts on the Gerdy tubercle on the lateral tibial condyle, as well as the lateral border of the patella and the lateral patellar retinaculum. Pain usually occurs at the lateral femoral epicondyle, but it also may be present at the greater trochanter. During flexion and extension of the leg, the ITB moves over the lateral femoral epicondyle, causing friction. In runners or sports that require repeated flexion and extension of the knee, especially in internal rotation, an athlete may complain of a snapping hip sensation as the ITB irritates the greater trochanteric bursa (4,9,21,22). Frequently, the athlete notices symptoms with changes in training patterns, such as increasing distance running or adding hill or stair workouts. Symptoms often occur reproducibly with specific activities or specific distances in running. As inflammation continues, the athlete's gait may be affected. On physical examination, the Ober test for tight hip abductors is usually positive. Treatment is conservative, involving icing, stretching, such as the hip abduction "teapot" stretch (Fig 35.8), antiinflammatory medication, massage, and myofascial therapy

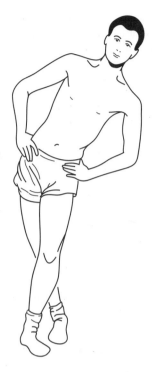

FIG. 35.8. Iliotibial band "teapot" stretch. After acute inflammation of the iliotibial band has subsided, rehabilitative stretching can be performed. The stretch depicted here resembles the "teapot" figure created by children in kindergarten. The child stands upright or uses the wall for balance. The symptomatic leg is extended and adducted behind the asymptomatic leg. The athlete flexes the trunk laterally away from the affected hip until a stretch is felt on the symptomatic hip. To increase the stretch, the arms may be held overhead, which will increase the lateral flexion at the trunk. This stretch should be performed gently and not beyond the point of pain. It should be held for 10 to 15 seconds.

(23). In rare refractory cases, the ITB may be released surgically.

Greater Trochanteric Bursitis

When the ITB repetitively rubs across the greater trochanter, it can cause an overuse syndrome in which the greater trochanteric bursae become inflamed. As with iliotibial band syndrome, this condition is generally seen in runners, especially in those who run on banked or uneven surfaces, but it can be seen in any sport that involves running. It also can be seen in athletes who have a leg length discrepancy. Tenderness to palpation that can be reproduced by actively moving the hip from extension into flexion is found over the greater trochanter,. Sometimes a snapping hip sensa-

tion can be palpated. Treatment includes relative rest (i.e., avoiding running), activity modification, icing, and stretching. If pain persists, injection of the bursae with an anesthetic may help to relieve pain. In older athletes, the anesthetic may be combined with a corticosteroid for longer-term antiinflammatory activity.

Psoas Tenosynovitis

Another cause of snapping hip that presents with anterior hip or groin pain is a tenosynovitis of the iliopsoas tendon near its insertion on the lesser trochanter or a "catch" of the iliopsoas tendon as it passes the iliopectineal eminence (1,9). Treatment consists of stretching exercises in hip abduction and external rotation; ultrasound, which should be used with caution in the pediatric age group; deep heat; and antiinflammatories.

Snapping Hip

Iliotibial band syndrome, greater trochanteric bursitis, and iliopsoas tenosynovitis, which were described above, can all be causes of a "snapping" or "catching" hip. Acetabular labral tear is a less common cause of intermittent catching of the hip. With a labral injury, the athlete presents with a deep, sharp hip pain and a catch or a giving way sensation in the hip. Tenderness is observed with internal rotation and extension of the hip. A click is present on the Thomas test. The Thomas test is performed with the contralateral hip flexed while the symptomatic hip is moved from full flexion to full extension. An acetabular labral tear can be diagnosed by magnetic resonance arthrography or by arthroscopy (3). Definitive treatment requires arthroscopy.

Piriformis Syndrome

The piriformis muscle can irritate the sciatic nerve by the sciatic notch, due to the close anatomical association. This creates symptoms of burning or tingling in the buttocks or the posterior thigh. An area of palpable tenderness is usually found in the buttock area between the ischium and greater trochanter. Posterior thigh paresthesias may also be present, and the ability to do a straight leg raise may be limited (21). Resisted external rotation may worsen the pain. Treatment includes icing and stretching.

Lumbar disc herniation in an adolescent can be difficult to distinguish from piriformis syndrome because both disorders can present with pain localizing to the hip. Limited range of motion of the lumbar spine and lumbar paravertebral spasms are usually present with lumbar disc herniation and not with piriformis syndrome.

Meralgia Paresthetica

Another nerve irritation that can occur around the hip and radiate down the thigh is irritation of the lateral femoral cutaneous nerve where it is adjacent to the anterior superior iliac spine. After sustaining a traumatic blow to the hip close to the anterior superior iliac spine in sports such as soccer or gymnastics (from hitting uneven parallel bars incorrectly), the athlete may complain of numbness, pain, or tingling that extends down the anterior lateral thigh. This sensory nerve irritation also can be seen in athletes wearing tight fitting clothing, as this places pressure on the nerve. Treatment consists of rest, activity or clothing modification to relieve pressure on the nerve, and the use of antiinflammatory agent (16).

Prevention

To prevent the occurrence of acute, chronic, and overuse injuries in the pediatric athlete's pelvis and hips, a periodic assessment of flexibility is important, and prophylactic stretching should be prescribed where necessary to decrease traction stress on the immature skeleton and tissues. The prudent course involves monitoring changes in the intensity, duration, terrain, or equipment of the athlete's training schedule, especially during times of growth spurts, because changes in these factors have been associated with injury.

Nontraumatic Hip Pain

When pediatric athletes complain of hip, thigh, or knee pain and present with a limp, other conditions besides traumatic injuries need to be considered. Some conditions that need to be considered are Legg–Calvé–Perthes disease, a slipped capital femoral epiphysis, transient synovitis, neoplasms, septic arthritis, and rheumatoid arthritis (24).

Legg–Calvé–Perthes Disease

Legg-Calvé-Perthes disease is a disorder in which ischemic necrosis of the proximal femoral epiphysis with later resorption is seen. A child with this condition may have a limp that worsens after activity and he or she may complain of hip, groin, knee, or inner thigh pain (1,25). The pain may interfere with sports activity. Pain may be present intermittently for days to months, or the click may have the classic presentation of a painless limp. It usually occurs in males between

4 and 8 years of age, although it may be seen in the 2-year-old to 13-year-old age range. The ratio of occurence of males to females is approximately 5 to 1. The disease can occur bilaterally approximately 10% of the time. The child may have muscle spasm, limited abduction, and internal rotation (26). The pathogenesis includes the interruption of the blood supply to the femoral head with ischemic necrosis, collapse, and later repair (25). The amount of residual deformity depends on the amount of epiphysis that is involved, the patient's age, and how promptly the diagnosis is made (26).

When the clinician is assessing the child for this disorder, he or she should observe the child's gait in a hallway and should examine the child for limb length discrepancy both by assessing iliac crest height standing and by supine tape measurement from the ASIS to the medial malleolus, as well as noting range of motion, hip rotation, and hip palpation. Frog leg lateral and anteroposterior (AP) radiographs can be used to confirm the diagnosis (Fig. 35.9). Early in the course of the illness, the ossified section of the femoral head appears smaller than the opposite side. A crescent-shaped line may be present on the lateral radiograph. After new bone growth, the femoral head has an abnormal shape and size. If the plain radiographs are initially negative but clinical suspicion is still high, MRI can be used to detect ischemic necrosis or a bone scan can be used to confirm diagnosis (7).

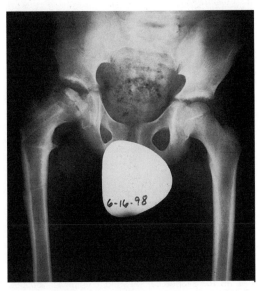

FIG. 35.9. Legg–Calvé–Perthes disease. Legg–Calvé–Perthes disease shows ischemic necrosis of the proximal femoral epiphysis.

This disorder is usually a self-limited process that lasts between 2 and 4 years (25). Treatment is directed toward reducing the child's pain and synovitis and lessening hip stiffness plus femoral head containment within the acetabulum to minimize deformation of the femoral head. If this disorder is left untreated, it predisposes the patient to disabling osteoarthritis as an adult. Pain reduction is usually achieved by the use of nonsteroidal antiinflammatory medication and activity restriction and/or modification; however, crutches or bed rest are sometimes indicated. To contain the femoral head, the child is braced or casted with the proximal femur in abduction. The epiphysis can remodel properly when the forces on it are decreased; this is accomplished by putting the femoral epiphysis in the acetabulum in an abducted and internally rotated position (26). The child may undergo a proximal femoral osteotomy or pelvic osteotomy that is performed

surgically, if conservative therapy is unacceptable or if a progressive femoral head deformity is occurring. The extent and timing of return to sports participation depends on the severity of involvement of the femoral head, the subsequent healing progression, and proper joint space preservation. The prognosis for recovery and unrestricted sports participation after treatment is extremely good for the majority of these children.

Slipped Capital Femoral Epiphysis

Another disorder in the differential diagnosis of Legg-Calvé-Perthes is slipped capital femoral epiphysis (SCFE), a growth plate injury that requires emergent orthopedic attention. SCFE is the most common nontraumatic hip disorder in adolescents, yet it is frequently missed. It can be associated with endocrine disorders, such as hypothyroidism, or with

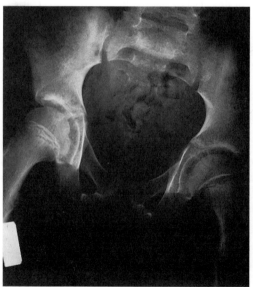

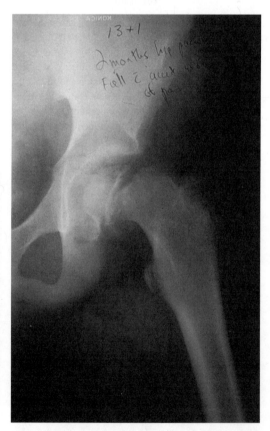

A   B

FIG. 35.10. Slipped capital femoral epiphysis. Slipped capital epiphysis demonstrates posterior and inferior slippage of the proximal femoral epiphysis on the metaphysis (femoral neck) through the physeal plate. The radiograph appears as an ice cream scoop falling off of the cone. **A:** Anteroposterior view. **B:** Frog leg lateral view.

renal osteodystrophy, although it more commonly is idiopathic. It frequently occurs in obese children, and 20% to 40% of these cases occur bilaterally. This disorder is usually seen between the ages of 11 and 16 years, with a peak incidence at 11.5 years of age for boys and at 13.0 years of age for girls (25). It is approximately 1.5 times as common in boys than in girls. When it does occur in girls, it usually is seen before menses have begun.

SCFE is caused by many factors, such as the hormonal changes of adolescence, puberty-related changes in physeal architecture and orientation, and obesity, which decrease physeal strength. These factors, plus the stress of weight-bearing forces and muscle pull on the proximal femur, exceed the strength of the capital femoral epiphysis. During adolescence, the thickness of the physis is increased, and its anchoring perichondral ring thins. SCFE occurs during the early adolescent growth spurt when the physeal plate between the femoral head and neck weakens; it is defined as posterior and inferior slippage of the proximal femoral epiphysis on the metaphysis (femoral neck) through the physeal plate. On radiographs, the femoral head appears to have slipped downward and backward, like a scoop of ice cream that has fallen off an ice cream cone (Fig. 35.10). Although the term "slipped capital femoral epiphysis" implies that the femoral epiphysis is displacing from its location on top of the metaphysis, a more accurate description is that the proximal femoral metaphysis displaces superiorly and anterolaterally (upward and forward) on the femoral epiphysis. The upper femoral epiphysis actually stays positioned within the acetabulum, but this arrangement gives the epiphysis the appearance of having slipped posteriorly and inferiorly (25–27).

Diagnosis of Slipped Capital Femoral Epiphysis

The most common symptoms of SCFE are pain and limp. The symptoms may be present and may be poorly localized for weeks to months. Pain may present as medial thigh, knee, or groin pain, and, less frequently, as hip pain due to the referred pain patterns from the anatomic innervation of the hip. Sometimes a vague history of trauma that precedes the onset of symptoms is present. The pain is usually present with walking, and it is worsened by running, jumping, cutting, or pivoting maneuvers. The pain is described as a dull ache, which usually does not radiate. The athlete may notice that he or she has difficulty performing in usual sports or even the activities of daily living, such as tying shoes (27). Due to the

variable presentations of pain, the diagnosis of SCFE is often enigmatic. The delay in diagnosis and treatment translates to a worse prognosis. If the patient has minimal SCFE, the signs and symptoms may also be minimal, with pain only on extremes of motion, limited loss of internal hip rotation, and a mild, altered gait. As the SCFE becomes worse, the patient's limp becomes more visible, and his or her leg is externally rotated. In addition to the loss of internal rotation of the affected hip, decreased flexion also occurs. The patient cannot touch the anterior thigh to his or her abdomen because, when flexed, the hip externally rotates. If the condition has been present for a while, leg shortening and thigh atrophy may have occurred. The knee examination is usually normal.

In a patient with stable SCFE, AP and frog leg lateral pelvic radiographs should be taken to confirm the diagnosis. Early in the disorder, the AP radiograph may appear normal; therefore, taking the lateral view is important. The patient may be in such great pain that sometimes only the AP view can be taken, and the lateral view, if it is taken, should be done cross table so that the physis is not displaced by the patient's attempt to do a frog leg lateral.

Treatment of Slipped Capital Femoral Epiphysis

The goals of treatment of SCFE are the permanent prevention of further epiphyseal displacement and enabling closure of the physis. Making an early diagnosis is helpful in achieving these goals. Of extreme importance is restricting the patient who has been diagnosed with SCFE from weight bearing and *immediately* referring him or her to an orthopedic surgeon for definitive treatment (27). Although several options exist for treatment of a stable SCFE, "most orthopedic surgeons currently recommend *in situ* fixation with a single screw" (27). Postoperatively, the athlete faces an average of 4 to 6 weeks of limited toe touch weight bearing on crutches. Return to sporting activities, including contact sports, can be made when the physis has closed. Degenerative arthritis in the affected limb will usually develop slowly over several decades. Although most orthopedic surgeons suggest internal fixation for an unstable SCFE, there is little agreement on which method is preferred. Unstable SCFEs have a much higher chance of avascular necrosis, due to disruption of the blood supply, which predisposes the patient to early arthritis and deterioration of the hip. Children with severe joint deterioration may require total joint replacement at a young age. Fortunately, over 90% of SCFEs are stable, and they have an excellent prognosis, including return to play within several months for most sports (27).

Summary

In summary, when a child presents with knee or hip pain, the differential diagnosis includes the following: developmental disorders, such as hip dysplasia, Legg–Calvé–Perthes disease, and slipped capital femoral epiphysis; inflammatory disorders, such as septic arthritis, acute transient synovitis, juvenile arthritis, and osteomyelitis; neoplastic tumors; and congenital structural abnormalities. Keeping hip disorders in mind is especially important when a child or adolescent presents with knee or thigh pain, even in the absence of hip pain.

THIGH

Soft Tissue Injury to the Thigh

Soft tissue injuries to the thigh include muscle strains of the hamstrings, quadriceps, or adductors; contusions; myositis ossificans; compartment syndrome; and neoplasm. Muscle strains can be graded as follows: grade I, minimal muscle disruption; grade II, tearing with significant hemorrhage; and grade III, complete disruption of the muscle and loss of function (19,21). Musculotendinous strains have been described with the classic symptom triad of tenderness to palpation, pain with resistance, and pain upon passive stretching. General treatment of muscle strains includes ice, compression, and rest from pain-producing activities (19,28–30). When inflammation subsides, the rehabilitation progresses from gentle stretching to low intensity strengthening and gradual return to sport-specific activities.

If a young athlete sustains a direct blow to the anterior thigh, the injury may result in a quadriceps hematoma. This type of injury should be closely monitored and managed with compression of the affected area, and the knee should be maintained in flexion. Heat, ultrasound, whirlpool therapy, and vigorous range-of-motion exercises may worsen this injury. Before the athlete makes a full return to sports participation, he or she should have normal quadriceps flexibility, strength parity between the quadriceps of the injured and uninjured legs, normal hip strength and flexibility, and normalized quadriceps to hamstring isokinetic testing (28). After strength and agility are restored, the athlete can return to full sports activities, but he or she should wear protective padding to lessen the risk of reinjury. The return to

sports participation usually takes 3 to 6 weeks (19), and the athlete should be monitored for any recurrence of pain.

Quadriceps Strains

Quadriceps strains are muscle belly tears that occur when the quadriceps are overstretched while contracting or rapidly decelerating, such as occurs when ending a sprint or missing a kick and kicking the ground or an opponent instead of the ball. They are most commonly seen in soccer, rugby, football, and track. The rectus femoris is the muscle that usually tears, commonly at its midsubstance, while the vastus lateralis and intermedius rupture in the upper and middle third of the muscle. The quadriceps tendon may rupture off the superior pole of the patella and the ligamentous patella (the infrapatellar common tendon). In skeletally immature athletes, instead of a ruptured tendon, the tibial apophysis is more likely to be avulsed. Although some quadriceps extensor motion from the lateral and medial retinacular bands may be seen, an individual with a quadriceps tendon rupture will be unable to perform a straight leg raise test. Treatment of quadriceps strains utilizes the principles of rest, ice, compression, and elevation (RICE) and rehabilitation (Fig. 35.11), similar to that described below for contusions. For complete tears of the quadriceps tendon, surgical repair is usually recommended.

Thigh Contusion

With a grade III (severe) contusion, the athlete should be kept on bed rest, with the thigh wrapped and iced. If continued swelling occurs after several hours of RICE therapy or if pain is escalating, the possibility of a developing compartment syndrome

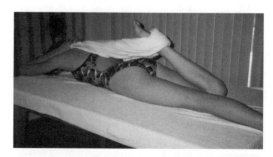

FIG. 35.11. Quadriceps exercise. In a prone position, with the knee flexed, the athlete attempts to extend the knee actively against autoresistance and then relaxes the leg, while passively pulling the leg into flexion with a towel.

should be considered. When good range of motion is present, isometric quadriceps strengthening can begin, followed by progressive resistance exercises. When the athlete is pain free and he or she has full range of motion, a gradual return to running may begin. Before a full return to sports participation, the athlete should have normal quadriceps flexibility, strength parity between the quadriceps of the injured and uninjured legs, normal hip strength and flexibility, and normalized quadriceps to hamstring isokinetic testing (28). After the athlete's strength and agility are restored, he or she can return to full sports activities, but protective padding should be worn to lessen the risk of reinjury. The return to sport usually takes 3 to 6 weeks (19), and the athlete should be monitored for any recurrence of pain. One of the concerns with regard to quadriceps contusion is that it can lead to the complications of myositis ossificans, if it is left untreated or if progressive bleeding occurs.

Myositis Ossificans Traumatica

One troublesome sequela of a muscle contusion is myositis ossificans traumatica (MOT). This condition is a type of heterotopic ossification that occurs within a hematoma in muscle tissue, usually after blunt trauma, such as a blow to the quadriceps in contact sports. It has been reported in about 10% to 20% of thigh contusions (31). Risk factors for the development of MOT include the severity of the initial injury; reinjury during the healing phase; delay in the treatment of muscle injury; the use of heat, ultrasound, or massage in treatment of the acute injury; a history of previous MOT; and surgery before the MOT lesion matures (1,31). The pathophysiologic mechanism for MOT is unknown. The MOT lesion looks similar to a bony callus, and, on biopsy, it may appear histologically identical to osteogenic sarcoma, so eliciting an accurate history of trauma is crucial. The most commonly involved muscles are the anterior and lateral quadriceps, followed by the upper arm brachialis muscle (31). The MOT lesion may occur from days to weeks postinjury. Typical findings include localized erythema, swelling, tenderness, increased warmth in the affected area, and possibly a palpable mass. The athlete may have decreased range of motion in an adjacent joint, and he or she may develop a fever. Initial radiographs following the injury will usually be negative, but they may show a fluffy density in the soft tissues near the bone at about 2 to 4 weeks after the injury. The MOT lesion can mature into lamellar bone over the next 6 to 12 months (Figs. 35.12 and 35.13), or it may resorb.

If the MOT is identified early, it is treated by rest, ice, application of a compression wrap, and non-

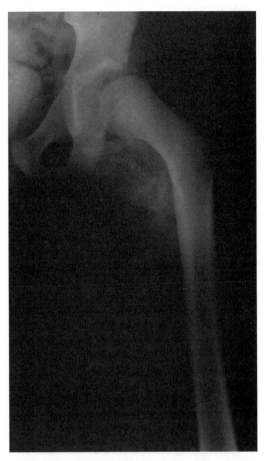

FIG. 35.12. Myositis ossificans traumatica. Myositis ossificans traumatica (MOT) is new bone formation in muscle following injury. After acute injury, MOT is a soft tissue mass, and it later develops into extraskeletal ossification that is visible on radiography. The MOT lesion pictured here occurred around the hip of a 12-year-old boy after hip dislocation.

steroidal antiinflammatory medication. Heat, ultrasound, massage, and aggressive range of motion should be avoided. Once the inflammation decreases, gentle range-of-motion exercises, both active and passive, can be initiated. Surgical excision is rarely indicated for the treatment of MOT, unless significant pain or loss of range of motion persists for 12 to18 months (31). If excision is performed before the lesion is mature, MOT may reoccur. Patient may return to full sports activity with protective padding in place, when the MOT affected area is nontender, full range of motion of affected muscle has been demonstrated, and the muscle's strength is about 85% to 90% of the uninjured side (31). The full return to sports participation usually takes between weeks to

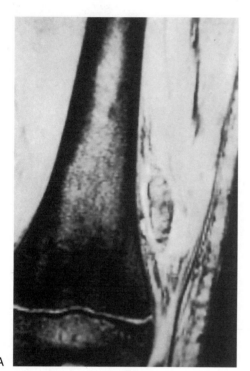

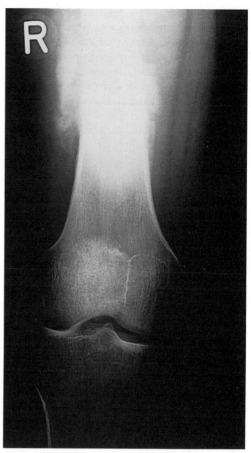

A   B

FIG. 35.13. Osteosarcoma. Myositis ossificans traumatica lesions **(A)** can radiographically appear similar to osteosarcoma **(B)**. Eliciting any history of trauma is helpful when trying to evaluate the lesions radiographically. The osteosarcoma in the distal femur pictured in **(B)** occurred in a 17-year-old girl with no history of trauma who noticed a mass in her thigh. The osteosarcoma lesion is attached to bone, in contrast to an ossified soft tissue mass, such as myositis ossificans. (Figure 35.13A is taken from Fu FH, Stone DA, eds. *Sports injuries: mechanisms, prevention, and treatment.* Philadelphia: Lippincott Williams & Wilkins, 2001, with permission.)

several months. Protective padding should be used for at least 6 months postinjury to avoid reinjury and subsequent MOT.

Hamstring Muscle Strains

Muscle strains are relatively uncommon in children in comparison to similar injuries in adults. Injuries to musculotendinous units most commonly occur at the apophyses in children. When muscle strains do occur, they usually happen during eccentric (lengthening) muscular contraction, such as is seen in the hamstrings, which span two joints, making them subject to stretching at more than one point (32,33). The hamstrings decelerate the swinging leg in gait and running,

and they contract with the quadriceps to stabilize the knee. Hamstring injuries commonly are seen in sports in which the athlete rapidly accelerates, such as rugby, track and field, football, and soccer. When athletes are not properly warmed up or if they have decreased flexibility, muscle strength imbalance relative to the quadriceps, or fatigue, they risk the possibility of hamstring injury (33,34). Having suffered a previous hamstring injury also increases the risk of reinjury.

The athlete with a hamstring strain usually complains of posterior thigh pain during or after running and during other activities involving eccentric contraction. On physical examination, swelling and tenderness are usually noted at the area of injury, and, sometimes, a palpable gap can be felt. The most com-

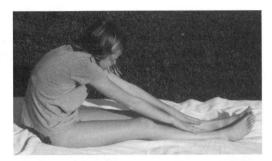

FIG. 35.14. Hamstring stretches. The sit and reach hamstring stretch is performed by sitting with the legs in front and grabbing the legs as far down as possible. The chest is pulled toward the knees. The stretch is held for 6 to 10 seconds.

mon site of hamstring injury is the musculotendinous junction. In skeletally immature athletes, the ischial apophysis may be avulsed, for which a surgical consultation may be required. Most hamstring strains respond to nonsurgical, conservative treatment that in-

cludes rest, ice, and compression. An athlete may ambulate without crutches with a grade I injury. With grade II (moderate) and III (severe) injuries, the athlete should be on crutches until pain-free walking is achieved. As pain subsides, the athlete should begin gentle active and passive stretching (Figs. 35.14 to 35.16) and early light range-of-motion exercises and should then progress to full weight bearing as tolerated. Cross training activities, such as swimming and cycling (if the tear is not at the pressure area of the bicycle seat), are good exercises that allow the athlete to maintain cardiovascular fitness. When pain-free range of motion has been achieved, a gradual running program may be resumed.

Hamstring strains may require long periods of convalescence—about 2 weeks for a grade I strain, 2 to 4 weeks for a grade II strain, and up to about 12 weeks for a grade III strain—before a full return to sports participation can occur. This can be quite frustrating for the athlete, the parents, and the clinician, so emphasizing cross training during rehabilitation and maintaining a positive attitude are important during recovery.

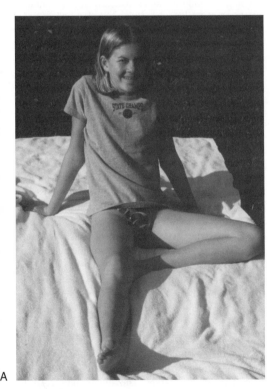

A

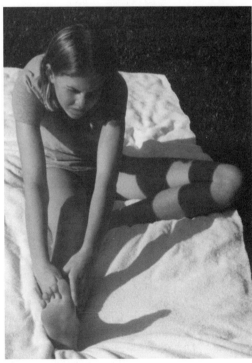

B

FIG. 35.15. Hurdler hamstring stretch. **A:** The hurdler stretch is performed with one leg extended, and the opposite leg is flexed at the knee and abducted at the hip so that the foot is resting on the inside of the other leg. **B:** The hamstring is stretched by grasping the legs as far down as possible. The stretch is held for 10 seconds.

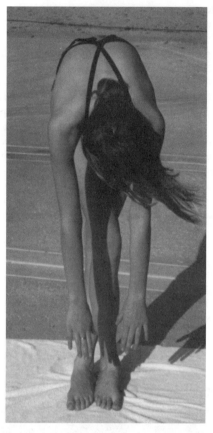

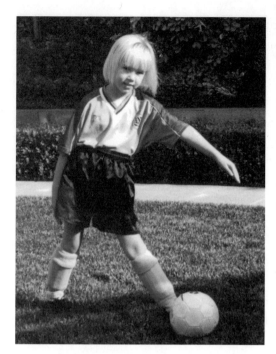

FIG. 35.17. Adductor strain. One mechanism for developing an adductor strain pictured here is extreme abduction of the leg while trying to kick a ball.

FIG. 35.16. Standing crossed hamstring stretch. The standing crossed hamstring stretch is performed by crossing the legs when standing, bending forward, and reaching down the legs as far as possible. The back leg should remain straight. The front knee may bend slightly.

Adductor Strains

Injuries to the thigh adductor muscles are common, and they are described in sports such as soccer, tennis, football, horseback riding, volleyball, water skiing, hockey, and running (11,19,31). Mechanisms of injury for the adductors are overstretch of the groin during excessive abduction of the leg (Fig. 35.17) and, more commonly, forced abduction of the thigh while performing an adduction maneuver (e.g., the leg gets kicked outward while the athlete is trying to kick a ball or the athlete changes direction quickly when running). In these latter descriptions, the muscle is performing a strong eccentric contraction, instead of the concentric contraction that was intended (11).

The athlete with an acute adductor strain usually feels a painful pulling sensation in the groin, and he or she may feel a pop or ripping sensation at time of injury. Associated pain, warmth, and possibly swelling are felt in the affected area. Adductor strains span the spectrum, ranging from an athlete who continues to participate with a low-grade strain to the athlete who is limping or who is unable to walk with a more severe strain. The groin is tender to palpation with an acute adductor strain. Often, associated ecchymosis of the medial thigh, which results from hemorrhage tracking down the thigh postinjury, is present. Resisted abduction and adduction and passive stretching will usually aggravate the pain. The goals of treatment are to relieve pain, diminish swelling, and restore range of motion. Treatment consists of RICE for an acute injury and progresses to gentle range of motion after the first 12 to 24 hours (19,31). Compression shorts can be used, or the area can be wrapped in a hip spica wrap to apply compression (19). After a few days, passive stretching and isometric exercises can be added (Figs. 35.18 and 35.19). Surgery may be indicated in cases of an acute complete tear or for a symptomatic chronic strain that has been refractory to therapy. The athlete may return to full sports participation after the range of motion is normal and strength is 90% when compared to the uninjured leg (19).

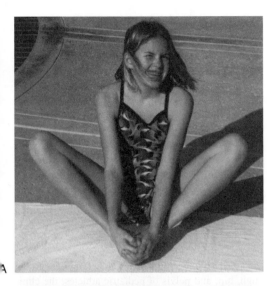

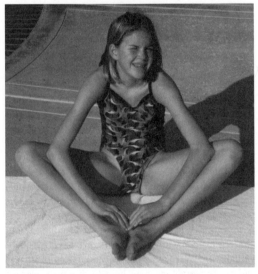

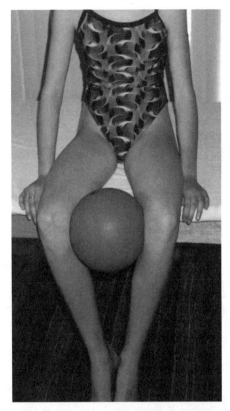

FIG. 35.19. Adductor exercise: seated ball squeeze. The athlete sits on a table with a ball between the knees and squeezes the ball for 6 to10 seconds.

FIG. 35.18. Groin stretch. The groin stretch is performed in seated position with soles of feet together. **A:** The athlete rests elbows on knees and grasps the ankles. **B:** The athlete presses down on knees with the elbows until a groin stretch is felt.

Groin Pain

Acute groin pain usually occurs with sports that involve kicking, cutting, and running, such as in soccer, football, and racquet sports. The most common causes of groin pain are musculotendinous strains of the following five muscles, which constitute the adductor group: the adductor longus, adductor brevis, adductor magnus, gracilis, and pectineus (Fig. 35.20). However, in pediatric athletes, avulsion fractures are more common than muscular strains. Other musculotendinous injuries that may occur and that present with groin pain are disruptions of the rectus abdominus (a spine flexor), the rectus femoris, the iliopsoas (a hip flexor), and the sartorius, as well as tears or dehiscence in the conjoined tendon (11,31). Additional musculoskeletal causes of groin pain were discussed above, including bursitis, a slipped capital femoral epiphysis, Legg–Calvé–Perthes disease, osteitis pubis, and stress fractures of the pelvic rami or femoral neck. Referred pain from the knee or spine or a herniated nucleus pulposus may also present as groin pain.

When evaluating musculoskeletal causes of groin pain, checking the athlete's flexibility may be helpful, because individuals with decreased flexibility and tight hamstrings, quadriceps, or abductors may present with groin pain (31). The treatment of musculotendinous groin injuries was discussed in the section titled "Adductor Strains."

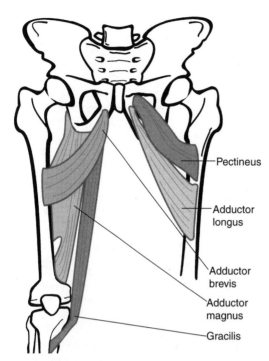

FIG. 35.20. Adductors of the hip and thigh. The adductors of the hip and thigh are the adductor longus, adductor brevis, adductor magnus, gracilis, and pectineus. (Drawn by DeEtte DeVille, M.D. Adapted from Brukner P, Bradshaw C, McCrory P. Obturator neuropathy: a cause of exercise-related groin pain. *The Physician and Sports Medicine* 1999;27:62–64, with permission.)

Nonmusculoskeletal causes of groin pain must be considered in the differential diagnosis, if the history is not consistent with a musculoskeletal cause. Some genitourinary medical diagnoses that should be contemplated in the athlete with groin pain are testicular torsion or rupture, urinary tract infection, renal stones, ovarian cysts, inguinal hernias, pelvic inflammatory disease and sexually transmitted diseases, epididymitis, hydroceles, and testicular neoplasms. Lymphadenopathy or arthritis may also present with groin pain.

Another cause of groin pain is nerve entrapment. In this scenario, the athlete complains of a burning pain that radiates in the distribution of the nerve. Nerves in the groin that may become entrapped by inflammation, injury, or scarring are the obturator, the ilioinguinal, and the genitofemoral nerves (11). These are treated with local anesthetic infiltration to the area around the nerve.

PATHOLOGIC DISORDERS

Several types of bone tumors are seen in the femur (e.g., osteoid osteoma and osteosarcoma) and cartilage (e.g., benign enchondroma and exostosis and neoplastic osteochondroma and chondrosarcoma). The child with osteoid osteoma presents with an aching thigh or hip or groin pain, which contrasts to the child with osteosarcoma, who may be asymptomatic. As "Imaging the Pediatric Hip" in this chapter discusses, radiographic imaging of injuries to identify these lesions is prudent, especially when the history of injury does not correlate with the extent of the physical findings.

PREVENTION

To aid in prevention of overuse injuries in the thigh, hip, and pelvis of pediatric athletes, the clinician should be aware of factors that predispose the athlete to injuries so that he or she can provide appropriate counsel to the athlete. Both apophyseal areas of active growth cartilage and periods of rapid growth can predispose the pediatric athlete to injury. Growth cartilage, such as that found in the apophyses, is predisposed to repetitive stress injury, such as apophysitis. More rapid changes in long bone length compared to that of the associated muscle–tendon attachments may result in muscle imbalance or inflexibility and may predispose the athlete to injury, particularly during the adolescent growth spurt. Other factors, such as musculoskeletal alignment abnormalities in the athlete, can also lead to injuries (5). Training errors can be another contributing factor in injuries. Improving the athlete's level of conditioning and ensuring that training programs have adequate variation in frequency, intensity, duration, and rest and/or recovery time may help to diminish overuse (5) and other growth-related injuries.

REFERRAL DECISIONS

When treating pediatric patients with thigh, hip, and pelvis injuries, some disorders (e.g., hip dislocation; femoral shaft and neck fractures; traumatic pelvic fractures; displaced pelvic fractures; septic arthritis [for drainage]; Legg–Calvé–Perthes disease; malignancy; and slipped capital femoral epiphysis) warrant prompt referral to an orthopedic surgeon consultant.

Other patients who may benefit from orthopedic consultation are those with significantly displaced apophyseal avulsion fractures and those for whom conservative treatment for avulsion fractures has failed, as well as patients with strains, sprains, a snapping hip (especially if intraarticular pathology is suspected), trochanteric bursitis, noninfectious arthritis, nondisplaced pelvic fractures that failed to heal in 12 weeks, and nonhealing meralgia paresthetica (lateral femoral cutaneous nerve syndrome). Other indicators for further evaluation include night pain, pain at rest, or a sudden increase in the severity of pain. In meralgia paresthetica that is unresponsive to treatment, further evaluations for pelvic or abdominal masses that can create similar symptoms should be considered. Orthopedic consultants also may provide guidance on management, rehabilitation, and return-to-play decisions in challenging cases.

RETURN-TO-PLAY DECISIONS

In pediatric athletes with thigh, hip, and pelvis injuries, care should be taken to minimize the risk of reinjury before the athlete is permitted to return to full athletic participation. Sometimes an athlete may become pain free before an injury has totally healed, such as with a mild apophyseal avulsion injury. The risk of reinjury or further apophyseal displacement is high if the athlete has not regained full strength and function of the injured muscles. In the 5-phase rehabilitation program described by Metzmaker and Pappas (6), the athlete may return to full athletic competition only when he or she has regained full strength and integration of the injured muscles that are needed for the athletic requirements of the sport (15).

In cases of fractures of the femoral neck, subtrochanteric femoral fractures, and stable pelvic fractures, the athlete may return to sport after full healing is demonstrated by radiograph and the patient has regained full lower extremity strength and range of motion. Patients with femoral neck fractures who meet these criteria can return to sports participation with internal fixation hardware in place. In athletes who have had a reduction of a hip dislocation, a gradual return to sports can occur after 3 months (following approximately 6 weeks of protected weight bearing and 6 weeks of additional rehabilitation), as long as no associated complications, such as avascular necrosis or myositis ossificans, have occurred. Athletes who have stress fractures of the femoral neck may cross train with swimming and bicycling with protected weight bearing. When healing occurs, athletes may return to sports participation if they are pain free. Osteitis pubis can be recalcitrant to treatment, and this condition may take as long as 9 months to heal before the athlete is pain free and can be allowed to return to the sport. In young children with Legg–Calvé–Perthes disease, high impact activities are restricted until the healing phase. An orthopedic consultant can help direct rehabilitation. In athletes with apophysitis, a return to sport is possible in about 4 to 6 weeks, if no pain recurs.

In thigh contusions, the athlete may return to sport after full strength has been regained and if myositis ossificans is absent. Hip strains of muscle tendon units can be treated with a graded rehabilitation program before a full return to sports participation. The graded program progresses from rest and ice for 48 hours to passive range of motion for 1 week, followed by 1 to 3 weeks of isometric exercises and cycling to regain strength and flexibility. Rehabilitation progresses to isotonic and isokinetic exercises by 3 to 4 weeks postinjury, and the return to sports is seen at 4 and 6 weeks. Thigh strains of the quadriceps and hamstrings are initially treated with RICE, followed by the use of a stretching and strengthening program for injured muscles. Isometric and conditioning exercises for 2 to 4 weeks progress to isotonic and isokinetic rehabilitation exercises by 4 to 6 weeks postinjury, followed by sport-specific rehabilitation exercises prior to the athlete's return to full sports participation (15). The return to sports may take longer than 8 weeks, particularly for hamstring injuries.

CONCLUSION

The increased numbers of pediatric and adolescent participants in sports has created a need for clinicians to consider the specific demands placed on the athlete's immature skeleton when evaluating injuries and prescribing treatment. The young athlete is at risk for physeal and nonphyseal skeletal injuries, as well as soft tissue injuries to the hip, thigh, and pelvis. With prompt accurate diagnosis of these injuries, the athlete can begin a treatment program directed at getting the athlete back to active sports participation.

REFERENCES

1. Paletta GA, Andrish JT. Injuries about the hip and pelvis in the young athlete. *Clin Sports Med* 1995;14:591–627.
2. Morrissy RT, Weinstein SL, eds. *Lovell and Winter's pediatric orthopaedics*, 4th ed. Philadelphia: Lippincott-Raven Publishers, 1996.
3. O'Kane JW. Anterior hip pain. *Am Fam Physician* 1999;60:1687–1696.
4. Wojtys EM. Sports injuries in the immature athlete. *Orthop Clin North Am* 1987;18:689–708.
5. DiFiori JP. Overuse injuries in children and adolescents. *The Physician and Sports Medicine* 1999;27:75–89.
6. Metzmaker JN, Pappas AM. Avulsion fractures of the pelvis. *Am J Sports Med* 1985;13:349–358.

7. Myers MT, Thompson GH. Imaging the child with a limp. *Pediatr Clin North Am* 1997;44:637–658.

8. Duffey TP, Hershman E, Sanders RA, et al. Investigating the subtle and obvious causes of hip pain. *Patient Care* 1997;31:76–99.

9. Waters PM, Millis MB. Hip and pelvic injuries in the young athlete. *Clin Sports Med* 1988;7:513–526.

10. Parris HG, Sallis RE, Anderson DV. Traumatic hip dislocation: reducing complications. *The Physician and Sports Medicine* 1993;21:67–74.

11. Ruane JJ, Rossi TA. When groin pain is more "than just a strain." *The Physician and Sports Medicine* 1998;26: 78–103.

12. Devas MB. Stress fractures of the femoral neck. *J Bone Joint Surg Br* 1965;47:728–738.

13. Devas MB. Stress fractures in children. *J Bone Joint Surg Br* 1963;45:528–541.

14. Johnson AW, Weiss CB, Wheeler DL. Stress fractures of the femoral shaft in athletes—more common than expected. *Am J Sports Med* 1994;22:248–256.

15. Stanitski CL, DeLee JC, Drez D, eds. *Pediatric and adolescent sports medicine.* Vol. 3. Philadelphia: WB Saunders, 1994.

16. Weiker GG, Munnings F. Selected hip and pelvis injuries—managing hip pointers, stress fractures and more. *The Physician and Sports Medicine* 1994;22: 96–106.

17. Weiker GG, Munnings F. How I manage hip and pelvis injuries in adolescents. *The Physician and Sports Medicine* 1993;21:72–82.

18. Cook PC, Leit ME. Issues in the pediatric athlete. *Orthop Clin North Am* 1995;26:453–464.

19. McKeag DB, Hough DO, eds. *Primary care sports medicine.* Dubuque, IA: Brown & Benchmark, 1993.

20. Swain R, Snodgrass S. Managing groin pain even when the cause is not obvious. *The Physician and Sports Medicine* 1995;23:55–66.

21. Reid DC, ed. *Sports injury assessment and rehabilitation.* Philadelphia: Churchill Livingstone, 1992.

22. Aronen JG, Chronister R, Regan K, et al. Practical conservative management of iliotibial band syndrome. *The Physician and Sports Medicine* 1993;21:59–69.

23. Fredericson M, Guillet M, DeBenedictis L. Quick solutions for iliotibial band syndrome. *The Physician and Sports Medicine* 2000;28:53–68.

24. Price CT, Moon BS. The limping child: an age-based approach to evaluation. *J Musculoskeletal Med* 1997; 14:32–45.

25. Koop S, Quanbeck D. Three common causes of childhood hip pain. *Pediatr Clin North America* 1996;43: 1053–1066.

26. Gerberg LF, Micheli LJ. Nontraumatic hip pain in active children: a critical differential. *The Physician and Sports Medicine* 1996;24:69–74.

27. Loder RT. Slipped capital femoral epiphysis. *Am Fam Physician* 1998;57:2135–2142.

28. Webber A. Acute soft tissue injuries in the young athlete. *Clin Sports Med* 1988;7:611–624.

29. Arrington ED, Miller MD. Skeletal muscle injuries. *Orthop Clin North Am* 1995;26:411–422.

30. Thorton JJ. Pain relief for acute soft tissue injuries. *The Physician and Sports Medicine* 1997;25:108–114.

31. Hasselman CT, Best TM, Garrett WE. When groin pain signals an adductor strain. *The Physician and Sports Medicine* 1995;23:53–60.

32. Saperstein AL, Nicholas SJ. Pediatric and adolescent sports medicine. *Pediatr Clin North Am* 1996;43: 1013–1033.

33. Best TM, Garrett WE. Hamstring strains expediting return to play. *The Physician and Sports Medicine* 1996; 24:37–44.

34. Snider RK, ed. *Essentials of musculoskeletal care.* Rosemont, IL: American Academy of Orthopaedic Surgeons, 1997.

36

Knee and Leg Injuries

David T. Bernhardt

The knee is literally and figuratively the pivotal hinge joint for many sporting activities. Whether a young athlete is running, kicking, jumping, swimming, or dancing, many different types of stress or strain may lead to either acute or chronic injury of the knee. These injuries may affect the exercising patterns of the youngster, but they may also influence attending school, standing in the church choir, or walking the grocery aisles with parents. This chapter reviews the epidemiology of knee injuries in the skeletally immature athlete; provides a brief overview of knee anatomy while highlighting the unique aspects of the growing athlete; discusses in detail the clinical evaluation, including the history and physical examination; and recaps the specific in-office diagnoses that one must consider when examining the young athlete with knee pain.

KNEE INJURIES

Anatomy

The knee consists of four bones—the femur, tibia, fibula, and patella—and three articulations—the patellofemoral, tibiofemoral, and tibiofibular. The osseous structures are structurally held together by a combination of ligaments, a joint capsule, and large dynamic muscle groups that transverse the joint. The epiphyses of the distal femur and proximal tibia are present at birth. The proximal fibular epiphysis and patellar ossification center, however, are not present until 3 or 4 years of age.

The medial collateral ligament (MCL) and the lateral collateral ligament (LCL), along with the arcuate ligament and an extension of the popliteus muscle, provide significant support to the knee. The MCL provides stability to valgus stress, and it connects the femur and tibia on the medial side of the knee. The distal femoral physis acts as the proximal attachment of the MCL in the skeletally immature athlete. The MCL and medial meniscus share common fibers, and they can be injured concurrently. The LCL connects the lateral femoral condyle to the proximal fibula, and it does not share fibers with the lateral meniscus. The LCL, along with musculotendinous constraints, provides protection against varus stress.

The anterior cruciate ligament (ACL) originates from the posteromedial aspect of the medial femoral condyle and inserts on the interspinous area of the tibia. The ACL primarily resists anterior displacement of the tibia and secondarily stabilizes the knee against rotational movement, as well as against medial and lateral stress. The posterior cruciate ligament (PCL) originates from the lateral aspect of the medial femoral condyle and inserts on the back of the tibia. The PCL acts to resist posterior displacement of the tibia on the femur.

The medial and lateral meniscus are C-shaped collagenous structures that act to cushion the femur as it rests on the tibia. The blood supply to the meniscus is tenuous, even in adolescents, as the outer one-third of each meniscus (the vascular zone) receives most of the blood supply originating from branches of the geniculate artery.

Extension of the knee is provided primarily by the quadriceps muscles that join to become the quadriceps tendon above the patella and the infrapatellar tendon (or patellar tendon) below the patella. The infrapatellar tendon inserts on the tibial tubercle apophysis in the young athlete and, later on, in the tibial tuberosity in the older athlete.

Flexion of the knee is the main function of the posterior and medial muscle groups, which include the biceps femoris, the semimembrinosis and semitendinosis, the gracilis, and the sartorius. The semimembrinosis, semitendinosis, and sartorius tendons all attach on the anterior superior aspect of the medial tibia, forming the pes anserine tendinous complex, which augments the medial stability to the knee.

Epidemiology

The risk of physical injury is inherent with participation in any athletic or recreational activity. Sports and recreational activities account for greater than one-third of all injuries to children between 5 and 19 years of age (1). Knee injuries are the most frequently reported injury, according to a prospective cohort study of Hawaiian high school athletes (2).

Acute knee injuries are seen commonly in football, basketball, soccer, hockey, and alpine skiing. Overuse knee injuries, such as patellar tendinitis, Osgood–Schlatter, and patellofemoral stress syndrome (PFSS), are more commonly seen in jumping and running sports.

Studies of gender differences show that females are more likely to suffer a knee injury than are their male counterparts in the same sports of basketball and soccer, with a significant portion of the difference related to ACL injuries. The National Athletic Trainers Association study of high school basketball players showed that the knee injury rate is 44% higher for girls, the surgery rate is twice as high for girls, and the ACL surgery rate is four times as high as that for boys' teams (3). Among varsity high school basketball players in Texas, the ACL injury rate and the knee injury rate, in general, were both higher for females (4).The risk of knee injury was more than twice as high for girls than it was for boys, and the risk of ACL injury was almost four times higher for girls in this population.

Similar to total injury rates, the incidence of knee injuries increases with increasing age and skill level. A study of ACL injuries among Norwegian soccer players showed that the rate for higher-level men was 0.41 per 1,000 game hours, whereas the incidence for the lowest level was 0.11 per 1,000 game hours (5).

Many hypothetical reasons for the gender differences have been proposed and investigated, but no single cause has been proven.

Chronic anterior knee pain is the bane of both sports medicine physicians and pediatricians. Whether the anterior knee pain is secondary to Osgood–Schlatter disease, patellar tendonitis, or PFSS, anterior knee pain is a common presenting complaint among young patients.

History

When evaluating the young athlete who complains of knee pain, the practitioner must determine whether the condition is due to an acute injury. For the acutely injured knee, the most compelling question then becomes that of the mechanism of injury. A description of a classic mechanism of injury can often make the diagnosis. Unfortunately, many adolescents have a difficult time recalling or explaining how the injury may have occurred. Therefore, the clinician may have to rely on others, such as athletic trainers, coaches, teammates, and parents, who might have witnessed the injury in order to gain a full picture of the mechanism of injury. The mechanism of injury can then give the clinician an idea of which structures were injured (Table 36.1).

Specific mechanisms of injury often assist the clinician when the physical examination is limited in the acute setting due to patient guarding and possible swelling. For example, a lineman who tackles a running back, causing a direct force to the outside of the knee (valgus stress), may cause injury to the MCL. A noncontact injury that involves sudden stopping or pivoting (hyperextension) often results in an ACL injury.

A history of acute severe swelling may be suggestive of a hemarthrosis secondary to an ACL tear, patellar dislocation, or fracture. However, the lack of significant swelling does not necessarily rule out injury to these structures. Many young athletes and their families are trained in the basics of acute injury treatment (rest, ice, compression, and elevation [RICE]), and thus the young athlete may not develop severe swelling, even with a significant injury.

Clinicians need to inquire about any episodes of instability (Table 36.2). Instability means that the athlete experiences spontaneous episodes of giving way, usually associated with pivoting activity secondary to an injury to the ACL or recurrent patellar subluxation. Sometimes the athlete will experience significant patellar pain with quadriceps contrac-

TABLE 36.1. *Mechanism of injury and injured structures*

Mechanism of injury	Injured structure
Hyperextension	ACL +/– meniscus
Valgus stress (direct force to outside of knee)	MCL +/– medial meniscus +/– ACL
Varus stress (direct force to inside of knee)	LCL
Twisting	Meniscus or dislocation of patella
Direct blow to anterior tibia	PCL

Abbreviations: ACL, anterior cruciate ligament; LCL, lateral collateral ligament; MCL, medial collateral ligament; PCL, posterior cruciate ligament.

TABLE 36.2. *Questions which should be asked by clinician*

Acute knee injuries
  How did this injury occur?
  Did immediate swelling occur at the time of injury?
  Do you feel like your knee has been giving out since the injury?
  Have you experienced any catching or locking type of symptoms?
  Do you have a history of other previous injuries to your knee?
Chronic knee pain
  How long have you had knee pain?
  Where is the pain most severe?
  What does the pain feel like?
  What activities aggravate the pain—activities of daily living versus athletic activities?
  Have you noticed any redness, warmth, or swelling?
  Have you noticed any other joint pain?
  Have you noticed any other symptoms—ill-defined rashes, fevers, chills, sweats, or weight loss?
  Does your family history include rheumatologic diseases, such as rheumatoid arthritis or lupus?

tion, and, through reflex quadriceps inhibition, he or she may experience a similar feeling of giving way.

A history of catching or locking suggests the presence of a loose body or a meniscal tear. Catching is considered to be the feeling of gravel or pebbles that interferes with motion. Locking is defined as the inability to extend the knee fully. Contrary to what is seen in adults, youngsters who suffer from a meniscus tear often have a history of a previous injury.

In contrast to the patient with an acute knee injury, the athlete with chronic knee pain often requires a more in-depth history for both the initial evaluation and subsequent follow-up visits. The history in both acute and chronic knee pain must include questions regarding previous knee injuries. As opposed to the diffuse pain that is observed with acute knee injuries, the patient with chronic knee pain may be able to localize that pain.

Classic anterior knee pain usually presents as an achy knee, with pain that is worse with the activities of daily living, including going up stairs, rising from a seated position, and kneeling. Sitting for long periods of time also may aggravate this condition.

Swelling that is associated with chronic knee pain suggests a possible meniscal injury, patellar subluxation, an osteochondral lesion, a rheumatologic condition, or a neoplastic process.

A history of redness or warmth suggests an infectious or rheumatologic process. Further questioning regarding trauma; other infectious sources, including tick bites; and the family history, are warranted (Table 36.2).

Physical Examination

An organized physical examination focusing on the knee is the next step when evaluating the knee. An or-ganized examination should parallel the examination done on all other joints, including inspection, range of motion, strength, ligamentous laxity, palpation, and special tests.

The general inspection of the knee looks for any gross deformity or obvious effusion in which the fluid is seen in the sulcus medial to the patella (Fig. 36.1). By inspecting the patient while both supine and standing, any alignment abnormalities, such as tibial torsion, femoral anteversion, or pes planus, may be noted. Finally, with the patient seated, the presence of any patellar tracking as the knee extends fully from 90 degrees of flexion should be noted. A patella that rides laterally towards the terminal extension suggests subluxation.

Strength should be assessed with both isometric and concentric contraction of the quadriceps and hamstring muscles. Reflex quadriceps inhibition with patellar pain may result in a unilateral quadriceps atrophy on the affected side.

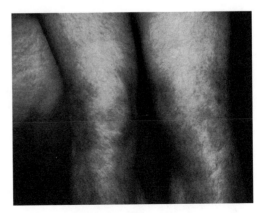

FIG. 36.1. Knee effusion.

TABLE 36.3. *Physical examination tests for ligamentous laxity*

Ligament to test	Examination maneuver	How to perform	Other tests
ACL	Lachman	Anterior translation of tibia, with knee in 15–20 degrees of flexion	Pivot shift
MCL	Valgus stress	Top hand acts as a fulcrum on outside of knee, stressing MCL in both full extension and 20 degrees of flexion	—
LCL	Varus stress	Top hand acts as a fulcrum on inside of knee, stressing LCL in both full extension and 20 degrees of flexion	—
PCL	Tibial sag	Tibia plateau not easily palpated with tibia displaced posteriorly	Posterior drawer Reverse pivot shift

Abbreviations: ACL, anterior cruciate ligament; LCL, lateral collateral ligament; MCL, medial collateral ligament; PCL, posterior cruciate ligament.

Assessment of ligament sprains is sometimes difficult for the inexperienced clinician. To simplify, each of the four ligaments (ACL, MCL, LCL, and PCL) has a test that corresponds to each ligament that is to be tested (Table 36.3). The Lachman test is the most sensitive test for determining laxity in the ACL. (Fig. 36.2). The Lachman test is conducted with the knee in approximately 20 degrees of flexion; a positive test is noted with more than 3 mm of asymmetry when compared to the uninjured knee or by the absence of an endpoint on the injured knee. Other tests, such as the pivot shift, can also be used to assess ACL laxity; however, these tests are technically more difficult to perform, and they often do not add much to the basic examination. Varus and valgus stress tests are used to evaluate the laxity of the LCL and the MCL, respectively. PCL injury is rare. PCL laxity is difficult to determine, but it should be suspected if the history is consistent with a PCL injury and with the inability to palpate the

medial and lateral tibial plateau when the knee is flexed at 90 degrees.

All joints have special tests to determine the presence of injury to structures specific to that joint. In the knee, the McMurray test is used to determine injury to the meniscus. The knee is flexed completely by the examiner. Internal and external rotation of the tibia during the subsequent extension places stress on the meniscus. A tender medial or lateral joint line, in addition to a painful click during this procedure, suggests the existence of an injury to the meniscus.

Palpation is the last aspect of the examination. Tenderness over the MCL or LCL suggests the possibility of injury to these structures. Tenderness directly over the physis may signal the possibility of an injury to an open growth plate in the skeletally immature athlete, and it should indicate the need for further radiographs. In chronic anterior knee pain, the specific diagnosis often depends on the location of the pain (Fig. 36.3). For example, tenderness over the tibial tuberosity often confirms the diagnosis of Osgood–Schlatter disease, whereas tenderness over the patellar tendon suggests "jumpers' knee" or patellar tendinitis.

Imaging

The standard four views that can be obtained to evaluate a knee injury include an anteroposterior, a lateral, a tunnel, and a patellar view. The anteroposterior and lateral views demonstrate femoral alignment and most supracondylar and intraarticular fractures. The tunnel view, which is taken with the knee flexed to 45 degrees, is needed when looking for an osteochondral lesion or loose bodies. A patellar view evaluates the patellar alignment, a patellar

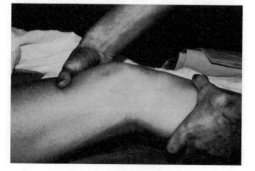

FIG. 36.2. Lachman test.

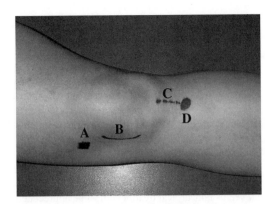

FIG. 36.3. Diagnosis of anterior knee pain depends on point of maximal tenderness. **A:** Adductor tubercle (site of tenderness associated with patellar subluxation). **B:** Medial facet (site of tenderness associated with patellofemoral stress syndrome). **C:** Patellar tendon (site of maximal tenderness associated with patellar tendinitis). **D:** Tibial tuberosity (site of maximal tenderness associated with Osgood–Schlatter).

fracture, and patellar osteochondral lesions. Several different patellar views exist, and they have different eponyms that are dependent on the knee flexion angle. Patellar subluxation is more easily demonstrated between 30 and 45 degrees of flexion.

Indications for radiographs include an obvious open fracture or penetrating trauma. Other major indications include a large effusion, the loss of range of motion, and an inability to bear weight. Indications for obtaining radiographs include a mechanism of blunt trauma or a fall, a patient age of less than 12 years, and the inability to walk four weight-bearing steps in the emergency department (6). Using on these criteria, only one significant fracture was missed in patients who otherwise would not have received radiographs, yielding a sensitivity of 99% and a specificity of 60% in this study (6).

Acute Knee Injuries

Anterior Cruciate Ligament Injuries

The ACL consists of two major bundles—the posterolateral and the anteromedial. The ACL originates on the posterior part of the medial surface of the lateral femoral condyle, and it inserts on a wide depressed area anterolateral to the anterior tibial spine.

Injury to the ACL is recognized as one of the most common major knee injuries incurred in athletics. The mechanism of injury is often a noncontact decel-

eration that involves hyperextension and either internal or external rotation.

Historically, the diagnosis is suggested by the appropriate mechanism of injury and a loud pop. Rapid swelling may be reported, although the acute application of ice and compression may decrease the degree of swelling. In cases of chronic ACL deficiency, recurrent episodes of giving way are associated with pivoting.

On examination, a positive Lachman test is the most specific finding. A large hemarthrosis, along with patient guarding, may make conducting this examination difficult in the acute situation. Therefore, a repeat examination after the swelling subsides may be necessary to establish the diagnosis.

The differential diagnosis for acute hemarthrosis includes an osteochondral fracture, patellar dislocation or subluxation, and a meniscus tear. Diagnostic knee arthroscopic findings in children between the ages of 7 to 18 years who had acute traumatic knee hemarthroses showed a high incidence of intraarticular lesions, including ACL and meniscal tears (7). In a more recent study including adults, the majority (85%) of hemarthroses were ACL tears (8).

Plain radiographs are often normal, but, in younger patients, they must be obtained to rule out a possible tibial spine avulsion. Magnetic resonance imaging (MRI) is often obtained to confirm the diagnosis or to establish the diagnosis when the physical examination is equivocal. The sensitivity and specificity of MRI are 90% and 67%, respectively, for detecting ACL injury (9).

Tear of the ACL can occur in the midsubstance of the ACL or, less frequently, at the tibial attachment. Similar to the pattern observed in adults, a high frequency of associated meniscal pathology is also found in younger patients. Because of the high incidence of possibly repairable meniscal tears, many orthopedists recommend the early use of MRI to provide further guidance for treatment decisions. Skeletally immature athletes with isolated ACL tears may be advised to avoid pivoting sports until physeal closure, at which time ACL reconstruction can be more safely pursued. For athletes with associated meniscus tears, early repair of the meniscus tear is advocated with a delay in ACL reconstruction until physeal closure occurs. For skeletally immature athletes who do not wish to modify their athletic activity, an increasing number of orthopedists has begun reconstructing the ACL with good results (10,11).

Most active patients who participate in pivoting sports have the ligament reconstructed approximately 3 to 4 weeks (at a minimum) after the injury to allow swelling to decrease and full range of motion prior to surgery. Athletes with an isolated ACL tear may modify their lifestyles to avoid pivoting type sports and can rehabilitate the knee through functional stabilization. If repeat instability can be avoided, the lower long-term damage to the meniscus results in better long-term knee health.

Reconstruction usually involves using a bone–patellar–bone or hamstring tendon autograft to reconstruct the ACL. Studies of these procedures show that more than 85% achieve good to excellent results.

Medial Collateral Ligament Injuries

Injury to the MCL occurs when a valgus force is applied to the knee while the lower leg is in external tibial rotation. This injury may be a noncontact twisting type of injury, or it can be the direct result of blunt trauma to the lateral side of the joint. The athlete will usually describe pain over the medial aspect of the knee.

On examination, isolated injury to the extraarticular MCL rarely results in a large effusion. A large hemarthrosis with valgus stress is often associated with the "terrible triad" of injuries to the ACL, MCL, and medial meniscus. In the skeletally immature athlete, the possibility of a physeal injury or an epiphyseal fracture must be considered in cases of a large effusion.

Collateral ligament injuries are usually graded on the basis of pain and laxity. A grade I injury is characterized by significant pain but no laxity with valgus stress testing. A grade II injury has some laxity compared to the other uninjured side, but a firm endpoint can be described. A grade III injury is the most severe, and it shows significant laxity without detection of a firm endpoint with valgus stress testing.

Treatment for isolated collateral ligament tears generally is nonoperative. Even isolated grade III lesions are treated with immobilization, followed by range-of-motion and functional stabilization.

Although many collegiate and professional football teams have players wear braces to prevent or reduce the severity of knee injuries, no conclusive evidence supports their use, and, in some studies, braces actually increase the frequency of injury in certain positions (12). Therefore, practitioners should not advocate their routine use for the pediatric and adolescent age groups.

Lateral Collateral Ligament Injuries

Injuries to the LCL are rare among skeletally immature athletes. Injury occurs when a varus stress is applied to a knee in internal tibial rotation. Similar to the MCL, the LCL is extraarticular, so little swelling is associated with isolated injury. However, the LCL is not as closely opposed to the meniscus, and, therefore, associated injuries to the lateral meniscus are rare.

Injuries to the posterolateral ligamentous complex are also rare. These injuries can occur with a sudden anteromedial force that brings the nearly fully extended joint into forced hyperextension. Although specific tests can be useful in the physical examination when attempting to diagnose posterolateral instability, these are often difficult to perform, and subtle abnormalities that may influence the choice of surgical versus nonsurgical treatment must be appreciated. Therefore, any athlete with a mechanism of injury that raises concern, in addition to tenderness in the posterolateral or lateral ligamentous complexes, should be referred for orthopedic consultation.

Posterior Cruciate Ligament Injury

The PCL is made up of two bands, anterolateral and posteromedial. The PCL attaches to the lateral portion of the medial femoral condyle, proximally, and to the depression on the posterior tibia between the tibial plateaus, distally. The PCL functions to prevent posterior translation of the tibia on the femur at all flexion angles.

Injury to the PCL is rare in children and adolescents. The mechanism of injury classically is a direct posterior force to the anterior tibia while the knee is flexed, such as occurs when a child falls off a bike. Severe hyperextension injuries may result in a PCL tear, although the ACL fails first.

The physical examination may show a positive posterior drawer test or posterior sagging of the tibia. Both of these findings can be quite subtle. Once again, if a PCL injury is strongly suspected, the athlete should be referred to an orthopedist.

Treatment of this condition is controversial, and many factors must be considered. The results of PCL reconstruction are less predictable than those of the ACL.

Meniscal Injuries

The meniscus plays a fundamental role in load transmission and shock absorption in the knee. It also functions in maintaining joint congruity, stability, lubrication, nutrition, and proprioception. In a study of patients who underwent a complete meniscectomy at the age of 16 years or younger (average follow-up at 21 years of age), 71% reported persistent pain; 68%, stiffness; 54%, swelling; and 41%, giving way; with only 27% reporting a complete lack of symptoms (13).

Anatomical differences exist between the medial and lateral menisci. The lateral meniscus covers more of the tibial plateau, and it is more circular in shape and more mobile than its medial counterpart. The medial meniscus is more firmly attached to the deep fibers of the MCL at the periphery.

The majority of the meniscus is avascular, receiving nutrition through diffusion. The perimeniscal capillary plexus from the geniculate artery supplies the peripheral aspect of the menisci. Attention to the vascular supply to the outer one-third is essential when considering potential healing with meniscal repair versus partial meniscectomy in treatment of these injuries.

Although they are thought to be rare, the exact incidence of meniscal injuries in children is unknown. Most meniscal injuries in the younger population involve high-energy activities, and, therefore, they are seen more commonly in adolescence.

A history of a twisting injury, with or without an associated pop, is classic for a meniscus tear. Persistent catching or locking, swelling, and pain also suggest the diagnosis. Joint line tenderness and swelling are the most common signs. The painful click with full flexion, as described by McMurray, often is not easily demonstrated, and the clinician must instead rely on the subtle finding of pain with full flexion, in conjunction with other signs and symptoms, to make the diagnosis.

The location and type of tear greatly influence the surgical treatment plan. A small vertical or radial tear in the vascular one-third is usually amenable to repair. Failure rates have been shown to be as low as 10% in some series. An unstable, ACL-deficient knee usually has a higher failure rate because of its recurrent instability. Results are better in ACL-reconstructed knees, due to knee instability and the bleeding associated with surgery, which results in a fibrin clot that stimulates healing.

Partial meniscectomies are sometimes necessary for larger tears that involve the less vascular area of the meniscus. Referral to a surgeon who is comfortable with meniscus repair is in the best interest of the athlete and the long-term function of his or her knee.

Patellar Instability

Complete dislocation of the patella usually results in a lateral displacement of the patella from the femoral trochlea or groove that persists until it is reduced by extending the knee. Valgus stress with a forcible contraction of the quadriceps muscle commonly is the mechanism of injury. The feeling of a pop that is associated with a sensation of patellar instability and acute swelling is reported in the history. The physical examination should show a large hemarthrosis with patellar tenderness, especially medially, and patellar apprehension (Fig. 36.4).

Reduction of the acute dislocation involves knee extension and gentle medial pressure along the lateral patella. Immobilization for comfort, followed by aggressive rehabilitation and a patellar tracking brace, is usually recommended.

Recurrent patellar subluxation is marked by transient, self-reducing, and partial displacement of the patella from the femoral groove. Patellar hypermobility and apprehension are evident on the physical examination. A more subtle finding is lateral tracking of the patella on active motion from 90 degrees of flexion to full extension. Plain radiographs may be normal in both conditions, especially after reduction. Patellar views may demonstrate subluxation, tilting of the patella, or a hypoplastic femoral groove that predisposes the patella to tracking problems. Treatment is quite similar to acute dislocation, with aggressive rehabilitation and the use of a patellar tracking brace.

Overuse Injuries

Patellofemoral Stress Syndrome

Anterior knee pain is the most common overuse injury affecting athletes, both young and old, and it accounts for frequent visits to the sports medicine physician's office. Symptoms can be vague, and the physical signs may be minimal. The condition has previously been termed chondromalacia patellae, describing a pathologic entity that involves softening or thinning of the articular cartilage under the patella. In

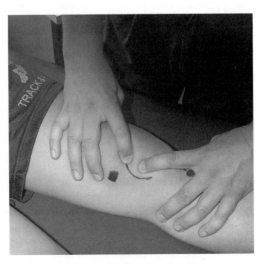

FIG. 36.4. Patellar apprehension.

most young patients, this pathologic finding is not seen, which results in an ambiguous nomenclature for describing this vague anterior knee pain (14). The use of the term "syndrome" is most appropriate, due to the common historical features and physical findings without a demonstrable cause or pathologic finding (15).

Historically, the athlete with PFSS often describes the insidious onset of dull, achy knee pain that is worse with activity, that seemingly surrounds the patella, but that is difficult to localize. Stair climbing usually results in worsening pain. Prolonged sitting or a "positive theatre sign" results in an exacerbation of symptoms. Biomechanically, this is thought to be secondary to increased contact between the patella and femur. Direct pressure on the patella with kneeling or squatting also reproduces the symptoms. Usually, minimal swelling, if any, occurs. "Giving way" may be described by the young athlete, and this phenomenon is possibly the result of reflex quadriceps inhibition.

Common physical examination findings include relative quadriceps atrophy, which is demonstrated by having the patient isometrically contract the quadriceps muscle while laying supine with the knee extended. Vastus medialis weakness or poor tone is often evident when compared to the other knee. Pain with isometric quadriceps contraction localizes the etiology to the patella. Patellar compression, palpation under the medial facet of the patella, and patellofemoral crepitation are all nonspecific findings, but they can help support the diagnosis.

The exact etiology for this condition is unknown, but it may be multifactorial. Biomechanical factors have been implicated, including a higher incidence among patients with femoral anterversion, tibial torsion, and foot hyperpronation. Poor hamstring and quadriceps flexibility has also been associated with this anterior knee pain (16). In a group of adult-aged runners with patellofemoral pain, factors related to knee pain included quadriceps weakness, increased weekly running mileage prior to becoming symptomatic, and a increased angle biomechanically between the hip, knee, and foot (17). Plain radiographs are often normal, and they are thus unnecessary when evaluating this condition. The patellar views are usually normal, but they may show malalignment findings similar to those seen in patellar subluxation. Refractory cases and the presence of effusion, catching, locking, or chronic pain are all indications for plain radiographs to rule out other diagnostic possibilities.

Treatment for this condition usually involves relative rest, ice, and antiinflammatories for pain control, in addition to rehabilitation that focuses on stretching of the hamstring muscles and strengthening the quadriceps muscles. Relative rest consists of avoiding activities that cause a significant increase in pain but allowing activities that are tolerable or that do not increase symptoms. A structured exercise program that involves progressive isometric quadriceps contraction over a 3-month period has been shown to be highly effective in adolescents (18). The main cause of persistent pain is noncompliance with the rehabilitation protocol. Placing an emphasis on the importance of an exercise program, combined with some behavior modification to increase compliance, may be necessary to motivate the young athlete to perform the exercises. Malalignment issues are difficult to address. For athletes with a relatively brief duration of symptoms, treatment with exercises alone may be sufficient, and changes of alignment may produce other problems. For more chronic pain, orthotic treatment may help to reduce the forces on the medial knee. A patellar tracking brace also may be useful when some component of patellar maltracking is suspected. As the athlete's symptoms improve, functional rehabilitation can progress to a gradual return to practice and competition.

Osgood–Schlatter Disease

Osgood–Schlatter disease, or tibial tubercle apophysitis, is a common affliction of the skeletally immature athlete. A Finnish study (19) reported an incidence of almost 13%, with a higher frequency among those subjects who participated in sports. Although this study reported the condition to be more common among boys, the popularity of girls' sports today might cause these findings to be disputed if the study was repeated.

First described by Osgood (20) in 1903, this lesion is caused by the traumatic disruption of a portion of the cartilaginous tibial apophysis by stresses at the insertion of the patellar tendon. The condition is a classic overuse traction apophysitis with pain and swelling that occurs over the area of greatest tensile force where the patellar tendon inserts. Calcification of the apophysis usually begins around 8 or 9 years of age in girls and between 11 and 12 years of age in boys. Complete fusion of the tuberosity usually occurs over the next 2 years.

The diagnosis is based on the history and physical examination. The insidious onset of achy knee pain over the area of the distal patellar tendon insertion in a young athlete is classic. The physical examination reveals point tenderness directly over a prominent tibial tubercle. For an athlete with bilateral symptoms and the classic history and physical examination, plain radiographs are not necessary. For athletes with unilateral symptoms, a lateral radiograph may be obtained to assess the possibility of malignancy and to reassure the family as to the diagnosis.

Several different treatment options have been reported (21,22), but none have demonstrated any advantage to the standard treatment of relative rest, ice, strapping, and hamstring flexibility exercises (23). Most sports medicine physicians and orthopedists concur that continued participation, even while symptomatic, does not increase the risk for avulsion of the tibial tubercle. In a series of tibial tuberosity fractures in adolescents, the contralateral knee was more often symptomatic for Osgood–Schlatter disease than was the side in which the fracture actually occurred (24).

Sindig–Larsen–Johanssen Disease

Sindig–Larsen–Johanssen disease is another apophysitis involving an apophysis at the distal pole of the patella. Clinical manifestations include pain and point tenderness over the distal pole of the patella, along with radiographic findings of an unfused apophysis at the distal pole of the patella. Treatment of this condition is similar to other causes of anterior knee pain, including relative rest, ice, and hamstring and quadriceps stretching.

Tendinitis

Patellar tendinitis, iliotibial band (ITB) tendonitis, and quadriceps tendinitis all result from overuse in running and jumping sports. This inflammatory condition is thought to result from repetitive tensile forces that cause microscopic shearing of the tendon tissue that is beyond the body's ability to repair the damage. Usually, these conditions present with the insidious onset of pain and tenderness over the affected tendon. Patellar tendinitis, or "jumpers' knee," is seen most frequently. ITB tendinitis is frequently observed among cyclists. Treatment for most tendinitis is rest, in addition to antiinflammatory medications, stretching, and progression to a strengthening program as symptoms improve.

Osteochondritis Dissecans

Osteochondritis dissecans (OCD) is a condition that results in the "quiet necrosis" of osteochondral lesions; it usually involves the distal femoral condyle, but it can occur in any other osteochondral area as well. In the knee, the lateral aspect of the medial femoral condyle is the most commonly affected area. However, the lateral femoral condyle and patella can also be affected. In almost one-third of patients, the lesions may be bilateral.

Patients usually present with chronic soreness and stiffness deep within the joint. Clicking, catching, and giving way may be reported. The physical examination is usually nonspecific. Subtle findings may include tenderness on the affected femoral condyle and an effusion. However, in many patients, the physical examination will be completely normal.

The key to making the diagnosis is by obtaining plain radiographs. A crater-like defect, with or without fragments, is the usual finding (Fig. 36.5). Often, these lesions are visible only on the posteroanterior (PA) tunnel views, and, therefore, these views should be part of any routine radiographic series for a patient with knee pain. If the defect is evident on plain radiographs, MRI is often required to evaluate the size and stability of the lesion. MRI is also useful when trying to determine whether to use a conservative versus a surgical approach to these lesions. Prognostic factors that favor conservative management include young age (skeletally open physis), small lesions, and lesions with no evidence of edema on MRI scans. Management decisions should minimally involve consultation with an orthopedic surgeon. Conservative management usually involves complete rest for an extended period of time, until the lesion shows evidence of radiographic healing.

LEG INJURIES

Overuse injuries to the lower leg include shin splints, stress fractures, and chronic exertional compartment syndrome. The young endurance athlete often suffers from vague lower leg pain that is difficult

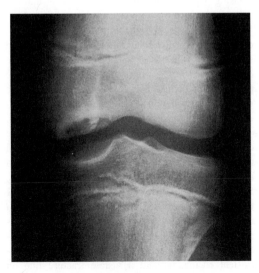

FIG. 36.5. Osteochondritis dissicans radiograph.

for the primary care provider to evaluate. This chapter attempts to differentiate these three fairly common conditions by a discussion of their history, physical examination, and diagnostic imaging so that the proper diagnosis can be made and the appropriate therapy is prescribed.

Medial Tibial Stress Syndrome or Shin Splints

Medial tibial stress syndrome (MTSS) (also known as periostitis, shin splints, or soleus syndrome) is a common affliction of the running and jumping athlete that results in chronic dull pain in the distal aspect of the tibia (25). This condition is not well understood, but it is thought to result from repetitive microtrauma. Most sports medicine practitioners feel that repetitive stress to the fascial attachment of the soleus on the tibia results in inflammation of either the fascia or periosteum.

Both intrinsic and extrinsic risk factors may predispose an athlete to this condition. Intrinsically, tight heel cords, midfoot hyperpronation and excessive tibial torsion may all place an undue force on the medial aspect of the tibia. Extrinsically, training errors (e.g., rapidly increasing training intensity or duration), poor medial shoe support, or training on hard banked surfaces can all predispose an athlete to overuse problems, including MTSS.

Typically, athletes with MTSS present with aching pain over the anteromedial aspect of the distal third of the tibia. The pain is usually described as a dull ache of varying intensity that is worse both at the beginning and end of activity. With continued activity and worsening symptoms, the athlete may experience increasing pain with activities of daily living that becomes more severe with practice or competition.

Diffuse tenderness over the distal third of the medial tibia that is often bilateral is the main finding on examination. Pain may be located directly on the edge of the medial tibia or over the soft tissue, in close proximity, or both. An inspection for other intrinsic risk factors also should be conducted during the physical examination.

Plain radiographs should be obtained when more chronic symptoms, worsening symptoms, or focal tenderness are evident on the examination in order to ascertain the possibility of a tibial stress fracture. Bone scan or MRI may be necessary to evaluate either condition further. Bone scan reveals a fusiform longitudinal area of tracer uptake at the posteromedial distal third of the tibia (26). MRI is just as sensitive and is more specific than bone scan; diffuse periosteal edema, without a visible fracture line on T2-weighted images, is the hallmark finding (27).

Treatment must emphasize the modification of training errors and a control of some of the intrinsic biomechanical risk factors through the choice of shoe wear, inserts, and rehabilitation. Relative rest from running through biking, swimming, or aqua jogging decreases stress on the area. Controlling excessive pronation through shoe wear or semirigid noncustom or custom orthotics helps decrease the stress on the medial tibia. Gastrocnemius and soleus stretches improve heel cord flexibility. Strengthening of the soleus and the posterior tibialis is important for correcting any strength deficits that may result from chronic pain. Ice and antiinflammatory medications may be used, as necessary, for comfort only. Surgical periosteal cauterization may be attempted if the symptoms persist despite prolonged conservative management.

Stress Fractures

Stress fractures of the tibia are thought to be the end stage in the MTSS spectrum. Prolonged and repetitive loading exceeds the bone's ability to remodel, leading to a microscopic fracture that results in more focal pain and tenderness.

The causes are very similar to MTSS in terms of training errors and biomechanical factors. Other intrinsic factors to consider include menstrual irregularity, disordered eating, and decreased calcium intake, which may predispose the athlete to osteoporosis. Although athletes in general may have a higher bone mineral density than their nonathletic counterparts, the bone mineral density needed to withstand the rigors of physical training required of or demanded by some young athletes is unknown. Therefore, a detailed menstrual and dietary history should be taken for any female athlete who presents with a stress fracture.

Clinically, an athlete with a stress fracture presents very similarly to one with shin splints. Pain over the tibia with running that improves with rest and that progresses in severity with increased pounding is the usual history. On physical examination, however, the athlete with a stress fracture typically demonstrates localized point tenderness on the tibia, commonly somewhere on the proximal two-thirds. Palpation may reveal an uneven tibial edge, which suggests recurring bone formation. Percussion on the bone from a more distant site may cause pain at the fracture site. Tenderness over the proximal tibia should never be assumed to be pes anserine bursitis in a young athlete. A stress fracture or some other type of etiology (e.g., malignancy) should be considered for any athlete with pain in this area.

Diagnostic imaging should be obtained in any athlete who has persistent focal tenderness for more than 2 to 4 weeks. Two weeks is generally the earliest time in which radiographic findings can first become evident. AP, lateral, and two oblique films increase the yield, and they may obviate the need for a bone scan or MRI. Periosteal bone formation is the pathognomic finding for a stress fracture. Bone scan or MRI will demonstrate the findings much earlier than conventional radiographs. Bone scan reveals a focal localized area of tracer uptake, whereas MRI demonstrates increased edema within the marrow, in addition to a visible fracture line.

Treatment involves complete rest from impact activity. A removable cast or walking boot is sometimes used for comfort. Cross training on a stationary bicycle or other aerobic nonimpact exercise equipment is permitted as pain improves. The return to the sport usually takes 6 to 8 weeks, but some midshaft fractures may take longer. Biomechanical factors, such as pronation or tibial torsion, may be addressed with shoe inserts or new footwear prior to the resumption of impact exercise. When the athlete does return to the sport, he or she must do so in a relatively gradual fashion in order to prevent a recurrence of the stress fracture.

Chronic Exertional Compartment Syndrome

Chronic exertional compartment syndrome is classically characterized by an inadequacy of the musculofascial compartment size, thus producing chronic and recurring pain that is made worse by activity.

A large series characterized the malady as mainly affecting active runners whose median age was 20 years; however, this syndrome may also be seen in racquet sports, gymnastics, skating, fencing, and swimming (28). As the median age is 20 years, adolescent athletes are not exempt from this problem. Adolescents, more so than younger athletes, are susceptible to this condition based on its the pathogenesis. Increased muscle bulk from training and increased blood flow to the muscles with physical conditioning must occur for the pressure in the compartment to increase. A tight fascia surrounding the muscles prevents them from expanding and results in the obstruction of blood flow, ischemia, and pain.

Consistent reproduction of localized pain with exertion is the hallmark symptom. The pain may be described as an ache, discomfort, tightness, or as having a sharp quality. The symptoms usually start 10 to 15 minutes into a conditioning session. Paresthesias in the feet and weakness may accompany the pain. The physical examination is usually normal, thus making the history even more important in the attempt to make the diagnosis. Pain is usually localized to the compartment that is affected; the anterior and lateral compartments are most frequently affected (28).

A definitive diagnosis can only be made by measuring the pressure inside of the muscle compartment both before and after exercise. A pressure greater than 15 mm Hg at rest and greater than 30 mm Hg immediately after exertion is diagnostic.

Treatment usually consists of either complete restriction from exercise, which is helpful (but only temporary) in most cases, or referral to a surgeon for compartment fasciotomy, which is curative without complication in 90% of cases (28). Following surgery, therapeutic strengthening exercises, as well as a gradual return to a conditioning program, should be prescribed.

Other Causes of Lower Extremity Pain

Lower extremity pain may be caused by the usual nonsports related conditions, including thrombophlebitis, osteomyelitis, cellulitis, a tumor, and intermittent claudication. Therefore, as with other conditions, the practitioner must consider nonsports-related conditions when treating an athlete with lower extremity pain. Similarly, other nonathletic causes of knee pain must be considered, including infectious and autoimmune causes and malignancy. Finally, in the pediatric-aged athlete, the clinician must never forget that hip pain may refer to the knee, so a detailed examination of the hip should be included in the initial evaluation.

REFERENCES

1. Bijur PE, Trumble A, Harel Y, et al. Sports and recreation injuries in US children and adolescents. *Arch Pediatr Adolesc Med* 1995;149:1009–1016.
2. Beachy G, Akau CK, Martinson M, et al. High school sports injuries: a longitudinal study at Punahou School: 1988–1996. *Am J Sports Med* 1997;25:675–681.
3. Powell JW, Barber-Foss KD. Sex-related injury patterns among selected high school sports. *Am J Sports Med* 2000;28:385–391.
4. Messina DF, Farney WC, De Lee JC. The incidence of injury in Texas high school basketball: a prospective study among male and female athletes. *Am J Sports Med* 1999;27:294–299.
5. Bjordal JM, Arnoy F, Hannestad B, et al. Epidemiology of anterior cruciate ligament injuries in soccer. *Am J Sport Med* 1997;25:341–345.
6. Seaberg DC, Yealy DM, Lukens T, et al. Multicenter comparison of two clinical decision rules for the use of radiography in acute, high-risk knee injuries. *Ann Emerg Med* 1998;32:8–13.
7. Stanitski CL, Harvell JC, Fu F. Observations on acute knee hemarthrosis in children and adolescents. *J Pediatr Orthop* 1993;13:506–510.

8. Adalberth T. Magnetic resonance imaging, scintigraphy, and arthroscopic evaluation of traumatic hemarthrosis of the knee. *Am J Sports Med* 1997;25:231–237.

9. Munshi M, Davidson M, MacDonald PB, et al. The efficacy of magnetic resonance imaging in acute knee injuries. *Clin J Sports Med* 2000;10:34–39.

10. Parker AW, Drez D, Cooper JL. Anterior cruciate ligament injuries in patients with open physes. *Am J Sports Med* 1994;22:44–47.

11. Andrews M, Noyes FR, Barber-Westin SD. Anterior cruciate ligament allograft reconstruction in the skeletally immature athlete. *Am J Sports Med* 1994;22:48–54.

12. Albright JP, Powell JW, Smith W, et al. Medial collateral ligament knee sprains in college football: effectiveness of preventive braces. *Am J Sports Med* 1994;22:12–18.

13. Wroble RR, Henderson RC, Campion ER, et al. Menisectomy in children and adolescents: a long-term follow-up study. *Clin Orthop* 1992;279:180–189.

14. Cascells W. Gross pathological changes in the knee joint of the aged individual: a study of 300 cases. *Clin Orthop* 1978;132:225.

15. Landry GL. Patellofemoral stress syndrome: a common but complex problem. *Compr Ther* 1988;14:21–28.

16. Smith AD, Stroud L, McQueen C. Flexibility and anterior knee pain in adolescent elite figure skaters. *J Pediatr Orthop* 1991;11:77–82.

17. Messier SP, Davis SE, Curl WW, et al. Etiologic factors associated with patellofemoral pain in runners. *Med Sci Sports Exerc* 1991;23:1008–1015.

18. O'Neill DB, Micheli LJ, Warner JP. Patellofemoral stress: a prospective analysis of exercise treatment in adolescents and adults. *Am J Sports Med* 1992;20: 151–155.

19. Kujala UM, Kvist M, Heinonen O. Osgood–Schlatter's disease in adolescent athletes: retrospective study of incidence and duration. *Am J Sports Med* 1985;13: 236–240.

20. Osgood RB. Lesions of the tibial tubercle occurring during adolescence. *Boston Med Surg J* 1903;148: 114–116.

21. Thomsen JEM. Operative treatment of osteochondritis of the tibial tubercle. *J Bone Joint Surg Am* 1956;38: 142–148.

22. Glynn MK, Regan BF. Surgical treatment of Osgood–Schlatter's disease. *J Pediatr Orthop* 1983;3: 216–219.

23. Levine J, Kashyap S. A new conservative treatment of Osgood–Schlatter disease. *Clin Orthop* 1981;158: 126–128.

24. Ogden JA, Tross RB, Murphy MJ. Fractures of the tibial tuberosity in adolescents. *J Bone Joint Surg Am* 1980;62:205–215.

25. Fick DS, Albright JP, Murray BP. Relieving painful "shin splints." *The Physician and Sports Medicine* 1992;20:105–113.

26. Holder LE, Michael RH. The specific scintigraphic patterns of shin splints in the lower leg. *J Nucl Med* 1984; 25:865–869.

27. Fredericson M, Bergman AG, Hoffman KL, et al. Tibial stress reaction in runners: correlation of clinical symptoms and scintigraphy with a new magnetic resonance imaging grading system. *Am J Sports Med* 1995;23: 472–481.

28. Detmer DE, Sharpe K, Sufit RL, et al. Chronic compartment syndrome: diagnosis, management and outcomes. *Am J Sports Med* 1985;13:162–170.

37

Ankle Injuries

Mark E. Lavallee and James R. Clugston

Ankle injuries are common in pediatrics, comprising 10% to 30% of sports-related injuries (1). The clinician must remember that most pediatric patients still have open ossification centers. These growth centers are often weaker than the supporting ligaments or tendons. When traumatic force is applied to the pediatric ankle, this relative weakness results in a higher frequency of bony injury than that seen in adult populations.

ANKLE ANATOMY

The ankle is a relatively small joint that transmits substantial stresses through the foot to the ground.

Bones

The ankle is composed of two long bones, the tibia and fibula, and two elliptical bones, the calcaneus and talus. They combine to form an arch, or "mortise," over the talus (Fig. 37.1). Because the fibula extends further distally than the tibia, the rate of fibular fractures may be higher than that of tibia fractures (see "Ankle Fractures" below). The distal fibula also sits slightly more posterior than the distal tibia. The talus is a wedge-shaped bone that articulates with the malleoli superiorly, the calcaneous inferiorly, and the navicular and cuboid distally. Also of note is the fact that the talus is wider anteriorly than posteriorly. This creates greater stability for the ankle in dorsiflexion, compared to the ankle in plantarflexion. Despite the wedged shape of the talus, it has the ability to remain in equal proximity to both sides of the malleoli from plantarflexion to dorsiflexion (2). This is accomplished by the slight internal rotation of the tibia and the slight external rotation of the fibula during dorsiflexion. The elasticity of the tibiofibular ligaments permits this movement.

The closure of the epiphyseal plates has a bearing on where and what injury occurs with trauma to the ankle. The primary care physician should note that fusion of the tibial epiphyseal plate begins in the central portion of the physis and spreads medially. The lateral tibia epiphyseal is the last portion to fuse. Complete fusion of the tibia takes approximately 18 months (3), and, as por-

tions of the epiphyseal plate fuse, they become areas of relative strength. These differences in strength along the epiphyseal plate are responsible for unusual pediatric fractures, such as juvenile Tillaux and triplane fractures, which result from ankle trauma during growth plate closure (4).

Ligaments

The ankle bones are held together by multiple ligaments that are important for the stability and mobility of the ankle. The medial and lateral ligaments support the ankle against excessive eversion and inversion (see Figs. 37.11 and 37.12), while allowing maximal flexion and extension.

The lateral ligaments may be injured in an inversion overload (Fig. 37.2). The anterior talofibular ligament (ATFL) is the weakest and the most commonly injured of these ligaments. The posterior talofibular ligament (PTFL), calcaneofibular ligament (CFL), and ATFL all originate from the distal fibula inferior to the physis.

Medially, the broad deltoid ligament stabilizes the medial malleolus from excessive eversion by connecting the tibia to the talus (Fig. 37.3). The deltoid ligament is split into the following segments: tibio-calcaneal, posterior tibiotalar, anterior tibiotalar, and the tibionavicular. Usually, a deltoid ligament injury occurs with failure of the talofibular ligaments and/or the tibiofibular ligaments. Deltoid injuries are also frequently associated with fracture of the distal tibia or fibula (2).

The ankle syndesmosis between the tibia and fibula is composed of ligamentous structures, the anterior tibiofibular ligament (ATiFL), the posterior tibiofibular ligament (PTiFL), and the interosseous membrane (Fig 37.1). The interosseous membrane is a sheet-like membrane running the entire length of the lower leg.

Muscles

Ankle motion is driven by 13 muscles. The gastrocnemius and soleus are the principal plantar flexors. Dorsiflexion when the foot is inverted is ac-

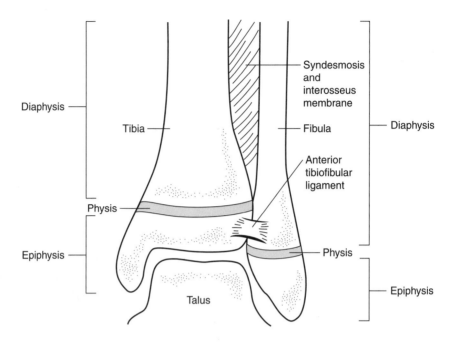

FIG. 37.1. Mortise of the left ankle.

complished by the tibialis anterior, while the extensor digitorum longus dorsiflexes the foot when it is everted. Both the peroneus longus and brevis muscles accomplish eversion in plantarflexion and dorsiflexion. The main inverter of the foot when it is dorsiflexed is the tibialis anterior muscle, and the tibialis posterior muscle is the main inverter when the foot is plantarflexed (5).

ANKLE FRACTURES

Physeal Fractures

Pediatric ankle fractures are classified according to the anatomy of the fracture pattern. In 1963, Salter and Harris classified physeal fractures as five types (see Chapter 26, Fig. 26.3) (6). This system is the most accepted and widely used classification system,

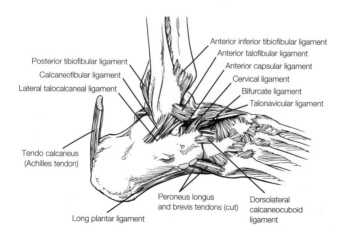

FIG. 37.2 Lateral ligaments of the ankle. (From Ferkel RD, The foot and ankle. In: Whipple TL, ed. *Arthroscopic surgery*. Philadelphia: Lippincott–Raven, 1996, with permission.)

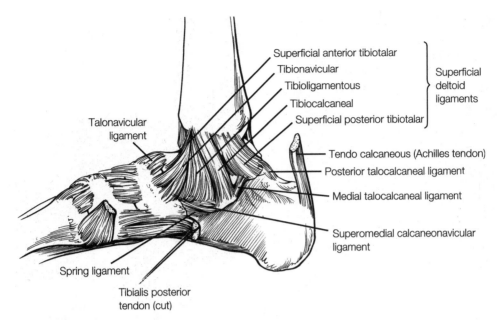

Talonavicular ligament

Superficial anterior tibiotalar

Tibionavicular

Tibioligamentous

Tibiocalcaneal

Superficial posterior tibiotalar

} Superficial deltoid ligaments

Tendo calcaneous (Achilles tendon)

Posterior talocalcaneal ligament

Medial talocalcaneal ligament

Superomedial calcaneonavicular ligament

Spring ligament

Tibialis posterior tendon (cut)

FIG. 37.3. Medial ligaments of the hindfoot. The fibers of the deltoid ligament provide stability to the medial aspect of the ankle. (From Ferkel RD. The foot and ankle. In: Whipple TL, ed. *Arthroscopic surgery.* Philadelphia: Lippincott-Raven, 1996, with permission.)

and it is useful for predicting outcomes and formulating treatment plans.

Tibia physeal fractures including both the proximal and distal physes are the most common physeal fractures of the lower extremity (2). Fibula physeal fractures are also quite common. Both of these physes produce significant contributions to the length of the lower leg, with the distal tibial physis contributing 45% of the tibia's final length and the distal fibular physis producing 40% of the fibula's adult length (2).

Salter–Harris Type I Fractures

Tibia

Type I fractures of the distal tibia are rare in the athletic pediatric population (7), and they are thought to occur at a younger age (<10.5 years of age, on average) than do other tibial physeal fractures (8). Instead, they are more commonly seen in neurologically impaired children or among children who have been abused (4). These fractures are difficult to diagnose, and they are often mistaken for ankle sprains. Some physeal fractures that are diagnosed as Salter–Harris type I fractures may actually result from type V crushing injuries (see "Salter–Harris Type V Frac-

tures" below) (2). The patient with a type I tibial fracture presents with pain and swelling about the ankle, often without any deformity. Full range of motion is possible, but it may be decreased secondary to pain. Initial radiographs typically show only soft tissue swelling, but they may show widening of tibial physis or displacement of the epiphysis relative to the tibial metaphysis (Fig. 37.4). Treatment usually consists of 4 weeks in a below-the-knee walking cast. This relieves pain and restores the growth plate to the normal thickness. The patient should be reevaluated in 6 months to monitor for growth arrest of the tibia (4).

Fibula

Type I fractures of the distal fibula are the most common ankle fractures in children (8). Despite their high incidence, they are often misdiagnosed as ankle sprains or are missed entirely. The mechanism of injury is usually external rotation of the foot and ankle. Patients will characteristically have pain over the lateral malleolus and swelling directly over the fibular physis. The "goose egg" is often diagnostic for fibular Salter–Harris type I fractures. Radiographs may show widening of the fibular physis and soft tissue swelling about the physis. These fractures respond well to 3 to 6 weeks of immobilization in a short-leg walking cast (7).

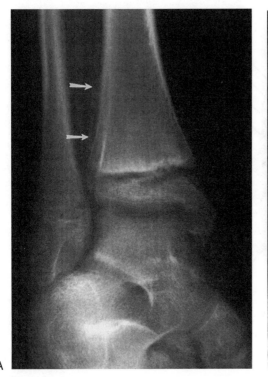 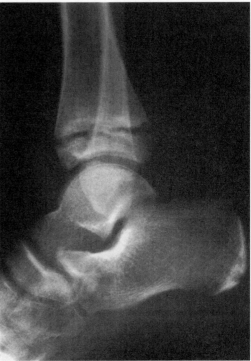

A   B

FIG. 37.4. Mortise **(A)** and lateral **(B)** views of an injured right ankle taken 3 weeks later show a healing Salter–Harris I fracture of the tibia with irregularity of the growth plate and periosteal new bone (*arrows*) along the tibia. (From Berquist TH, ed. *Radiology of the foot and ankle*, 2nd ed. Philadelphia: Lippincott Williams & Wilkins, 2000, with permission.)

Salter–Harris Type II Fractures

Tibia

This is the most common distal tibial physeal fracture. It results from external rotation while the ankle is in fixed supination. This fracture is often accompanied by a distal, but nonphyseal, fibula fracture. These fractures cause swelling and pain, and, unlike type I tibia fractures, they present with ankle deformity. These fractures are sometimes mistakenly diagnosed when a Salter–Harris type IV fracture is present (see discussion of medial tibia fractures in "Salter–Harris Type IV Fractures" below). Treatment consists of a long-leg cast that is flexed to 30 degrees for 2 to 3 weeks, followed by 4 weeks in a short-leg walking cast (4).

Fibula

Type II fractures of the distal fibula are rare (7); when seen, they should be treated similarly to type II tibia fractures.

Salter–Harris Type III Fractures

Tibia

Two kinds of Salter–Harris type III fractures of the distal tibia—medial and lateral—are observed. The pathophysiology of each type depends on the closing patterns of the distal tibial physis. As was mentioned earlier (see "Anatomy" above), the distal tibial physis first closes centrally, then medially, and finally laterally.

The medial type III fracture occurs in young children whose tibial growth plate has not begun to close. Supination-inversion forces to the ankle shear the fibular epiphysis, allowing the talus to strike the medial malleolus and producing a type III fracture. These fractures, as well as medial type IV fractures, are the most likely to produce deformities from growth arrest of all ankle physeal fractures (2). The child will present with pain over the medial malleolus, and, if the fibula has been fractured, he or she will also have pain over the lateral malleolus. Closed reduction is usually possible, but this treatment option requires weekly radiographic follow-up to ensure that no displacement occurs during

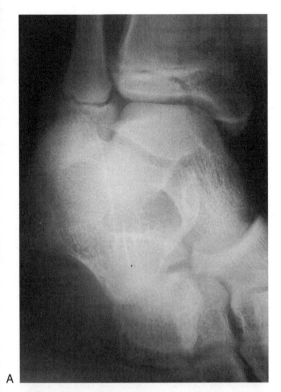

A

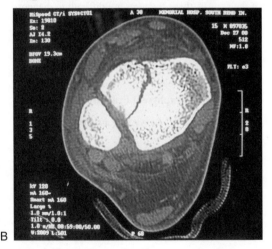

B

FIG. 37.5. A: Juvenile Tillaux fracture. **B:** Computerized tomography of juvenile Tillaux fracture.

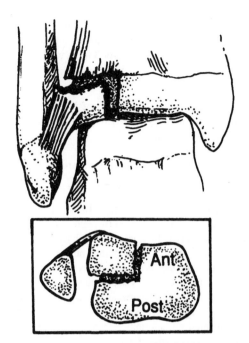

FIG. 37.6. Juvenile fracture of Tillaux (Salter–Harris type III lateral fracture). Abbreviations: Ant, anterior; Post, posterior. (From Craig EV, ed. *Clinical orthopaedics.* Philadelphia: Lippincott Williams & Wilkins, 1999, with permission.)

The lateral type III fracture of the distal tibia physis (juvenile Tillaux fracture) occurs in children whose tibial growth plate has closed medially but remains open laterally. This fracture is referred to as the juvenile fracture of Tillaux, and its healing is the most unpredictable of all ankle epiphyseal fractures (7) An external rotational force applied to the partially closed physis causes the ATiFL to avulse the lateral portion of the tibial epiphysis (Figs. 37.5 and 37.6), which corresponds to the portion of the distal tibia physis that is still open (3). The patient will present with minimal swelling, minimal deformity, and local tenderness at the anterior lateral joint line, contrary to an ankle sprain in which the tenderness generally is found below the joint (3). If displacement is small, visualizing this fracture on radiographs may be difficult. Depending on the size of the avulsed fragment, the risks of growth arrest, angular deformity, and ankle osteoarthritis are increased (4). Usually, however, growth disturbance is rare because this fracture occurs near the end of growth (3). Closed reduction under anesthesia, followed by percutaneous fixation, may be attempted if the fragment displacement is less than 2 mm. Most of these fractures, however, will require open reduction and fixation (7). After reduction, the patient should be

the first 2 weeks. These patients are placed in an above-the-knee, non–weight-bearing cast initially (4). Failure to reduce the interfragmentary gap to less than 2 mm has been associated with growth arrest and deformity (9). If such a gap remains after closed reduction, open reduction with internal fixation should be performed (3,4).

placed in an above-the-knee cast with 30 to 40 degrees of knee flexion for 3 weeks; this is followed by a below-the-knee walking cast for 3 more weeks (4).

Fibula

Salter–Harris type III fractures of the fibula are extremely rare, and they usually require open reduction and internal fixation (3).

Salter–Harris Type IV Fractures

Tibia

Similar to Salter–Harris type III fractures of the tibia, both medial and lateral (triplane fracture) tibial Salter–Harris type IV fractures are observed.

As with the type III medial tibial physis injury, type IV fractures of the medial tibial physis are rare, and they are usually caused by supination–inversion forces to the ankle. These fractures, as well as medial type III fractures, are the most likely of all ankle physeal fractures to produce deformities from growth arrest (2). When the metaphyseal fragment is small, it may not be recognized on radiographs, so these injuries are frequently misdiagnosed as Salter–Harris type II fractures (2). This misdiagnosis may result in inadequate treatment, which leads to asymmetric growth arrest and varus deformity (2). Treatment usually consists of open reduction and internal fixation followed by 3 weeks in an above-the-knee, non–weight-bearing cast. This is followed by 3 weeks in an above-the-knee walking cast.

Lateral type IV injuries to the distal tibial physis are referred to as triplane fractures. They are believed to be caused by the external rotation of a supinated and plantarflexed foot. The fracture line extends from the articular surface, through the epiphysis, to the physis and through the tibial metaphysis in the coronal, sagittal, and frontal planes (Figs. 37.7 and 37.8). These are often difficult to recognize on plain radiographs, and computerized tomography (CT) scanning may be required for evaluation. They often appear as Salter–Harris type II on lateral projection or as type III fractures on anteroposterior (AP) radiographs. Triplane fractures tend to occur at younger ages than juvenile fractures of Tillaux because fewer physeal plates have closed and the fracture plane may travel a greater distance along the physis until it reaches a portion that has closed.

Triplane fractures usually produce two bone fragments in adolescent patients and three or more fragments in preadolescent children (2). As with juvenile Tillaux fractures, most cases of triplane fracture occur when the growth plates are nearing closure, so growth arrest is not a big concern. The propensity of these fractures to lead to osteoarthritis and chronic pain is a matter of concern. Anatomic reduction of the articular surface is, therefore, mandatory. After successful reduction, the fracture sites are stabilized with pinning. The extremity is placed in a short-leg cast for 6 to 8 weeks, with weight bearing allowed at 3 to 4 weeks (3).

Fibula

Salter–Harris type IV distal fractures of the fibula are rare; they usually require open reduction and internal fixation (3).

Salter–Harris Type V Fractures

These types of fractures are extremely rare, and they are believed to result from crush injuries (6). The premature closure of the growth plates that is seen with these fractures may result from factors related to immobilization secondary to treatment (10). Regardless of their cause, these fractures are difficult to diagnose because the initial radiographs are often normal. In most cases, the diagnosis is made retrospectively after premature arrest of the growth plate occurs in a previously injured epiphyseal plate (4).

Nonphyseal Fractures

Proximal Lower Leg Fractures

Tibia

Proximal tibia fractures usually are not related to ankle injury. They usually require evaluation by an orthopedist, and they should be considered for open reduction and internal fixation if any displacement or comminution of the fracture is found.

Fibula

These fractures often accompany ankle injuries, and they may be classified as either stable or unstable.

FIG. 37.8. Triplane fracture of a 15-year-old boy who jumped from a tree and hurt his ankle. **A:** The frontal view shows a vertical fracture extending sagittally through the epiphysis and horizontally along the lateral physis (*arrows*) and suggests a Salter–Harris type III fracture. The medial part of the physis is closed. **B:** The lateral view shows a fracture that extends through the metaphysis along the coronal plane (*arrows*) and suggests a Salter–Harris type II fracture. The findings are typical of a triplane fracture. (From Kirks DR, ed. *Practical pediatric imaging: diagnostic radiology of infants and children*, 3rd ed. Philadelphia: Lippincott-Raven, 1997, with permission.)

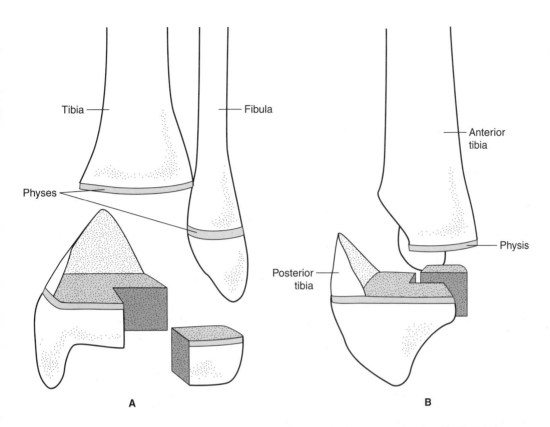

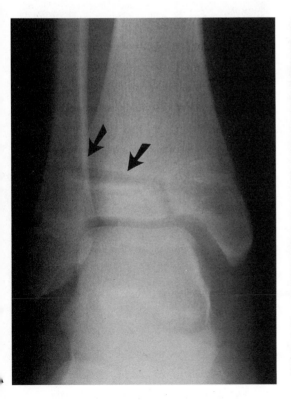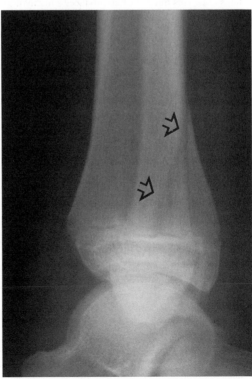

FIG. 37.7. Salter–Harris type IV lateral tibia (triplane) fracture. **A:** Anteroposterior view. **B:** Medial view.

B

Trauma to the lateral aspect of the lower leg or a severe ankle sprain that disrupts the syndesmosis membrane are common mechanisms of injury. Closed reduction is usually attempted, but, because the fibula is essentially a non–weight-bearing bone, some amount of displacement can be tolerated. Stable proximal fibula fractures are managed with a cast or a supporting splint for 3 to 4 weeks, followed by gradual return to athletics after 8 weeks (11).

Unstable proximal fibular fractures often occur just distal to the fibular head, and these are known as *Maisonneuve* fractures. This location is the weakest and thinnest part of the fibula. *Maisonneuve* fractures may remain undiagnosed when the proximal lower leg is not examined, especially with radiographs that do not include the proximal lower leg following severe ankle injuries. Additional views should be obtained in severe ankle injuries where this type of fracture is suspected. With this fracture, the ATiFL and PTiFL are usually disrupted via a rapidly dorsiflexed foot. The forces are transmitted upward through the syndesmosis membrane, and they exit through the proximal fibula (Fig. 37.9). When a clinician is viewing ankle radiographs, he or she must suspect the presence of a *Maisonneuve* fracture if the mortise joint space is not equal among the medial, horizontal, and lateral portions (12). This fracture often produces a highly unstable ankle joint (12). *Maisonneuve* fractures frequently require open reduction with internal fixation if the fibula is severely displaced, if the mortise joint space is abnormal, or if the ankle is unstable. If the ankle joint is stable, the fracture can be treated in a long-leg cast for 2 weeks, followed by a short-leg cast for 3 to 4 more weeks. Return to play usually is seen 6 to12 weeks after injury or 2 to 6 weeks after immobilization.

Distal Lower Leg Fractures

Four common distal lower leg nonphyseal fractures—the non-displaced lateral malleolar fracture, the displaced lateral malleolar fracture, the bimalleolar fracture, and the trimalleolar fracture—involve the ankle. The nondisplaced lateral malleolar fracture is treated conservatively with casting for 4 to 6 weeks. Gradual resumption of athletics is possible at approximately 12 weeks (11). Distal fractures of the lateral malleolus that are displaced usually mandate open reduction and internal fixation (Fig. 37.10). A cautious return to athletics is possible after 16 weeks.

Bimalleolar fractures, which are fractures through both the lateral and medial malleolus, also are often considered unstable fractures (Fig. 37.11). If these fractures are displaced or unstable, the patient must undergo open reduction and internal fixation. Postoperatively, non–weight-bearing healing, ranging from 4 to 8 weeks, with early motion and a cautious return to athletics at 16 to 20 weeks is recommended (11).

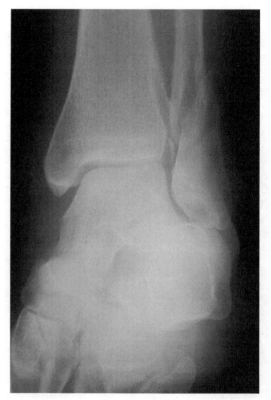

FIG. 37.10. Displaced distal fibular fracture.

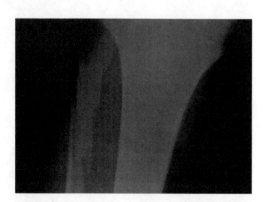

FIG. 37.9. Anteroposterior view of proximal tibia and fibula showing Maisonneuve fracture. (From McGlamry ED, Banks AS, Downey MS, eds. *Comprehensive textbook of foot surgery,* 2nd ed. Vol. 3. Philadelphia: Williams & Wilkins, 1992, with permission.)

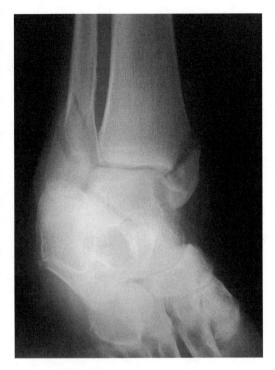

FIG. 37.11. Tibia-fibula fracture.

A trimalleolar fracture involves both malleoli and the posterior portion of the tibial plafond. It is considered an unstable fracture, and it should be referred to an orthopedist for open reduction and internal fixation.

General Considerations in Pediatric Ankle Fracture Management

When the clinician is evaluating a possible ankle fracture, he or she should perform the following steps (Table 37.1). The examination should begin away from the most tender site and should move toward the area of most discomfort. Particular attention should be paid to the distal tibia and fibula because these are the most common areas of injury in the lower extremity of children (4). The physical examination is often as useful as

radiographs in diagnosing a fracture (e.g., "goose bump" in Salter–Harris type I fibula fractures).

Not all ankle injuries require radiographs. The decision to obtain these should be based on findings in the physical examination, such as deformity and bony tenderness, and on the Ottawa ankle rules where appropriate (Table 37.2). The Ottawa ankle rules have traditionally been applied to patients with closed growth plates (usually those who are older than 15 years of age), but, recently, they have been successfully applied to pediatric patients with open growth plates (13). Many physicians continue to take a more cautious approach, and they obtain radiographs in any patient with open physes who has significant ankle pain and tenderness, who walks with a limp, or who cannot bear weight (14). Radiographs should always include at least three views of the ankle—AP, lateral, and oblique. Mortise views also may be helpful. CT scanning and/or plain tomography may be needed in the juvenile fracture of Tillaux and in triplane fractures for diagnosis and subsequently for confirmation of appropriate reduction (7).

In children with open physes, the primary care physician must realize that any physeal injury has the potential to cause growth arrest and subsequent deformity. Growth arrest is thought to occur from callus formation that produces a bony bridge or attachment across the physis, thus compressing the cartilage columns of the physis. If this happens, the callus is replaced by bone. Fortunately, especially in young children, the cartilage column may be strong enough to overcome the bony bridge, which allows normal bone elongation to continue (2). Because of the possibility of growth arrest after physeal injury, careful follow-up until physeal closure is achieved is imperative. Some authors recommend follow-up examinations and radiographs every 6 months for 2 years after the injury (3).

TABLE 37.1. *Assessment of the acutely fractured ankle*

- Note the mechanism and time of injury.
- Check neurovascular status distal to the ankle immediately.
- Note the amount of swelling, deformity, and the integrity of the skin.
- Gently palpate all bones of the lower leg, ankle, and foot.

TABLE 37.2. *Ottawa ankle rules*

When a patient presents (within 10 d) with an injured ankle, radiographs of the injured ankle should be obtained if any **one** of the following is positive:
(a) Adults (>55 yr) *or* children (<5 yr) with open growth plates
(b) Pain to palpation over the distal 6 cm of posterior one-third of either malleoli
(c) Pain to palpation over the base of the 5th metatarsal
(d) Pain to palpation over the navicular
(e) Inability to bear weight (could not take five consecutive steps) immediately after injury

From Stiell IG, Greenburg GH, McKnight RD, et al. Decision rules for the use of radiography in acute ankle injuries: refinement and prospective validation. *JAMA* 1993;269:1127–1132, with permission.

In addition to growth arrest and deformity, complications seen in pediatric fracture management include compartment syndrome, reflex sympathetic dystrophy, and peroneal nerve injury.

ANKLE SPRAINS

Ankle sprains are the most common athletic injury in both adults and children (15). Older children with closed growth plates get ankle sprains more frequently than their younger counterparts.

Mechanism of Injury

The three main mechanisms of injury of the ankle are inversion, eversion, and dorsiflexion. The most common is inversion injury (85%), which is responsible for lateral ankle sprains (16). This occurs when the foot is plantarflexed and inverted (Fig. 37.12).

Medial ankle sprain, which affects the deltoid ligament, is usually caused by plantarflexion with eversion (Fig. 37.13). This allows the unsupported medial aspect of the athlete's foot to drop downward, thus stressing the deltoid ligament.

The last major type of ankle sprain is the infamous syndesmosis, or "high" ankle sprain. This injury occurs with rapid dorsiflexion and eversion, and it accounts

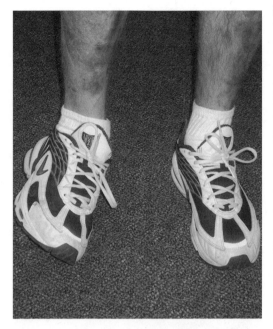

FIG. 37.13. Ankle eversion.

for 10% of all ankle sprains (17). This is often seen when a child jumps from a considerable height or slides into a stationary base (e.g., second base). In dorsiflexion, the widest part of the talus is forced into the mortis joint. If this occurs rapidly and with enough force, the syndesmosis membrane between the tibia and fibula may be damaged. When an external rotational force is applied, the ATiFL and the PTiFL may rupture. Once this occurs, the syndesmosis membrane, which runs like a sheet between the whole length of the tibia and fibula, may tear. This is the most serious type of ankle sprain because it leaves the ankle mortis unstable. Surgery in the form of a syndesmotic or compression screw across the mortise may be necessary to maintain joint integrity and stability. Syndesmosis sprains often take twice as long to heal as other ankle sprains.

Presentation

Almost universally, initial pain and some swelling are seen (Fig. 37.14). The more involved sprains—those with completely torn ligaments and swelling—actually may have minimal pain because of complete transection of the nerves of the injured ligaments. Reflex inhibition of the peroneal muscles due to pain may cause the joint to become stiff and functionally unstable and may involve the loss of proprioception. The five stages of healing in ankle sprains are shown in Table 37.3.

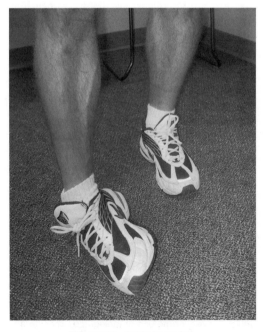

FIG. 37.12. Ankle inversion.

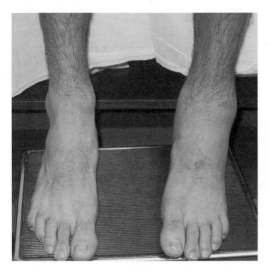

FIG. 37.14. Left ankle sprain, grade II.

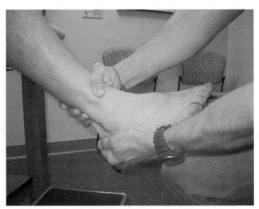

FIG. 37.15. Anterior drawer test.

Physical Examination

Gross deformities, asymmetry, effusion, or ecchymosis may indicate a more complex injury (i.e., fracture and/or dislocation). Effusion above the ankle capsule may signify a syndesmotic or high ankle sprain.

The two hinged joints of the ankle—the talar mortise and the subtalar joint—should be assessed for range of motion. A soft endpoint with inversion of the foot is consistent with a lateral ankle ligamentous injury. A hard endpoint when the foot is dorsiflexed, thus limiting its range of motion, may be consistent with an os trigonium fracture or a displaced talar dome osteochondral defect.

Palpation of the lateral and medial malleoli is crucial for helping to rule out ankle fractures. In addition, the Achilles and its insertion into the calcaneus and the peroneus brevis and its insertion into the base of the fifth metatarsal should be assessed to rule out avulsion injuries. The joint spaces, especially the talonavicular, talocuboid, and mortise, should be palpated. In addition, the proximal fibula and the fibular head should be palpated to aid in discerning whether a Maisonneuve fracture is present.

The following are special tests that can help discern which ligament may have been injured.

1. *Anterior drawer.* This test checks the integrity of the ATFL and the anterior aspects of the deltoid ligament. The patient is seated with his or her leg over the side of the examination table. The clinician holds the lower leg with one hand and places the other hand under the heel, with the thumb across dorsum of midfoot (Fig. 37.15). Then, the foot is distracted anteriorly. A positive test reproduces pain over the ATFL, while demonstrating significant laxity (>2 mm of anterior translation by radiography and >5 mm clinically), when compared to the unaffected ankle.

2. *Talar tilt.* This test checks the integrity of the CFL or the midsubstance of the deltoid ligament. The clinician holds the lower leg with one hand. With the other hand under the heel, the thumb and forefinger are placed on either side of the talus and the foot is inverted to stress the CFL or everted to stress the deltoid ligament (Fig. 37.16). A positive test reproduces pain and demonstrates significantly more ligamentous laxity, when compared to the nonaffected side.

3. *Dorsiflexion and or external rotation maneuver.* This test assesses the integrity of the syndesmosis ligament and mortise. With one hand, the clinician holds the lower leg over each malleolus. With the other hand, he or she dorsiflexes and externally rotates the foot. A positive test reproduces pain, and, in severe cases, the malleoli may actu-

TABLE 37.3. *Different phases of ankle ligament healing*

Phase	I	II	III	IV	V
Day	1	2–5	5–14	15–21	>21
Stage of healing	Immediate	Acute inflammation	Subacute	Rapid progression	Final rehabilitation

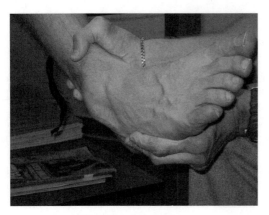

FIG. 37.16. Talar tilt test.

ally be felt to separate. If this test is positive, the proximal fibular rock test should be performed.

4. *Proximal fibular head rock test.* This test is used to look for a Maisonneuve fracture of the proximal fibula. With one hand, the clinician gently but firmly rocks the fibular head. If the test produces pain, it is positive, and radiographs are warranted.
5. *Tib–fib malleolar squeeze test.* This test checks for syndesmosis sprain. Both distal malleoli are squeezed between the clinician's thumb and forefinger. If the test evokes pain, it is positive.
6. *Thompson test.* This test checks for Achilles tendon rupture. The patient should lie prone with the knee flexed to 90 degrees. The middle third of the calf should be squeezed. If the foot does not plantarflex, the Achilles tendon has been ruptured.
7. *Kleigers test.* This test assesses the integrity of the deltoid ligament. The foot is everted in the coronal plane. A true positive reproduces pain over the deltoid ligament. This test is often confused with the dorsiflexion and/or external rotation test because they both use the talus as a "wedge."

Grading Scale

Ankle sprains are usually graded by one of two grading scales. One scale rates the sprain by which ligaments are injured, while the other scale looks at the general integrity of the ankle joint. Both scales are based on physical examination findings, and both progress from the least serious grade of 1 to the most severe grade, which is 3. The scale used to grade the injury must be specified, or confusion may result (Tables 37.4 and 37.5).

Differential Diagnosis

Many other diagnoses are possible with a painful ankle (Table 37.6). Tarsal coalition secondary to limited subtalar motion and sinus tarsi syndrome may both present with acute ankle pain (18). Tenderness, specifically over the ligaments and not the physes, probably represents a true sprain.

Treatment

Initial treatment in the acute setting follows the well-established PRICE (protection, rest, ice, compression, and elevation) protocol. First, the patient should be *protected* from further injury. This refers not to taping or bracing but to the cessation of activities or athletic events, which could cause further damage. Relative *rest* is important. This can last for a few minutes or up to a few weeks, depending on the injury. For moderate to severe cases, crutches are often used until weight bearing is less painful (19). Cryotherapy or *ice* has been shown to be extremely helpful, not only in decreasing swelling but also in decreasing pain perception. *Compression* via tape or elastic wrap helps to minimize swelling, especially when the patient is ambulatory. *Elevating* the ankle above the level of the heart also prevents or reduces swelling when it occurs. Nonsteroidal antiinflammatory drugs (NSAIDs) often are used for pain control. In grade 3 sprains, NSAIDs are not recommended for the first 24 hours because of their weak antiplatelet effect, in view of the possibility of complete ligament ruptures in which more bleeding or swelling may occur (19). Often a grade 3 or severe ankle sprain will not only require crutches for an ex-

TABLE 37.4. *Grading scales of ankle sprains*

Ligament integrity scale	
I. Minimal	None of ligaments appear totally torn; one or two ligaments may be involved
II. Moderate	Two or three ligaments involved; one ligament may be totally torn
III. Severe	Unstable; two or three lateral ligaments appear torn
Joint integrity scale	
I. Stable with pain	Minimal to mild swelling
II. Mildly unstable with pain	Good endpoint; swelling
III. Grossly unstable with or without pain	No endpoint; notable effusion

TABLE 37.5. *Physical findings in ankle sprains*

Signs and symptoms	Grade 1	Grade 2	Grade 3
Tendon	No tear	Partial tear	Complete tear
Loss of function	Minimal	Some	Great
Pain	Minimal	Moderate	Severe[a]
Swelling	Minimal	Moderate	Severe[b]
Ecchymosis	Rare	Frequently	Yes
Difficulty weight bearing	No	Usually	Almost always

[a]Sometimes minimal pain is seen, due to transection of regional nerves in severe cases.
[b]A torn ankle capsule may not allow a severe amount of swelling to accumulate.
From Wexler RK. The injured ankle. *Am Fam Physician* 1998;57:474–480, with permission.

tended period of time, but it may also mandate the use of an ankle–foot orthosis and, rarely, that of a short-leg cast (20). Prolonged immobilization of ankle sprains is counterproductive (21).

The next phase of treatment of an ankle sprain should consist of the following three basic stages: range of motion, strengthening, and proprioception. Many minor ankle sprains may preserve the range of motion, but grade 2 and 3 sprains often have considerable swelling, resulting in decreased range of motion. Once the range of motion of the ankle is improving, strengthening exercises may be started. These exercises may include isometric exercises using pillows, concentric contractions using resistance cords, and eccentric contractions using weights. Proprioceptive retraining of the Golgi body–tendon apparatus of the injured ankle ligaments is often overlooked, which possibly contributes to an increase in reinjury rates of the ankle.

Return to Play

An injured patient should not be allowed to return to play until this can be accomplished safely, without a significant risk of worsening the injury. Bracing has been shown to improve proprioception, and it is recommended for the previously sprained ankle. Once an athlete has recovered range of motion, strength, and proprioception in the injured joint, he or she can progress from walking to jogging to running and cutting. A full return to play can then be made.

Complications

Although most patients with ankle injuries return to full activity within 4 to 8 weeks, 20% to 40% of adult patients have persistent pain and symptoms (22). Talar dome osteochondral lesions occur in 6.8% to 22% of ankle sprains (21). Some reasons for delayed recovery are the functional instability caused by chronic CFL or AFTL laxity, as a result of nerve injury from a subluxing peroneal tendon, or because of peroneal muscle weakness, pain secondary to impingement, the presence of a pathologic tumor, or poor proprioception (22).

OVERUSE INJURIES

Pediatric "overuse" injuries of the ankle are less common than they are in adults. Overuse injuries result from repetitive microtrauma, and they occur when the involved structure is stressed beyond its ability to repair itself. These injuries include (a) stress fractures of the talus, distal tibia, and distal fibula; (b) tendonitis of the flexor hallucis longus, Achilles, anterior tibialis, posterior tibialis, and peroneal tendons; (c) apophysitis of the Achilles–calcaneus attachment (Sever disease); (d) osteochondritis dissecans of the talar dome (see Chapter 38); (e) anterior and posterior ankle impinge-

TABLE 37.6. *Differential diagnosis in acute ankle trauma*

Fractures	Dislocations	Other ligaments	Tendon injury
Salter–Harris	Subtalar	Dorsal talonavicular	Achilles
Fibular shaft	Talonavicular	Sinus tarsi syndrome	Peroneal subluxation
Maisonneuve		Talocalcaneal coalitions	
Proximal 5th metatarsal		Calcanealcuboid coalitions	
Anterior process of calcaneus			
OCD of talar dome			
Os trigonium fracture			

Abbreviation: OCD, osteochondral defect.

ment; and (f) bursitis of the retrocalcaneal and anterior ankle bursa. The primary care sports medicine physician should consider these conditions in any patient who presents with a history of chronic overuse.

Treatment of overuse injuries is almost always non-surgical. Rest and activity modification are the most important components of treatment. The PRICE principles are helpful, but they are not as useful in the treatment of chronic overuse injuries as they are in the management of acute injuries. Pain and inflammation reduction with NSAIDs and, occasionally, corticosteroid injection are sometimes necessary. Unweighting (i.e., the use of harnesses in physical therapy or pool therapy) or restriction from weight bearing may also be required. Physical rehabilitation, including stretching, strengthening, and balance training, are often helpful, and these may be accomplished in formal physical therapy sessions or in a less supervised setting. Successful treatment of chronic overuse injuries requires patience and a thorough understanding of the problem from the patient, parents, coaches, and physician. Communication between these parties is paramount for a successful outcome.

REFERENCES

1. Perlman M, Leveille D, DeLeonibus J, et al. Inversion lateral ankle trauma: differential diagnosis, review of the literature, and prospective study. *J Foot Surg* 1987; 26: 95–135.
2. Connolly JF. *Fractures and dislocations: closed management*. Philadelphia: WB Saunders, 1995.
3. Cummings RJ. Distal tibial and fibular fractures. In: Rockwood CA, Wilkins KE, Beaty JH, eds. *Fractures in children*, 4th ed. Philadelphia: Lippincott-Raven, 1996: 1377–1428.
4. Crawford AH. Fractures and dislocations of the foot and ankle. In: Green NE, Swiontkowski MF, eds. *Skeletal trauma in children*. Philadelphia: WB Saunders, 1998: 505–575.
5. Simons S. *Personal communication*, 2000.
6. Salter RB, Harris WR. Injuries involving the epiphyseal plate. *J Bone Joint Surg Am* 1963;45:587–621.
7. Sullivan, JA. Ankle and foot injuries in the pediatric athlete. In: Stanitski CL, Delee JC, Drez D, eds. *Orthopedic sports medicine*. Vol. 3. Philadelphia: WB Saunders, 1994:441–455.
8. Spiegel PG, Cooperman DR, Laros GS. Epiphyseal fractures of the distal ends of the tibia and fibula. A retrospective study of 237 cases in children. *J Bone Joint Surg Am* 1978;60:1046–1050.
9. Kling TF Jr, Bright RW, Hensinger RN. Distal tibial physeal fractures in children that may require open reduction. *J Bone Joint Surg Am* 1984;66:647–657.
10. Peterson HA, Burkhart SS. Compression injury of the epiphyseal growth plate: fact or fiction? *J Pediatr Orthop* 1981;1:377–384.
11. Stanish WD. Lower leg, foot, and ankle injuries in young athletes. *Clin Sports Med* 1995;14:651–668.
12. Marsh JS, Daigneault JP. Ankle injuries in the pediatric patient. *Curr Opin Pediatr* 2000;12:52–60.
13. Plint AC, Bulloch B, Osmond MH, et al. Validation of the Ottawa ankle rules in children with ankle injuries. *Acad Emerg Med* 1999;6:1005–1009.
14. Ganley TJ, Flynn JM, Pill SG, et al. Ankle injury in the young athlete: fracture or sprain? *J Musculoskeletal Med* 2000;17:311–325.
15. Garrick JG. The frequency of injury, mechanism of injury, and epidemiology of ankle sprains. *Am J Sports Med* 1977;5:241–242.
16. Tropp H, Askling C, Gillquist J. Prevention of ankle sprains. *Am J Sports Med* 1985;13:259–262 .
17. Fouts D. Ankle injuries: current recommendations for diagnosis and treatment. *Fam Pract Recertification* 1998; 20:56–72.
18. Omey ML, Micheli LJ. Foot and ankle problems in the young athlete. *Med Sci Sports Exerc* 1999;31:S470–S486.
19. Wexler RK. The injured ankle. *Am Fam Physician* 1998; 57:474–480.
20. Lane S. Severe ankle sprains. *The Physician and Sports Medicine* 1990;18:43–51.
21. Wolfe M, Uhl T, Mattacola C, et al. Management of ankle sprains. *Am Fam Physician* 2001;63:93–104.
22. Grana WA. Chronic pain after ankle sprain. *The Physician and Sports Medicine* 1995; 23:67–79.

38

Foot Injuries

Stephen M. Simons and Brian K. Sloan

Pediatric patients often present with foot problems that often are not related to athletic participation. Much of the foot pathology that is encountered occurs as part of normal childhood development. The increase in sport participation among the pediatric population undoubtedly has contributed to the proportional increase in foot problems in this subgroup of patients. The topics covered in this chapter provide the primary care physician with an understanding of the problems that may occur in athletics or in normal childhood development.

FOREFOOT PROBLEMS

Juvenile Hallux Valgus

Juvenile hallux valgus is a deformity of the first metatarsophalangeal joint (MTPJ) that is characterized by medial deviation of the first metatarsal and lateral deviation and rotation of the great toe, the consequence of which are a prominent MTPJ. The reported incidence varies widely, ranging from infrequent to 39% of school-aged girls (1,2). Some authors believe the problem is rare before the age of 10 years, while others have witnessed bunions as early as 1 month of age (3,4).

Hallux valgus often remains stable until 10 to 14 years of age, at which time the deformity begins to accelerate. This rapid acceleration is thought to occur when a critical angle of the hallux valgus has been exceeded (5). The following two radiographic measurements are often used to assess bunions: intermetatarsal angle (IM) and metatarsalphalangeal (MTP) angle. IM is the angle formed by lines that bisect the first and second metatarsals. Lines that bisect the first metatarsal and the proximal phalanx of the hallux form the MTPJ angle. A greater than normal IM angle is present in both the affected and unaffected feet of children with hallux valgus (6).

Etiology

The etiology of hallux valgus is probably multifactorial. A genetic predisposition is seen, and most adults with bunions recall having the condition since adolescence (7,8). Various factors, such as metatarsus varus, pes planus, ligamentous laxity, and tight Achilles, are associated with bunions (9). Shoes are often blamed for initiating or causing bunions to progress (10). However, this assertion does not explain the bunions of preambulatory patients, and it was not supported by a study conducted by Groiso (4).

Presentation

Patients seek consultation for pain over the MTPJ, painful callosities, deformity of the great toenail, and an inability to find shoes that can accommodate the widened forefoot. Many patients remain asymptomatic, and appearance may be the only reason the patient requests help. Bunions are often a source of greater concern for the parents than they are for adolescents. The examination reveals prominent MTPJ, occasional bursitis, and other associated foot deformities.

Treatment

Conservative care can be utilized, but results are uncertain. Observation may be the best approach for the asymptomatic patient. Controlling excessive pronation with orthotic devices has been proposed, but this approach was not supported in a 3-year longitudinal study by Kilmartin et al. (11). Groiso (4) showed that a thermoplastic splint that was applied at night and that was supplemented with exercises reduced either the IM angle or the MTPJ angle in half of the study participants. The splint is molded around the midfoot, and it has a flange that extends to the great toe. This flange, when it is wrapped around the lateral side of the toe, provides a varus force to the toe. Passive MTPJ capsular stretches and active abductor hallucis exercises also may have contributed to the study's success (4).

Surgical intervention should be delayed until bone maturation is complete (12,13). Bunion recurrence is unpredictable when surgery is pursued prior to growth plate closure (3). A discussion of the variety of specific surgical techniques, however, is beyond the scope of this text. Some authors strongly recommend the use of in-shoe orthotic devices postoperatively, but their long-term prophylactic value remains unproven (3,13).

Freiberg Disease

Freiberg disease, also known as Freiberg infraction, is considered an osteochondrosis of the metatarsal heads. Several hypotheses that have been proposed to explain this unusual problem are as follows: acute trauma, repetitive microtrauma to subchondral bone, and aseptic necrosis (14). Smillie (15) has contended that a structurally weak foot with a short varus or hypermobile first metatarsal predisposes patients to the development of Freiberg infraction. A vascular insult has been theorized by Viladot and reviewed by Katcherian (16), who described the following five phases: (a) mechanical compression of the arteries to the metatarsal head; (b) spasm of the arteries; (c) spasm that gives rise to ischemia of the epiphysis; (d) prolonged compression that leads to occlusion of the vessels; and (e) granulation tissue that brings new blood supply to the epiphysis, causing bone to resorb, remodel, and collapse and leaving a sequela of arthrosis of the MTPJ.

Incidence

The true incidence of Freiberg disease is not known, since many cases may remain asymptomatic and may be noted only incidentally on radiographs that are performed for other indications. This is the only osteochondrosis that is more common in females than in males. Females to male incidence ratios vary from 1 to 1 to 11 to 1, with an average of 5 to 1 (16). The age range for reported cases is 8 to 77 years, but most are identified between ages 11 and 17 years; the average age is 24 years (16). The second metatarsal is the site that is most often affected, followed by the third metatarsal. This condition is unilateral 93.4% of the time.

Presentation

Symptomatic patients usually present with pain and limitation of movement at the MTPJ. Quite often, the pain is simply vague forefoot pain. Some patients will remain pain free for years and, possibly, even permanently. An inciting event, such as athletic trauma or high-heeled shoes, may unmask this problem. Examination reveals periarticular swelling, a reduced range of motion with pain on the extremes of motion, tenderness, soft tissue thickening, and, in some cases,

plantar callosities. The metatarsal head will become palpably enlarged (16).

Staging

Radiographic findings correlate with the pathologic stage, not with physical complaints. Several staging classifications have been proposed (14,17,18). The radiographic stage, however, cannot predict the eventual course of the patient's progress. This staging may be helpful for description and treatment options.

Treatment

Critical evaluation of conservative versus surgical management is lacking. Smith et al. (19) briefly mention 13 of 28 patients that were seen over a 6-year span who improved with nonoperative treatment. Explicit details of the care given to these patients is absent. Omer (20) recommends two phases of conservative care. The first is protected immobilization. This consists of using a short-leg cast with the option of adding crutches so that the patient is non–weight-bearing. Following immobilization, shoe modifications with metatarsal pads or bars or, alternatively, an insertable orthosis may be used to distribute the body weight proximal to the metatarsal heads. The patient then progressively returns to full weight-bearing activity. Injections, physical therapy, and low dose antibiotics also are proposed, but less supportive evidence is found for these measures (16).

The patient should be referred to surgery when incapacitating symptoms persist in spite of conservative care. Surgical treatment focuses on reducing symptoms, while minimizing the advent of transfer lesions to adjacent MTPJs. Joint debridement is the least destructive surgery, but it does nothing to alter the course of the disease. Recently, Maresca et al. (14) presented an arthroscopic approach to debridement, with good results. Other surgical options include metatarsal head excision, dorsal osteotomy, proximal phalanx base excision, and joint replacement. All these procedures may improve symptoms, but joint function suffers as a result. Dorsiflexion osteotomy is favored by Katcherian (16) for the younger, more active patient.

Turf Toe

Turf toe is a debilitating injury to the first MTPJ. This injury has been known of for some time but was first described in 1976. It was associated with an increase in playing time on artificial synthetic surfaces (21). Although these injuries are traditionally associated with American football, they are not limited to this sport. Turf toe can occur in soccer, basketball, rugby, or any other activity that stresses the first MTPJ (22). Epidemiologically, no objective evidence appears to indicate that children are more or less predisposed to turf toe than is the adult population.

Mechanics

Traumatic dorsiflexion of the MTPJ occurs when the forefoot is fixed on the ground and the heel is raised or when forcible lateral deviation of the great toe occurs, such as when "cutting." These events cause a traction or stretch injury to the plantar joint capsule. A compression injury to the dorsal articular surface of the MTPJ may also accompany this traction injury to the ligaments. Softer (i.e., more flexible) shoes provide less resistance to the external forces acting at the MTPJ (23). Artificial turf surfaces are suspected to harden with time, which may contribute further to this aggravating injury (24). In addition, the athlete's intrinsic foot structure may predispose him or her to turf toe. The excessively pronated pes planus foot or the athlete with hallux valgus theoretically may have a greater risk of valgus injury to the medial side of the MTPJ (25).

Presentation

Athletes with turf toe present with a swollen, red first MTPJ. The history may involve a single event or, less commonly, multiple, cumulative events. Often the athlete is unable to run or even to walk without a visible limp. Examination of the joint reveals edema, erythema, and restricted range of motion. Careful palpation of the sesamoids should be performed to rule out the presence of a fracture or an isolated injury to these accessory ossicles.

Clanton and Ford (26) classified turf toe into three grades. Clinically, a grade 1 injury displays minimal pain, swelling, and disability with nearly normal range of motion. This represents a minor stretch injury to the capsuloligament complex. A grade 2 injury demonstrates somewhat greater pain, swelling, ecchymoses, and disability. Pathologically, a partial tear has occurred. Grade 3 injuries represent complete disruption of the capsule and ligament structures. The tearing most often occurs on the metatarsal side of the joint. The patient exhibits severe pain, swelling, ecchymosis, and an inability to bear weight.

Imaging

Radiographs are not necessary to diagnose this clinical entity, but they may be warranted to rule out a sesamoid or metatarsal fracture and to evaluate joint congruity. Comparison views with the contralateral foot can be helpful. Stress radiography, arthrography, and bone scintigraphy are not usually necessary for guiding clinical management. Magnetic resonance imaging (MRI) is also not indicated in most circumstances, but it may help in clarifying the exact tissue that has been injured in cases that do not improve according to clinical expectations.

Treatment

The basic goals of treatment include limiting stress, preventing further injury, and enabling a return to competition. The initial management utilizes the principles of protection, rest, ice, compression, and elevation (PRICE). The use of compressive dressings and early non–weight-bearing range of motion are important for reducing swelling and hastening the return to sport. Grade 3 injuries are best treated with a non–weight-bearing approach and the use of crutches for a few days. Increased support to the MTPJ can be accomplished with the use of a stiffer athletic shoe that has an insole with rigid stainless steel forefoot or by application of a custom-molded orthosis with a Morton's extension (26). Surgical referral is indicated after 6 weeks if the injury fails to respond to conservative treatment.

Return to Sports

A premature return to sports participation can lead to recurrence and a further delay for the athlete in returning to play. The athlete is often at risk for such recurrence, as this problem seems trivial to many coaches, players, and parents. Generally, in order to be able to return to play, athletes should have minimal pain, and they should be able to push off the affected side without difficulty with the use of the appropriate taping or shoe modifications. Clanton and Ford (26) utilized their grading system to guide treatment and return-to-sport decisions. The athlete with a grade 1 injury may be allowed to play within his or her pain tolerance if the toe is taped to limit dorsiflexion. Athletes with grade 2 injuries must rest for 3 to 14 days. Grade 3 injuries require 2 to 6 weeks of rest. Rehabilitation should progress to gradual weight bearing and return to play only after the athlete has achieved complete range of motion and pain-free running. Extensive injury to the MTPJ may result in degenerative changes to the joint that progress to a hallux rigidus.

Middle Metatarsal Stress Fractures

The original "march fracture," which was described in 1855 by Briethaupt, refers to middle metatarsal stress fractures. The incidence of these stress fractures in the athletic population is second only to that of tibial stress fractures. Over 90% of metatarsal stress fractures occur to the middle three metatarsals. Ground-reactive forces and associated bending strain on the second metatarsal are 6.9 times greater than the force that is applied to the first metatarsal (27). The second metatarsal is possibly more susceptible to stress fracture because it is inherently more rigid. The base of the second metatarsal is recessed into the midfoot, and it is entirely flanked by the cuneiforms. Muscular fatigue to the long flexors of the toes can also contribute to the high loading forces on the second metatarsal (28). Risk factors in children include, but are not limited to, amenorrhea or oligomenorrhea, heavy training, poor footwear, and high-risk sports. Metatarsal stress fractures are associated more frequently with pes planus, in contrast to the tibial stress fracture, which is associated with a pes cavus foot structure. Second metatarsal base stress fractures are unique, and they will be discussed separately in the following section.

Clinical History

The patient with a metatarsal stress fracture often complains of poorly defined forefoot pain. Usually, the pain begins intermittently with weight bearing, and it eases after activity ceases. Eventually, the pain persists with activities of daily living and even becomes symptomatic without weight bearing. The focus of pain eventually narrows to the site of the fracture.

Examination

Often the forefoot appears normal, but it can exhibit mild generalized swelling. Subtle swelling may be detected by the loss of definition of the borders of the extensor tendons. Tenderness to the metatarsal can be elicited by palpating the head, neck, and shaft of the metatarsal with firm pressure that is applied dorsally and to the plantar simultaneously. This, however, lacks specificity as tendinitis or a soft tissue injury may also be tender with this examination. Pain at the fracture site can be evaluated by an axial load. The examiner's thumb is placed on the plantar aspect of the metatarsal head while the toes are dorsiflexed. A direct axial load is applied by pushing the metatarsal towards the rear foot. Reproducing the patient's pain at a site away from that of the direct pressure is suggestive of a stress fracture. The tuning fork test can also suggest the possibility of a stress fracture; however, the sensitivity of this test is unknown. Finally, a firm, bony mass can be palpated at the site of an older or maturing stress fracture.

Imaging

Plain radiography performed in the first week or two is usually normal. At 2 to 3 weeks, however, a periosteal reaction surrounds the fracture site. A distinct fracture line may be seen occasionally. Although the use of a technetium bone scan for an active adolescent is rarely necessary in the clinical setting, focal uptake on the scan confirms the presence of a stress fracture. Nuclear imaging can show the increased uptake at the fracture site at 1 to 2 days after injury.

Treatment

The principal treatment consists of adequate rest from the offending activity. Metatarsal stress fractures usually heal sufficiently within 4 to 6 weeks. In one study of 19 metatarsal stress fractures in 51 runners, the clinical healing time was 7 weeks. The symptoms should be monitored, and return-to-sport activity should be allowed when the patient no longer has pain with walking and local tenderness is resolved. The temporary use of crutches, followed by the use of a stiff-soled shoe, can be helpful for the particularly painful stress fracture (29).

Prevention

A gradual return to training is required to avoid a stress fracture recurrence. Some athletes may benefit from the use of a custom-molded orthotic. Although, theoretically, the empiric use of an orthotic is compelling mechanically, hard evidence for its efficacy in injury prevention is lacking. The custom orthotic that has a cutout depression under the fractured metatarsal may enhance the force distribution so that it is away from the injured metatarsal.

Second Metatarsal Base Stress Fracture

The second metatarsal base is subject to a stress fracture—known as a dancer's fracture—that occurs almost exclusively in ballet dancers (30–32). The *en pointe* position of the ballet dancer has been proposed as the cause of these unusual stress fractures. The anatomical rigidity of the second metatarsal base, the tremendous compressive loads from the *en pointe* position, and the traction from the tibialis posterior and peroneous longus during weight-bearing plantarflexion all contribute to this unique fracture. The classic Morton foot, which has a short first metatarsal, also predisposes the individual to this fracture (33).

Dancers present with an insidious onset of midfoot pain. Examination reveals tenderness to the base of the second metatarsal. A provocative maneuver to elicit pain is to have the patient assume a releve position on the balls of the foot (33). Radiographs of the foot should be supplemented by a special posterior–anterior or plantar–dorsal view (32). The tuning fork test lacks the sensitivity to diagnose the stress fracture accurately; however, if it is positive, the test can suggest that a cortical interruption is present. Brukner et al. (33) suggest that the MRI is preferable for differentiating a stress fracture from a stress reaction.

Treatment consists of rest in a short-leg walking cast or a wooden shoe. The average time for the athlete's return to dance is 6 weeks after the diagnosis was made. A gradual return-to-activity program is prudent.

Iselin Disease

Iselin disease is a traction apophysitis to the secondary ossification center on the proximal fifth metatarsal. This apophysis appears at about 9.7 years of age in females and 12.1 years of age in males. Fusion to the shaft of the metatarsal takes place at approximately 11.6 years of age in females and 14.2 years of age in males (34).

Active adolescents present with pain to the lateral side of the foot and tenderness over the proximal fifth metatarsal. The presence of acute trauma is not necessary, as this injury usually is a result of overuse. An inversion ankle injury may be an inciting event. Activities that require running, jumping, and cutting maneuvers also predispose the athlete to this malady. Examination reveals a proximal fifth metatarsal that is enlarged when compared to that of the uninvolved foot. Soft tissue swelling and erythema may be present. Resisted eversion utilizing the peroneus brevis elicits pain. Oblique view x-rays may show an enlarged apophysis and fragmentation of the secondary ossification center. A bone scan often is unnecessary, but, if obtained, it will demonstrate increased radioactive uptake at the apophysis (35).

This rare condition is probably underreported. It is most often mistaken for a fracture. A typical fracture line, however, is transverse to the long axis of the metatarsal, whereas the apophyseal line is parallel. The apophyseal line does not extend proximally to the cubometatarsal joint or medially to the fourth–fifth metatarsal joint. Lehman et al. (35) suggest that this line is always self-limiting and that it resolves upon skeletal maturity, but Canale and Williams (34) reported a case that was persistently symptomatic at the age of 20 years.

Treatment consists of the cessation of aggravating activities, immobilization as needed to control pain, and physical therapy to improve strength and coordination. Early diagnosis and appropriate treatment

can achieve good results and can avoid long-term sequelae.

Proximal Fifth Metatarsal Fractures

In addition to Iselin disease, the proximal fifth metatarsal is subject to three distinct fractures. Two of these are acute, and the third is a chronic overuse injury. The two distinct acute fractures are (a) an avulsion fracture to the tuberosity of the fifth metatarsal and (b) an acute fracture at the metaphysis and diaphysis junction within 1.5 cm of the tuberosity, which is also known as the Jones fracture. The third fracture is a stress fracture that occurs to the most proximal 1.5 cm of the diaphysis (36). Seven structures attach to the proximal fifth metatarsal, and a precise knowledge of anatomy is helpful for understanding the injuries to this area. The most proximal part of the tuberosity is primarily composed of cancellous bone that is well vascularized. Relatively avascular cortical bone appears distal to the tuberosity. This reduced vascularity contributes to the poor healing of all fractures other than the simple proximal tuberosity avulsion.

Avulsion Fractures

Avulsion fractures involve only the tip of the fifth metatarsal tuberosity. Although this injury traditionally was thought to be a traction injury caused by the peroneus brevis, a lateral band of the plantar fascia is now thought to be responsible for the avulsion (37). A dynamic pull from the peroneus brevis is unlikely to cause this fracture, as the proneus brevis actually attaches distal to the usual transverse fracture line. These fractures usually heal without complications. A stiff-soled shoe or a cast shoe may be used for a brief period of time. A boot walker or a below-the-knee cast is used only for significant pain relief. The athlete may return to activity as symptoms allow. The return to full activity usually occurs by 4 to 6 weeks postinjury.

Jones Fractures

Sir Robert Jones described his own acute fracture, which he sustained while dancing around a tent pole at a military party (38). A Jones fracture is an acute fracture that is directed transversely and that is located at the metaphyseal–diaphyseal junction; it does not extend distal to the articular facet between the fourth and fifth metatarsals. To avoid confusion, the term Jones fracture should be reserved for acute fractures at this location that are no greater than 1.5 cm distal to the metatarsal tuberosity. This fracture occurs with running, jumping, and cutting maneuvers that place the foot in a plantarflexed position while applying an adduction force to the forefoot.

Acute Jones fractures lack an antecedent history of lateral foot pain. Oblique radiographs demonstrate a fresh fracture line without intramedullary sclerosis and, possibly, only slight cortical hypertrophy. Nonoperative treatment with 4 to 6 weeks of non–weight-bearing immobilization, followed by a walking cast or boot for another 4 weeks, is usually effective. Follow-up radiographs are necessary to demonstrate healing. Fractures that do not heal may require longer immobilization in a cast or surgical fixation (39). Competitive athletes should be offered early intramedullary screw fixation to ensure a quicker return to activity.

Proximal Diaphysis Stress Fractures

A fracture to the proximal fifth metatarsal diaphysis merits considerable attention as these fractures are notorious for delayed union or nonunion (40). There is confusion in the literature regarding their classification, epidemiology, and management because true Jones fractures are also often seen in the presence of these diaphyseal fractures. Torg et al. (41) proposed a useful classification system for initial management decisions regarding these fractures. Type I fractures occur in the previously asymptomatic patient. Although they are clinically acute, these are early stress fractures. Radiographs show a slight periosteal reaction but no medullary sclerosis. A type II fracture has a history of prior pain or known fracture. X-rays reveal a well-demarcated fracture line and some evidence of cortical hypertrophy and medullary sclerosis. Patients with type III fractures report a history of repeated trauma, and a distinct fracture nonunion with complete obliteration of the medullary canal is seen on x-ray.

A number of authors (41–44) have recommended treatment protocols for these stress fractures. Type I fractures in the nonathlete should be treated conservatively with non–weight-bearing cast immobilization for 6 to 8 weeks and should be followed radiographically for signs of healing. Persistent nonunions can be treated surgically if the nonsurgical management fails. Although Type I may be managed nonsurgically, in the athlete, the best course of action is surgical treatment to effect a quicker return to the sport and to minimize the potential for

the presence of a persistent fracture line. Type II fractures can be treated nonsurgically, but this choice of treatment requires prolonged immobilization with its attendant problems (39). Any athlete with a type II fracture should undergo surgical management. In this procedure, a cannulated percutaneous screw is placed through a proximal incision and into the medullary space. The screw is countersunk and is allowed to remain in place following fracture healing. Some authors allow immediate weight bearing; the return to full activity occurs in 6 to 8 weeks. Type III fractures are managed similarly to the type II fracture; however, the surgical management may include drilling of the medullary canal prior to screw fixation or bone grafting. The postoperative return to activity is delayed if a bone graft is conducted.

In summary, proximal fifth metatarsal stress fractures inherently have the potential for a delayed union or nonunion with persistent clinical symptoms. Early recognition, referral to the appropriate consultant, appropriate management, and a cautious return to activity is absolutely necessary for athletes with these uncommon fractures.

MIDFOOT PROBLEMS

Posterior Tibial Tendinitis

Etiology

The posterior tibial tendon is subject to significant eccentric loading with each step. The skeletal shape of the foot is the primary determinant of the integrity of the medial longitudinal arch. However, the posterior tibial muscle provides dynamic secondary support to the descending arch upon contact and into midstance. Tendinitis may occur when the athlete rapidly alters training, uses old or inadequate shoes, or exhibits an excessively pronated foot that predisposes the body to posterior tibial stresses. Children do not show a higher predilection than adults for developing posterior tibial tendon dysfunction. Of note is the fact that the left foot is particularly susceptible to this tendinitis when training on a track. The body lean that occurs going into left turns dynamically stresses the posterior tibial tendon.

Clinical Presentation and Treatment

The young athlete usually presents with pain along the course of the tendon, most often between the medial malleolus and the insertion site on the base of the first metatarsal. This pain is aggravated by continued or increased sports activity, and it is relieved with rest. Examination of the tendon demonstrates occasional swelling, tenderness, and pain with resisted inversion and/or plantarflexion. The differential diagnosis includes flexor hallucis longus and flexor digitorum longus tendinitis, tarsal tunnel syndrome, an occult fracture to the talus or sustentaculum tali of the calcaneus, and a symptomatic accessory navicular bone. Treatment consists of the principles of PRICE; relative rest; and attention to biomechanical contributors (e.g., extreme flatfoot and supportive shoes). A "motion control" type of shoe resists the heel eversion that accompanies arch collapse. The stable rear foot materials and construction of these type of shoes shoes provide a buttress that supports the rear foot and allows less collapse of the arch. Use of a custom orthotic control for the foot may be helpful.

Posterior Tibial Tendon Rupture

A posterior tibial tendon rupture occurs rarely in the pediatric population. Previous corticosteroid injections probably predispose the tendon to rupture (45,46). Relative hypovascularity of the tendon posterior and distal to the medial malleolus also increases the risk that this tendon will undergo degenerative changes and rupture (47). Acquired collapse of the medial longitudinal arch and difficulty performing a toe rise on the affected foot suggest the presence of a posterior tibial tendon rupture.

Peroneal Tendinitis

The peroneal tendons area also subject to tendinitis and occasional rupture. As occurs with the posterior tibial tendon, the patient usually experiences pain between the lateral malleolus and the tendon insertions. Peroneus longus involvement can create pain on the lateral side of the foot, as well as along the tendon course across the plantar aspect of the foot. Examination demonstrates tenderness along the course of the tendon and worsened pain with resisted foot eversion and plantarflexion. Crepitance may be palpable along the tendon sheath. Treatment consists of rest, ice, nonsteroidal medications, and gentle stretching. An evaluation of biomechanical issues may be helpful.

Pediatric Flatfoot

Most often, the child or adolescent has an asymptomatic flexible flatfoot that does not require intervention. A rigid flatfoot, which caused by a congenital vertical talus, is usually diagnosed at a young age and is not a likely consideration in an athlete (Fig. 38.1). The rigid flatfoot that is caused by tarsal coali-

tion is discussed below in "Tarsal Coalitions." The flexible flatfoot may or may not be symptomatic. Based on a comparison of shod and predominantly unshod societies, the adult prevalence of flatfoot symptoms is not influenced by whether shoes are worn (48). Moreover, Rao and Joseph (49) demonstrated a decreasing prevalence of flatfoot with age and a higher prevalence of flatfoot in children who wore shoes compared to those who were unshod.

The flexible flatfoot should be examined in non–weight-bearing and weight-bearing positions. In a non–weight-bearing position, the clinician assesses the passive range of motion of the ankle, subtalar, and midtarsal joints, as well as the strength of the muscles operating the foot. The flexible flatfoot usually shows a normal arch in this non–weight-bearing position. When the foot is in a weight-bearing position, it is put through a series of maneuvers to evaluate the subtalar joint and muscular function. When the patient rises onto the toes, heel varus and a good arch structure are seen. The maneuver of rolling to the outside and then the inside of the foot is used to assess the subtalar motion. Standing on the heel confirms that the Achilles is of adequate length. The individual's gait should also be assessed to search for neuromuscular causes of flatfoot. Radiographs are rarely necessary.

Treatment first focuses on providing reassurance to the parents. Most adolescent flatfeet either improve with age or do not predict symptomatic flatfoot in adulthood. Treatment of the symptomatic flatfoot is less conclusive. The results of studies evaluating the wearing of corrective shoes or orthotic

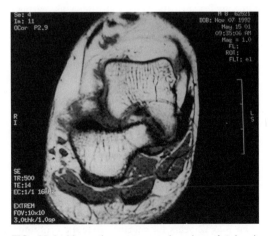

FIG. 38.1. Magnetic resonance imaging of talocalcaneal fibrous union of the middle facet in an 8-year-old boy. Clinically rigid flatfoot with progressive weight-bearing foot pain.

inserts have not been convincing in achieving an alteration of the patient's foot structure or clinical picture (50). However, Aharonson et al. (51) used medial wedges to restore the normal weight-bearing distribution through the foot. In the normal foot, only 4% of weight is borne through the middle of the foot. Flatfoot imposes from 17% to 30% of the weight bearing to the middle of the foot. The medial wedges used in this laboratory study nearly normalized the midfoot weight-bearing forces in the flatfooted condition. Clinical outcomes, however, were not studied. Because of the uncertainty of the benefits of using expensive shoe modifications or corrective orthotic inserts, a prudent first approach is the use of inexpensive, off-the-shelf arch supports or orthotic devices. Surgical management of flexible flatfoot is rarely indicated. A variety of surgical procedures have been tried, but many complications were reported. Sullivan (50) argues that the risks of these complications do not justify surgery for conditions that usually resolve into a functional, pain-free foot in adulthood.

Tarsal Coalitions

Tarsal coalition, as the name implies, is an osseous, fibrous, or chondral connection between two or more tarsal bones. The most plausible explanation for a tarsal coalition is failure of mesenchymal segmentation. As the condition has a familial tendency, it is thought to be due to an autosomal dominant inheritance (52,53). The prevalence is probably less than 1%, and it occurs bilaterally in 50% to 60% of those affected (53,54). The coalition is now believed to occur between the talus and calcaneus, particularly the middle facet (48.1% of the time), and between the calcaneus and navicular (43.6% of the time) (54).

Presentation

The obligatory subtalar joint restriction creates abnormal motion in adjacent joints, thereby contributing to the development of a painful foot. This restriction and the accompanying abnormal motion surface when the child or adolescent increases their play or sporting activities. Symptom onset correlates with the coalition ossification. This happens between the ages of 3 to 5 years for talonavicular coalitions, from 8 to 12 years for calcaneonavicular coalitions, and between 12 and 16 years for talocalcaneal coalitions. Often, these are the ages of presentation, although sometimes the patient will be much older.

The patient complains of vague rear foot pain that is aggravated by activity or prolonged standing. An ankle sprain or another traumatic injury may precede symptom onset. Many patients remain asymptomatic indefinitely, or symptoms may not surface until they are much older.

The examination usually reveals a flatfoot, a heel valgus, and an abducted forefoot or "too many toes" sign. The subtalar joint motion is restricted. This restriction can be appreciated upon passive heel movement by the examiner and also by the patient's limited ability to invert the heel on toe raise. These maneuvers usually are also accompanied by pain. The patient is often unable to stand on the lateral side of the foot.

Imaging

Plain radiographs are the initial choice of imaging when a tarsal coalition is suspected. Ideally, a standing anteroposterior (AP) and a lateral view, as well as a 45-degree oblique view, are obtained. The AP view will not identify the most common tarsal coalitions, but it can visualize the less common coalition types. The lateral view is useful for identifying the secondary signs of coalition, including the presence of talar beaking, which is a traction spur to the superior–anterior surface of the talar head. Other secondary signs of coalition include prolongation of the lateral process of the calcaneus, which is known as the "anteater" sign; narrowing of the subtalar joint; and a concave undersurface to the talus (55).

Computerized tomography (CT) should be performed to clarify any questionable radiographs and to determine precisely the location and the extent of coalition (56,57). Coronal and axial images are usually adequate for diagnosing a coalition. Talocalcaneal coalitions are usually seen best on coronal images in which a bony bar bridges the middle facet. If the connection is nonosseous, the middle facet may be narrowed, and reactive cystic and hypertrophic changes of the subchondral bone may be demonstrated (57). Wechsler et al. (58) compared CT to MRI in 10 feet with clinically suspected tarsal coalitions. The CT successfully demonstrated four of five calcaneonavicular coalitions and two cartilaginous coalitions, but it failed to identify one fibrous coalition and it incorrectly diagnosed two fibrous and one osseous coalition as cartilaginous. CT also correctly identified two osseous talocalcaneal coalitions, but it failed to depict two fibrous coalitions. The authors concluded that CT has limitations in the depiction of fibrous coalitions. Emery et al. (59) also compared CT to MRI and found

97.5% agreement between the two techniques. These authors suggested that MRI offered little advantage over CT, and they recommended the latter, as CT is less costly (59). Sakellariou and Claridge (52) concurred that CT remains the gold standard for evaluating tarsal coalitions and that MRI should be performed only with compelling clinical and plain radiographic implications of coalition in the face of a normal CT. Radionucleotide bone scans have been suggested as a screening tool in the evaluation of tarsal coalitions (60,61). However, bone scans are too nonspecific to be diagnostic, although they can be used to focus further CT or MRI study.

Treatment

Many tarsal coalition cases are found by happenstance while the clinician is evaluating the patient for some other condition. These asymptomatic cases can be managed with simple observation and follow-up if the condition is discovered during the growth years (62). If the individual has pain, conservative measures should be tried initially. These efforts include activity modification, shoe modification, and medial wedge or orthotic therapy to minimize the need for subtalar motion. An "airsplint" ankle brace may also be used to provide increased subtalar stability. Intermediate efforts may be tried for those who do not respond to this first stage of conservative care. This can consist of a short-leg walking cast for 4 to 6 weeks, followed by orthotic support and/or ankle bracing. If this fails, Sakellariou and Claridge (52) suggest a second round of casting and a rigid custom-made ankle–foot orthosis.

Surgical treatment for the talocalcaneal coalition differs from that for the calcaneonavicular coalition. The surgical choice is resection of the coalition versus arthrodesis. McCormack et al. (63) reviewed the clinical results of the talocalcaneal middle facet resection in the feet of nine patients 10 years after surgery. All continued to have a good clinical result, with no pain recurrence and the maintenance of motion. Middle facet resection is an option for maintaining subtalar motion. This course is probably useful only for the younger patient. Arthrodesis is possible for the patient with recalcitrant pain, but he or she must understand the potential for degenerative changes to adjacent joints later in life. Calcaneonavicular coalitions can be resected at any age; however, the greater the degenerative change is in older patients, the less likely the procedure is to succeed. In this procedure, the extensor digitorum brevis is interposed into the defect created by the bridge resection.

If the patient is given the opportunity to maintain tarsal joint mobility but the attempt still fails with ongoing pain, triple arthrodesis is the final surgical choice.

Navicular Stress Fractures

A tarsal navicular stress fracture is an underappreciated injury, which is probably more prevalent than the current epidemiologic studies report. Brukner et al. (64) reported that 73% of these fractures occur in track and field athletes, specifically in sprinting and middle distance running. This fracture is also reported in basketball, football, soccer, racket sports, field hockey, gymnastics, and ballet (65). Bennell and Brukner (66) compiled 18 epidemiologic studies encompassing 2,254 stress fractures. The incidence of tarsal navicular stress fracture ranged from 0% in a few studies to 28.6% in one track and field study.

The cause of navicular stress fractures is not clear. Several presumed contributors to this injury have been identified. Overuse and training errors are common to both the novice and elite athlete. In addition, the middle third of the tarsal navicular has diminished vascularity (67). Shear forces through the middle third of the proximal navicular are also probably contributory. During the stance phase of gait, the talar head is laterally positioned (supinatory), relative to the navicular on footstrike, and then it quickly moves to a medial or pronatory position on midfoot loading. The head then moves back to a lateral position during the resupination of the foot. Thus, the navicular bone is subject to a bow-springing action over the course of each loading event. No clear foot structure, whether excessively pronated or supinated, has been statistically proven to predispose the individual to navicular stress fractures. The only clinically relevant examination finding was a preponderance of poor ankle dorsiflexion that was seen in 13 of 15 patients (65).

The clinical history reveals an insidious onset of dorsal midfoot pain, and it sometimes includes ankle pain. The pain radiates medially along the arch or, sometimes, laterally to the cuboid. The pain is worsened with weight-bearing activities, and it can be relieved with just a few days of rest, only to recur, however, upon resumption of activity. The poorly defined pain and the lack of clinical suspicion for this injury contribute to a delayed diagnosis. An individual who has symptoms that are present for 4 months or longer is common (68). The history should focus on identifying significant changes in the training regime. Inspection of the foot is usually not helpful, as swelling or ecchymoses is rarely seen. Careful palpation is the key when the examiner suspects this injury. The talonavicular joint can be identified easily by locating the navicular tuberosity and then moving the palpating finger proximally while inverting and everting the foot. The talar head is present with the foot everted, and it then disappears when the foot is inverted. This important landmark then helps the examiner isolate the navicular. This is followed by moving the examining finger to the dorsum of the navicular to isolate the "N" spot. This location, as proposed by Khan (68), is often the only tender focus. Another physical finding with untested predictive value is hopping on the affected foot, while it is held in an equinus position (i.e., hopping on the toes). In the presence of a stress fracture, this provocative maneuver will cause pain (69).

Imaging begins with plain radiography; this injury, however, rarely causes radiographic abnormalities. A sufficient level of clinical suspicion should direct the clinician to the use of technetium bone scan. Isotope recovery is easily isolated to the entire tarsal navicular. Further clarification with a CT scan can be helpful for management decisions (Fig. 38.2). Thin slice CT cuts oriented to the plane of the talonavicular joint show a progression of bone change. A curvilinear fracture that often begins dorsally is directed in a plantar direction. A late diagnosis can lead to a com-

pletely transected navicular, in which the fracture extends totally from the dorsum to the plantar aspect of the bone. A dense sclerotic rim often encompasses the fracture line and portends the chronic nature of this stress fracture.

Treatment of the tarsal navicular stress fracture is controversial. Most fractures can heal well with conservative measures (68). However, a high incidence of delayed union or fracture nonunion is reported. Controversy exists over the best conservative management and what constitutes the surgical candidate. Continued weight bearing without sports activity, as is often prescribed for other stress fractures, has met with a high incidence of failure (67,68). Quirk (69), former president of the American Orthopaedic Foot and Ankle Society, suggests the following protocol for the conservative management of tarsal navicular stress fractures:

- Six weeks on crutches with a below-the-knee non–weight-bearing cast.
- Removal of cast and reexamination of the "N" spot. If continued tenderness is present, return the patient to the cast for another 2 weeks.
- The cast is removed, and a careful gradual return to supervised weight-bearing activity occurs.

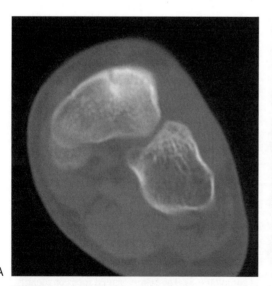
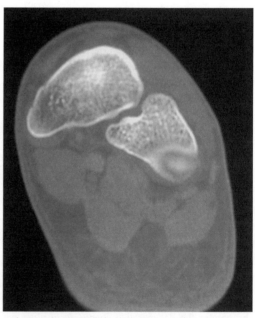

A   B

FIG. 38.2. Tarsal navicular stress fracture. **A:** Computed tomography of tarsal navicular stress fracture in a 13-year-old soccer player and cross country runner. Note predictable location of this stress fracture in the dorsal cortex (middle one-third). **B:** Same individual following 6 months of nonoperative management, as outlined in the text. Some residual bony sclerosis is seen, but resolution of frank fracture line has occurred.

A repeat CT or bone scan often is not helpful. Management decisions, thus, are best made based on examination findings. Persistent symptomatic nonunion necessitates surgical fixation with a bone graft and screw placement across the fracture site.

The patient must be forewarned about the prolonged recovery and the painstakingly slow return to sports participation. This can help avert unrealistic expectations of an earlier return to sports activity in those individuals who are unfamiliar with the clinical course of stress fractures. The average time to return to play is 5.6 months (68). Injury prevention has focused on improving gastroachilles flexibility and on the use of custom-molded shoe orthoses. Frequent shoe changes are suggested.

Lisfranc Injuries

History

The Lisfranc joint is the eponym given to the tarsometatarsal joint. During the Napoleonic era, the joint often became injured when cavalry troops got their feet caught in the stirrups while falling off of horses. The French field surgeon Jacques Lisfranc (1790–1847) became famous for the speed at which he could amputate feet through the tarsometatarsal joint. The decreased use of horses in daily life has caused a dramatic decrease in the number of cases of vascular complications resulting from fracture–dislocations of the tarsometatarsal joint (70,71).

Dislocations and fracture–dislocations through the Lisfranc joint are uncommon injuries. The annual incidence approaches one case per 55,000 persons per year (72,73). This injury is even rarer in the pediatric patient. However, the true extent of injury is often missed. Furthermore, devastating sequelae can result from misdiagnosis or incorrectly prescribed treatment.

Anatomy

The tarsometatarsal articulation (the Lisfranc joint) is formed by the three cuneiform bones, the cuboid bone proximally, and the bases of the five metatarsals distally. The second metatarsal base has a dovetail shape, and it is recessed into a mortise that is created by the surrounding cuneiforms. This articulation is the "key" to the stability of the Lisfranc joint (73,74). Transverse ligaments join the bases of the adjacent metatarsals with one exception—no ligamentous attachment is seen between the bases of the first and second metatarsals. However, the second metatarsal articulates with the medial cuneiform at its medial base with an oblique ligamentous attachment that is termed the Lisfranc ligament (75). The Lisfranc ligament and the mortise created by the base of the second metatarsal are the main stabilizers of the entire tarsometatarsal articulation.

Mechanism of Injury

The most common reported mechanisms of injury are related to slips, falls, athletics, and motor vehicle accidents (74,76,77). Some authors use the term "Lisfranc joint complex" when referring to injuries that involve the Lisfranc joint, as well as the cuboid, navicular, and cuneiform bones (78). The anatomic complexity at the Lisfranc joint complex leads to multiple injury patterns. Sprains are the most common injury, with the midfoot sprain representing the least severe injury (79).

Direct forces to the Lisfranc joint result in injuries to the dorsum of the foot in a crushing or blow type injury. The direct mechanism is more uncommon than the indirect (75). Crush injuries involving the tarsometatarsal joint displace the metatarsals plantarward, causing a variety of dislocation patterns depending on the vector of the force and the position of the foot. The bones and soft tissue overlying the Lisfranc joint are susceptible to injury with this force, which makes the consideration of both compartment syndrome and vascular disruption involving the dorsalis pedis artery imperative when one is evaluating patients with this mechanism of injury.

The indirect mechanism is more commonly seen. Wilson (80), in his clinical survey of 20 patients and his experimental cadaveric study of 11 feet, demonstrated that the foot must be in plantar flexion at the time of the injury because, in dorsiflexion, the strain falls on the ankle. Forced plantarflexion, which is usually combined with rotation, can occur in the following three ways: longitudinal compression, a backward fall with the foot entrapped, and a fall on the point of the toes (75). A load applied to the heel when the foot is plantarflexed is a mechanism by which a football player might sustain this injury—for instance, he might be on his knee attempting to get up when he then is "piled on" by opposing players. Dancers also may sustain an injury to the tarsometatarsal joint when *en pointe*. If a dancer loses his or her balance while *en pointe* and falls forward, the joint compresses in an axial direction with the toes flexed, causing the injury.

Abduction injuries also can occur. With the hindfoot stationary, the forefoot is forcefully abducted, producing lateral displacement of the metatarsals and an associated fracture of the metatarsal base (81).

Clinical Examination

Misdiagnosis of Lisfranc injuries is common, and it can lead to significant chronic disability. The physical findings of a Lisfranc injury, especially those resulting from an indirect mechanism, are often subtle and nonspecific. Typical signs and symptoms include pain, swelling, and an inability to bear weight. Swelling usually is localized over the midfoot region. Palpation will often reveal tenderness along the tarsometatarsal articulations, and force applied to this area may elicit medial or lateral pain. Since the dorsalis pedis artery courses over the proximal head of the second metatarsal, vascular compromise should be ruled out by a thorough examination that includes an assessment for acute compartment syndrome. When the clinician is considering the possibility of a Lisfranc complex injury, comparing the injured extremity to that of the contralateral limb in order to find the subtle differences between normal and abnormal is helpful.

The functional status of the foot also should be evaluated. The presence of an antalgic gait, an evaluation of the medial longitudinal arch for flattening, and the ability to bear weight on tiptoes should prompt one to consider the possibility of an injury to the tarsometatarsal joint (73,77).

Imaging

Plain radiographs should be ordered for those patients presenting with possible Lisfranc complex injuries. These radiographs should be carefully reviewed because the injuries are often subtle. If possible, weight-bearing views should be ordered, including the AP, 30-degree oblique, and lateral views. The most consistent relationship seen in radiographs of the normal foot is the alignment of the medial edge of the base of the second metatarsal with the medial edge of the second cuneiform on the AP or oblique view (72).

Other consistent findings on radiograph include continuity between the second and third intermetatarsal space with the space found between the lateral and middle cuneiforms on oblique views. In addition, the lateral border of the third metatarsal shaft should form a straight line with the lateral border of the lateral cuneiform, and the medial border of the fourth metatarsal should be continuous with the medial border of the cuboid on the oblique view (82). Finally, a metatarsal should never be more dorsal than its respective tarsal bone on the lateral view (83).

CT scanning can help to clarify further the extent of lesions, the size of which may be missed on standard radiographs. Other advantages of CT are seen when evaluating patients with midfoot pain. The patient does not need to be weight bearing to conduct the diagnostic test. Furthermore, the optimal visualization of even small abnormalities, which are easily obscured on plain radiographs, can be used for the best possible assessment of even small deformities. Moreover, the interposition of soft tissues can be seen easily on CT scans. Finally, the quality of a reduction is readily controlled, even when a plaster cast is in place.

Treatment

Early recognition and proper treatment of Lisfranc complex injuries is imperative for the prevention of a poor functional outcome (73). The goal in treating tarsometatarsal fracture dislocations is the reestablishment of a painless, stable, and functional foot, with the precise anatomic reduction necessary to reduce future disability (72).

If the clinical evaluation indicates the probability of a mild or moderate sprain and the radiograph shows no diastasis, the use of immobilization is suggested (84). Treatment consists of a short-leg walking cast, a removable short-leg orthotic, or a non–weight-bearing cast for 4 to 6 weeks until symptoms have resolved (85).

After a period of immobilization, ambulation, and rehabilitation, exercises should be instituted progressively. If symptoms persist, ordering repeat weight-bearing radiographs is indicated.

Surgical treatment is indicated for any cases with fractures, dislocation, or diastasis that involve the Lisfranc joint. The method of repair is the subject of controversy. Some orthopedists prefer closed fixation using Kirshner wires, whereas others feel that this does not hold the anatomic position and fixation. Wiring is unlikely to be successful in cases of soft tissue interposition and severe comminution or if a diastasis is found between the medial and intermediate cuneiform bones, thus suggesting the interposition of the tibialis anterior tendon (86). Current thinking on the management of Lisfranc joint injury tends towards the use of open reduction and internal fixation (87). A study by Arntz et al. (88) reported on 41 tarsometatarsal injuries that were treated with open reduction and internal fixation using screws. The authors concluded that precise reduction was achievable and that 95% of patients had good or excellent functional recovery. Most authors advocate postoperative immobilization for a period of 4 to 6 weeks in a below-the-knee non–weight-bearing cast.

Köhler Disease

Köhler disease is an osteochondrosis of the tarsal navicular bone that was first described in 1908 (89). The etiology is unknown, but speculations about the existence of abnormalities in the developing ossification center flourish. Waugh (90) suggested that delayed ossification during childhood leads to the irregular appearance seen in adults. These changes may be due to normal weight-bearing forces. Ischemia secondary to compression of the vessels traversing the cartilage-to-bone transition is thought to cause the pain that is typical of this disease.

Prevalence

Williams and Cowell (91) estimate that up to 30% of males and 20% of females from the ages of 2 to 9 years have irregular ossification of the tarsal navicular. Only a fraction of these children are symptomatic. The mere presence of irregular ossification in an asymptomatic patient does not indicate that the patient has Köhler disease. Typical symptoms and radiographic bone density changes are both necessary for a diagnosis of Köhler disease.

Presentation

Children present with a limp and vague pain to the medial midfoot. Swelling may or may not be present, and tenderness is usually found directly over the navicular. Occasionally, erythema to the overlying skin is observed. Radiographs show an increased bone density, a decreased length in the dorsoplantar projection, a loss of trabecular pattern, and apparent fragmentation of the tarsal navicular. Distinguishing radiographic abnormalities from normal changes of bone growth in a symptomatic patient may be difficult. Bone scintigraphy may be helpful for early diagnosis (92). The absence of radioisotope uptake is consistent with the ischemia that is thought to characterize this disease.

Treatment

Treatment goals focus on the prompt resolution of symptoms. Although several treatments have been utilized, they differ only by the length of time to symptom improvement. These treatments do not alter the eventual outcome. Most patients enjoy complete symptom resolution and radiographic restoration of normal bone architecture. Williams and Cowell (91) compared 8 weeks of short-leg cast with noncasting. The group treated with a cast improved in an average of 2 to 3 months, whereas the untreated group required 15 months to resolve the symptoms. Devine and Van Demark (93) reported a single case that improved with arch supports. Ippolito et al. (94) compared casting to arch supports and found that weight-bearing plaster casts rendered patients asymptomatic after 3 months. Arch supports provided only palliative care and averaged 7 months to pain resolution.

Regardless of treatment type, Köhler disease remains a mild, self-limiting disease of childhood. The patients can be expected to have a normal foot at adulthood, with an eventual reconstitution of the tarsal navicular and a complete recovery of function (95). Athletes with Köhler disease should refrain from activity during the active stage of the disease; they may then resume activity once the symptoms have resolved.

REARFOOT PROBLEMS

Sever Disease

In 1912, Sever (96) described heel pain due to inflammatory injury to the calcaneal apophysis. This condition is sometimes called "Osgood–Schlatter disease" of the heel because it is a traction injury to the secondary calcaneal ossification center (97). This ossification center appears between 6 and 8 years of age in most children. The growth plate is C-shaped and vertically oriented, as the lateral radiograph demonstrates (Fig. 38.3). Achilles insertion to this secondary ossification center provides the potential for large shearing forces at the growth plate. Fusion most often occurs between the ages of 12 and 15 years.

Etiology

The cause of this syndrome is a combination of musculotendinous inflexibility as a result of recent rapid skeletal growth with an increased athletic workload. Biomechanical maladies, such as pes planus and pes cavus, are also suggested to predispose the individual to the stresses that cause Sever disease.

Presentation

The young athlete complains of intermittent or continuous heel pain that correlates with his or her level of physical activity. The heel pain can be unilateral, but it most often is bilateral. The male to female preponderance is 3 to 1 (98). Most children present between the ages of 8 and 12 years, with boys later than girls; however, the reported age range for presentation can extend from 7 to 15 years. A recent growth spurt preceding presentation reinforces clinical suspicion for this diagnosis. These children generally do not experience night pain.

On examination, erythema and swelling are usually absent. The patient's gait may be normal or antalgic. When the patient stands on tiptoe, the pain may be worsened. Side-to-side heel compression or the "squeeze test" usually elicits pain over the lower one-third of the posterior calcaneus (97). Heel cord tightening can be appreciated in most cases. Radiographic imaging is usually not necessary. The fragmented and sclerotic appearance of the C-shaped apophysis is normal and thus is not diagnostic. Radiographs may be performed to rule out other possible causes of heel pain.

Treatment

The initial management includes rest, ice, and heel lifts or viscoelastic heel cups. Adequate rest from sports activity is the cornerstone of recovery. The time to symptom-free activity is generally about 2 months, but it can take as long as 6 months. Micheli and Ireland (98) used a combination of gastroachilles stretching exercises, dorsiflexion strengthening exercises, and a soft orthotic or plastizote heel support. The use of nonsteroidal antiinflammatory medicines and shoes with good support, as well as the avoidance of barefoot walking, may be helpful. More aggressive immobilization with a short-leg cast or a boot walker may be nec-

essary for cases that do not improve with these strategies. A dorsiflexion splint, applied at night, may facilitate pain relief and may help to maintain flexibility (99). Return-to-sport activities are permissible when symptoms allow.

Preventing recurrence is enhanced with a few simple strategies. Stretching; strengthening exercises; high quality shoes; a gradual return to activity; icing after sports activity; and reducing duration, intensity, and frequency of sports participation if symptoms occur all aid in keeping the athlete on the playing field. Sever syndrome resolves without long-term sequelae upon skeletal maturation and the fusion of the ossification center to the body of the calcaneus.

Osteochondral Lesions of the Talus

Osteochondritis dissecans (OCD) of the talar dome is a common cause of chronic ankle pain in children and adolescents (100). The talar dome is the most frequent site of appearance for OCD, although the head of the talus may be involved (101). Sports that involve frequent starting, stopping, and cutting are more susceptible to repetitive ankle injuries, and these are the sports in which OCD is most often seen. Pathologically, OCD is a collapse to subchondral bone at vulnerable articular locations (102). If further injury occurs, the condition progresses to bone fragmentation of the talar articular surface. The term "osteochondritis dissecans of the ankle" was coined by Kappis (103) in 1922, when he noticed the similarities between the lesions that occurred in the knee with those seen in the ankle.

Etiology

The etiology of OCD of the talus is uncertain. Suggested causes of this disease include endocrinopathies, vascular insults, infection, and trauma (104). The most important factor appears to be repetitive trauma to a subchondral bone (102). The landmark study, which was conducted by Berndt and Harty (105) in 1959, concluded that the lesion is caused by trauma and that it is actually a transchondral fracture of the talar dome. In this analysis of 200 cases from the literature that also considered 24 of their own patients and cadaver specimens, the authors concluded that both medial and lateral lesions could be attributed to trauma to the ankle. This trauma most commonly was an inversion stress. They developed a four-stage radiologic classification system that, with subtle modification, is still in use today (Table 38.1).

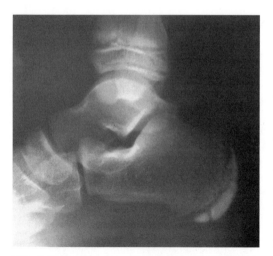

FIG. 38.3. Sever calcaneal apophysitis. Radiographic findings are nonspecific. Possible bony sclerosis at the margins of the physis.

A study conducted by Canale and Beaty (106) showed that 68% of patients had symptoms that began in the second decade of life. In this study of 31 lesions, 14 were medial, 16 were lateral, and one was central. All had a previous history of trauma.

Diagnosis

Most patients will recall spraining an ankle, although this original injury may have been relatively trivial. Ankle pain is the usual presenting complaint. If the lesion has progressed to fragmentation, then mechanical symptoms (e.g., locking, catching, clicking, or popping) will occur (100). Examination for tenderness to the anterior ankle at the talar dome is best accomplished with the foot in plantarflexion. Swelling may also be present.

Carefully scrutinized radiographs of the ankle can reveal OCD lesions (Fig. 38.4). Anderson et al. (107) reported that nearly 50% of OCDs identified by scintigraphy, CT, or MRI are not visible on plain radiographs. Oblique and plantarflexed views that avoid tibial overlap show the lesion better than do the standard ankle views. Bone scintigraphy can be quite sensitive, but it is nonspecific. CT scan can be insensitive in detecting stage I subchondral fractures, but it may be used to document progression of more advanced lesions. MRI has become the gold standard for staging OCD lesions. De Smet et al. (108) believed that MRI could assist clinical decision making by differentiating lesions that were stable from those that were not and that therefore require surgery (108). Taranow et al. suggested that MRI is sufficient for determining the bony component of an OCD but that it is inadequate for assessing the condition of the cartilage (Table 38.2).

Arthroscopy is used for further staging of the OCD cartilage into "viable and intact" (grade A) or "breached and nonviable" (grade B). Taranow suggested that this clarification of cartilage condition is necessary for the determination of the success of conservative versus operative treatment.

Treatment

Nonoperative treatment can be successful for stage I and some stage II lesions. Immobilization, followed by prolonged non–weight-bearing management, can be used during the acute stages (109). The young athlete with a stage I lesion may only need to withdraw from sporting activities for the symptoms to resolve. Stage III medial lesions are generally more stable than stage III lateral lesions; therefore, a trial of conservative therapy for medial lesions is warranted. Stage III lateral lesions often fail to resolve with conservative therapy, but, nonetheless, nonoperative care should be attempted in the adolescent population.

Several surgical treatments are available for OCD, including excision of the fragment, excision and curettage with drilling, excision and curettage without drilling, cancellous bone grafting, osteochondral transplantation, or internal fixation of the fragment. No randomized, controlled trials have been conducted to compare the different types of treatment. Tol et al. (110) reviewed the literature in an attempt to compare the results of treatment strategies for OCD of the

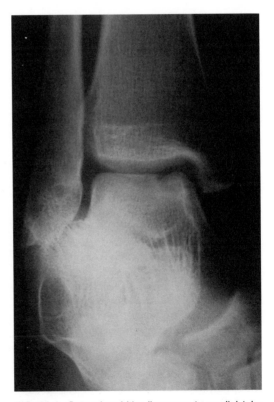

FIG. 38.4. Osteochondritis dissecans to medial talar dome.

TABLE 38.1. *Four-stage radiological classification system of osteochondritis dissecans*

Stage I	Localized trabecular compression
Stage II	Incompletely separated bone fragment
Stage IIA	Formation of subchondral cyst
Stage III	Undetached, undisplaced fragment
Stage IV	Displaced or inverted fragment

TABLE 38.2. *Magnetic resonance imaging bone classification*

Stage I: subchondral compression or bone bruise, appearing as high signal on T2–weighted image
Stage II: subchondral cysts that are not seen acutely
Stage III: partially separated or detached fragments *in situ*
Stage IV: displaced fragments of bone

talus. The success rate of nonoperative treatment was 45%. The success rate of excision alone was 38% in 39 patients. Excision and curettage involves excising the loose body and curetting the surrounding necrotic tissue with the use of an open surgical technique or arthroscopy. In 11 studies with 141 patients, this mode of treatment was 78% successful. The best results were obtained by excision, curettage, and drilling to the subchondral bone. This technique, which was reported for a total of 135 patients in 16 studies, enjoyed a success rate of 85%. Other operative treatment strategies include cancellous bone grafting, osteochondral transplantation, and fixation. Hangody et al. (111) reported excellent results in 11 patients with OCD who were treated with autologous grafts from the ipsilateral knee.

Plantar Fasciitis

Plantar fasciitis is an extremely common and painful condition that, if untreated, can become chronic and degenerative. It is a clinical condition characterized by pain and tenderness that is localized to the plantar surface of the heel. More than 2 million Americans receive treatment each year for heel pain, and most have plantar fasciitis (112). This problem afflicts adults more commonly than children; nonetheless, it does occur in adolescents. It is seen in both sedentary and active people. While its exact cause is not always easily identifiable, a few associated factors include obesity, excessive walking or running, middle age, and biomechanical disorders, such as pes planus, pes cavus, and a tight Achilles tendon (113). The incidence of plantar fasciitis among runners is 10%; however, the current opinion is that from 50% to 70% will sustain injury to the plantar fascia as a result of their sport at some time in their life. Multiple retrospective studies show that this condition affects women more often than men. Synonyms for plantar fasciitis include heel pain syndrome, heel spur syndrome, subcalcaneal pain syndrome, and calcaneal periostitis. When the clinician suspects plantar fasciitis, the possibility of seronegative spondyloarthropathies (e.g., ankylosing spondylitis and Reiter syndrome) should be entertained in the appropriate populations.

Mechanism of Injury

The plantar fascia is the most important structure for dynamic arch support. It provides secondary stability to the midfoot, it absorbs forces in the midtarsal joints, and it aids in raising the arch of the foot (114). Plantar fasciitis is an overuse injury. It results from repetitive microtrauma to the plantar fascia at the calcaneal attachment site. This results in inflammation of the plantar fascia and the perifascial structures. The presenting picture of plantar fasciitis can also be caused by nerve entrapment. Surgical resection of the medial calcaneal nerves supports this assertion because relieving the entrapment improves symptoms. Louisia and Masquelet (115) reported that the inferior calcaneal nerve (ICN), a branch of the lateral plantar nerve, is the nerve that is responsible for heel pain. Any tissue hypertrophy anterior to fascial attachment may cause entrapment of the ICN. This hypertrophy could result from inflammation secondary to the repetitive microtrauma mentioned above.

History

The patient with plantar fasciitis will present with a complaint of heel pain. Upon further questioning, he or she typically will localize this pain to the anterior medial aspect of the heel (116). The patient typically will describe the pain as a deep, aching type of pain. The pain will be worse with the patient's first steps in the morning or after prolonged rest, such as occurs following sitting or riding in a car. As the patient takes a few steps, the pain moderates, only to worsen again after prolonged standing or a long walk or run. The pain is of gradual onset, so any pain that is associated with known trauma or that is of acute onset is not characteristic of the pain seen with plantar fasciitis. These latter findings should point the clinician towards a different diagnosis. Furthermore, plantar fasciitis is not associated with swelling, weakness, numbness, or paresthesias. In addition, no radiation of pain to the legs should occur. Initially, the patient may be able to continue with daily activity, but, as the pain worsens, he or she may difficulty in tolerating even weight bearing.

Examination

Examination of the plantar fascia begins with inspection, although usually no swelling, ecchymoses, or external signs of injury are visible. The clinician should palpate the plantar aspect of the foot to identify the exact location of pain. Tenderness is typically located along the anterior medial aspect of the heel, although, not uncommonly, tenderness is absent at the time of the examination. The pain may be exacerbated by dorsiflexing the MTPJs or the ankle. A Tinel sign performed over the tarsal tunnel—medial, posterior, and inferior to the medial malleolus—may be helpful, but this is not diagnostic for the nerve entrapment caused by tarsal tunnel syndrome, which is part of the differential diagnosis in patients with heel pain. A short (i.e., tight) plantar fascia is detected by comparing hallux dorsiflexion while the foot is plantarflexed and relaxed to the the hallux motion that is available when the forefoot is loaded in a dorsiflexed position. This latter foot posture simulates tension on the plantar fascia in the late propulsive phase of gait. A general biomechanical examination, with particular attention to excessive pronation, supination, and Achilles inflexibility, will identify factors that contribute to plantar fascia stress. Evaluation of shoe integrity and wear patterns may provide the clinician with important clues as to the etiology of the pain.

Diagnostic Studies

Plantar fasciitis generally is diagnosed clinically. If the history and examination deviates from the classic plantar fasciitis picture, further investigation is appropriate. Lateral projection radiographs can identify fractures, spurs, bone tumors, and possibly other rheumatologic disorders. The presence of a horizontal bone spur is thought to be incidental, and it is not the cause of heel pain for most patients (117). If the lateral films are not diagnostic and the clinician is dealing with an atypical presentation, a triple-phase bone scan may be performed. A positive bone scan for plantar fasciitis shows increased uptake at the origin of the plantar fascia. One study performed by Intenzo et al. (118) identified a linear appearance of increased uptake along the medial ventral surface of the calcaneus on the blood-pooled images, while an increased uptake within the inferior calcaneal surface was found anteriorly on the static images. This pattern differs from the images that would be seen with a calcaneal stress fracture. This stress fracture would instead show focally increased activity on both the blood-pooled and delayed scans.

Two other imaging options include ultrasound and MRI. Cardinal et al. (119) showed plantar fascial thickening of 5.2 mm in symptomatic patients versus that of 2.9 mm in asymptomatic patients. They also showed a hypoechoic plantar fascia in 84% of symptomatic patients, with no reduction in signal in asymptomatic patients. In the study conducted by Gibbon and Long (120), abnormal echogenicity of the plantar fascia was found in 78% of patients who had plantar fasciitis. MRI findings in plantar fasciitis include a thickened plantar fascia, as well as thickened perifascial soft tissues and tendons (121).

Other diagnostic studies may include blood work, such as an erythrocyte sedimentation rate and a rheumatoid panel. These studies should be reserved for the patient with an atypical presentation or when the clinician suspects other possible etiologies.

Treatment

A conservative approach to plantar fasciitis treatment is successful in 90% of cases. The patient should be advised that successful conservative treatment may take a long time. Generally speaking, the longer the patient has had the heel pain, the longer he or she will take to heal. Initial treatment strategies include rest from the offending activity, stretching, supportive shoes, the application of ice, and the use of antiinflammatory medication. A complete rest from sports activity may be necessary for the severely symptomatic patient. Relative rest by reducing training volume, intensity, duration, and frequency may allow continued sports participation without the complete cessation of activity. This compromise regarding the rest effort should be abandoned if it is not successful.

Stretching is directed to the gastroachilles complex. Improved sagittal plane dorsiflexion at the ankle reduces arch collapse and plantar fascial stress in the midstance of gait cycle. Chandler and Kibler (122) outlined an excellent rehabilitation program that focuses on regaining the individual's range of motion and strength symmetry.

Passive stretch that is applied to the plantar fascia at night can be achieved with some form of night splints. Batt et al. (123) achieved excellent results with an average treatment time of 12.5 weeks. Powell et al. (124) used a crossover, prospective, randomized design to demonstrate improved clinical results in a group of recalcitrant cases of plantar fasciitis. Eighty-eight percent of these patients improved during 1 month of night splint use. Mizel et al. (125) also showed an improvement among 77% of patients with the use night splints, although, in this study, a steel shank and an anterior rocker bottom that were applied to the shoe were also used. A commercially made night splint is available, but a molded fiberglass splint that is applied with an elastic bandage is considerably less expensive. The foot is held in 5 degrees of dorsiflexion while the fiberglass dries. If a ski boot or cowboy boot is available, some physicians will actually use these to achieve similar nighttime dorsiflexion without the expense of a night splint.

If these initial treatments fail to remedy the patient's pain, the use of corticosteroid injections can be considered. Anatomical landmarks and the point of maximal pain are usually used clinically to determine the site of injection, but Dasgupta and Bowles (126) suggested that scintigraphic localization can assist the clinician in finding the optimal site for injection. Miller et al. (127) demonstrated the efficacy of a single steroid injection for the relief of heel pain, but they acknowledged that the injection may not provide permanent relief. Injections can lead to fat pad atrophy and the rupture of the plantar fascia (128,129). Acevedo and Baskin (130) estimated that 10% of patients suffer rupture of the plantar fascia following one injection of steroids. The average time to rupture, following injection, was 10 weeks according to their research. The athlete often feels tremendous pain relief following the injection. They may then feel quite tempted to return to the sport quickly and aggressively. However, a cautious return to sports activity after several weeks of rest is prudent. The athlete should be advised of the increased risk of plantar fascia rupture and the risk of early return to sports participation. Alternatively, the application of dexamethasone by iontophoresis provides a noninvasive method for prompt pain relief (131). This quick relief of pain may be useful for the athlete who is interested in an aggressive return-to-play protocol. In this study, which was conducted by Gudeman et al. (131), no complications were observed, but the long-term effects on patients were not reported.

Other options for treatment include the use of custom orthotics to assist with biomechanical problems (132). Pfeffer et al. (133) found that a prefabricated silicone insert was more effective and much less expensive than a custom orthosis in the first 8 weeks of treatment.

Patients for whom prolonged conservative treatment fails may consider a surgical release. Most published reports involve adult patients, and surgery is rarely indicated for the adolescent population. Surgical procedures include the partial release of the plantar fascia and decompression of the nerve to the abductor digiti quinti (134). Although surgical release of the plantar fascia may provide early heel pain relief, biomechanical consequences are seen with the loss of the plantar fascia (135). These sequelqae are

supported by anatomical studies that show subsequent arch collapse and increased tarsal joint movements (136–138). An MRI study conducted by Yu et al. (121) demonstrated the presence of persistent plantar fasciitis, peroneal and posterior tibial tendinitis, flexor digitorum brevis edema, and/or cuboid stress fracture in patients who had undergone plantar fascia release 22 months earlier. These results reinforce the need of exhausting all possible nonsurgical treatments before considering the release of the plantar fascia.

MISCELLANEOUS PROBLEMS

Accessory Ossicles

Kruse and Chen (139) revealed that 36% of all foot radiographs demonstrate the presence of identifiable accessory bones. Although accessory bones are rarely symptomatic, they are often confused with fractures. The accessory navicular in the adolescent and the os trigonum following trauma are the accessory bones that are most commonly described as causing pain (139). Other accessory bones that are occasionally seen are the os intermetatarseum and the os vesalii.

Os Trigonum

The os trigonum is located at the lateral tubercle of the posterior process of the talus bone. It can appear either separate from, or fused to, the talus. The os trigonum, which is found in 3% to 20% of the population, is unilateral in two-thirds of individuals. Debate continues regarding the etiology of this accessory ossicle. Many support the theory that the os trigonum is an independently formed ossicle originating from a secondary ossification center, while others claim that it is a fracture of an already fused os trigonum. Usually, a secondary ossification center will appear between the ages of 8 and 11 years, and it unites with the talus within 1 year of its appearance. The following three mechanisms of formation have been proposed by McDougall (140): (a) lack of fusion of the secondary ossification center, (b) lateral tubercle and posterior tibia impingement that causes a stress fracture, and (c) trauma that causes acute fracture. A fourth possibility includes the avulsion of the posterior talofibular ligament from the lateral tubercle (141). The lateral tubercle has been classified by Watson and Dobas (142) into the following four classes:

1. Asymptomatic, with the normal appearance of the lateral tubercle;
2. Enlarged tubercle;
3. An accessory bone that has been irritated by chronic repetitive trauma;

4. An accessory bone that has a cartilaginous or synchondrotic bridge with the talus and that is susceptible to fracture due to injury.

Clinical Presentation

The history may elicit symptoms that began following a single trauma, or it may include the insidious onset of posterior ankle pain. Patients may give a history of prior ankle sprain. Ballet dancers can suffer posterior impingement syndrome caused by compression of the posterior talofibular ligament and the posterior aspect of the ankle capsule (143). The pain may increase with running, jumping, descending stairs, or other activities that force the foot into plantarflexion. Physical signs include swelling to the posterior ankle, tenderness in the retrocalcaneal space, and pain with active or passive use of the flexor tendons that course near the os trigonum.

Lateral radiographs of the ankle are most useful when interpreted in conjunction with AP views; mortise views also are recommended (141). Distinguishing os trigonum from a lateral tubercle fracture can be difficult. Since the os trigonum is often unilateral, comparison views are unreliable. In acute fractures, the bony fragment may have a rough anterior surface and a smooth posterior surface. An os trigonum, on the other hand, would be expected to appear as round or oval and to be smooth circumferentially, similar to the appearance of an old fracture (144). Bone scans also may be helpful in the evaluation of os trigonum (145).

Treatment

Initial treatment for both an acute fracture and a chronic injury is 4 to 6 weeks of immobilization. Range of motion of the first MTPJ should be initiated following casting to prevent the adhesion of the flexor hallucis longus tendon. The athlete should pursue a gradual return to sports activity, while minimizing participation in the previously offending activity. Surgical excision of the os trigonum remains an alternative for patients who fail to respond to conservative care.

Accessory Navicular

The accessory navicular bone, which is present in 4% to 21% of the population, is located at the medial or posteromedial aspect of the navicular tuberosity. This bone, which is also called the prehallux, accessory scaphoid, os tibiale externum, os naviculare secundarium, and navicular secundum, is not radiographically seen until the 9 to 10 years of age. The symptomatic accessory navicular is more common in women than in men. Whether the accessory navicular bone is related to the tibialis posterior tendon or to the navicular tuberosity has created much controversy. Some argue that the os tibiale externum is attached to the tendon, while others claim that a relationship with the navicular tuberosity exists. Several classification schemes based on the anatomic location have been proposed (146–148).

Clinical Presentation

Medial side foot pain is the most common complaint that is associated with symptomatic accessory navicular bones. Pain may be worse at the end of the day, and it may be present at rest. Weight bearing, walking, running, athletic activity, and shoes may all aggravate the area and may cause increased discomfort. A history of trauma may or may not be present. Examination usually reveals a prominent bulge on the medial side of the foot that often gives the appearance of extreme arch collapse and excessive pronation. Significant skin calluses or soft tissue inflammation also may be present.

Radiographs show a medial navicular eminence that is best visualized on a lateral oblique view. In cases of a bilateral accessory navicular, a bone scan may be useful. Symptomatic accessory naviculars will be "hot," while asymptomatic accessory naviculars should not show increased uptake. Miller et al. (149) also noted that MRI may reveal a bone marrow edema pattern (BMEP) in patients with symptomatic accessory navicular bones. BMEP may be indicative of chronic stress and/or osteonecrosis, and it can furnish an objective basis for the management plan.

Treatment

Conservative treatment to delay surgery consists of alterations of footwear, in addition to the use of exercises for the intrinsic muscles of the foot and the lateral thigh rotators (150). Orthotic devices should be designed to reduce tensile forces on the tibialis posterior while avoiding an increase in local irritation. The patient may be placed in a short-leg walking cast for 4 to 6 weeks. Antiinflammatory medications, rest, and the application of felt along the medial longitudinal arch may help to reduce the symptoms. Acute pain reduction may be achieved with corticosteroid injection, followed by immobilization for approximately 2 to 3 weeks. When conservative treatment fails, excision of the accessory navicular, the synchondrosis, or the prominent navicular tuberosity, with or without tendon transposition, should be considered (150–152).

Os Intermetatarseum

The os intermetatarseum is a relatively common accessory bone that is proximally located in the first and second intermetatarsal space. It can be divided into three basic types as follows: free-standing, articulating, and fused (153). A free-standing intermetatarseum is completely independent with no osseous or articular connections to any other structure. An articulating intermetatarseum forms a synovial joint with the first or second metatarsal or the first cuneiform. The fused type forms "spurs." These are recognizable as large osseous projections that are directed between the first and second metatarsal space. Two main hypotheses exist to explain the origin of the os intermetatarseum. One describes the intermetatarseum as a true accessory bone, and the other claims that the os intermetatarseum represents a supernumerary bone and that it is a form of central polydactyly (153).

Clinical Presentation

The presenting symptom is pain, which is usually found on the dorsum of the foot near the bases of the first and second metatarsals or the first cuneiform. Pain may be elicited by weight bearing or upon palpation of the dorsum of the foot in these areas. Henderson (154) suggested that an os intermetatarseum creates a wedge in the first metatarsal interspace that contributes to a hallux valgus. Standard radiographs of the foot may demonstrate this accessory bone.

Treatment

The usual course of management may consist of conservative measures, including rest (refrain from weight bearing), ice, nonsteroidal antiinflammatory drugs, and shoe alterations. If these modalities do not offer relief, surgical excision is required.

Os Vesalianum

An os vesalianum, which is situated at the proximal end of the fifth metatarsal in the peroneus tendons, may be formed by the failure of a secondary ossification center to fuse to the metatarsal (Fig. 38.5) (155). An ossification center is apparent in this location between 10 and 12 years of age, and it fuses to the shaft of the fifth metatarsal by the age of 15 years. In children, the os vesalianum should be differentiated from the proximal fifth metatarsal apophysis.

REFERENCES

1. American Academy of Orthopaedic Surgeons. *Orthopaedic knowledge update 3. Home study syllabus.* Park Ridge, IL: The American Academy of Orthopaedic Surgeons, 1990.
2. Cole AE. Foot inspection of the school child. *J Am Podiatr Assoc* 1959;49:446–454.
3. Scranton PE Jr, Zuckerman JD. Bunion surgery in adolescents: results of surgical treatment. *J Pediatr Orthop* 1984;4:39–43.
4. Groiso JA. Juvenile hallux valgus: a conservative approach to treatment. *J Bone Joint Surg Am* 1992;74:1367–1374.
5. Hardy RH, Clapham JCH. Observations on hallux valgus: based on a controlled series. *J Bone Joint Surg Br* 1951;33:376–391.
6. Kilmartin TE, Barrington RI, Wallace WA. Metatarsus primus varus: a statistical study. *J Bone Joint Surg Br* 1991;73:937–940.
7. Johnston O. Further studies of the inheritance of hand and foot anomalies. *Clin Orthop* 1959;8:146–159.
8. Piggott H. The natural history of hallux valgus in adolescence and early adult life. *J Bone Joint Surg Br* 1960;42(4):749–760.
9. Kalen V, Brecher A. Relationship between adolescent bunions and flat feet. *Foot and Ankle* 1988;8:331–336.
10. Coughlin MJ, Mann RA. *The pathophysiology of the juvenile bunion.* Instructional course lectures, The American Academy of Orthopaedic Surgeons. Park Ridge, IL. 1987;36:123–136.
11. Kilmartin TE, Barrington RL, Wallace WA. A controlled prospective trial of foot orthosis for juvenile hallux valgus. *J Bone Joint Surg Br* 1994;76:210–214.

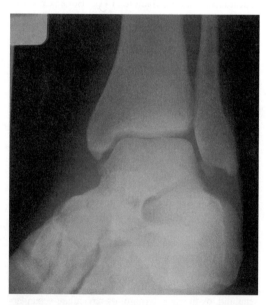

FIG. 38.5. Os vesalianum inferior to the fibula. Variable location. May be seen often at base of the fifth metatarsal and confused for fracture or secondary ossification center.

12. Ball J, Sullivan JA. Treatment of the juvenile bunion by Mitchell osteotomy. *Orthopedics* 1985;8:1249–1252.
13. Geissele AE, Stanton RP. Surgical treatment of adolescent hallux valgus. *J Pediatr Orthop* 1990;10:642–648.
14. Maresca G, Adriana E, Falez F, et al. Arthroscopic treatment of bilateral Freiberg's infraction. *The Journal of Arthroscopic and Related Surgery* 1996;12: 103–108.
15. Smillie I. Freiberg's infraction (Koehler's second disease). *J Bone Joint Surg Br* 1955;39:580.
16. Katcherian DA. Treatment of Freiberg's disease. *Orthop Clin North Am* 1994;25:69–81.
17. Gauthier G, Elbaz R. Freiberg's infraction: a subchondral bone fatigue fracture. A new surgical treatment. *Clin Orthop* 1979;142:93–95.
18. Thompson F, Hamilton W. Problems of the second metatarsophalangeal joint. *Orthopedics* 1987;10: 83–89.
19. Smith TWD, Stanley D, Rowley DI. Treatment of Freiberg's disease: a new operative technique. *J Bone Joint Surg Br* 1991;73:129–130.
20. Omer G. Primary articular osteochondroses. *Clin Orthop* 1981;158:33–41.
21. Bowers KD Jr, Martin RB. Turf-toe: a surface related football injury. *Med Sci Sports Exerc* 1976;8:81–83.
22. Jennings D, Gissane C. Turf-toe: super league toe [Letter]. *Br J Sports Med* 1997;31:164.
23. Hockenbury RT. Forefoot problems in athletes. *Med Sci Sports Exerc* 1999;31:S448–S458.
24. Bowers KD Jr, Martin RB. Impact absorption: new and old Astroturf at West Virginia University. *Med Sci Sports Exerc* 1974;6:217–221.
25. Rodeo SA, O'Brien S, Warren RF, et al. Turf-toe: analysis of metatarsophalangeal joint sprains in professional football players. *Am J Sports Med* 1990;18: 280–285.
26. Clanton TO, Ford JJ. Turf toe injury. *Clin Sports Med* 1994;13:731–741.
27. Gross TS, Bunch RP. A mechanical model of metatarsal stress fracture during distance running. *Am J Sports Med* 1989;17:669–674.
28. Sharkey NA, Ferris L, Smith TS, et al. Strain and loading of the second metatarsal during heel-lift. *J Bone Joint Surg Am* 1995;77:1050–1057.
29. Sullivan D, Warren RF, Pavlov H, et al. Stress fractures in 51 runners. *Clin Orthop* 1984;187:188–192.
30. Michelli LJ, Sohn RS, Soloman R. Stress fractures of the second metatarsal involving Lisfranc's joint in ballet dancers: a new overuse of the foot. *J Bone Joint Surg Am* 1985;67:1372–1375.
31. Harrington T, Crichton KJ, Anderson IF. Overuse ballet injury of the base of the second metatarsal. *Am J Sports Med* 1993;21:591–598.
32. O'Malley MJ, Hamilton WG, Munyak J, et al. Stress fractures at the base of the second metatarsal in ballet dancers. *Foot Ankle Int* 1996;17:89–94.
33. Brukner P, Bennell K, Matheson G. *Stress fractures*. Victoria, Australia: Blackwell Science, 1999:175–178.
34. Canale ST, Williams KD. Iselin's disease. *J Pediatr Orthop* 1992;12:90–93.
35. Lehman RC, Gregg JR, Torg E. Iselin's disease. *Am J Sports Med* 1986;14:494–496.
36. Brukner P, Bennell K, Matheson G. *Stress fractures*. Victoria, Australia: Blackwell Science, 1999
37. Richli WR, Rosenthal DJ, Avulsion fractures of the

38. Jones R. Fractures of the base of the 5th metatarsal bone by indirect violence. *Ann Surg* 1902;34:697–700.
39. Zogby RG, Baker BE. A review of nonoperative treatment of Jones fracture. *Am J Sports Med* 1987;15: 304–307.
40. Dameron TB. Fractures and anatomical variations of the proximal portion of the 5th metatarsal. *J Bone Joint Surg Am* 1975;57:788–792.
41. Torg JS, Balduini FC, Zelko RR, et al. Fractures of the base of the fifth metatarsal distal to the tuberosity : classification and guidelines for non-surgical and surgical management. *J Bone Joint Surg Am* 1984;66: 209–214.
42. Delee JC, Evans JP, Julian J. Stress fracture of the fifth metatarsal. *Am J Sports Med* 1983;11:349–353.
43. Zelko RR, Torg JS, Rachun A. Proximal diaphyseal fractures of the fifth metatarsal-treatment of the fractures and their complications. *Am J Sports Med* 1979; 7:95–101.
44. Weinfeld SB, Hadda SL, Myerson MS. Metatarsal stress fractures. *Clin Sports Med* 1997;16:319–338.
45. Woods L, Leach RE. Posterior tibial tendon rupture in athletic people. *Am J Sports Med* 1991;19:495–498.
46. Simpson RR, Gudas CJ. Posterior tibial tendon rupture in a world class runner. *J Foot Surg* 1983;22:74–77.
47. Frey C, Shereff M, Grenidge N. Vascularity of the posterior tibial tendon. *J Bone Joint Surg Am* 1990;72: 884–888.
48. Sachithanandam V, Joseph B. The influence of footwear on the prevalence of flat foot: a survey of 1846 skeletally mature persons. *J Bone Joint Surg Br* 1995;77:254–257.
49. Rao UB, Joseph B. The influence of footwear on the prevalence of flat foot: a survey of 2300 children. *J Bone Joint Surg Br* 1992;74:525–527.
50. Sullivan JA. Pediatric flatfoot: evaluation and management. *J Am Acad Orthop Surg* 1999;7:44–53.
51. Aharonson Z, Arcan M, Steinback TV. Foot-ground pressure pattern of flexible flatfoot in children, with and without correction of calcaneovalgus. *Clin Orthop* 1992;278:177–182.
52. Sakellariou A, Claridge RJ. Review: tarsal coalition. *Orthopedics* 1999;22:1066–1076.
53. Leonard MA. The inheritance of tarsal coalition and its relationship to spastic flat foot. *J Bone Joint Surg Br* 1974;56:520–526.
54. Stormont DM, Peterson HA. The relative incidence of tarsal coalition. *Clin Orthop* 1983;181:28–36.
55. Sullivan JA. Pediatric flatfoot: evaluation and management. *J Am Acad Orthop Surg* 1999;7:44–53.
56. Warren MJ, Jeffree MA, Wilson DJ, et al. Computed tomography in suspected tarsal coalition: examination of 26 cases. *Acta Orthop Scand* 1990;61:554–557.
57. Newman JS, Newberg AH. Congenital tarsal coalition: multimodality evaluation with emphasis on CT and MR imaging. *Radiographics* 2000;20:321–332.
58. Wechsler RJ, Schweitzer ME, Deely DM, et al. Tarsal coalition: depiction and characterization with CT and MR imaging. *Radiology* 1994;193:447–452.
59. Emery KH, Bisset GS, Johnson ND, et al. Tarsal coalition: a blinded comparison of MRI and CT. *Pediatr Radiol* 1998;28:612–616.
60. Deutsch AL, Resnick D, Campbell G. Computed to-

fifth metatarsal: experimental study of pathomechanics. *Am J Roentgenol* 1984;143:889–891.

mography and bone scintigraphy in the evaluation of tarsal coalition. *Radiology* 1982;144:137–140.

61. de Lima RT, Mishkin FS. The bone scan in tarsal coalition: a case report. *Pediatr Radiol* 1996;26:754–756.

62. Vincent KA. Tarsal coalition and painful flatfoot. *J Am Acad Orthop Surg* 1998;6:274–281.

63. McCormack TJ, Olney B, Asher M. Talocalcaneal coalition. *J Pediatr Orthop* 1997;17:13–15.

64. Brukner P, Bradshaw C, Khan KM, et al. Stress fractures: a review of 180 cases. *Clin J Sport Med* 1996;6: 85–89.

65. Brukner P, Bennell K, Matheson G. *Stress fractures.* Victoria, Australia: Blackwell Science, 1999.

66. Bennell KL, Brukner PD. Epidemiology and site specificity of stress fractures. *Clin Sports Med* 1997; 16:179–196.

67. Torg JS, Pavlov H, Cooley LH, et al. Stress fractures of the tarsal navicular: a retrospective review of twenty-one cases. *J Bone Joint Surg Am* 1982;62:700–712.

68. Khan KM, Fuller PJ, Brukner PD. Outcome of conservative and surgical management of navicular stress fracture in athletes. *Am J Sports Med* 1992;20: 657–666.

69. Quirk R. President's guest lecture. Stress fractures of the navicular. *Foot Ankle Int* 1998;19:494–496.

70. Quenu E, Kuss G. Etude sur les luxations du metatarse. *Reb Chir* 1909;39:281.

71. Taussig G, Hautier S. Les fractures-luxations de l'articulation de Lisfranc. *Ann Chir* 1969;23:1131–1141.

72. Englanoff G, Anglin D, Hutson HR. Lisfranc fracture-dislocation: a frequently missed diagnosis in the emergency department. *Ann Emerg Med* 1995;26:229–233.

73. Mantas JP, Burks RT. Lisfranc injuries in the athlete. *Clin Sports Med* 1994:13:719–730.

74. Aitken AP, Poulson D. Dislocations of the tarsometatarsal joint. *J Bone Joint Surg* 1963;45: 246–260.

75. Renstrom Per AFH, Kannus P. Injuries of the foot and ankle. In: DeLee JC, Drez D, eds. *Orthopedic sports medicine,* 1st ed. Philadelphia, WB Saunders, 1992: 1753–1755.

76. Cassebaum WH. Lisfranc fracture-dislocations. *Clin Orthop* 1963;30:116–129.

77. Faciszewski T, Burks RT, Manaster BJ. Subtle injuries of the Lisfranc joint. *J Bone Joint Surg Am* 1990;72: 1519–1522.

78. Myerson MS, Fisher RT, Burgess AR, et al. Fracture dislocations of the tarsometatarsal joints: end results correlated with pathology and treatment. *Foot Ankle* 1986;6:225–242.

79. Curtis MJ, Myerson M, Szura B. Tarsometatarsal joint injuries in the athlete. *Am J Sports Med* 1993;21: 497–502.

80. Wilson DW. Injuries of the tarso-metatarsal joints. Etiology, classification and results of treatment. *J Bone Joint Surg Br* 1972;54:677–686.

81. Wiley JJ. The mechanism of tarso-metatarsal joint injuries. *J Bone Joint Surg Br* 1971;53:474–482.

82. Kazian JD, Karlin JM, Scurran BL, et al. Lisfranc's fracture-dislocation: a review of the literature and case reports. *J Am Podiatr Med Assoc* 1991;81:531–539.

83. Leenan LP, van der Werken C. Fracture-dislocations of the tarsometatarsal joint, a combined anatomical and computed tomographic study. *Injury* 1992;23: 51–55.

84. Burroughs K, Reimer C, Fields K. Lisfranc injury of the foot: a commonly missed diagnosis. *Am Fam Physician* 1998;58:118–124.

85. Heckman JD. Fractures and dislocations of the foot. In: Rockwood CA, Green DP, Bucholz RD, eds. *Rockwood and Green's fractures in adults,* 3rd ed. Vol. 2. Philadelphia: Lippincott-Raven, 1991:2140–2151.

86. Hardcastle PH, Reschauer R, Kuscha-Lissberg E, et al. Injuries to the tarsometatarsal joint. Incidence, classification and treatment. *J Bone Joint Surg Br* 1982;64: 349–356.

87. Buzzard BM, Briggs PJ. Surgical management of acute tarsometatarsal fracture dislocation in the adult. *Clin Orthop* 353;125–133.

88. Arntz CT, Veith RG, Hansen ST Jr. Fractures and fracture dislocations of the tarsometatarsal joint. *J Bone Joint Surg Am* 1988;70:173–181.

89. Kohler A. A frequent disease of individual bones in children, apparently previously unknown. *Muench Med Wochenschr* 1908;55:1923.

90. Waugh W. The ossification and vascularization of the tarsal navicular and their relation to Kohler's disease. *J Bone Joint Surg Br* 1958;40:765.

91. Williams FA, Cowell HR. Kohler's disease of the tarsal navicular. *Clin Orthop* 1981;158:53–59.

92. Gips S, Ruchman RB, Groshar D. Bone imaging in Kohler's disease. *Clin Nucl Med* 1997;22:636–637.

93. Devine KM, Van Demark RE Sr. Kohler's osteochondrosis of the tarsal navicular: a case report with twenty-eight year followup. *SDJ Med* 1989;42:5–6.

94. Ippolito E, Ricciardi Pollini PT, Falez F. Kohler's disease of the tarsal navicular: a long term follow-up of 12 cases. *J Pediatr Orthop* 1984;4:416–417.

95. Borges JL, Guille JT, Bowen JR. Kohler's bone disease of the tarsal navicular. *J Pediatr Orthop* 1995;15: 596–598.

96. Sever JW. Apophysitis of the os calcis. *N Y Med J* 1912;95:1025–1029.

97. Madden CC, Mellion MB. Sever's disease and other causes of heel pain in adolescents. *Am Fam Physician* 1996;54:1995–2000.

98. Micheli LJ, Ireland ML. Prevention and management of calcaneal apophysitis in children: an overuse syndrome. *J Pediatr Orthop* 1987;7:34–38.

99. Crosby LA, McMullen ST. Heel pain in an active adolescent? Consider calcaneal apophys

100. Marsh JS, Daigneault JP. Ankle injuries in the pediatric population. *Curr Opin Pediatr* 2000;12:52–60.

101. Dolan AM, Mulcahy DM, Stephens MM. Osteochondritis dissecans of the head of the talus. *Foot Ankle Int* 1997;18:365–368.

102. Koch S, Kampen WU, Laprell H. Cartilage and bone morphology in osteochondritis dissecans. *Knee Surg Sports Traumatol Arthrosc* 1997;5:42–45.

103. Kappis M. Weitere Beitrage zur traumatisch-Mechanischen entstehung der "spontanen" Knorpelablosungen (sogen. Osteochondritis dissecans). *Deutsche Zschr Chir* 1922;171:13.

104. Pizzutillo P. The osteochondroses. In: Sullivan JA and Grana WA, ed. *The pediatric athlete: guidelines to participation.* Park Ridge, IL: American Academy of Orthopedic Surgeons, 1990.

105. Berndt AL, Harty M. Transchondral fractures of the talus. *J Bone Joint Surg Am* 1959;41:988–1029.

106. Canale ST, Beaty JH. Osteochondral lesions of the

talus. In: Hamilton WC, ed. *Traumatic disorders of the ankle*. New York: Springer-Verlag New York, 1984.

107. Anderson IF, Crichton KJ, Grattan-Smith T, et al. Osteochondral fractures of the dome of the talus. *J Bone Joint Surg Am* 1989;71:1143–1152.

108. De Smet AA, Fisher DR, Burnstein MI, et al. Value of MR imaging in staging osteochondral lesions of the talus (osteochondritis dissecans): results in 14 patients. *AJR Am J Roentgenol* 1990;154:555–558.

109. Huguera J, Laguna R, Peral M, et al. Osteochondritis dissecans of the talus during childhood and adolescence. *J Pediatr Orthop* 1998;18:328–332.

110. Tol JL, Struijs PAA, Bossuyt PMM, et al. Treatment strategies in osteochondral defects of the talar dome: a systematic review. *Foot Ankle Int* 2000;21:119–126.

111. Hangody L, Kish G, Karpati Z, et al. Treatment of osteochondritis dissecans of the talus: use of the mosaicplasty technique- a preliminary report. *Foot Ankle Int* 1997;18:628–634.

112. Pfeffer G, Bacchetti P, Deland J, et al. Comparison of custom and prefabricated orthoses in the initial treatment of proximal plantar fasciitis. *Foot Ankle Int* 1999; 20:214–221.

113. Tisdel C , Donley B, Sferra J. Diagnosing and treating plantar fasciitis: a conservative approach to plantar heel pain. *Cleve Clin J Med* 1999;66:231–235.

114. Kim W, Voloshin AS. Role of the plantar fascia in the load bearing capacity of the human foot. *J Biomech* 1995;28:1025–1033.

115. Louisia S, Masquelet AC. The medial and inferior calcaneal nerves: an anatomic study. *Surg Radiol Anat* 1999;21:169–173.

116. Glaser V. Osteoarthritis, shoulder impingement, cervical radiculopathy, plantar fasciitis. *Patient Care* 1999; July:176–202.

117. Schepsis A, Leach R, Gorzyca J. Plantar fasciitis. *Clin Orthop* 1991;266:185–196.

118. Intenzo C, Keith W, Chan P, et al. Evaluation of plantar fasciitis by three-phase bone scintigraphy. *Clin Nucl Med* 1991;16:325–328.

119. Cardinal E, Chhem RK, Beauregard CG, et al. Plantar fasciitis: sonographic evaluation. *Radiology* 1996;201: 257–259.

120. Gibbon W, Long G. Ultrasound of the plantar aponeurosis. *Skeletal Radiol* 1999;28:21–26.

121. Yu JS, Spigos D, Tomczak R. Foot pain after a plantar fasciotomy: an MR analysis to determine potential causes. *J Comput Assist Tomogr* 1999;23:707–712.

122. Chandler TJ, Kibler WB. A biomechanical approach to the prevention, treatment and rehabilitation of plantar fasciitis. *Sports Med* 1993;15:344–352.

123. Batt ME, Tanji JL, Skattum N. Plantar fasciitis: a prospective randomized clinical trial of the tension night splint. *Clin J Sport Med* 1996;6:158–162.

124. Powell M, Post WR, Keener J, et al. Effective treatment of chronic plantar fasciitis with dorsiflexion night splints: a crossover prospective randomized outcome study. *Foot Ankle Int* 1998;19:10–18.

125. Mizel MS, Marymont JV, Trepman E. Treatment of plantar fasciitis with a night splint and shoe modifications consisting of a steel shank and anterior rocker bottom. *Foot Ankle Int* 1996;17:732–735.

126. Dasgupta B, Bowles J. Scintigraphic localisation of steroid injection site in plantar fasciitis. *Lancet* 1995; 346:1400–1401.

127. Miller RA, Torres J, McGuire M. Efficacy of first-time steroid injection for painful heel syndrome. *Foot Ankle Int* 1995;16:610–612.

128. Leach RE, Jones R, Silva T. Rupture of the plantar fascia in athletes. *J Bone Joint Surg Am* 1978;60: 537–539.

129. Sellman JR. Plantar fascia rupture associated with corticosteroid injection. *Foot Ankle Int* 1994;15: 376–381.

130. Acevedo J, Baskin J. Complications of plantar fascia rupture associated with corticosteroid injection. *Foot Ankle Int* 1998;19:91–97.

131. Gudeman SD, Eisele SA, Heidt RS Jr, et al. Treatment of plantar fasciitis by iontophoresis of 0.4% dexamethasone. A randomized, double-blind, placebo-controlled study. *Am J Sports Med* 1997;25:312–316.

132. Kwong PK, Kay D, Voner RT, et al. Plantar fasciitis: Mechanics and pathomechanics of treatment. *Clin Sports Med* 1988;7:119–126.

133. Pfeffer G, Bacchetti P, Deland J, et al. Comparison of custom and prefabricated orthoses in the initial treatment of proximal plantar fasciitis. *Foot Ankle Int* 1999; 20:214–221.

134. Sammarco GJ, Helfrey RB. Surgical treatment of recalcitrant plantar fasciitis. *Foot Ankle Int* 1996;17: 520–526.

135. Murphy GA, Pneumaticos SG, Kamaric E, et al. Biomechanical consequences of sequential plantar fascia release. *Foot Ankle Int* 1998;19:149–152.

136. Thordarson DB, Kumar PJ, Hedman TP, et al. Effect of partial versus complete fasciotomy on the windlass mechanism. *Foot Ankle Int* 1997;18:16–20.

137. Arangio GA, Chen C, Kim W. Effect of cutting the plantar fascia on mechanical properties of the foot. *Clin Orthop* 1997;339:227–231.

138. Kiaoka HB, Luo ZP, An KN. Effect of plantar fasciotomy on stability of arch of foot. *Clin Orthop* 1997; 344:307–312.

139. Kruse RW, Chen J. Accessory bones of the foot: clinical significance. *Mil Medicine* 1995;160:464–467.

140. McDougall A. The os trigonum. *J Bone Joint Surg Br* 1955;37:257.

141. Le TA, Joseph PM. Common exostectomies of the rearfoot. *Clin Podiatr Med Surg* 1991;8:601–623.

142. Watson CA, Dobas DC. The os trigonum: discussion and a case report. *Arch Podiatr Med Surg* 1976;3:17.

143. Hamilton WG, Geppert MJ, Thompson FM. Pain in the posterior aspect of the ankle in dancers. *J Bone Joint Surg Am* 1996;78:1491–1500.

144. Martin BF. Posterior triangle pain: the os trigonum. *J Foot Surg* 1989;28:312–318.

145. Bellemans J, Reynders-Frederix PA, Stoffelen D, et al. Os trigonum and soleus tertius anomaly. *Acta Orthop Belg* 1993;59:412–414.

146. Chater EH. Foot pain and the accessory navicular bone. *Ir J Med Sci* 1962;442:471–475.

147. Bareither DJ, Muehleman CM, Feldman NJ. Os tibiale externum or sesamoid in the tendon of tibialis posterior. *J Foot Ankle Surg* 1995;34:429–434.

148. Sella EJ, Lawson JP. Biomechanics of the accessory navicular synchondrosis. *Foot Ankle* 1987;8:156–163.

149. Miller TT, Staron RB, Feldman F, et al. The symptomatic accessory tarsal navicular bone: assessment with MR imaging. *Radiology* 1995;195:849–853.

150. Macnicol MF, Voutsinas S. Surgical treatment of the

symptomatic accessory navicular. *J Bone Joint Surg Br* 1984;66:218–226.

151. Ray S, Goldberg V. Surgical treatment of the accessory navicular. *Clin Orthop* 1983;177:61–66.

152. Veitch JM. Evaluation of the Kidner procedure in treatment of symptomatic accessory tarsal scaphoid. *Clin Orthop* 1978;131:210–213.

153. Case DT, Ossenberg NS, Burnett SE. Os intermetatar-

seum: a heritable accessory bone of the human foot. *Am J Phys Anthropol* 1998;107:199–209.

154. Henderson RS. Os intermetatarseum and a possible relationship to hallux valgus. *J Bone Joint Surg Br* 1963; 45:117–121.

155. Jahss MH. *Disorders of the foot and ankle: medical and surgical management*, 2nd ed. Philadelphia: WB Saunders, 1991:69–71,1477–1479.

39

Special Problem Areas

James L. Moeller and Sami F. Rifat

Although no sport is associated with a unique set of injuries, some injuries have a tendency to occur more frequently in certain sports. This section discusses several injuries and conditions that are associated with many popular individual and team sports.

RUNNING

Running is an incredibly popular recreational and team sport around the world. Each year, millions of American children take to the streets or the track as a part of organized school and club teams. While runners do not suffer from any unique injury, several injuries and conditions are commonly encountered.

Runners, like most athletes, do not want their training and competition to be interrupted by injury. They also dislike prolonged periods of inactivity that may be required for injury rehabilitation. Physicians who care for runners should keep this in mind and, if possible, should devise a treatment regimen that protects the injured area but allows modified training or cross training to continue.

Medical Issues

Inadequate Nutrition

Prolonged or distance running places a great deal of stress on the child and adolescent body. Adequate fuel intake is therefore essential. In general, a well balanced diet adequately meets the nutritional needs of young athletes (see Chapter 4). Athletes should select their diet from a variety of wholesome foods, and they should consider the routine use of a multivitamin as the only supplementation of any benefit. Unfortunately, many young athletes do not eat a balanced diet, and they may thus suffer from one or more nutritional deficiencies. Inadequate iron, protein, and/or calcium intake are the most common nutritional deficiencies in the young runner.

Anemia can result from low iron levels that can be due to blood loss in the gastrointestinal tract, hemoly-sis and, in women, menses. A thorough evaluation of the young athlete noted to be anemic is warranted so that other medical causes of anemia can be excluded. If an evaluation by the primary care physician determines that the cause is related solely to iron deficiency, simple supplementation is the only intervention that is required.

Many adolescents do not consume adequate amounts of calcium in their diet, so they may require supplementation. The National Institute of Health Expert Panel recommends 1,200 to 1,500 mg of calcium per day for individuals from 11 to 24 years of age (1). Calcium is important for normal bone metabolism, and, if the dietary intake of calcium is inadequate, bone mineral density may decrease, placing the runner at an increased risk for developing a stress fracture.

Adequate calcium intake is particularly important in women because of the relationship between physical activity, estrogen levels, and calcium absorption. Peak bone deposition in women usually occurs in their late 20s or early 30s. Therefore, adequate calcium intake during adolescence is essential for optimizing the peak bone density.

Menstrual Dysfunction

Menstrual abnormalities are common in female endurance athletes. Menstrual dysfunction includes amenorrhea (both primary and secondary), oligomenorrhea, a shortened luteal phase, and anovulation. All of these abnormalities of menstrual cycles can occur as a result of the stress of running. The etiology of menstrual dysfunction in most young female endurance athletes, including runners, is generally multifactorial. A common component that is often noted is the decreased secretion of gonadotropin-releasing hormone (GnRH) from the hypothalamus. Because estrogen is essential for normal bone metabolism, prolonged menstrual dysfunction may lead to osteoporosis. Menstrual irregularities and osteoporosis may be compounded in many young female athletes by their disordered eating patterns. The combination of menstrual dysfunction, osteoporosis, and disordered eating is often termed the "female athlete triad" (see Chapter 13).

Despite the strong association between menstrual dysfunction and endurance training, the confirmation of the etiology of menstrual dysfunction remains a diagnosis of exclusion. The diagnosis and treatment of menstrual dysfunction is discussed in Chapter 13. Successful management of menstrual dysfunction in the young runner is dependent on decreasing the training and increasing the body weight. The reluctance of most athletes to comply with these recommendations often poses a significant clinical challenge.

Overtraining

Overtraining is often manifested in young runners by a complex of symptoms, including fatigue, irritability, and sleep disturbance. This condition often occurs when the young athlete increases his or her training intensity or duration. The physical examination and laboratory studies are typically normal. Often, the young athlete may feel depressed or angry before intervention due to the fact that his or her performance has plateaued (see Chapter 9). After the presence of systemic and depressive illness has been ruled out, the young runner should be urged to decrease his or her activity level, to focus on proper nutrition, and then to advance training slowly. The assistance of a sports psychologist in the care of these athletes is often a useful adjunct for successful management.

Gastrointestinal Problems

Approximately 25% of all runners will experience some sort of gastrointestinal disturbance. Pain, cramps, diarrhea, and heartburn are the most common symptoms reported by young runners. Exercise increases acid secretion in the gastrointestinal tract that may manifest as nausea, vomiting, or heartburn. Precompetition anxiety may exacerbate the hypersecretion. After other medical causes have been excluded, the athlete may benefit from a trial of an H-2 blocker or a proton pump inhibitor.

Gastroesophageal reflux with delayed gastric emptying is also a common gastrointestinal problem in runners, and it is managed with a treatment regimen similar to those noted above. Gastrointestinal hemorrhage has been reported in young endurance athletes, but this is usually self-limiting and it generally resolves within 3 days.

Other Medical Concerns

Other medical conditions, such as heat-related illness and/or injury, exercise-induced bronchospasm (EIB), and exercise-induced syncope, can occur in runners. These concerns are discussed elsewhere in this text.

Musculoskeletal Issues

Overuse Injury

Overuse is the most common injury mechanism among runners. Overuse injuries are often described as belonging to one of four types (2). In a type I injury, the athlete experiences pain after running, which sometimes makes relating the activity to the symptoms difficult for the athlete. In a type II overuse injury, the athlete experiences pain during activity, but no decrease in performance is seen; a type III injury, however, involves a decrease in performance. Finally, type IV overuse injuries are characterized by continuous pain (3).

Training errors account for approximately 80% of all overuse musculoskeletal injuries in runners. Simply doing too much too soon and too quickly causes injury. Abrupt increases in training intensity, duration, or frequency are the most common causes of overuse injury. Inadequate rest and nutrition contribute to these injuries. Changes in the running surface (soft to hard) or route (flat to hills) are examples of other common training errors.

In runners, the majority of chronic or overuse injuries involve the lower extremity, and approximately half of these affect the knee.

Patellofemoral Pain Syndrome

Patellofemoral stress syndrome (PFSS) is the most common injury seen among runners. The cause is multifactorial, possibly involving abnormal patellar tracking, muscle imbalance, or other biomechanical factors. This syndrome is also a frequent consequence of overtraining.

PFSS is characterized by anterior knee pain that is usually aggravated with kneeling, squatting, or stair climbing (descending is worse than ascending). The individual will often notice discomfort with prolonged sitting, which is often referred to as the "theater sign." Treatment of this symptom complex is usually conservative, consisting of relative rest, ice, analgesics, and rehabilitation programs that include vastus medialis obliquus (VMO) strengthening and lower extremity flexibility training. The VMO is a dynamic stabilizer of the patella, and any strength deficiency of the VMO may increase the risk that PFSS might develop in a runner. Depending on the severity of the symptoms, the runner will need to modify the training regimen (i.e., decrease its intensity or duration) or cross train with a nonpainful physical activity, such as biking or swimming.

Iliotibial Band Syndrome

Iliotibial band friction syndrome is a common problem in runners. It occurs when a tight iliotibial band is repeatedly rubbed over the prominence of the lateral femoral condyle at the knee. Runners typically complain of lateral knee pain that begins during a run and becomes progressively worse until the activity ceases. Physical examination findings vary widely. In less severely affected cases, runners with this condition may have physical examinations that are entirely normal. In more advanced cases, tenderness is found over the lateral femoral condyle, and a tight iliotibial band is noted when the examiner performs an Ober test. Treatment consists of relative rest, cross training, ice, and stretching. For more severely affected cases, physical therapy regimens that include phonophoresis or iontophoresis may be beneficial.

Medial Tibial Stress Syndrome

Medial tibial stress syndrome is another common problem among runners. This clinical entity probably accounts for the majority of cases known as "shin splints." The term "shin splints" simply refers to pain occurring between the knee and the ankle, and, by itself, it is not a discrete clinical entity. Medial tibial stress syndrome is a painful condition that is caused by irritation or inflammation of the periosteum and underlying bone that results from the repetitive stress of running or some other physical activity.

Runners with medial tibial stress syndrome typically complain of pain over the middle third of the medial aspect of the tibia. This area is often diffusely tender along the posteromedial aspect of the bone. Medial tibial stress syndrome can be associated with high arched feet and excessive pronation. Radiographs of the tibia are negative in medial tibial stress syndrome. However, in the early stages of this syndrome, a negative radiograph does not exclude the possibility of a tibial stress fracture. If a tibial stress fracture is a suspected, a radionucleotide bone scan should be obtained because routine radiographs often fail to detect stress fractures.

Treatment of medial tibial stress syndrome consists of relative rest, ice, cross training with low impact or nonimpact exercise, and lower extremity flexibility exercises. Because medial tibial stress syndrome may progress to, or be coincident with, a tibial stress fracture, careful instructions should be provided to the runner and his or her parents with regard to close monitoring of the signs and symptoms that may signal a need for additional evaluation and more aggressive management. The young athlete may attempt a gradual return to running when the symptoms have resolved.

Exertional Compartment Syndrome

Exertional compartment syndrome represents a painful condition in which intracompartmental pressure in one or more of the compartments in the leg increases during running. If intracompartmental pressure becomes excessive, normal compartmental processes are compromised, and muscle function, vascular circulation, and nerve function may be affected. Typically, the runner experiences pain that occurs at a specific point during exercise (e.g., at 1 mile). As the runner continues, pain symptoms progress until he or she is eventually forced to discontinue the training or competitive event. The symptoms usually resolve completely within several minutes of initiating rest. If nerve function is compromised, the individual may experience weakness, numbness, and tingling. If vascular structures are affected, the lower extremity may appear swollen, red, blue, or cold.

The examination may be unremarkable. Some individuals may have muscle tenderness or evidence of muscle herniation, which appears as a mass or bulge. The lower extremity may feel firm when compared to the unaffected side. The measurement of intracompartmental pressure can establish the diagnosis. Initial treatment consists of ice, relative rest, massage, and stretching. Unfortunately, conservative treatments are not always effective, and surgical fasciotomy may be needed. The success of surgery varies, depending on which compartment is affected. The best results are obtained with release of the anterior compartment, followed by that of the lateral, the superficial posterior, and, finally, the deep posterior compartments.

Stress Fractures

Lower extremity stress fractures are common in runners. Runners experience approximately 70% of

TABLE 39.1. *Sites of lower extremity stress fractures in runners*

Site	Percent (%)
Tibia	34
Fibula	24
Metatarsal	18
Femur	14
Pelvis	6
Miscellaneous	4

all stress fractures seen in athletes. Table 39.1 shows the distribution of lower extremity stress fractures in runners (4).

A young athlete with a stress fracture complains of localized pain that is aggravated by running or any weight-bearing activity. The runner will often complain of pain at rest and at night. Point tenderness at the site of the stress fracture is a common finding in the physical examination. Swelling, bruising, or a palpable enlargement of the bone may also be noted. Plain radiographs, although they are highly specific, are not highly sensitive for detecting stress fractures. Two-thirds of plain radiographs are negative initially, and only one-half of all stress fractures ever become visible on radiographs. Consequently, a nucleotide bone scan is the most definitive imaging tool for this condition.

The treatment of a stress fracture is generally conservative (4). Most rehabilitative protocols consist of rest, protected ambulation with crutches (if appropriate), ice, and analgesics. When the individual becomes asymptomatic, he or she may begin a gradual return to activity. Stress fractures at certain high-risk locations (Table 39.2) warrant referral to

TABLE 39.2. *High risk stress fractures*

Femur
  Neck
Patella
Tibia
  Transverse shaft, "dreaded black line"
Tarsal bones
  Navicular
  Cuneiform
Metatarsals
  5th metatarsal—"Jones fracture"
Pelvis
  Inferior pubic ramus
Lumbar spine
  Par interarticularis (spondylolysis)
  Facet
Calcaneus

a sports medicine specialist for definitive treatment.

Apophysitis

The tendinous insertion at a bony growth center is known as an apophysis. The insertion represents a structurally vulnerable point, and thus it is at risk for injury. When overuse precipitates irritation at one of these sites, the resulting clinical condition is an apophysitis. This condition occurs only in the skeletally immature athlete.

Common sites of apophysitis in a runner include the tibial tubercle (Osgood–Schlatter disease), the calcaneus (Sever disease), the anterior superior iliac spine (ASIS), and the iliac crest. The diagnosis and treatment of these injuries are discussed elsewhere in this text.

Other Overuse Conditions Affecting Runners

Young runners are at risk for other lower extremity overuse injuries, including tendinopathies at the quadriceps, patellar, and Achilles tendons. These have been discussed elsewhere in this text, and their treatment does not vary significantly in a runner.

Acute Injury

Although the majority of injuries affecting the young runner are overuse in nature, some acute injuries do occur.

Apophyseal Avulsions

Apophyseal avulsions can occur in sprinting athletes. These injuries are caused by a sudden, violent muscle contraction. Apophyseal avulsions always should be suspected in the skeletally immature sprinter, and the appropriate radiographs should be obtained. Table 39.3 describes several apophyseal avulsion fractures that are seen in the sprinting athlete.

Treatment of apophyseal avulsion fractures consists of protected weight bearing, ice, analgesics, and rest. These injuries typically take several weeks to heal. Activity may be slowly resumed once radiographic evidence of healing is seen, the area is no longer tender, and passive motion without pain is observed in the physical examination. Widely displaced avulsion fractures and symptomatic nonunions may require surgical repair.

TABLE 39.3. *Sites and signs of common avulsion injuries in runners*

Site	Tendon insertion	Physical findings
Anterior superior iliac spine (ASIS)	Sartorius	Tender ASIS Pain with resisted sartorius testing Pain with resisted hip flexion
Ishium	Hamstring	Pain with straight leg raise Pain with resisted knee flexion Tender ischial tuberosity
Lesser trochanter	Iliopsoas	Pain with flexion and extension of hip against resistance Pain with rotation of hip against resistance
Anterior inferior iliac spine	Rectus femoris	Pain with rectus femoris testing Pain with resisted hip flexion

Muscle Strains

Muscle strains are more likely to occur in the skeletally mature athlete. As the bone matures, the musculotendinous unit becomes the "weakest link" in the kinetic chain, and it subsequently has an increased risk of injury. Like apophyseal avulsion fractures, these injuries are more common among sprinters because of the explosive movement and high tension placed on the musculature in these events. The hamstrings and quadriceps are most commonly affected.

Initial treatment of muscle strains consists of rest, assisted ambulation (as necessary), ice, and gentle range of motion. As the young athlete's symptoms improve, stretching to regain or to improve baseline flexibility and strengthening exercises are added. Of crucial importance is the fact that the sprinting athlete must regain full range of motion and normal strength prior to his or her return to full activity, so that the risk of reinjury is reduced.

CYCLING

Millions of children take to the roads on their bicycles each year, and injuries due to cycling accidents are a major cause of visits to emergency rooms and physician offices. Most are recreational cyclists, using their bikes only as a means of transportation. Other forms of cycling, such as touring (distance riding), mountain biking, bicycle motocross (BMX), and stunt riding, can increase the risk of overuse and serious acute injury.

Medical Issues

Head Injuries

Head injuries are common in cycling. In an accident, if the cyclist's head endures a significant impact with the pavement or hard ground, a variety of injuries ranging from contusions and lacerations to concussions, skull fractures, and intracranial hemorrhage can occur. Higher speeds on the bike create greater injury forces; however, injuries that occur at low rates of speed can also be extremely serious. The consistent use of helmets by every child every time he or she gets on a bike is highly recommended. The use of helmets has significantly lowered the incidence of serious head injury in cyclists.

Simple contusions can be treated with ice. The initial treatment of lacerations includes direct pressure over the wound. While ice may decrease blood loss by causing vasoconstriction, direct pressure should be the first intervention. Scalp lacerations may bleed profusely, and primary closure is often needed. Facial lacerations may leave a cosmetically unsatisfactory outcome if they are allowed to heal by secondary intention. Decisions on the treatment of facial lacerations (e.g., sutures, skin glue, adhesive strips) should be made on a case-by-case basis.

Treatment of concussions is based on the severity of the injury. Many different grading systems for concussion are found, but none is considered to be the "gold standard." Minor concussions can be followed in the outpatient setting, while more serious injuries may require hospitalization for observation and diagnostic testing. Chapter 28 includes a full discussion of concussions.

Dermatology

Painful callous formations over the ischial tuberosities are commonly known as saddle sores. Various degrees of skin irritation may also be present. Padding of the bike saddle and the use of padded shorts may prevent or relieve the pain associated with this problem. If a contact or irritant dermatitis is also present, corticosteroid creams may be of benefit.

Nerve Injuries

Palmar hand numbness in the fourth and fifth fingers is a common complaint in avid cyclists. This ulnar neuropathy is caused by the direct pressure of the handlebars against the ulnar nerve at the Guyon canal. This injury is worsened by the repetitive impacts absorbed by the hands when a cyclist is riding on rough ground. Padded grips and gloves will decrease the impact forces, and thus they can be helpful in treating or preventing this problem. Newer handlebar designs also help alleviate pressure on the ulnar nerve.

The repetitive shocks absorbed at the wrist can also lead to carpal tunnel syndrome. Irritation of the median nerve at the wrist causes the classic symptoms of wrist pain, hand pain, burning, numbness, and weakened grip strength. The examination reveals atrophy of the thenar musculature and positive Tinel and Phalen tests. Wrist splints may be helpful, but most cyclists find them cumbersome to wear while riding.

Male Genitourinary Problems

Male cyclists may experience penile numbness due to pudendal nerve compression. Although this is anxiety-provoking, the problem is generally not serious. Thinner hard seats and long periods of time in the saddle are the causes. Changes in seat position, frequent standing during rides, or the use of a newly designed seat that relieves pressure on the pudendal nerve are appropriate and effective interventions.

Testicular torsion occurs most frequently in the neonatal and adolescent periods. In the older child and adolescent, it has been associated with cycling. Scrotal pain and swelling are the hallmarks of torsion. The physical examination may reveal an elevated testicle. No change in discomfort with elevation of the testicle above the level of the symphysis pubis (negative Prehn sign) increases the suspicion of testicular torsion, but this test is not extremely reliable. Scintigraphy or a Doppler ultrasound evaluation may be needed to confirm the diagnosis. Rapid urology referral is recommended.

Musculoskeletal Issues

Acute Injuries

Fractures of the forearm, wrist, and clavicle occur frequently from falls in cycling. Treatment of the fracture varies, depending upon location, the amounts of displacement or angulation, the growth plate involvement, and so forth. Pediatricians and other pri-mary care providers can adequately treat many fractures, but, if the clinician is uncomfortable with basic fracture care, referral to a sports medicine physician should be considered. Orthopedic surgery referral should be obtained for complicated fractures.

Other acute injuries, such as shoulder dislocation, do occur as a result of cycling, but these are relatively less common.

Overuse Injuries

Cyclists, especially those participating in competitive events, are likely to sustain overuse injuries. Most injuries involve the lower extremities, particularly the thigh and knee. Seat height may play a role in the development and treatment of some of these problems; however, no "appropriate seat height" is generally accepted as of yet.

Anterior Knee Pain

Many potential causes of anterior knee pain exist in children, any of which can be brought on or exacerbated by bicycle riding. The most common of these problems are Sinding–Larsen–Johansson disease (SLJ), Osgood–Schlatter disease, and PFSS.

Although SLJ is not truly a "disease," it is a cause of anterior knee pain that most commonly strikes children in the preteen years. It is more common in males than in females. Traction on the immature inferior pole of the patella causes pain at that site that is exacerbated by activity and relieved by rest. Persistent traction may lead to calcification and ossification. The physical examination reveals tenderness at the junction of the inferior pole of the patella and the patellar tendon. The remainder of the knee examination should be unremarkable. Radiographs may show varying degrees of calcification and/or ossification; however, in younger patients with a recent onset of symptoms, the radiographs are usually negative. Signs and symptoms of this overuse injury usually spontaneously resolve within 12 to 18 months. Raising the height of the bicycle seat can assist resolution of this process. Ice, nonsteroidal antiinflammatory drugs (NSAIDs), quadriceps stretching, and other activity modifications may help alleviate some of the symptoms.

Osgood–Schlatter disease is an extremely common cause of anterior knee pain in late preteen and early teenaged children. Traction at the tibial tubercle causes irritation, swelling, and pain at this apophysis. The patient presents with pain and swelling at the tibial tubercle. These signs and symptoms are easily confirmed on direct examination of the affected area. The remainder of the knee examination is typically normal. In general, radiographs are not helpful, as even a normal tubercle apophysis may appear fragmented on a lateral radiograph. Treatment is similar to that for SLJ. Older adolescents who are skeletally mature do not suffer from SLJ or Osgood–Schlatter disease. Once the apophyses can withstand the forces imparted by the quadriceps, these forces are transmitted to, and are more prone to cause irritation in, the weakest link in the kinetic chain, the patellar tendon. Consequently, patellar tendonitis is a common cause of anterior knee pain in the mid to late teenage group. Quadriceps stretching, ice, massage, NSAID use, seat height adjustment, and a patellar knee sleeve with a superior buttress pad are useful in treating this disorder.

PFSS is probably the most common cause of anterior knee pain in most age groups. Pain develops because of friction between the subpatellar chondral surface and the trochlea of the femur. The patient presents with a complaint of anterior knee pain that is often described as being located along the sides of the patella, under the patella, and between the patella and femur. The pain is typically worse with activity, but it may be especially worse after spending prolonged period in a sitting position. Normal daily activities, such as ascending and/or descending stairs, kneeling, squatting, and getting up from a seated position, may be painful.

The examination reveals a ligamentously stable joint that is painful with grind testing, in which the examiner holds the patella down against the femur, while the patient activates the quad complex. Pain, with or without crepitus, is a positive test. The patient also may report pain with palpation of the patellar facets. Poor medial quadriceps muscle strength, genu valgum, tibial torsion, and foot pronation are physiologic factors that may increase the risk or severity of PFSS. In cycling, a low seat position and the consistent use of high gears are risk factors for developing this pain syndrome. Vastus medialis obliquous (i.e., medial quadriceps) strengthening, ice, massage, NSAID use, and seat height adjustment should be used as initial therapeutic interventions. A patellar knee sleeve with buttress padding may help some patients, and its use should be considered.

Iliotibial Band Syndrome

Iliotibial band syndrome (ITBS) is a cause of lateral knee pain in cyclists. This entity is more common in the late adolescent age group than it is in younger individuals. It is a friction syndrome that develops due to repetitive motion of the ITB over the lateral femoral condyle. When the knee is in extension, the ITB is positioned anterior to the condyle. When the knee is flexed, the ITB crosses the condyle to a posterior position. Patients present with lateral knee pain, and they have tenderness over the lateral femoral condyle that is worsened with knee flexion and/or extension. The Ober test is positive. Treatment includes ice, massage, NSAIDs, ITB stretching, and activity modification. If the bike seat is too high, the knee achieves a greater extension angle, increasing the athlete's likelihood of developing ITBS. This condition may be prevented or ameliorated by keeping the seat in a lower position.

General Recommendations

Every bike rider, regardless of age and biking experience, should wear a helmet every time he or she rides. Limiting distractions (e.g., avoiding the use of personal listening devices) may decrease the likelihood of acute injuries. Cyclists expect drivers to treat them with respect and to follow the rules of the road. Cyclists also should learn the rules of safe cycling, especially in situations in which different types of vehicles are sharing the same roadway. Cyclists should respect other cyclists and other drivers and should make defensive riding a priority for safe travel. Finally, to avoid overuse injuries, the bike needs to fit the rider, and his or her equipment needs to be maintained in good working order.

SKATING

Many forms of skating are enjoyed today. Ice skating can be recreational or sport related (e.g., ice hockey, figure skating, and speed skating). Many children and adolescents inline skate for both recreation and competition. Although the skating motion is similar in all of these activities, injury patterns vary between the specific sports.

Medical Issues

Exercise-Induced Bronchospasm

Although medical and musculoskeletal problems vary, depending on the specific sport, EIB is a common medical problem encountered in all forms of ice skating.

EIB is frequently encountered in athletes who practice and compete in cold, dry climates. Airway hyperreactivity occurs shortly (6 to 10 minutes) after the onset of intense activity. Ninety percent of children with underlying asthma will demonstrate an exercise-induced component, but this entity can also exist in people without baseline asthma (incidence is approximately 10%). Children with environmental allergies also have an increased risk of EIB (5).

Most commonly, the young athlete will present with a history of cough, shortness of breath, wheezing, and/or chest tightness that occurs shortly after the onset of strenuous activity. When the individual is examined in the office, the cardiopulmonary examination is likely to be normal. An in-office exercise challenge may bring on symptoms and physical findings, although the ambient temperature, humidity, and physical challenge may be insufficient to trigger signs and symptoms of EIB.

Although many physicians feel that treatment based on history is appropriate, the diagnosis and treatment may be more precise when both baseline and exercise-challenged pulmonary function testing (PFT) is obtained prior to initiating interventions. The reasons for testing are twofold as follows: (a) testing may identify a child with underlying asthma who may benefit from long-term, as opposed to pre-exercise, treatment and (b) other conditions (e.g., cardiac diseases, other lung diseases, vocal cord dysfunction, gastroesophageal reflux disease) may mimic EIB. Peak flow testing, although it is less accurate, can be done in the office, and it is often substituted for the full PFT. A baseline PFT should be performed, and, when appropriate, a postexercise (6-minute to 10-minute exercise challenge at 85% of maximal predicted heart rate) test also should be conducted. A drop of 15% or more in forced expiratory volume at 1 second (FEV_1) is diagnostic of EIB. If the testing facility does not have the ability to perform an appropriate exercise challenge test, a methacholine challenge can be utilized. Typically, a β-agonist is then given to ensure a return to the baseline PFT levels.

A short-acting inhaled β-agonist (e.g., albuterol) that is used 15 to 30 minutes prior to exercise is the medication intervention for this condition. Other medications, such as longer acting β-agonists (e.g., salmeterol) and inhaled mast cell stabilizers (e.g., cromolyn sodium), are also effective. In patients with underlying asthma, inhaled corticosteroids should be considered a mainstay of long-term therapy. Newer agents, such as leukotriene inhibitors, are proving to be quite helpful in the treatment of asthma, and their effectiveness in the treatment of EIB has shown promise. A more thorough discussion of EIB is found in Chapter 18.

Musculoskeletal Issues

Muscle strains are the most common musculoskeletal problem encountered in skating. The power of skating is generated mainly from the hip, gluteal, and thigh (i.e., hamstring and quadriceps) musculature, and the adductor musculature then assists in bringing the legs back to a midline position. Typically, the muscles are injured when they are being stretched while trying to contract.

Young skaters often present with pain in a particular muscle region, rather than in an individual muscle. Direct palpation of the muscle group and muscle contraction against resistance causes tenderness. Weakness may or may not be present. Young athletes have many apophyses located throughout the pelvis. The relative bony weakness of these areas necessitates a cautious, yet thorough, examination. Strong muscle contraction can avulse these bony areas. A pelvic bony avulsion is treated with periods of rest (and often crutch ambulation) prior to the onset of rehabilitation; most muscle strains, however, can be treated aggressively with active rehabilitation.

ICE HOCKEY

Ice hockey is a collision sport. Because of this, traumatic medical and musculoskeletal injuries are frequently encountered. In the United States, younger age groups have eliminated body checking in an attempt to lower the rate of injury. Checking from behind also has been ruled an illegal tactic in an attempt to protect young athletes against cervical spine injuries. Equipment changes have eliminated some problems; however, many children do not wear the proper equipment when they are playing on a pond or backyard rink.

Medical Issues

Head Injuries

Closed head injuries are more frequently being recognized in hockey players. Even though helmets are considered mandatory equipment at all levels of organized hockey, the numbers of reported concussions have increased. This increased incidence may possibly be due to an increased awareness of this problem among parents, coaches, and physicians. The advent of the seamless glass that surrounds many rinks today may also be a factor, as this type of glass may be more rigid and less forgiving to contact. Chapter 28 contains a full discussion of concussions.

Facial Injuries

The incidence of eye, facial, and dental injuries due to hockey have decreased since the introduction of the protective facemask and the mandatory use of mouth guards in youth hockey. Once a quite common cause of trips to local emergency centers, these injuries are now seldom seen.

Genitourinary Injuries

The padding in properly fitting hockey pants provides a degree of protection for the kidneys. Flack jackets can be worn for added flank protection. Renal contusions do occur in youth ice hockey in spite of the regulation requiring the use of protective gear. When renal contusion is documented by hematuria and a physical examination, conservative management is most often indicated. Most cases resolve with time and observation. Testicular trauma is a risk primarily if the athlete is not wearing a protective cup.

Musculoskeletal Issues

Contusions

Contusions are one of the most common musculoskeletal injuries encountered in ice hockey, due to the contact and collision nature of the game (6). While these types of injuries are highly common, they can be severe enough to warrant extensive medical care. The puck is a 6-oz piece of vulcanized rubber that can reach speeds of over 75 mph in youth hockey. The force generated by this object can easily result in contusions in both protected and unprotected soft tissue structures. Contact with the boards, the goal structure, an opponent's hockey stick, and an opposing player are other common causes of contusions in young hockey players. Careful examination of the injured area should be performed as soon as possible after the injury to assess the severity and depth of the contusion. Superficial contusions require only close observation and protection from further injury. Deeper and more extensive contusions, particularly those in the quadriceps and biceps, also require close observation and protection because these injuries may be associated with hematoma formation in the muscle groups. Aggressive management, including immobilization and compression, may be required to prevent the development of myositis ossificans in the injured muscle.

Fractures

Extremity fractures are relatively uncommon in ice hockey, compared to other youth sports. The two most common mechanisms of fracture are falls and contact with other players, equipment, and the barriers surrounding the rink.

Clavicle fractures are among the more common fractures seen in hockey. Most midshaft clavicle fractures, even with displacement, can be treated with a sling, a figure-of-eight splint, or a combination of the two. Proximal one-third and distal one-third fractures should be evaluated by a sports medicine or an orthopedic surgical specialist. Fractures associated with skin or neurovascular compromise should be treated by an orthopedic surgeon.

Fractures to the facial bones, especially the mandible and the nasal bones, are encountered in ice hockey at all levels of play. The severity of the injury and the presence or absence of injury to the adjacent organs (i.e., the teeth or eyes) will determine the necessity and appropriate direction of subspecialty referral. The proper and consistent use of facemasks will decrease this risk.

Acromioclavicular Sprains

Acromioclavicular (AC) sprain injuries are more common in the older adolescent athlete. AC sprains occur when the top of the shoulder makes contact with another player, the boards, or the ice, thus driving the shoulder inferiorly. The clavicle strikes the first rib and stops its motion, while the acromion sustains further inferior displacement. This forceful motion places varying degrees of stress on the coracoacromial, coracoclavicular, and AC ligaments.

A stretch injury of the coracoacromial ligament with no displacement of the AC joint is classified a type I injury. Type II injuries show a mild to moderate displacement of the clavicle. Injuries are classified as type III when the clavicle is completely displaced from the acromion (7). Type I, II and III injuries can be treated conservatively if no significant overlying skin damage or neurovascular compromise of the affected extremity is present. The athlete must be made aware of the possibility that this injury may result in a noticeable defect, and the physician should confirm that the final cosmetic appearance is acceptable to the patient. Treatment of AC separations consists of applying a sling for comfort, ice, and antiinflammatory or analgesic medication use. Residual problems with joint stiffness and limited range of motion may be decreased if the athlete begins range-of-motion exercises early in rehabilitation. Initially, passive range-of-motion exercises should be performed below the pain threshold level. As range of motion improves and the discomfort level decreases, active range of motion across a wider range can be initiated. When range-of-motion exercises can be performed in a relatively pain-free fashion through the entire functional range of the joint, strengthening exercises may be initiated.

Special AC pads can be worn under the usual shoulder pads upon return to play in order to improve the athlete's comfort and possibly to decrease the risk of additional injury. AC injuries that have prolonged symptoms, neurovascular compromise, significant associated soft tissue damage, and special return-to-play considerations will often prompt the primary care physician to refer the young athlete to a sports medicine specialist. The more serious type IV, V, and VI injuries all should be referred to an orthopedic surgeon for treatment.

FIGURE SKATING

Many figure skaters begin skating lessons that include long hours of practice at a very young age. Overuse injuries are common, and they are similar, in some ways, to the overuse injuries seen in dancers. Acute injuries typically occur due to falls. The lower extremity injuries seen in figure skating are relatively sports-specific because of the structural characteristics of the boots that are worn. As in many sports in which the judging of the competition includes a subjective component of style and image, athletes who compete in the sport of figure skating are at risk for the development of eating disorders.

Medical Issues

Eating Disorders

Anorexia nervosa and bulimia nervosa are encountered commonly in sports where aesthetics is important for judging purposes (see Chapter 9). These sports include, among others, gymnastics, diving, and figure skating.

An athlete who suffers from anorexia nervosa has a symptom complex that includes several of the following characteristics: (a) refusal to maintain body weight at or above a minimally normal weight for age and height (85% of expected weight); (b) intense fear of gaining weight or becoming fat, even though the patient is underweight; (c) altered body image; and (d) amenorrhea in postmenarcheal females (8). The prevalence of anorexia nervosa is about 1% in the adolescent and young adult female population. The actual incidence of anorexia nervosa in specific sports, at specific ages, is difficult to determine.

Bulimia nervosa is more prevalent in the general population than it is in these athletes (1% to 3%); however, as in the case of anorexia nervosa, the incidence of bulimia nervosa among young male and female skaters is difficult to determine. The diagnostic criteria for bulimia nervosa include the following: (a) recurrent episodes of binge eating, characterized by eating a larger than "normal" amount of food in a discrete period of time and a sense of lack of control over eating during the episodes; (b) recurrent inappropriate compensatory behavior in order to prevent weight gain (e.g., self-induced vomiting, laxative use); (c) occurrence of the above activities, on average, at least twice weekly for 3 months; (d) self evaluation that is unduly influenced by body shape and weight; and (e) an occurrence of the disturbance that is not exclusively confined to episodes of anorexia nervosa (8).

Coaches and parents may unknowingly put their young athletes at risk for developing an eating disorder by inadvertent remarks. As with many elite young athletes, many young ice skaters tend to be perfectionists and overachievers. A coach or parent may make what he or she perceives as a simple comment, such as "Your skating dress is getting a little tight." In intensely competitive young athletes, an innocuous sounding comment such as that may actually cause a young skater to experience feelings of self-doubt and fear of losing acceptance in the sport because his or her weight is outside of an acceptable range.

Once a primary care sports medicine physician recognizes an eating disorder, the nutritional status and the overall health of the young athlete are of utmost importance. Anorexia nervosa and bulimia nervosa should be considered potentially life-threatening conditions. Treatment needs to be started immediately and aggressively. Behavioral therapy and nutritional interventions should be initiated as part of a multidisciplinary approach to treatment.

Musculoskeletal Issues

Back Pain

In adults, most back pain complaints are due to either muscular strain or disc pathology. Empiric treatment can often be initiated safely. If symptoms fail to improve, a more specific diagnostic workup is then initiated. Back pain in a child or adolescent, however, should prompt an early aggressive workup to identify an underlying cause prior to the initiation of significant therapeutic interventions.

Spondylolysis is the most common cause of low back pain in active adolescents who seek medical attention for pain (9).

Repetitive hyperextension activities are felt to be the primary cause of this injury. The stress of landing multiple jumps and layback spins puts the posterior elements of the spinal column at risk for injury, especially in young athletes. While spondylolysis is more likely to occur in boys than in girls, sponylolisthesis, a bilateral spondylolysis that results in anterior or posterior slippage of the adjacent vertebral segments, is more common in girls. A family history of spondylolysis or the presence of spina bifida occulta are considered additional risk factors for the development of this condition.

Young athletes who have spondylolysis usually present with unilateral low back pain. Less often, they may experience bilateral symptoms. In most cases, no radiation of discomfort, no radicular symptoms, no loss of bowel or bladder control, and no history of fevers, sweats, chills, or unexplained weight loss are present. The young athlete may have a history of trauma, due to their physically active lifestyle. Pain is typically worsened by activity, especially that which involves an upright position or hyperextension activities. The discomfort often is partially relieved by rest.

Physical examination of the young athlete's lower back usually reveals tenderness in the paravertebral muscles. Lateral bending, rotation to the side of the injury, and hyperextension of the lower back, especially while the athlete is standing on one leg (stork test), may all increase the patient's pain. When the history and physical examination are consistent with spondylolysis, radiographs should be obtained. Many lesions can be identified on anteroposterior (AP) and lateral projections alone; however, oblique views are useful when looking for radiolucent changes at the neck region of the "Scotty dog" (see Chapter 30). AP views also are helpful in determining the presence of spina bifida occulta, and the lateral view is necessary for diagnosing spondylolisthesis. A radiolucent defect on standard radiograph examination does not determine whether the lesion is active or if it is already in the healing phase. In order to determine the age and stage of healing of the injury, a radionucleotide bone scan should be obtained. If further studies are indicated, computerized tomography (CT) or magnetic resonance imaging (MRI) may provide the clinician with additional information about the bony lesion or the presence or absence of soft tissue lesions.

Active spondylolysis lesions are managed conservatively. Initial management of these lesions involves restricting the athlete from activity in competition, practice, and training that involves hyperextension and other movements of the lower back. Ice and/or heat may provide comfort, and these modalities can be used alone or in a contrast pattern. Acetaminophen or NSAIDs also can alleviate the discomfort. A rehabilitation program that incorporates lower extremity flexibility with an abdominal strengthening and trunk stabilization program can be initiated. If these initial measures are unsuccessful, bracing with a thoracolumbarsacral orthosis may be needed. Bracing should be used in conjunction with the rehabilitation regimen outlined above. Following successful rehabilitation of spondylolysis, activities should be introduced at an extremely low level of intensity, with a slow progression to full activity. Primary care physicians who do not regularly treat spondylolysis should strongly consider referring patients to a sports medicine physician.

Spondylolisthesis presents with clinical symptoms similar to spondylolysis. A lateral radiograph is used to determine the degree of anterior or posterior displacement of the adjacent vertebral bodies. The progression of spondylolisthesis should be closely monitored during an adolescent's maximum linear growth stage due to the increase risk of vertebral body displacement during this period. Many patients with a grade I injury (less than 25% displacement) are asymptomatic, and these individuals can compete normally without symptoms or long-term problems. Larger degrees of displacement may require a thoracolumbarsacral orthosis, and, if the degree of displacement increases or neurological compromise develops, surgical intervention may be necessary.

Fibular Stress Fractures

Stress fractures in the lower leg are common in many sports, including ice skating. In the lower leg, the tibia bears the majority of force compared to the fibula. For this reason, tibial stress fractures are quite common in upright sports that involve running and jumping; however, primary care physicians need to be cognizant of the possibility for fibular stress fractures in figure skating. Most of these injuries occur in the area of the fibula that corresponds to the top of the skating boot. The compressive force of the skating boot at this location is thought to play a role in the development of fibular stress fractures. An additional factor is the fact that figure skaters, unlike other jumping athletes, do not jump straight up and down. Take off and landing occur while leaning on either the inside or outside of the foot, known as inside and outside edges of the skate blade, respectively. Outside edge activities place increased stress on the peroneal musculature and fibula and contribute to the risk of fibular stress fracture. Other risk factors for the development of fibular stress fractures in young skaters include poor diet (primarily poor calcium and vitamin D intake), abnormal foot mechanics, poor jumping and/or landing mechanics, muscle imbalances, improperly fitting boots, and menstrual irregularities.

Patients with fibular stress fractures present with lateral lower leg pain that is worsened by activity and relieved by rest. In more severe cases, routine daily activities may cause discomfort. Usually, no specific history of trauma to the area is seen. The patient may report soft tissue swelling with this type of injury, but, less often, the individual reports ecchymosis, erythema, and paresthesias or other evidences of neurovascular compromise. Palpation of the affected area during the physical examination reveals tenderness along the fibula that may mimic isolated peroneal muscle and/or tendon tenderness. Significant swelling along the surface of the fibula increases the likelihood that a stress fracture is present. Testing muscle strength against resistance may provoke tenderness in the affected area; however, a positive finding in this component of the physical examination may not be helpful for differentiating between a stress fracture of the fibula and simple soft tissue injuries to muscles and tendons in the lower leg. Use of a tuning fork to elicit tenderness with vibratory stimulus may provide additional evidence of the presence of stress fracture.

Radiographs should be obtained whenever fibular pain is present. Periosteal thickening, periosteal elevation, or the presence of a cortical lucency are all positive radiographic findings that are consistent with the presence of a stress fracture. If radiographs are negative but symptoms persist or the clinical index of suspicion for a fibular stress fracture remains high, a bone scan should be obtained. A definitive diagnosis confirming the presence or absence of a stress fracture of the fibula is of great importance because the treatment for stress fracture differs drastically from that of muscle strains and tendinopathies. When these are treated inappropriately, the young athlete may experience an adverse outcome (e.g., progression to a completed fibular fracture). If a stress fracture progresses to a complete fracture, he or she may have to add a prolonged period of immobilization and inactivity to the rehabilitation regimen.

Treatment of fibular stress fractures includes addressing factors that may play a role in the development of this lesion and removing the athlete from activities that result in high stress to the injured bone. If the patient has pain with routine activity, restriction to non–weight-bearing or partial weight-bearing activity may be of benefit. To facilitate healing of the fracture,

however, crutches should be weaned as soon as the pain permits because weight bearing stimulates bone metabolism. The young athlete may begin progressing to more vigorous physical activity when the signs and symptoms of the stress fracture have resolved and when he or she is able to perform routine activities of daily living in a pain-free manner. During this rest period, the athlete should be encouraged to remain as physically active as possible by engaging in activities that do not cause pain to the injured area. This continuing physical activity prevents deconditioning both from a muscular and a cardiovascular standpoint. These activities may include bicycling, swimming, water running, and some resistance training. Once the decision to return to sports activity has been made, activities should start at low intensity, with a slow progression back to full activity.

Muscle Strains and Tendinopathy

Muscle strains and tendonitis (perhaps, more appropriately, tendinosis) are extremely common overuse injuries in figure skaters. Although a great deal of the power for skating and jumping is generated from the hip, gluteal, and thigh musculature, the foot and ankle plantar flexors also play a large role in the development fo speed and the fine control of jumping and landing. For this reason, the muscles and tendons involved in foot and ankle plantarflexion are exposed to a high degree of eccentric activity, as well as a high risk of injury. These muscles and tendons include the gastrocnemius and soleus muscles that make up the Achilles tendon. They also include the tibialis posterior, flexor hallucis, the flexor digitorum muscles and tendons on the medial side of the ankle, and the peroneal longus and brevis muscles and tendons on the lateral side of the ankle.

Many muscle and tendon injuries can be treated aggressively with rehabilitation while the athlete continues to skate at a decreased level of intensity. A general program of muscle stretching and endurance training is initiated as soon as pain permits. Pain, swelling, and inflammation can be treated with a combination of compression, elevation, ice, and NSAIDs. Activities should be performed below the soreness threshold, which can be remembered by the mnenomic REST. (*REST* = *r*esume *e*xercise below the *s*oreness *t*hreshold). In more severe cases, electrical stimulation and ultrasound may be beneficial. In cases in which the signs and symptoms of injury are severe and more refractive to these interventions, iontophoresis or phonophoresis may prove helpful.

Malleolar Bursitis

An interesting entity described almost exclusively in figure skaters is malleolar bursitis. Typically, bursae do not develop over the malleoli; however, adventitial bursae may develop in this region if the ankle is exposed to consistent stress and friction forces. Because of long hours in the skating boot, a great deal of friction develops over the malleoli, and some skaters will develop such an adventitial bursa. This bursa can grow large enough to cause the skating boot to fit improperly, which worsens the friction, creating an inflammatory cycle. Many skaters present with this problem as a result of the swelling, rather than pain.

The diagnosis of maleolar bursitis is usually straightforward. Neither a history of trauma to the affected area nor a significant history of pain are elicited. Fluctuant swelling is located directly over the malleolus. Radiographs are of limited value in making an accurate diagnosis. If infection of the bursa is suspected based on clinical signs and symptoms (e.g., pain, fever, erythema, adenopathy), the laboratory evaluation of the bursal fluid will assist in diagnosis and will aid in prescribing the correct antibiotic.

Malleolar bursitis does not respond well to simple conservative measures (10). Boot stretching to allow proper fit of the skate may be helpful, but this may not solve the problem entirely. Aspiration of the bursal fluid may be both diagnostic and therapeutic. After the area is appropriately prepared, a large gauge needle is used to aspirate the thick gelatinous fluid. The viscosity of the fluid may make aspiration through a small bore needle difficult or impossible. If the fluid is clear and no microscopic evidence of infection exists, a small amount of corticosteroid can be injected in an attempt to decrease the inflammation within the bursa. A pressure wrap should then be applied. Subsequently, ice and NSAIDs can be used to lessen the chance of fluid reaccumulation. Even with appropriate interventions, the risk of fluid reaccumulation is high, and surgical excision of the bursae may be required in more refractive cases.

INLINE SKATING

Inline skating is an activity performed by millions of children every day. The most common injuries associated with inline skating are falls on cement and asphalt that result in fractures, contusions, head injury, abrasions, and lacerations. Many of these injuries are not unique to inline skating, and they have been discussed in other chapters in this book. All children who engage in any type of roller skating, whether inline or parallel, should wear an approved helmet. Other protective equipment that is strongly recommended includes hard knee and elbow padding and wrist guards.

Musculoskeletal Issues

Growth Plate Fractures

Growth plate fractures are common in children and adolescents. The epiphyseal plate is the "weak link" in the skeletal system, and, as such, it is highly susceptible to injury. Severity of growth plate injury is based on the amount of growth plate involvement, as well as the presence or absence of fracture extension into the metaphysis or epiphysis. The Salter–Harris classification system (see Chapter 26, Fig. 26.3) is the generally accepted method of classification for these injuries (11). The higher the number corresponding to the injury is on the Salter–Harris scale, the greater the likelihood of complications and/or poor outcome.

Primary care physicians should feel comfortable treating most type I injuries. In the setting of the appropriate mechanism of injury, pain over an open growth plate is diagnostic of a growth plate fracture, even in absence of abnormal radiographic findings. In a nondisplaced Salter type I fracture, splinting may be all that is needed for appropriate treatment.

Primary care physicians with appropriate training and expertise may feel comfortable treating Salter type II and III injuries. Because of the increased risk of poor outcome, a sports medicine or orthopedic referral should be considered, unless the physician has sufficient experience with managing these categories of fractures. Most Salter type IV injuries and all Salter type V injuries should be referred to an orthopedic surgeon for evaluation and treatment. An incorrect diagnosis or improper treatment can lead to poor outcomes, including growth arrest of the affected extremity, in the pediatric population.

Wrist Fractures

A fall onto an outstretched arm is the classic mechanism of injury for many wrist problems, including fractures. Fractures of the distal radius and ulna are commonly encountered in inline skaters. The history of the injury typically includes a fall onto an outstretched arm and immediate pain in the arm or wrist. The child or parent may notice a gross deformity, although the majority of cases show no external evidence of a bony defect. The patient also may report numbness in the hand and wrist distal to the site of injury. A physical examination of the injured area reveals pain on palpation, and the examiner may detect a step-off or another palpable bony deformity and crepitus. The neurovascular status of the extremity distal to the point of injury should be tested carefully and documented. If a fracture is suspected, radiographs should be obtained prior to vigorous motion, stress, or strength testing.

Nondisplaced or minimally displaced fractures of the distal radius and/or ulna can be treated with cast immobilization. The choice of long-arm versus short-arm cast depends on the location and severity of the break. Risks, such as malunion and nonunion, should be discussed with the athlete and the athlete's parents. In skeletally immature athletes, the risk of growth arrest must also be discussed if the epiphyseal plate is involved. Repeat radiographs should be performed 4 to 6 weeks after the initial injury to document healing. Moderately to severely displaced fractures or fractures that involve compromise of the extremity distal to the point of injury should be reduced and should subsequently be managed by an orthopedic surgeon.

Scaphoid Fractures

Scaphoid fractures in the wrist deserve special attention because of the risk of malunion and nonunion. Because of this risk, these injuries should be treated by physicians who have a great deal of experience in fracture care. The most common mechanism of injury in scaphoid fractures is a fall onto an outstretched arm. Many young athletes who have sustained an injury to the wrist that has resulted in a fracture to the scaphoid present to the primary care physician with pain on the radial aspect of the wrist. Other signs and symptoms, such as bruising, swelling, numbness, and tingling, are less consistent. Pain with palpation in the anatomical snuffbox is a reliable physical finding that should alert the clinician to the possibility of a scaphoid fracture. If pain in this area is a consistent finding, radiographs should be obtained. If the radiographs are negative, the young athlete should be treated for a presumptive scaphoid fracture by the application of a short-arm thumb spica cast. Follow-up radiographs in 10 to 14 days may confirm the presence of healing. If the radiographs remain negative but the physical examination results are consistent with a scaphoid fracture, a bone scan or CT scan may be useful for confirming the diagnosis. If confirmed, casting should continue until healing is documented radiographically and/or clinically (12).

GYMNASTICS

Gymnastics is another sport that, even at the elite level, has many participants that are in the pediatric age range. The formal training programs and aggressive competitive schedules for these younger athletes predispose them to a variety of overuse injuries.

Medical Issues

Eating Disorders

Eating disorders are more commonly encountered in sports that are judged subjectively, including gymnastics. The diagnosis and management of anorexia nervosa and bulimia nervosa in young athletes were discussed in "Figure Skating" above. At the present time, significant differences in the pattern of eating disorders in young athletes in these sports categories are not apparent.

Musculoskeletal Issues

Back Pain

Gymnastics is consistently associated with the development of spondylolysis and spondylolisthesis in the young athletic population. Any young gymnast who presents with the complaint of low back pain should be considered as having one of these problems until proven otherwise. As with eating disorders, the diagnosis and management of spondylolysis and spondylolisthesis in young gymnasts does not differ significantly from the clinical approach discussed previously for young ice skaters.

Stress Fractures

Lower extremity stress fractures are common in running and jumping sports, including gymnastics. Stress fractures of the tibia are one of the most common stress fractures seen in young gymnasts, but fibular, calcaneal, navicular, and metatarsal stress fractures also occur. Because gymnasts use their arms in a weight-bearing function, upper extremity stress fractures may also occur. Risk factors in the development of these injuries include poor mechanics; inadequate diet, especially calcium and vitamin D intake; amenorrhea; and eating disorders.

As is commonly the case with stress fractures in other young athletes, the young gymnast typically presents with a complaint of pain that is worsened by activity and relieved by rest. At the onset of a stress fracture, pain may be noted late in the activity session. In cases in which the athlete continues to train, practice, or compete in spite of the presence of a stress fracture, the symptoms begin appearing earlier in the activity session. Many gymnasts continue to work out and compete, even with pain symptoms that are severe enough to interfere with normal daily activities. The physician will usually note tenderness over a discrete section of bone during the physical examination. Other symptoms, such as swelling, bruising, redness, and numbness, are usually absent. Depending on the part of the body that is examined, differentiating bone tenderness from soft tissue tenderness may be difficult. If muscle tenderness is present and the pain is worsened by passive stretching or resisted activation of the muscle group, a simple strain may be the etiology of the symptoms. Diffuse tenderness that is associated with any degree of neurovascular compromise should alert the examining physician to the possibility that an exertional compartment injury is present, and further evaluation, including manometric studies of the affected compartment, may be required.

Whenever a stress fracture is considered to be a diagnostic possibility, plain radiographs should be obtained. Often, the early radiographs are negative, so a bone scan is needed to make a definitive diagnosis. These tests should be undertaken prior to allowing the athlete to return to full participation.

Stress fractures in gymnasts are managed according to protocols that are similar to those used in other sports, such as ice skating. Rest and protection from further injury constitute the main initial components of therapy. For many stress fractures of the tarsal or metatarsal bones, 4 to 6 weeks in a shoe with a firm sole may be sufficient. Stress fractures with more severe symptoms or those found in young athletes who are unable or unwilling to rest and protect the affected extremity may require casting or the use of a walking boot. If the patient continues to have pain with ambulation, a non–weight-bearing period may be required. Stress fractures that fail to respond to initial interventions or that require additional consultation for return-to-play determinations should be referred to a sports medicine specialist.

Most tibial and fibular stress fractures can be treated adequately with rest alone. As with stress fractures of the tarsal and metatarsal bones, if normal ambulation causes pain, non–weight-bearing assisted ambulation may be required. Utilizing non–weight-bearing training and conditioning techniques, such as swimming, may prevent deconditioning in the young athlete.

Physicians who manage stress fractures in young athletes need to be aware of one important finding in

stress fractures of the mid tibia. A stress fracture along the anterior border of the tibia, particularly in the midshaft region, is a problematic injury that is associated with a high risk of progression to an unstable complete fracture. On lateral radiographs of the tibia, this stress fracture is recognized by the presence of "the dreaded black line." This radiolucent area represents an unresolved stress fracture. A normal tibia has a slight back bend shape, which places the anterior edge under tension. Tension side stress fractures at any location (the other common location is the femoral neck) should be referred immediately to an orthopedic surgeon for possible surgical fixation.

Gymnasts are more likely than athletes who engage in other sports to sustain stress fractures of the upper extremities. When managing gymnasts, the primary care physician should consider the arms, wrists, and hands as weight-bearing areas. In young gymnasts, a stress fracture of the bones of the upper extremity should be considered in the differential diagnosis of upper extremity pain.

The physical examination, the use of radiographs, and the need for bone scans are similar to the principles for managing the young athlete who has sustained a lower extremity stress fracture that were discussed above. Successful conservative treatment primarily consists of discontinuing arm weight-bearing activities. Symptoms that are refractive to conservative management regimens that include rest and protection from further injuries should be referred to a sports medicine specialist for further evaluation.

Foot and Ankle Tendinopathy

Foot and ankle tendinopathies are common in gymnastics, as well as in other sports, such as dance. Because gymnasts perform many of their floor exercise and balance beam maneuvers with the ankle held in a plantarflexion position, the muscles and tendons involved in plantarflexion are at risk for acute and overuse injuries. Structures that hold the ankle in plantarflexion include the Achilles tendon; the gastrocnemius and soleus muscles; the tibialis posterior; the flexor digitorum longus; and the flexor hallucis, longus, and peroneals.

Injury to these structures is especially prone to occur when eccentric loads are placed on the muscle–tendon unit. In general, eccentric contractions impart significantly more stress to the muscle tendon unit than does concentric activity.

Diagnosis of ankle and/or foot tendinopathy is based on a history of foot or ankle pain that is worsened by activity and relieved by rest. The physical examination signs and symptoms that are consistent with tendinopathy include tendon regions that may be swollen and tender to the touch. Passive stretching of the muscle group causes pain, as does resisted strength testing. Weakness may or may not be present. Primary care physicians must be aware of the fact that stress fractures may be part of the differential diagnosis, and, if so, the appropriate use of radiographs and nuclear medicine studies should be considered.

If the clinical diagnosis is limited to tendinopathy, conservative management is appropriate. A regimen that includes relative rest, stretching, ice, massage, and the appropriate use of NSAIDs is followed by the addition of strengthening, proprioception activities, and the slow reintroduction of sport-specific activities.

Wrist Pain

Wrist pain in a young gymnast may be a challenging diagnostic and therapeutic clinical problem for the primary care physician. Wrist pain, especially in the dorsum of the wrist, is a common complaint in the young gymnast who is participating aggressively in gymnastic training and competition. Aggressive repetitive activity with the wrists in a position of extreme extension and while supporting significant force loads results in most of the overuse wrist injuries in this sport. Most of these athletes describe an insidious onset to their discomfort and a lack of clinical signs (i.e., no swelling, redness, bruising, numbness, tingling, weakness). Many will continue to train and compete for months before presenting to the clinician, despite the presence of discomfort.

During the physical examination, the primary care physician often detects some swelling and decreased wrist extension in the young gymnast. General tenderness may also be found on palpation of the dorsum

of the wrist. The physical findings may remain nonspecific, and, in addition, the radiographs are frequently nondiagnostic. More extensive imaging (e.g., nuclear bone scan, MRI, and CT) studies may assist the physician in eliminating various aspects of the differential diagnosis.

The differential diagnosis of dorsal wrist pain in the gymnast includes, but is not limited to, acute fracture, stress fracture, tendinitis, capsular sprain, scapholunate dissociation, triangulofibrocartilage complex injury, and Kienböck disease (Table 39.4).

The treatment varies widely, depending upon the diagnosis, and it should be specific to the diagnosis. Wrist splinting, avoiding inciting activities, ice, stretching, strength training, and NSAIDs are often employed in the management regimen.

DANCE

General Considerations

Dancers represent a unique segment of the athletic population. They require strength, flexibility, and the ability to interpret music artistically. Dancers are known to be at significant risk for injury, and most report at least one injury per year (13). Compounding matters, dancers often strongly resist interrupting their performances or rehearsals to manage injury appropriately.

Most dancers begin training at a young age, with male dancers beginning their training at a later age than their female counterparts. Most dance training is highly structured, with little time allocated for rest and recuperation. As with most professional sports, the dance world functions on a pyramid system, where the most successful dancers occupy a few top positions and face continued competition from those below them.

TABLE 39.4. *Differential diagnosis of dorsal wrist pain in gymnasts*

Diagnosis	Pathophysiology	Physical finding	Diagnostic test finding
Acute fracture	Complete break	Pain over affected bone	Plain x-ray shows fracture line
Stress fracture	Overuse stress injury	Pain over affected bone	X-ray often normal; bone scan positive
Tendinitis	Tendon or peritendon microtears	Tenderness over affected tendon, worse with resisted strength testing	—
Scapholunate dissociation	Ligament tear	Positive Watson test	X-ray shows widening of the scapholunate junction
Triangular fibrocartilage complex tear	Cartilage tear	Pain in the ulna/triquetrum joint space	X-ray may show positive ulnar variance
Kienböck disease	Avascular necrosis of the lunate	Findings may be nonspecific	X-ray findings vary widely, based on stage of disease

Medical Issues

Menstrual Abnormalities

Of all the medical problems affecting dancers, perhaps the one most frequently encountered by the primary care physician is the presence of menstrual abnormalities. Menstrual abnormalities may be an isolated entity or they may be associated with eating disorders and osteoporosis. Delayed onset menses (primary amenorrhea) is frequently seen in young female dancers. Both primary and secondary amenorrhea may result from many hours of exhaustive training. Disordered eating may compound the severity of these menstrual abnormalities.

Disordered Eating

As was discussed with competitive ice skaters and similar to what is seen in other elite sports where body habitus is perceived to be a critical component of successful competition, bulimia and anorexia nervosa occur more frequently among dancers than they do in the general population. The risk of disordered eating increases with age, as young dancers enter more competitive dance formats in their teenage years. Disordered eating contributes to the demineralization of bone, osteoporosis, and the increased risk of stress fracture or injury.

Tobacco Abuse

The incidence of cigarette smoking is reported to be more prominent in the dance community. This, when combined with the fact that the adolescent female population is the fastest growing segment of new smokers, makes the dance population at particular risk. The exact reasons for the increased incidence of smoking in the dance population are not clear. One possible factor that may contribute to the increased incidence of smoking in this population of athletes is the perception that smoking is an effective method of weight control.

Musculoskeletal Issues

Acute Injuries

Few injuries are unique to dancers; however, due to the specific demands of dance, some injuries are seen in greater frequency. Common sites of injury for dancers are the spine, foot, and ankle.

Parathoracic Muscle Strains

Injuries to the scapular stabilization muscles (rhomboids, trapezius, and levator) in the parathoracic region are common among dancers. In males, these injuries may occur when the dancer lifts his partner and may result from inadequate upper body strength. Typically, the dancer reports pain in the region of the shoulder blades. The symptoms may be quite severe. Treatment is directed toward the relief of pain symptoms, and it consists of relative rest, ice, and analgesics. Rehabilitation programs utilize upper body conditioning programs in an effort to prevent further or repetitive injury. Massage and stretching also are useful adjunct therapies.

Lumbar Spondylolysis

Low back pain is a common complaint among dancers. In the young athlete, contrary to the adult, the diagnosis of lumbar strain should be considered a diagnosis of exclusion due to the greater frequency of other causes of low back pain. Lumbar spondylolysis is perhaps the most common cause of low back pain in the adolescent dancer who seeks medical attention. Unfortunately, this diagnosis often goes unrecognized. For this reason, low back pain in a child or adolescent athlete should always be evaluated thoroughly, and a definitive diagnosis should be obtained.

Lumbar spondylolysis, a stress injury to the pars interarticularis, is commonly encountered in young dancers. Increased lumbosacral lordosis that is caused by inadequate external rotation of the hips is believed to be a predisposing factor for the development of this stress-related injury in the dancer. A common sign of spondylolysis in the physical examination is back pain on hyperextension. Furthermore, the standing one leg hyperextension test (stork test) is frequently positive. Oblique radiographs of the lumbar spine may reveal a pars defect, although the well-trained eye may detect the abnormality on AP or lateral views. As was discussed with ice skaters, a negative radiograph does not exclude the possibility of spondylolysis. Conversely, radiographically apparent injuries do not necessarily indicate the presence of an active process because pars interarticularis fractures often heal with fibrous union, which may remain visible indefinitely. Because of this, a nucleotide bone scan with single-photon emission computer tomography (SPECT) may yield information that is more clinically relevant in adolescents with back pain. Nucleotide imaging studies will assist the clinician in determining whether the stress injury to the pars interarticularis is active (recent injury) or inactive (old injury).

The treatment of spondylolysis is usually conservative, and most dancers return to full activity. The treatment may include restrictions of dancing and other impact or extension activity of the back for a minimum of 4 to 6 weeks. Physical therapy protocols that consist of trunk stabilization exercises and programs that address flexibility deficits of the lower extremities are now considered standard treatment. Recently, the efficacy of bracing the lower back for spondylolysis has been questioned. When symptoms resolve, physical activity may be slowly and progressively resumed, adding the more stressful dance maneuvers last.

Cuboid Syndrome

Cuboid syndrome is a common, but often unrecognized, condition among dancers. This injury is believed to represent a small plantar subluxation of the cuboid tarsal bone. Dancers with this condition usually report a sudden onset of lateral midfoot pain that is often accompanied by the inability to bear weight. The dancer also often reports that he or she is unable to push-off. During the physical examination, the physician will usually elicit pain with dorsal pressure on the plantar aspect of the cuboid. Occasionally, the physician may note a shallow depression on the dorsum of the foot. Imaging studies usually are of little benefit in establishing the diagnosis. Treatment of this condition consists of ice, protected weight bearing, padding and/or taping, physical therapy, and manipulation. Manipulation of this subluxation has been reported to have a 90% success rate in the acute setting.

Chronic Injuries

Flexor Hallucis Longus Tendinitis

Flexor hallucis longus tendinitis is the most common site of lower extremity tendinitis in ballet dancers. The pain associated with this condition is located along the posterior medial aspect of the ankle behind the medial malleolus. Ballet dancers commonly present reporting pain when they are *en pointe*. The pain associated with this condition can be reproduced by a maneuver in which the examining physician flexes the great toe with the foot in the plantarflexed position. The tendon is usually tender to palpation, and it may develop crepitance or triggering (e.g., catching or locking of the flexor tendon in its sheath). Treatment consists of relative rest (reducing the amount of time spent *en pointe*) and the applica-

tion of ice. In more persistent cases, physical therapy may be appropriate. Though many cases resolve within several days, the more severe cases, which are characterized by triggering or crepitance, often take several weeks to resolve. The use of injectable steroids is the subject of discussion among sports medicine specialists. Referral to a sports medicine specialist for further evaluation and treatment is appropriate if this intervention is being considered. Severe cases or cases that do not respond to more conservative interventions may require a brief period of immobilization. Rarely, severe cases that include debilitating episodes of triggering may require surgical decompression of the tendon.

Posterior Ankle Impingement

This painful condition is caused by impingement of the os trigonum or the adjacent soft tissues in the posterior aspect of the ankle. The os trigonum is the nonunited lateral tubercle on the posterior aspect of the talus. It is a common anatomic finding that is seen in approximately 10% of the population; it is generally harmless and is usually asymptomatic. In dancers, however, posterior ankle impingement is quite common, as the foot is repetitively placed in plantarflexion, which pinches the os trigonum or adjacent soft tissues between the posterior lip of the tibia and the calcaneus. Dancers with this condition complain of posterior ankle pain. On physical examination, this pain can be reproduced with passive or active plantarflexion of the foot. Appropriate treatment consists of relative rest (avoidance of pointe work), ice, and physical therapy. Strengthening exercises that focus on the muscles that evert and invert the ankle are particularly helpful. Recurrent cases that are refractive to conservative interventions may necessitate surgical removal of the process or os trigonum.

FOOTBALL

Football is a collision sport with a relatively high incidence of injury in the young athletes who participate in this popular sport. Participants are vulnerable to a wide variety of medical and musculoskeletal conditions that may require intervention by the primary care physician. Each year about 1.5 million individuals participate in football. Estimates indicate that approximately 300,000 high school football players and half of all collegiate and professional players are injured to some extent during every football season. At the collegiate level, the injury rate is higher in spring football than that of the regular season. The knee, ankle, and shoulder are the most frequent sites of injury, while sprains, strains, and contusions are the most common types of injury.

Medical Issues

Neck Injury

Neck injuries have potentially catastrophic clinical outcomes. Any physician involved with the on-site coverage of high-risk events (e.g., football) should be familiar with the acute management of neck injury. This subject is discussed in Chapters 27 and 29.

Concussion

Concussion is defined as an alteration in mental status, with or without loss of consciousness, within minutes or hours of trauma to the head. According to current estimates, one in five high school football players will experience a concussion each season. Several classification schemes for describing the severity of concussions in athletes exist in the medical literature; however, no universal agreement regarding the grading of concussion has been achieved. Likewise, appropriate management of the acute injury and subsequent return-to-play decisions are the subject of ongoing study in the sports medicine community. Several key points that need to be included in the decision making process of the primary care physician are important to emphasize (See Chapter 27).

Loss of consciousness is not required to make the diagnosis of concussion (see Chapter 28). In fact, most concussions in football do not involve loss of consciousness. Symptomatic individuals who sustain concussive injury while still experiencing symptoms from a previous concussion, even if the second occurrence is relatively mild, may experience catastrophic brain swelling that is often referred to as "second impact syndrome." While true cases of second impact syndrome in athletic competition seem relatively uncommon, younger athletes are at greater risk than adult athletes for the development of catastrophic episodes of brain swelling with sequential episodes of head trauma. Every athlete who sustains a head injury that results in a concussion should be carefully evaluated and closely monitored until all symptoms have resolved, both at rest and during the resumption of physical activity.

Mild concussion, or "bell ringers," are the most common. Although classification systems vary, mild concussions typically involve no loss of consciousness. Mild disturbances in gait and coordination may be present. The individual should be carefully evaluated and monitored for the development of postconcussive symptoms, such as headache, nausea, vomiting, difficulty concentrating, photophobia, and amnesia. The symptoms of a mild concussion usually resolve within 5 to 15 minutes. Players who have alterations in mental status, either at rest or with the resumption of activity, that persist beyond 15 minutes from the time of the head trauma should be removed from competition for a minimum of 24 hours. All athletes who sustain a concussion, no matter what the degree, should be reexamined by a physician within 24 to 48 hours. The individual may return to participation when the symptoms have fully resolved.

More severe concussions involve a loss of consciousness and anterograde or retrograde amnesia. Typically, these individuals also are not allowed to return to competition for a minimum of 24 to 48 hours from the time of the head trauma. In the medical literature, return-to-play decisions in athletes who sustain either single or multiple concussions are controversial, and they are the subject of ongoing discussion and research.

Stingers and Burners

Stingers or burners are the most frequent neurologic injury in football. Many, if not all, football players have experienced this type of injury at some point in their careers. This injury is believed to be caused by either a transient brachial plexopathy or a nerve root traction injury. Typically, the athlete reports a burning or stinging pain, accompanied by numbness and tingling that originates in the supraclavicular region and radiates down the affected arm to the fingers. An associated transient weakness in the arm may be present. Burners and stingers typically do not involve significant neck pain or neck muscular stiffness. If these symptoms are present, the primary care physician should be more aggressive, and he or she should manage the injury as a potentially severe neck injury. The athlete typically will try to relieve the discomfort by trying to "shake it out." Since the superior portion of the brachial plexus that contains the C-5 to C-6 nerve roots is the area most commonly affected, the most common motor deficit is deltoid weakness. The degree of involvement of these neuronal components can be evaluated routinely by an assessment of the strength of shoulder abduction. Symptoms associated with stingers and burners usually resolve within minutes. If the symptoms persist, a further evaluation for more serious neck injury should begin, and appropriate precautions should be taken. The athlete may return to competition when the symptoms have resolved completely and the examination is normalized.

Additional evaluation is indicated for those individuals with recurrent stingers and those with symptoms that do not resolve within 24 hours. The initial evaluation consists of plain radiographs of the cervical spine. Other imaging studies, such as MRI of the cervical spine and/or brachial plexus, should be performed as clinically indicated. Electromyography (EMG) is of limited clinical use in the acute phase of this injury, and, since electromyographic abnormalities may persist for years despite full clinical recovery, EMG may be of limited use in assisting with return-to-play decisions. The incidence of and severity of stingers and burners may be reduced by appropriate preventive measures that include a shoulder and neck strength and conditioning program. In addition, aggressive coaching regarding proper tackling techniques is important in preventing this type of injury. Additional benefit may be gained from ensuring that equipment fits properly and from the use of possible additional protective equipment, such as neck rolls and collars.

Infectious Mononucleosis

Infectious mononucleosis (IM) is an acute self-limited disease that is caused by the Epstein–Barr virus. The primary concern with IM with regard to football and other collision sports is the potential for splenic enlargement and subsequent rupture secondary to contact during practice or competition (14). Although splenic rupture is rare, occuring in only 0.1% to 0.2% of all cases, it has lethal potential if unrecognized. Splenomegaly may not be apparent clinically on physical examination. Ultrasonography should be considered in young athletes when the primary care physician remains suspicious of splenomegaly in the young athlete with mononucleosis although the physical findings are inconclusive. Statistically, splenic rupture is more likely to occur between 4 and 21 days after the onset of the illness. The risk of rupture diminishes after 4 weeks from the onset of symptoms. Most sports medicine physicians agree that football players should be restricted from vigorous activity for a minimum of 3 weeks after the onset of symptoms. After 3 weeks, the athlete may resume light conditioning if no splenomegaly or splenic tenderness is present, the liver enzymes are normal, and the athlete is afebrile. If the athlete remains asymptomatic during the initial period of activity, he or she may return to contact and collision play after 4 weeks.

Musculoskeletal Issues

Musculoskeletal injuries are a relatively common occurrence in youth football. The knee, ankle, and shoulder are the most frequent locations of injury in young football players. The most frequent types of injury are sprains, strains, and contusions.

Knee Injuries in Football

Medial Collateral Ligament Injury

Injuries to the knee can be categorized into ligamentous, meniscal, and overuse types. Injury to the medial collateral ligament (MCL) is commonly encountered in football. The biomechanical mechanism of this injury is typically a direct impact to the lateral aspect of the knee that produces a valgus stress. After an injury to the MCL in a young athlete, the primary care physician will most likely detect pain along the medial aspect of the knee and pain with or without laxity. Laxity is especially apparent when the physician applies a valgus stress to the affected joint while the knee is maintained at 30 degrees of flexion. The greater the laxity with a valgus stress at 30 degrees of flexion, the greater is the degree of injury. The presence of even more serious injury is indicated when the physician detects laxity following the application of valgus stress with the knee at full extension.

Less severe injuries to the MCL are treated nonoperatively with protected weight bearing and ice. In addition, initial restricted range of motion with a subsequent progression to full range of motion that is followed by progressive resistance exercises are valuable components to the rehabilitation regimen. The resolution of symptoms will typically require 2 to 4 weeks of rehabilitation. When the athlete returns to play, a functional MCL brace may be of benefit in symptom control and may offer, in addition, a degree of protection from further injury. The degree to which prophylactic functional bracing will protect a young football player from initial or recurring injury has been a source of controversy in the pediatric sports medicine literature. Currently, most experts believe that prophylactic bracing is more effective for high-risk positions (e.g., offensive linemen) or at higher levels of competition (e.g., collegiate football).

Anterior Cruciate Ligament Injury

Injury to the anterior cruciate ligament (ACL) of the knee occurs from a twisting injury to the joint. This type of injury mechanism can occur with or without contact. The athlete usually reports hearing a "pop," followed by swelling of the affected knee that develops within a few hours of the incident. Physical examination of the injured joint usually reveals the presence of an effusion that is associated with a poor endpoint on the Lachman test, as well as a positive pivot shift test.

Individuals who wish to return to football usually require surgical reconstruction of the ligament. In an effort to provide the knee joint with improved long-term joint stability, reconstruction of the damaged ACL may also be indicated in skeletally mature young athletes. Persistent knee instability in individuals whose ACL is deficient, when accompanied by the high stresses placed on the knee during football, make conservative treatment unlikely to succeed. Furthermore, functional bracing of ACL-deficient individuals has not proven effective in the younger athlete.

Meniscal Injury

Meniscal injuries usually occur with a twisting mechanism, and they can be either associated with contact or noncontact mechanisms. Symptoms of joint pain and associated joint swelling usually develop within several hours of the injury. The young athlete will often report the sensation of "catching" in the affected knee. If the athlete cannot fully extend the knee or if the knee is "locked," a bucket handle meniscal tear should be suspected. The term "bucket handle" refers to a concentric tear in the meniscus in which a portion of the meniscus may be displaced into the joint. Bucket handle meniscus tears usually require prompt surgical attention. If the physical examination is equivocal, MRI may be utilized to confirm the diagnosis. Although conservative treatment may be initiated, most meniscal tears in young athletes require surgery.

Overuse Injury

Overuse injuries to the knee are common in football. Conditions such as PFSS and patellar tendonitis occur frequently in young football players. Treatment of these injuries is conservative, and it has been discussed previously in Chapter 36. As with all overuse injuries, prevention is the best form of treatment.

Shoulder Injuries in Football

Clavicle Fractures

A fracture of the clavicle is a common injury in football, and it is often managed by the primary care physician. These injuries usually occur as a result of a direct blow to the lateral aspect of the shoulder. Conservative treatment is usually successful, except in cases where the injury involves a fracture of the distal tip of the clavicle. This type of fracture will often require surgical fixation for proper healing to occur. A figure-of-eight harness or an arm sling may be used for comfort while the clavicle fracture is healing. The athlete may return to football when the fracture has healed and the athlete has regained normal strength in the affected shoulder and arm.

Acromioclavicular Injury

Injury to the AC joint is also a common shoulder injury in football. A fall or blow to the lateral aspect of the shoulder can cause shoulder separations. The young football player usually reports tenderness at the AC joint. The primary care physician may note a gross deformity or swelling at the site of the injury, depending on the degree of severity and the type of injury (7). The athlete generally experiences pain with horizontal adduction of the affected shoulder. Conservative treatment with ice, analgesics, and an arm sling for comfort is appropriate for the initial management of uncomplicated AC injuries. The athlete may return to competition when pain symptoms have resolved and strength and range of motion have returned. The return to football can be aided by padding the joint for additional comfort.

Glenohumeral Instability

Shoulder dislocation and subluxation commonly occur in football. Anterior shoulder dislocation is the most common mechanism of injury. This injury usually occurs when the shoulder is in abduction and external rotation. An experienced physician may gently reduce acute shoulder dislocations on the field. If the shoulder cannot be easily reduced on the field, the athlete should be transported to the emergency center for reduction. Radiographs should be obtained in those injuries in which the reduction is performed in the outpatient setting. Following reduction of the injured joint, sling immobilization should be employed for comfort. When pain symptoms have improved, rehabilitation should begin. Physical therapy focuses on the maintaining joint flexibility while increasing shoulder strength and stability. The young athlete and his or her family should be made aware of the risk of recurrence of this type of injury. Athletes who experience frequent recurrences of shoulder dislocation may require surgical intervention to stabilize the affected joint. The role of arthroscopic versus open repair for a

Bankart lesion with capsular shift is the subject of on-going discussion in the sports medicine literature.

Posterior shoulder dislocation is a less common injury in football, but it can occur in football linemen. The mechanism of this injury is a sudden load to the shoulder while it is in an adducted and internally rotated position. The acute treatment is similar to that for anterior dislocation, consisting of reduction. However, because of the increased risk of fracture that is associated with a posterior dislocation injury of the shoulder, obtaining radiographs of the affected joint prior to attempting reduction should be considered. Subsequently, management of the injury involves immobilization and rehabilitation protocols similar to those of anterior shoulder dislocation injuries. The role of surgical treatment is controversial with this type of injury as well.

Other Injuries to the Lower Extremity in Football

Hip Pointers

The term "hip pointer" is typically used to describe a contusion to the iliac crest. Skeletally immature athletes should be evaluated radiographically to rule out the possibility of apophyseal avulsion. Most hip pointers are treated conservatively with ice, analgesics, rest, and extra padding, and the athlete may return to play as symptoms resolve.

Thigh Contusions

Contusions to the quadriceps muscle occur as a result of a direct blow to the muscle. The athlete typically reports pain and loss of motion in the affected extremity. Occasionally, the primary care physician will detect a mass when conducting an examination of the affected area. On-field treatment of the injury consists of immobilization of the leg, with the quadriceps held in flexion to prevent or minimize hematoma formation. The athlete should be restricted to non–weight-bearing activity and the use of crutches and should be instructed to keep the affected extremity immobilized for at least 24 hours. Ice should be applied judiciously, and heat should be avoided. After the initial phase of treatment, gentle range-of-motion exercises and functional rehabilitation begin. The risk of myositis ossificans (heterotopic bone formation after deep muscle contusion) should be discussed with the athlete and his or her parents. The athlete may return to competition once range of motion and strength have returned to their preinjury levels and clinical resolution of the hematoma has occurred.

Turf Toe

Hyperextension or, less commonly, hyperflexion injury to the first metatarsalphalangeal joint may cause a painful injury that is referred to as turf toe. This injury was initially labeled "turf toe" because it more commonly is seen in play on artificial turf. The flexible footwear worn on artificial turf is believed to contribute to the relative increased frequency of this injury compared to that of natural grass and with the use of firmer soled shoes. The physical examination of the affected toe reveals tenderness at the first metatarsalphalangeal joint and pain with passive dorsiflexion. The individual usually reports pain with push-off. The radiographs are usually unremarkable, but avulsion fractures are occasionally detected. Consequently, if the symptoms are severe or persistent, radiographs may be required. Treatment of the injury usually consists of ice, activity as tolerated, and taping for support. Analgesics may also be helpful. More severe cases of turf toe may take several weeks to resolve. Return to play should begin progressively with the resolution of symptoms. Determination of playing status hinges on the athlete's ability to perform in light of his or her clinical symptoms (i.e., athletes may play despite continued discomfort).

SOCCER

Soccer is one of the most popular sports for young athletes in the United States. At the international level, soccer, which is known as football, is the sport that is played by the largest number of both young male and young female athletes. For people in the United States, soccer is an important component of physical exercise for over 12 million individuals. Three million young people are playing soccer in high schools and youth soccer associations. Because of the large number of young people participating in this sport, the pattern of injuries associated with soccer has been studied and reviewed by many authors and organizations (15).

Differences in the risk of injury to players are based on whether a young soccer player is competing in outdoor or indoor soccer. A higher risk of injury exists for athletes who are competing in indoor soccer. The reasons for this increased risk are not definitive; they may, however, include differences in playing surface, and they could be attibutable to the possibility of players colliding with the barriers that surround the playing field.

Approximately half of the injuries that are reported in young soccer players are the result of player-to-player contact, and 48% of these contact-related injuries are the result of tackling. Most of the injuries in youth soccer are minor soft tissue injuries and overuse injuries. While these injuries are not unique to youth soccer, several problem areas specific to soccer are worth examining.

Medical Issues

Head Injuries

Soccer is classified as a collision sport. Although the risk for catastrophic head and neck injuries is less than that seen in football, the on-field management of concussion and neck injuries requires an equivalent level of medical care when an injury occurs. Likewise, the return-to-play decisions following the recovery of an athlete who has sustained a head or neck injury are similar for athletes who are playing soccer to those for athletes involved in football.

Head injuries that result from a practice and competition technique referred to as "heading the ball" are a highly controversial area of concern in youth soccer. The extent to which heading the ball results in immediate cognitive loss in young athletes or the degree to which this technique results in cognitive delays later in life is being examined in several research centers internationally. One study has found that, in adult soccer players, the degree of cognitive loss is higher in players who use the technique more frequently (16). Whether younger soccer players who head the ball have a greater risk of cognitive loss than do adult players has not been established. Currently, many authors advise that young players minimize their use of this technique. No clinical evidence exists that indicates that any headgear used to reduce the force of the blow to the head from the soccer ball has the ability to reduce the risk of cognitive loss. Some sports medicine physicians have expressed concern that the use of headgear may actually increase the overall risk of injury by giving young players a false sense of security or invincibility that may result in a tendency to engage in more aggressive play. Likewise, the weight of the soccer ball may be implicated in the risk of cognitive loss. Many sports medicine physicians and youth soccer associations have recommended that smaller and lighter soccer balls be used in youth soccer practice and competition. Finally, no definitive evidence indicates that the risk of cognitive loss from heading the ball can be reduced by the use of "appropriate" or "correct" techniques.

Heat Injuries

Young soccer players appear to have risks of heat-related injuries that are similar to those of other young athletes. One variable of competition encountered with young soccer players can, however, increase the frequency and severity of heat-related injuries. Tournament competition often requires multiple games in a relatively short time frame. If the competition occurs when the environmental conditions include high heat and high humidity, young soccer players may become progressively at more risk for heat-related injuries as the tournament progresses. Physicians who provide medical coverage for these events should be extremely alert to the signs and symptoms of heat-related illness in these young athletes. They should also be highly proactive in assisting the parents, officials, and event organizers in providing adequate preventive measures. Finally, aggressive medical interventions should be initiated if a young soccer player begins developing signs and symptoms of heat-related illness.

Musculoskeletal Issues

The most common injuries that a primary care physician will encounter in young soccer players are soft tissue contusions, sprains, and strains. Fractures are relatively uncommon in comparison to the incidence of these minor injuries. Of all injuries reported in youth soccer, fractures account for less than 10%; these usually involve the lower extremity. No soccer-specific injury patterns in the lower extremities have been identified.

Medial Ankle Injuries

One type of injury that may be encountered more frequently in youth soccer than in other youth sports is medial ankle trauma. Ball handling techniques that consist of repetitive kicking utilizing the medial aspect of the foot and ankle are the most commonly used skills in soccer. Trauma to the medial aspect of the ankle can occur if the soccer player makes contact with a trapped ball or with another player's foot or ankle. While shin guards are routinely used to decrease the frequency and severity of lower extremity injuries, the medial aspect of the ankle is difficult to protect. Acute contusions to this area are managed by ice and/or cold compresses. Padding also may be utilized to protect the area during the healing phase and to reduce the risk of additional injury when the athlete returns to play. More severe injuries to the medial aspect of the ankle may require additional evaluation. Radiographs of the affected extremity should be considered if the severity of the injury prevents the athlete from ambulating, if tenderness extends from the medial malleolus distally to the forefoot and/or proximally to the mid tibia, or if signs and symptoms of the injury fail to resolve with appropriate initial management.

Calcaneal Apophysitis

One overuse injury that is commonly encountered in skeletally immature soccer players is calcaneal apophysitis (Sever syndrome). One of the major advantages that youth soccer has, relative to other youth sports, is the fact that the level of sustained activity contributes to cardiovascular fitness. Unfortunately, this amount of running also contributes to overuse injuries to the heel. Modifying shoes (e.g., minimizing the use of cleated shoes and using heel cups and/or full-foot orthoses to provide additional cushion) may reduce the incidence and severity of this condition.

Ophthalmologic and Orofacial Injuries

In Europe, a soccer-related injury to the eye is the most common cause of sports-related orbital blowout fracture (17). Fifty percent of soccer-related eye injuries result in hyphema. The risk of eye injuries in youth soccer has prompted several organizations to add soccer to the list of sports in which safety sport glasses with polycarbonate lenses are recommended for both practice and competition (18). The risk of orofacial and dental injuries in youth soccer is second only to that of young athletes who play basketball. The American Dental Association suggests that soccer players, like other young athletes, should use protective mouth gear during practice and competition to reduce the incidence and severity of orofacial and dental injuries (19).

Fatal and Catastrophic Injuries

One type of soccer-related injury may pose a disproportionately higher risk for fatal injury to these young athletes. The United States Consumer Product Safety Commission monitors fatal injuries resulting from traumatic contact with soccer goal posts. From 1979 through 1994, 30 serious injuries, 21 of which were fatal, have been reported either from collisions with, or as a result of soccer goals falling on, young athletes. Physicians should be aware that there are specific recommendations for ensuring that soccer goals are secured adequately during play and when they are not in use (20).

SUMMARY

Although no sport has an injurty that is truly unique, some sports are more closely associated with specific injuries than others. The ability to recognize those individuals at a higher risk for certain injuries, based on participation patterns, is important.

REFERENCES

1. Ulmry LD, McGowan JA, Shulman LE. Optimal calcium intake. *NIH Consensus Statement Online* 1994;12:1–31.
2. Fredericson M. Common injuries in runners. Diagnosis, rehabilitation and prevention. *Sports Med* 1996;21:49–72.
3. Puffer JC, Zachazewski. Management of overuse injuries. *Am Fam Physician* 1988;38:225–232.
4. Bennell KL, Brukner PD. Epidemiology and site specificity of stress fractures. *Clin Sports Med* 1997;16:179–196
5. Murphy S, ed. *Guidelines for the diagnosis and management of asthma.* NIH publication no. 97-4051. Bethseda, MD: National Institutes of Health, 1997.
6. Sim FH, Simonet WT, Melton LJ, et al. Ice hockey injuries. *Am J Sports Med* 1987;15:30–40.
7. Rockwood CA, Williams GR, Young DC. Injuries to the acromioclavicular joint. In: Rockwood CA, Green DP, Bucholz RW, eds. *Rockwood and Green's fractures in adults,* 3rd ed. Philadelphia: JB Lippincott Co, 1991: 1181–1251.
8. American Psychiatric Association. Eating disorders. In: *Diagnostic and statistical manual of mental disorders,* 4th ed. Washington, D.C.: American Psychiatric Association, 1994:539–550.
9. Micheli LJ, Wood R. Back pain in young athletes—significant differences from adults in causes and patterns. *Arch Pediatr Adolesc Med* 1995;149:15–18.
10. Brown TG, Varney TE, Micheli LJ. Malleolar bursitis in figure skaters: indications for operative and non-operative treatment. *Am J Sports Med* 2000;28:109–111.
11. Brown JH, Deluca SA. Growth plate injuries: Salter–Harris classification. *Am Fam Physician* 1992; 46:1180–1184.
12. Richard JR. Office orthopedics: thumb spica casting for scaphoid fractures. *Am Fam Physician* 1995;52: 1113–1119.
13. Solomon R, Brown T, Gerbino PG, et al. The young dancer. *Clin Sports Med* 2000;19:717–739.
14. Maki DG, Reich RM. Infectious mononucleosis in the athlete. Diagnosis, complications and management. *Am J Sports Med* 1982;10:162–173.
15. American Academy of Pediatrics Committee on Sports Medicine and Fitness. Injuries in youth soccer: a subject review. *Pediatrics* 2000;105:656–661.
16. Tysvaer A, Lochen E. Soccer injuries to the brain. *Am J Sports Med* 1991;19:56–60.
17. Jones N. Orbital blowout fractures in sport. *Br J Sports Med* 1994;28:272–275.
18. American Academy of Pediatrics Committee on Sports Medicine and Fitness and American Academy of Ophthalmology Committee on Eye Safety and Sports Ophthalmology. Protective eyewear for young athletes. *Pediatrics* 1996;98:311–313.
19. American Dental Association Counsel on Dental Materials. Mouth protectors and sports team dentists. *J Am Dent Assoc* 1984;109:84–87.
20. United States Consumer Product Safety Commission. *Guidelines for movable soccer goal safety.* Washington, D.C. United States Consumer Product Safety Commission, 1995.

Appendices

Appendix A
Interim History

SPORTS HEALTH RECORD: INTERIM HISTORY

This form may be used prior to participation in any new sport during the interval between preparticipation examinations. Positive responses should prompt a physical examination.

NAME _____ AGE _____ DATE _____

ADDRESS _____ PHONE _____

1. Over the next 12 months I wish to participate in the following sports:

 a. _____ b. _____ c. _____ d. _____

2. Have you missed more than 3 consecutive days of participation in usual activities because of an injury this past year? Yes ___ No ___

 If yes, please indicate:

 a. Site of injury _____

 b. Type of injury _____

3. Have you missed more than 5 consecutive days of participation in usual activities because of an illness or have you had a medical illness diagnosed that has not resolved in this past year? Yes ___ No ___

 If yes, please indicate:

 a. Type of illness _____

4. Have you had a concussion or been unconscious for any reason in the last year? Yes ___ No ___

5. Have you had surgery or been hospitalized in the past year? Yes ___ No ___

 If yes, please indicate:

 a. Reason for hospitalization _____

 b. Type of surgery _____

6. List all medications you are presently taking and what condition the medication is for.

 a. _____

 b. _____

 c. _____

7. Are you worried about any problem or condition at this time? Yes ___ No ___

 If yes, please explain: _____

 _____

 _____

 _____

I hereby state that to the best of my knowledge my answers to the above questions are correct.

_____ _____

Signature of athlete   Date

_____ _____

Signature of parent   Date

FIG A.1. Sports health record: interim history. (From Squire DL. Eating disorders. In: Mellion MB, ed. *Sports medicine secrets*, 2nd ed. Philadelphia: Hanley & Belfus, 1999:139–144, with permission.)

Appendix B
Preparticipation Physical Evaluation

Preparticipation Physical Evaluation

HISTORY

DATE OF EXAM _____

Name _____ Sex _____ Age _____ Date of birth _____

Grade _____ School _____ Sport(s) _____

Address _____

Personal physician _____ Phone _____

In case of emergency, contact

Name _____ Relationship _____ Phone (H) _____ (W) _____

Explain "Yes" answers below.
Circle questions you don't know the answers to.

	Yes	No
1. Have you had a medical illness or injury since your last check up or sports physical?	☐	☐
Do you have an ongoing or chronic illness?	☐	☐
2. Have you ever been hospitalized overnight?	☐	☐
Have you ever had surgery?	☐	☐
3. Are you currently taking any prescription or nonprescription (over-the-counter) medications or pills or using an inhaler?	☐	☐
Have you ever taken any supplements or vitamins to help you gain or lose weight or improve your performance?	☐	☐
4. Do you have any allergies (for example, to pollen, medicine, food, or stinging insects)?	☐	☐
Have you ever had a rash or hives develop during or after exercise?	☐	☐
5. Have you ever passed out during or after exercise?	☐	☐
Have you ever been dizzy during or after exercise?	☐	☐
Have you ever had chest pain during or after exercise?	☐	☐
Do you get tired more quickly than your friends do during exercise?	☐	☐
Have you ever had racing of your heart or skipped heartbeats?	☐	☐

	Yes	No
10. Do you use any special protective or corrective equipment or devices that aren't usually used for your sport or position (for example, knee brace, special neck roll, foot orthotics, retainer on your teeth, hearing aid)?	☐	☐
11. Have you had any problems with your eyes or vision?	☐	☐
Do you wear glasses, contacts, or protective eyewear?	☐	☐
12. Have you ever had a sprain, strain, or swelling after injury?	☐	☐
Have you broken or fractured any bones or dislocated any joints?	☐	☐
Have you had any other problems with pain or swelling in muscles, tendons, bones, or joints?	☐	☐

If yes, check appropriate box and explain below.

☐ Head	☐ Elbow	☐ Hip
☐ Neck	☐ Forearm	☐ Thigh
☐ Back	☐ Wrist	☐ Knee
☐ Chest	☐ Hand	☐ Shin/calf
☐ Shoulder	☐ Finger	☐ Ankle
☐ Upper arm		☐ Foot

13. Do you want to weigh more or less than you do now? ☐ ☐

Have you had high blood pressure or high cholesterol?

Have you ever been told you have a heart murmur?

Has any family member or relative died of heart problems or of sudden death before age 50?

Have you had a severe viral infection (for example, myocarditis or mononucleosis) within the last month?

Has a physician ever denied or restricted your participation in sports for any heart problems?

6. Do you have any current skin problems (for example, itching, rashes, acne, warts, fungus, or blisters)?

7. Have you ever had a head injury or concussion?

Have you ever been knocked out, become unconscious, or lost your memory?

Have you ever had a seizure?

Do you have frequent or severe headaches?

Have you ever had numbness or tingling in your arms, hands, legs, or feet?

Have you ever had a stinger, burner, or pinched nerve?

8. Have you ever become ill from exercising in the heat?

9. Do you cough, wheeze, or have trouble breathing during or after activity?

Do you have asthma?

Do you have seasonal allergies that require medical treatment?

Do you lose weight regularly to meet weight requirements for your sport?

14. Do you feel stressed out?

15. Record the dates of your most recent immunizations (shots) for:

Tetanus _____   Measles _____

Hepatitis B _____   Chickenpox _____

FEMALES ONLY

16. When was your first menstrual period? _____

When was your most recent menstrual period? _____

How much time do you usually have from the start of one period to the start of another? _____

How many periods have you had in the last year? _____

What was the longest time between periods in the last year? _____

Explain "Yes" answers here: _____

_____

_____

_____

_____

_____

I hereby state that, to the best of my knowledge, my answers to the above questions are complete and correct.

Signature of athlete _____   Signature of parent/guardian _____   Date _____

FIG. B.1. The history and physical evaluation forms. (From Smith DM, Kovan JR, Rich BSE, et al. *Preparticipation physical evaluation*, 2nd ed. Minneapolis: McGraw-Hill, 1997, with permission.) *Continued on next page.*

485

Preparticipation Physical Evaluation

PHYSICAL EXAMINATION

Name _____ Date of birth _____

Height _____ Weight _____ % Body fat (optional) _____ Pulse _____ BP _____ / _____ (___ / ___ , ___ / ___)

Vision R 20/ _____ L 20/ _____ Corrected: Y N Pupils: Equal _____ Unequal _____

	NORMAL	ABNORMAL FINDINGS	INITIALS*
MEDICAL			
Appearance			
Eyes/Ears/Nose/Throat			
Lymph nodes			
Heart			
Pulses			
Lungs			
Abdomen			
Genitalia (males only)			
Skin			
MUSCULOSKELETAL			
Neck			
Back			
Shoulder/arm			
Elbow/forearm			
Wrist/hand			
Hip/thigh			
Knee			
Leg/ankle			
Foot			

*Station-based examination only

CLEARANCE

☐ Cleared

☐ Cleared after completing evaluation/rehabilitation for: _____

☐ Not cleared for: _____ Reason: _____

Recommendations: _____
_____
_____

Name of physician (print/type) _____ Date _____

Address _____ Phone _____

Signature of physician _____, MD or DO

FIG. B.1. *Continued*

Appendix C
Preparticipation Physical Evaluation Clearance Form

Preparticipation Physical Evaluation
CLEARANCE FORM

☐ Cleared

☐ Cleared after completing evaluation/rehabilitation for: _____

Reason: _____

_____

_____

☐ Not cleared for: _____

Recommendations: _____

_____

_____

Name of physician (print/type) _____ Date _____

Address _____ Phone _____

Signature of physician _____, MD or DO

FIG. C-1. Preparticipation physical evaluation clearance form. (From Smith DM, Kovan JR, Rich BSE, et al. *Preparticipation physical evaluation*, 2nd ed. Minneapolis: McGraw-Hill, 1997, with permission.)

489

Appendix D
Growth Charts and Body Mass Indices

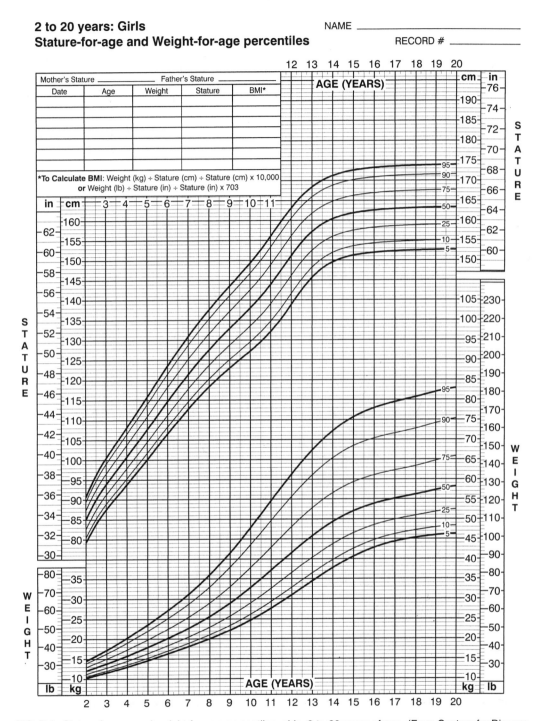

FIG. D.1. Stature-for-age and weight-for-age percentiles, girls, 2 to 20 years of age. (From Centers for Disease Control and Prevention. Available at http://www.cdc.gov/growthcharts/. Accessed June 2002, with permission.)

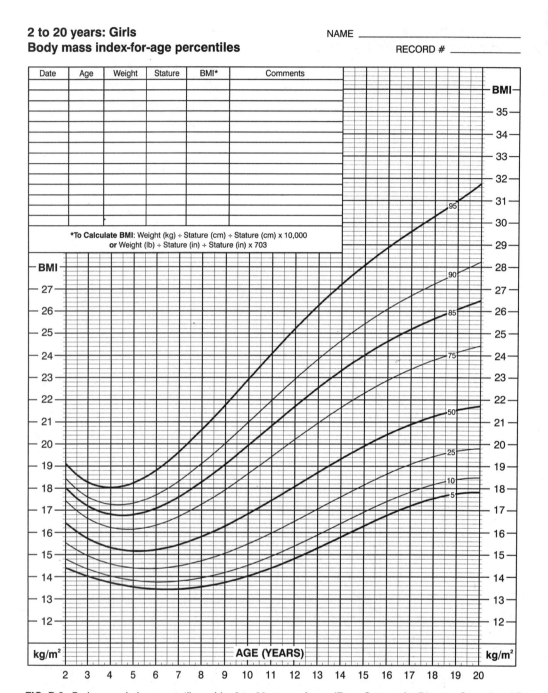

FIG. D.2. Body mass index percentiles, girls, 2 to 20 years of age. (From Centers for Disease Control and Prevention. Available at http://www.cdc.gov/growthcharts/. Accessed June 2002, with permission.)

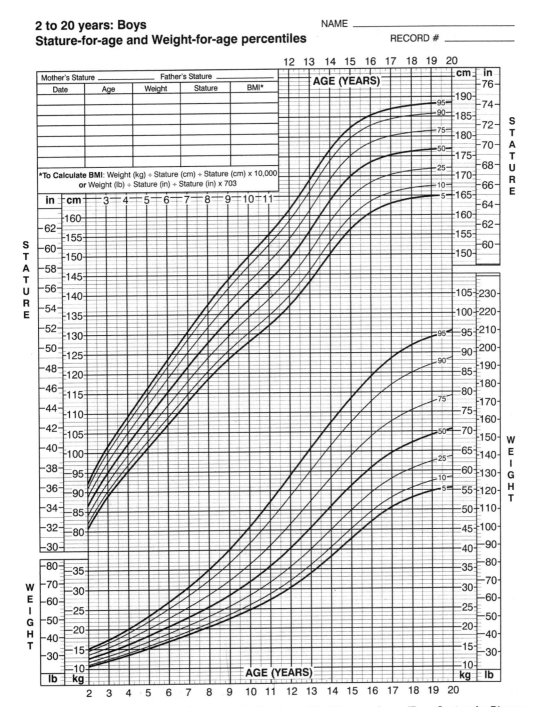

FIG. D.3. Stature-for-age and weight-for-age percentiles, boys, 2 to 20 years of age. (From Centers for Disease Control and Prevention. Available at http://www.cdc.gov/growthcharts/. Accessed June 2002, with permission.)

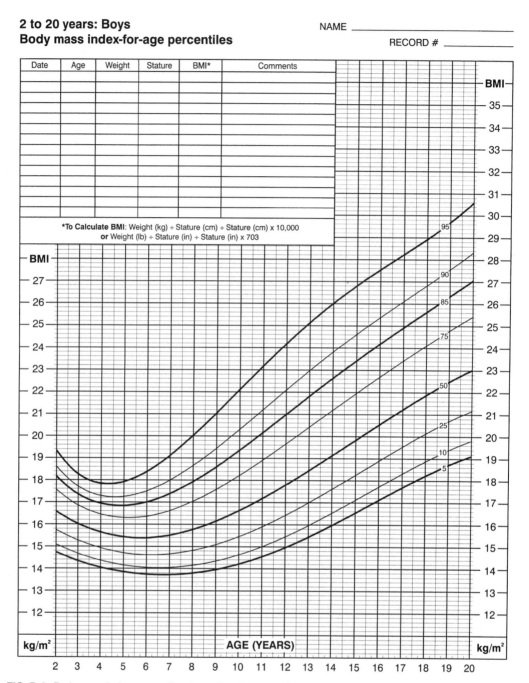

2 to 20 years: Boys
Body mass index-for-age percentiles

NAME _____

RECORD # _____

*To Calculate BMI: Weight (kg) ÷ Stature (cm) ÷ Stature (cm) x 10,000
or Weight (lb) ÷ Stature (in) ÷ Stature (in) x 703

FIG. D.4. Body mass index percentiles, boys, 2 to 20 years of age. (From Centers for Disease Control and Prevention. Available at http://www.cdc.gov/growthcharts/. Accessed June 2002, with permission.)

Appendix E

Position Stands of the American College of Sports Medicine

POSITION STANDS

The position stands are the official statements of the American College of Sports Medicine (ACSM) on topics related to sports medicine and exercise science. They are based on solid research and scientific data, and they are a valued resource for both professional organizations and governmental agencies. They are first published in the ACSM's scientific journal, *Medicine & Science in Sports & Exercise*. They are available online at http://www.acsm.org/positionStands.htm, and they include the following:

The Recommended Quantity and Quality of Exercise for Developing and Maintaining Cardiorespiratory and Muscular Fitness and Flexibility in Healthy Adults

Exercise and Physical Activity for Older Adults

AHA/ACSM Joint Statement: Recommendations for Cardiovascular Screening, Staffing, and Emergency Policies at Health/Fitness Facilities

ADA/ACSM Joint Statement: Diabetes Mellitus and Exercise

The Female Athlete Triad

Heat & Cold Illnesses During Distance Running

Exercise and Fluid Replacement

The Use of Blood Doping as an Ergogenic Aid

Weight Loss in Wrestlers

Osteoporosis and Exercise

Exercise for Patients with Coronary Artery Disease

Physical Activity, Physical Fitness, and Hypertension

The Use of Anabolic-Androgenic Steroids in Sports

Proper and Improper Weight-Loss Programs

The Use of Alcohol in Sports

CURRENT COMMENTS

The ACSM has developed a series of Current Comments, which are proactive statements concerning sports medicine and exercise science-related topics of interest to the public at large. They are written in language that is understandable, relevant, and helpful to the general public. The ACSM has developed Current Comments on the following:

- Anabolic Steroids
- Caffeine
- Chromium Supplements
- Corporate Wellness
- Creatine Supplementation
- Dehydration and Aging
- Eating Disorders
- Exercise and Age-Related Weight Gain
- Exercise and the Common Cold
- Exercise for Persons with Cardiovascular Disease
- Explosive Exercise
- Health-Related Fitness for Children and Adults with Cerebral Palsy
- Preparticipation Physical Exams
- Sickle Cell Trait
- Skiing Injuries
- Stress Fractures
- Vitamin and Mineral Supplements and Exercise
- Youth Strength Training
- Weight Loss in Wrestlers
- Women's Heart Health and a Physically Active Lifestyle

For a single copy of any one of the above, the reader should send a self-addressed, stamped envelope to the ACSM Public Information Department at P.O. Box 1440, Indianapolis, IN 46206. For all 20 Current Comments, send $2.50 or call 317-637-9200 to make a credit card order.

Appendix F

Postexposure Prophylaxis for Human Immunodeficiency Virus

STEP 1: Determine the Exposure Code (EC)

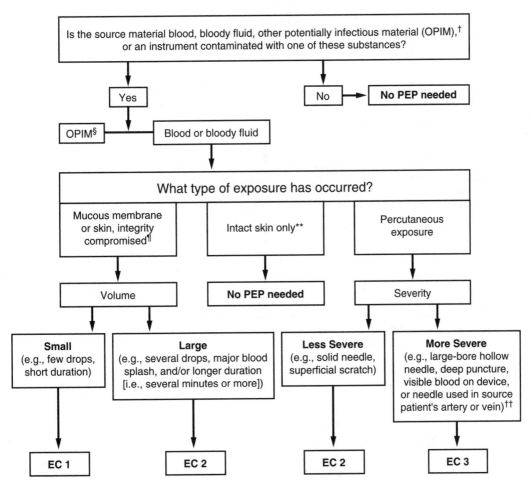

* This algorithm is intended to guide initial decisions about PEP and should be used in conjunction with other guidance provided in this report.

† Semen or vaginal secretions; cerebrospinal, synovial, pleural, peritoneal, pericardial, or amniotic fluids; or tissue.

§ Exposures to OPIM must be evaluated on a case-by-case basis. In general, these body substances are considered a low risk for transmission in health-care settings. Any unprotected contact to concentrated HIV in a research laboratory or production facility is considered an occupational exposure that requires clinical evaluation to determine the need for PEP.

¶ Skin integrity is considered compromised if there is evidence of chapped skin, dermatitis, abrasion, or open wound.

** Contact with intact skin is not normally considered a risk for HIV transmission. However, if the exposure was to blood, and the circumstance suggests a higher volume exposure (e.g., an extensive area of skin was exposed or there was prolonged contact with blood), the risk for HIV transmission should be considered.

†† The combination of these severity factors (e.g., large-bore hollow needle *and* deep puncture) contribute to an elevated risk for transmission if the source person is HIV-positive.

FIG. F.1. Recommendations for the Centers for Disease Control and Prevention of postexposure prophylaxis (PEP) of healthcare workers (HCW) exposed to human immunodeficiency virus (HIV). Abbreviation: AIDS, acquired immune deficiency syndrome. (From Centers for Disease Control and Prevention. Public Health Service (PHS) guidelines for the management of healthcare worker exposures to HIV and recommendations for postexposure prophylaxis. *MMWR* 1998;47;14–15, with permission.)

STEP 2: Determine the HIV Status Code (HIV SC)

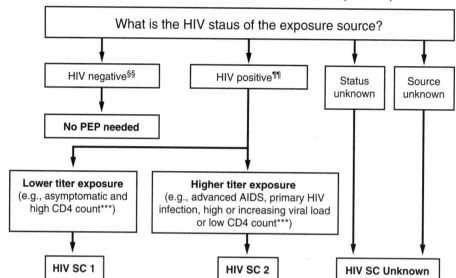

§§ A source is considered negative for HIV infection if there is laboratory documentation of a negative HIV antibody, HIV polymerase chain reaction (PCR), or HIV p24 antigen test result from a specimen collected at or near the time of exposure and there is no clinical evidence or recent retroviral-like illness.

¶¶ A source is considered infected with HIV (HIV positive) if there has been a positive laboratory result for HIV antibody, HIV PCR, or HIV p24 antigen or physician-diagnosed AIDS.

*** Examples are used as surrogates to estimate the HIV titer in an exposure source for purposes of considering PEP regimens and do not reflect all clinical situations that may be observed. Although a high HIV titer (HIV SC 2) in an exposure source has been associated with an increased risk for transmission, the possibility of transmission from a source with a low HIV titer also must be considered.

STEP 3: Determine the PEP Recommendation

EC	HIV SC	PEP recommendation
1	1	**PEP may not be warranted**. Exposure type does not pose a known risk for HIV transmission. Whether the risk for drug toxicity outweighs the benefit of PEP should be decided by the exposed HCW and treating clinician.
1	2	**Consider basic regimen**.††† Exposure type poses a negligible risk for HIV transmission. A high HIV titer in the source may justify consideration of PEP. Whether the risk for drug toxicity outweighs the benefit of PEP should be decided by the exposed HCW and treating clinician.
2	1	**Recommend basic regimen**. Most HIV exposures are in this category; no increased risk for HIV transmission has been observed but use of PEP is appropriate.
2	2	**Recommend expanded regimen**.§§§ Exposure type represents an increased HIV transmission risk.
3	1 or 2	**Recommend expanded regimen**. Exposure type represents an increased HIV transmission risk.
	Unknown	If the source or, in the case of an unknown source, the setting where the exposure occurred suggests a possible risk for HIV exposure, and the EC is 2 or 3, consider PEP basic regimen.

††† Basic regimen is four weeks of zidovudine, 600 mg per day in two or three divided doses, ***and*** lamivudine, 150 mg twice daily.

§§§ Expanded regimen is the basic regimen plus ***either*** indinavir, 800 mg every 8 hours, ***or*** nelfinavir, 750 mg three times a day.

FIG. F.1. *Continued*

Subject Index

Note: Page numbers followed by *f* indicate figures; those followed by *t* indicate tables